THE UTTAL TETRALOGY OF
COGNITIVE NEUROSCIENCE

Volume 1

THE PSYCHOBIOLOGY OF
SENSORY CODING

THE PSYCHOBIOLOGY OF SENSORY CODING

WILLIAM R. UTTAL

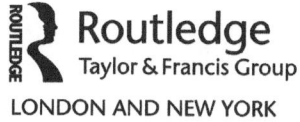

Routledge
Taylor & Francis Group

LONDON AND NEW YORK

First published in 1973

This edition first published in 2014
by Psychology Press

Published 2016 by Routledge
2 Park Square, Milton Park, Abingdon, Oxfordshire OX14 4RN
711 Third Avenue, New York, NY 10017

First issued in paperback 2015

Routledge is an imprint of the Taylor and Francis Group, an informa business

British Library Cataloguing in Publication Data
A catalogue record for this book is available from the British Library

ISBN: 978-1-84872-428-0 (Set)
ISBN 13: 978-1-138-98976-4 (pbk)
ISBN 13: 978-1-84872-429-7 (hbk)

Publisher's Note
The publisher has gone to great lengths to ensure the quality of this book but
points out that some imperfections from the original may be apparent.

Disclaimer
The publisher has made every effort to trace copyright holders and would
welcome correspondence from those they have been unable to trace.

THE PSYCHOBIOLOGY OF SENSORY CODING

WILLIAM R. UTTAL
University of Michigan

Harper & Row, Publishers
New York, Evanston, San Francisco, London

Sponsoring Editor: George A. Middendorf
Project Editor: Sandra G. Turner
Designer: Michel Craig
Production Supervisor: Robert A. Pirrung

THE PSYCHOBIOLOGY OF SENSORY CODING

Standard Book Number: 06–046737–1

Library of Congress Catalog Card Number: 73–15972

For Michan

CONTENTS

PREFACE

Why would anyone want to write a textbook? After having done so, I feel impelled to once again ask myself that question. The answer to which I return time after time is that there is a message to be delivered, and it is often difficult to make that message heard at the level of the senior experimental scientist; rather, it is to the young people who are beginning their careers in science to whom this book is mainly addressed—those graduate and advanced undergraduate students who have not yet crystallized their personal answers to some of the basic questions often ignored later in one's career.

Briefly, the message of this book is that the relationship between the neurophysiological and the behavioral is a researchable problem, particularly if one works in the domain of the sensory processes. An additional major premise of this work is that the real psychobiological sensory-coding issue is embodied in comparisons made between behavioral and neurophysiological responses rather than between the stimulus and either of these two response domains. Furthermore, it is clear that a more complex set of conceptual issues is involved in this combined aspect of the mind-body problem than either neurophysiology or behavior must deal with separately. An additional fact is that this psychobiological domain must be framed in a more multidimensional manner than is often implied by some of the more conventional textbooks. Finally (and delightfully), all workers in the field would agree with me that there are still many gaps in our knowledge concerning the neurophysiological coding of sensory processes.

Neither this book, nor any other in the foreseeable future, is going to tell the whole story of the psychobiology of sensory coding.

I hope it is not too extravagant to express my conviction that this field is one of the most exciting and interesting in modern science and yet also only one new facet of one of the grand and ancient issues in man's perpetual concern with his own nature. As such, its topical relevance in today's world is great in spite of the fact that some might feel that the world we live in has other more pressing needs. I believe in this work sufficiently to be convinced, however, that the world would gradually run out of its intellectual "fuel" if studies of this and other similarly "esoteric" fields were not pursued with all possible energy by a substantially large portion of our scientific community.

The subject matter of this book is broad, but it is not intended to be encyclopedic. Rather than an unending list of a host of experimental studies, I have tried, as judiciously as possible, to select the prime examples of research that make key points and then to present them in detail. In doing so, I am sure that I have missed quite a few important contributors, and I offer whatever apologies are appropriate. The content matter of this book must necessarily be selective. Topic selection has been influenced in large part, frankly, by what I am interested in as well as constrained and delimited by the main goal—a definition of the relationship between sensory neurophysiology and sensory psychophysics. Thus, some important material has been intentionally omitted or deemphasized.

This book is the culmination of a long-term plan. I suppose I first began thinking about doing it in graduate school, but I did not formally begin work on a manuscript until 1967. In the years that have elapsed, it has consumed a large portion of my energies and, as any author might note, there were times when I was not so sure that it ever would be finished. But it is now, and I present it to the community with a sense of completion, but also with a profound sense of obligation to all of those people who have contributed in one way or another to the development of the ideas expressed here or to the preparation of this volume. First, it is most appropriate for me to acknowledge the enormous debt that I owe my mentors at the Ohio State University. Professor Donald R. Meyer must bear the responsibility for having converted me from physics to physiological psychology and also for alerting me to the grandeur of the mind-body problem. Professor Philburn Ratoosh specifically whetted my appetite for the sensory sciences, and Professor Leo Lipetz introduced me to the delights of the neurophysiological approach. The influence of the late Professor Paul M. Fitts, both as a scientist and as a responsible human being, I hope will stick with me for the rest of my life.

More recently, I have had the advantages of support from a number of other colleagues and agencies. Parts of this book were written during visits away from the University of Michigan. I enjoyed the hospitality and support of the Laboratory of Sensory Sciences at the University of Hawaii in the winter of 1968—a glorious sun-drenched period for which I am especially grateful to Professor A. Leonard Diamond, who was the director at that time. In 1970–1971 I spent an extraordinarily productive and pleasant academic year among the wonderful people and stimulating intellectual environment of the Department of Psychology at the University of Western Australia. The cordiality and friendship of Professors John Ross and Aubrey Yates, Dr. Vincent DiLollo, and all of my other Australian friends made that year a memorable one both professionally and personally.

For the last decade at the University of Michigan, my research has been supported by the university, in particular the Mental Health Research Institute, and also by federal grants. I am particularly happy to acknowledge continued research support over the last nine years from the Psychobiology Branch of the National Science Foundation and, more recently, a National Institute of Mental Health Research Scientist Award.

I have also had the benefit of editorial comments from some very capable people. Professor Paul Witkovsky of the New York University did a Herculean job of providing advice (thus cleaning the "Augean Stables" of some early drafts) in a way which has made this a much better book than it would otherwise have been. Professor H. Philip Zeigler, editor of the Harper & Row Physiological Psychology Series, was indefatigable in his comments and advice over the entire period in which I worked on the book. George Middendorf, executive editor of the Harper & Row College Department, also "helped," to say the least, all of us over some of the rough spots. Others of my colleagues had read lesser portions or provided specific bits of advice, which I hope I have fully acknowledged in the text. Needless to say, however, none of these people can be held accountable for the deficiencies that certainly will be included even in the final version of this book.

The astute reader will also note the influence of many other workers with whom I am not personally well acquainted. I often know them only through their writings, and many of them rightfully deserve a more specific acknowledgment than is possible here. Ideas spread through the scientific community along paths that are sometimes hard to identify precisely, and I am sure that, especially in an effort such as this, the multiple effects of other people's work is both profound and quite clear. I hope that each has been adequately cited in the body of the text, although I am sure that there is no way in which this could be done completely. No omission was intentional, but no list of citations could be complete either. If they should ever read this book, such distinguished scientists as Theodore Bullock, Frank Geldard, Ragnar Granit, Henri Piéron, Walter Rosenblith, and Burton Rosner will be able to detect their influence on my general perspective. Perhaps most particularly, I have in many ways been influenced by the prolific and stimulating writing of the late Georg von Békésy who passed away this summer after a long and distinguished career. Many others share a sense of loss with me at his passing. To those others I may have missed, my apologies and gratitude for helping me toward an understanding of this subject matter.

Many students who have been through my course on sensory processes at the University of Michigan have also contributed, though unknowingly, to the development of this book. Their comments, discussions, as well as the vigorous controversies which somehow emerged even in this highly technical subject matter have all added to my understanding of this material and, I hope, to the quality of my presentation.

The manuscript of this book has been typed (and retyped so many times, it seems) by so many secretaries that some of their names have faded off into the past, but I am especially grateful for the dedicated efforts of Ms. Lynn Gore and Ms. Patricia Eaton who withstood the brunt of the most difficult final period of work on the manuscript. I am also indebted to Mr. Paul Laszlo and Ms. Maureen Powers who assisted and advised in the preparation of the figures.

Last but not least, my family, my wife, May, and three daughters, Taneil, Lynet, and Lisa, who have traveled with me to unfamiliar places or simply done without me on those evenings and weekends I became overly engrossed in the manuscript, not only have my affection and love but also my appreciation for making all of this possible. May, better than anyone else, you know that without you this never could have come about.

William R. Uttal

CHAPTER 1: AN ORIENTATION

I. INTRODUCTION

A. Psychology, Physiology, and Psychobiology

This book is about the acquisition and transmission of information patterns from the external environment to the central nervous system, where presumably these patterns become the substance of our mental life. It deals with a subject matter that thus transcends the conventional borders of neurophysiology and psychology as well as those of related disciplines such as anatomy and physics. From this diversity of substance has come both the richness of content and the major difficulty in the preparation of a satisfactory text of this sort. It is impossible to conceive of a single volume that would be capable of comprehensively covering the broad spectrum of theory and data that now make up such a vast literature. This present book, therefore, is selective and incomplete in a number of important ways. It has not been possible to comprehensively cover either the phenomena of sensory psychology or the abundant detail of sensory physiology to the depth desired. On the contrary, this book is built on a single axiom, and only material specifically relevant to that axiom has been included. That axiom states that the external world is represented within the organism by patterns of neural activity that, while the patterns themselves differ greatly from the external world in terms of the physical energies involved, do maintain some sort of an equivalence of pattern or organization, if not an isomorphism, of neural activity. The persistence of patterns of information, independent of the physical medium or specific neural dimension in which they exist, is the essential idea of the notion of neural *coding*.

To concretize this idea, let us consider a specific example of what it is that we mean by equivalence and isomorphism. Consider the problem of auditory pitch. Physical signals, varying primarily in the temporal characteristics of waves of compression and rarefaction of air pressure, are interpreted as sounds of different pitches by a listener. The original signal information is, in this example, in the form of the temporal pattern of the air wave. But as we shall see, these temporal information patterns are encoded largely by spatial distributions of activity in the inner ear. Thus, while the spatial neural patterns convey the same information and are hence equivalent, they are in no sense isomorphic (of the same shape), nor do they even possess the same dimensionality as the stimulus. Rather, they are encoded representations of the original pattern.

The concept of *coding* has in recent years come to be, for sensory studies in particular, the contemporary expression of a continuing intellectual perplexity: how does the body and its parts relate to, represent, or in some way provide a receptacle for the self-awareness that every man has of his own existence? We shall detail in later parts of this chapter the specific nature of this new outlook, but for the moment let us consider the problem of mind-body relationships in their more classical sense. The problem has been considered by some thoughtful philosophers (see, for example, Feigl, 1958) to be a question inadequately stated and inappropriately asked. Certainly, when one considers the fact that the *intrapersonal* self-awareness that all men seem to possess is not subject to *interpersonal* examination and comparison, the perplexities of how one can handle the problem of the construction of an internally consistent science of psychology appear substantial. But before one should be discouraged from attempting the task, it should be remembered that in fact most of our sciences—physical, biological, as well as behavioral—share this same difficulty. The physics of nuclear structure, for example, is a science in which the components under investigation can never be seen directly. We can only infer their existence (and transient indeed they may be) from the tracks of a bubble or spark chamber or even more abstractly from the necessity to balance an energy equation.

Astronomy shares this same dilemma. It appears that the facts surrounding the speed of light as an upper limit for the movement of either physical objects or energetic waves through space make travel to distant galaxies just as unlikely as a direct observation of one man's awareness by another. If the theory that there exists an upper limit of the speed of light is sustained in the future, we shall always be forced to limit our observations of the nature of distant universes to those measurements that can be made on the ancient light signals that have been traveling toward us in some cases for millions of years. It should be remembered that what we may be observing with telescopes now may long ago have ceased to exist. This temporal dilemma, at least, is a problem not faced by psychology. Psychology, a science whose proper content is the set of the inner awarenesses which Feigl (1958) refers to as *Raw Feels*, is therefore in no way unique from the point of view of invisible subject matter.

Psychology, as a science, has responded to the limitations on interpersonal comparison by emphasizing behavioral measures. This is often so, it seems to some, to the exclusion of the subject matter itself. But even though it seems clear that the great initiative for studying awareness or consciousness comes from the individual's self-awareness, nevertheless, in order to provide a reasonable foundation for replicable and organizable observations, it is to the *behavior* of others that we must turn for our experimental data. This methodological twist often obscures the fact that behavior is *not* the subject matter of the psychological sciences, but it is rather only an approach to the real content, which is represented by such symbolic terms as *consciousness, awareness, thought, perception,* or any of the other terms that have gained momentary popularity over the centuries. In the same vein, who would classify astronomy as either the study of telescopes or the study of ancient light? The objects of attention of most astronomers are planets, stars, and galaxies and not the instruments or measurements necessary to acquire information about these objects. Similarly, the objects of attention of psychology are thought, perceptions, sensations, and other aspects of conscious experience.

The other major approach to sensory science is the neurophysiological one. The objects of concern to this science are the processes that are performed by the specialized tissues and cells of the nervous system. From our particular frame of reference, that of the problem of sensory communication, the objects of attention are the physiological processes of the highly specialized nervous tissues responsible for the transduction, transmission, and integration of incoming information patterns. The scientific accomplishments of the last half century have made it quite clear that it is the brain and the other components of the nervous system to which we must look for a reductive explanation of psychological acts. It may be somewhat surprising to realize how recently in human history this idea gained a solid foundation. We still are all too apt, in the vernacular at least, to refer to the "heart" as the seat of emotional awareness.

There is another idea which has also been current in our modern infatuation with electrophysiological techniques. This idea is that a physiological investigation of the activity produced in the nervous system by peripheral stimuli is sufficient in itself to explain the coding processes of sensory systems. Such a notion is probably untrue. A substantial number of misconceptions have been introduced into our understanding of the mind-body problem by this overattentive concern with physiological recording. On the other hand, it is important not to minimize the enormous contributions that have been made using these techniques when they are placed within a psychological framework.

It is also true, however, that the psychological approach is, by itself, incapable of providing a definitive answer to problems of sensory coding. In fact, because of the intrinsic limitations of the two techniques when used separately, a combined approach has become more and more popular in recent years. This approach has gone under many names—biopsychology, neuropsychology, or physiological psychology, but we have chosen the term psychobiology as the one that seems most appropriate to the emphasis we shall place on the physiological substrates of sensory experience. Psychobiology represents a merger of techniques from both the psychological and the physiological laboratories. Indeed, we see today behavioral techniques being used by physiologists, and electrophysiological recording proficiency developed to a high level among people originally trained in psychology. It is often difficult to distinguish the original training of a practitioner of the new combined art.

The adoption of new techniques in either field reflects the increasing tempo of the interdisciplinary trend in many other sciences. But more important, in this particular field, it reflects the emerging awareness of the significant conceptual pressure that an integrated psychobiology of sensory activity exerts on our perspective of the classic mind-brain controversy. My aim in this book is to tie together the work of the psychologist and the neurophysiologist into a coordinated approach to the problems of sensory experience. Some have pointed out that the psychological approach is a necessary precursor to electrophysiological studies so that the neurophysiologist will know what there is to look for. Neurophysiologists have properly pointed out the inability of the psychological techniques to solve the problems of sensory representation within the "black box" of the closed organism. In fact, both points are correct, and just as a sensory psychology text that ignored the neurophysiological contributions would be meaningless in the terms of today's knowledge, similarly a text of sensory neurophysiology would be incoherent if it ignored the massive contributions of the psychophysical laboratories.

B. The Scope of "Sensory" Sciences

It is appropriate at this point that we attempt to define the field of inquiry with which we shall be concerned. Sensory processes in biological systems are defined, in large part, by an intrinsic directionality of the flow of information. The sensory system is designed, as we have said, to pick up patterns of information from the external world, transduce this information from any of a number of physical forms of energy to the electrochemical forces of neural activity, and transmit that pattern toward the complex central portions of the nervous system. The nature of the subsequent processing of sensory information by the higher nervous centers in the exquisitely complicated ways cataloged by the cognitive descriptors evolved by psychologists will not, by intent, be among the topics we shall consider. It is, of course, not possible to draw a sharp line of demarcation between the content of this book and that of these other areas of subjective activity. Indeed, as our understanding progresses, the line should be pushed further and further upward.

A cogent argument can be made that the "simpler" sensory processes, with which we shall concern ourselves, are in reality no simpler than the more complex processes. They may represent only a subset of cognitive functions which, for a number of reasons, are more susceptible to experimental control and probing. Furthermore, we must recognize that in defining the field to be covered by this book, we are specifically faced with the knotty problem of distinguishing between those subject matters that are usually classified as sensory and those that are usually classified as perceptual. It seems most appropriate to ignore any real difference between the two. Rather, for the purposes of this volume, we shall make a very artificial distinction. We shall talk about the sensory phenomena that are closely related to well-defined stimulus patterns and known or plausible neural mechanisms. We shall simply exclude from our discussion those more complex perceptions that are apparently based upon such complex neural interactions and weakly defined stimulus conditions that the reductive aspects of our science have not yet come to grips with them. For example, we shall not deal with the well-known fact that familiarity enhances word recognition. There is no physiological theory that can even begin to account for such a phenomenon.

The conceptual and anatomical straightforwardness of the sensory functions has been their great asset in establishing their preeminence in the reductionism of modern psychobiology. We understand information processing better in sensory systems in large part because they are much simpler in both anatomical and functional organization than the systems underlying, for example, such processes as problem solving. They are in some cases so simple that they can be considered characterizations or abstractions of the operation of more complex and general neural nets, just as simple invertebrate "model" nervous systems often help us to understand mammalian neural mechanisms. For this reason, through the study of sensory processes, we are often able to advance our knowledge not only of the immediate problems surrounding sensory coding, but also of the possible modes of action of the more complicated mechanisms.

We shall be looking at the sensory systems mainly in terms of their function of communicating information from the periphery toward the central nervous structures. This has been called, by some, communication in the *ascending* direction (the pun being associated with the notion of the "higher" centers of the brain), even though in some cases the "ascending" nerves may actually travel downward during at least part of their route. Others have used the term *afferent* emphasizing the inward-going direction of these communication links as distinguished from the *efferent* lines of the effector or motor systems. The word sensory is always used in this book as a synonym for either input, ascending, or afferent and not—as some would choose—as a synomym for simple perceptions. Thus, it is entirely consistent to speak of sensory neurophysiology or sensory coding without referring to the psychological connotations. However, this simple categorization is inadequate to handle some recent data. We shall be concerned with information processing between and among units of the afferent pathways in ways that require awareness of such concepts as feedback and reverberation. In fact, we shall also be concerned with some signal pathways that are intimately tied to the sensory systems but are patently efferent or descending. We refer here to observations which indicate that there is centrifugal (from the center) activity which operates to powerfully modulate the sensory input pattern.

From a more psychological point of view, the material with which we shall be most concerned will deal with those relatively simple awarenesses of relatively simple stimulus patterns. Psychophysical techniques are in a rapid stage of metamorphosis as the traditional techniques of measuring the responses to brief and transient unitary stimuli give way to more interestingly designed experiments with more elaborately patterned stimulus situations. But in spite of this, there is a clearly defined group of experimental paradigms, which will be seen to fit the problem area we have chosen for this book more closely than others involving other more complex, although equally interesting, stimuli. The key test of relevance will be: is a given sensory or perceptual phenomenon an input function with a plausible neural explanation?

As we have said, the main goal of this book is to integrate the two sets of data from psychology and neurophysiology into a unified discussion. In addition to selecting a circumscribed topic area—sensory processes—for consideration, we shall also be making a number of implicit assumptions in the development of this book, which should be overtly stated as fundamental premises. One of these premises is our point of view concerning the nature of the interaction between the psychological and the neurophysiological. Our approach is one that would certainly be classified within the general rubric of monisms. It is, explicitly, an expression of the belief that sensory activities, and for that matter all psychological activity, are ultimately reducible to the terms, linguistic and conceptual, of patterns of neural activity.

In addition to the premise of monism, which underlies our attempt to integrate the two approaches to the study of sensory processes—the psychological and the neurophysiological—we shall also attempt a synthesis at another level of discussion. Traditionally (Troland, 1930; Geldard, 1953; Wyburn, Pickford, and Hirst, 1964), sensory textbooks have been organized in chapters, which discuss one sensory modality at a time. Although Osgood (1953) and Corso (1967) do partially deviate from this tradition, we usually see conventional chapters on vision separated from those on audition, which are likewise separate from those on the chemical or somatic sensations. It is a further premise of the present work that there are general principles of sensory organization that can and should be emphasized independent of a specific modality. The processes of transduction or of transmission, for example, have features common to all the senses, and these commonalities become self-evident when all of the senses are discussed together. Similarly, the coding of sensory quantity, space and time, or even quality have so many common attributes among the different modalities that we believe it is meaningful to consider these dimensions free of the restrictions imposed by the limitation of our attention to a single modality at a time.

It is important to acknowledge at this point that this is not the first book to deviate from the traditional pattern of considering the senses separately. I have been particularly influenced by the writing of Henri Piéron, particularly as he presents his discussion of the sensory processes in his elegant treatise, *The Sensations* (1952).

II. VARIETIES OF SCIENTIFIC QUESTIONS AND APPROACHES

A. Some Thoughts on the Nature of Scientific Activity

As we have said, the general notion of coding provides a framework for consideration of the mind-body problem that is much more concrete than the purely philosophical speculations of the past. But, paradoxically, each of the experiments, which are performed in the belief that they are relevant to the problem of sensory coding, must be considered relatively insignificant and unimportant in itself. A sensory-coding experiment, like any other one, is important only in terms of its contribution to our general appreciation of the system we are studying and in direct relation to its ability to add to or modify the general outlook. It is all too easy, in a highly technological problem area such as this, to lose sight of the reason that experiments are performed and to overemphasize the techniques or resulting set of data. The end product of this scientific tunnel vision is wasted effort and resources. It is my belief that the reasons that physiological psychologists do their work are generally misrepresented by their own writings. It is incomplete to say that one is doing an experiment to determine the response function of a given receptor in the eye of the frog, for example, without some realization of the more general problems which surround that purely technical issue. There exists, in fact, a hierarchy of questions which are asked about any scientific issue. In general, those scientists who are unaware of the greater implications of the specific technical questions asked day to day in their laboratories must ultimately stagnate in a pool of trivial and pointless experimental manipulations. Not everyone has to be a full-time philosopher of science, but all technically oriented scientists must be aware of the conceptual implications of their work. We would all be better men and better scientists if there were a wider appreciation of the great issues that surround the small steps we make in our laboratories.

Coding theory, as it represents the major cutting edge into the mind-body problem, represents perhaps the pinnacle of man's contemporary intellectual efforts. There may be fields of science that have made greater technical progress, or ones in which the formal structure is better understood, but there is no other field that more clearly epitomizes the most human of endeavors—the analysis by man of his own intellect.

Just as the field is important, it is also diversified. It is obvious that no single professional scientist is fully capable of the mastery of all of the skills necessary to study the full range of sensory phenomena. Similarly, few of our great insights into sensory processes have been based on a single key experiment from a single approach. Most have been based on an intentional effort to integrate a variety of data bases into a single theoretical structure.

The point that is being made is that there is probably no one single "best" way to approach a problem like sensory coding. Indeed, there is probably no single strategy that can be applied to any subproblem in science which is uniquely capable of providing a solution. Platt (1964) calls for an increase in the technique of *hard inference* as the single approach to experimental research. Yet one cannot read the eloquent plea of Hebb (1959) for an eclectic approach to science without appreciating the value of multiple approaches to problems of interesting complexity. Perhaps the best argument for multiple approaches to scientific research is the inherent disorganization of the frontiers of science. The exciting cutting edge of scientific inquiry is not the precisely laid out studies explicated in the modern journal format, but the often confused and disorganized ideas of a

man working with an idea for the first time in human history. The simple
fact is that the meat of science is the formless and the unknown, and not
the known and collectively understood. As fast as new knowledge is exposed and integrated into a community perspective, it diminishes in importance and interest to any scientist worth his salt. The best scientists in
the business are the ones who eventually lose interest, become bored, and
move on to other new areas of inquiry. The role of each new discovery is
to change our world as it changes our perspectives and subtly alters our
approach to the next problem. Because of this unstructured chipping away
at the boundaries of our ignorance, I believe it remains a practical impossi-
bility to predetermine which will be the best strategy or to make long-range
advance plans in the truly explorative aspects of science.

If the process of science is to be considered from the point of view of
a search rather than as an accomplishment, if the content of science is to be
considered as the unknown rather than the known, then it is clear that
science can be best appreciated when it is formulated in terms of hierarchical series of questions rather than as answers or specific research
methods. These questions arise in many different ways. There are some
questions whose history is as long as man's and arose as soon as the unique
capability of man to concern himself with his relationship to the world
around him appeared. The emergence of self-awareness probably did not
substantially predate the awareness that there was a difference between a
living and dead organism that could apparently be explained only in terms
of some "thing" missing. The observation of the death of a member of one's
own species is a powerful force first toward asking questions about life
and death and then answering them in ways that do not violate the obvious
"fact" of one's own consciousness. Primitive considerations such as this
have evolved into the extremely intricate philosophies of the mind-brain
problem. The mind-brain problem is still of interest because it has not yet
been answered, not because its riddle has been solved. Physiological psychology, in particular, is formulated more in terms of the quest than in the
results. So these grand and historic questions can provide one set of motives
for the thrust of scientific inquiry.

But contemporary surprises and the unexpected findings of some accident of observation also provide a rich source of motivation for scientific
endeavor. This is very often associated with the introduction of a new
observational instrument. The invention of the microscope or of a new
electrophysiological recording instrument have both been extremely powerful situational factors in the development of new knowledge by exposing
a portion of our environment that had been unappreciated previously. The
laboratory use of computers promises to be equally important. New sciences spring up almost immediately as the world around us enlarges. The
questions of the past are reformulated in terms of new observations; new
approaches emerge that could never have been seriously considered solely
in terms of earlier speculations and less effective tools.

Another rich source of questions for science, which must not be
underestimated particularly in our own pragmatically oriented world, is the
search for the solution of specific problems that face mankind from time to
time. How can we cure this disease? How can we provide enough food for

our population? How can we build a device capable of operating at 4000°F? All of these issues, in addition to their applied engineering aspect, bring a larger group of people into contact with sets of natural phenomena. They thus increase the possibility of discovery as they open new vistas.

We can, therefore, discern three major sources of motivation for scientific research:

1. Classic issues of speculative philosophy.
2. The unexpected discovery from an undirected exploration of the general environment often due to the introduction of a new instrument.
3. The attempted elimination of some clearly identified obstacle to human comfort, health, or happiness.

It is unlikely that any of the three can be given priority in the past motivation of science. Nevertheless, it is possible to distinguish general stages in the development of any particular scientific inquiry. These stages must be considered only in their historical sense, for no individual scientist progresses rigidly through the sequence any more than any experiment actually fits into the rigid format of today's standard scientific journal article. Different scientists work at different levels of this paradigm at different times in history.

To illustrate the nature of the proposed hierarchy of levels of inquiry, let us consider a major problem within the field with which this book is concerned. We have chosen a scientific problem, which has really been motivated by all three of the sources mentioned above. The problem of *color vision* has had a long history. It originally was formulated in terms of the philosophical issues of the mind-brain problem. But later, the anomalies of color blindness were noted, and the facts of color addition were observed and formulated.[1] More recently applied technological motivations have led to additional effort to explain the phenomenon of color vision.

But whatever the source of the effort, the first question in the hierarchy is: how do we see colors? This is a question that is, however, rarely overtly asked by modern students of color vision. They are more often operating at a finer level. For example, the next lower echelon of questions might well be described in terms of different receptor theories. One might ask the question: are there separate red and green receptors? This is a relatively technical issue based upon a specific hypothesis or prejudgment about the nature of color receptors which has gone far beyond the general philosophical notions originally being considered.

Later, both historically and in the individual experience, even more detailed questions must be asked; for example, what is the nature of the interaction between the different kinds of receptors? Finally, we find the most specific questions of all formulated in terms of the solution of some

---

[1] The formularization of a specific series of rules is not, of course, a prerequisite for the implicit utilization of the rules of any subset of them. Artists have been aware of the laws of color and visual space and have been able to use both for tens of thousands of years without explicit formularization.

very specific issues of measurement. How can we measure some particular phenomenon? What is the effect of manipulating independent variable x? The hierarchy of questions might be carried on to even more detailed levels.

The important point is that there are two ways to consider such a hierarchy. The first is the historical one already expressed. As we gain more and more information about a specific problem, we tend to deal with more specialized subportions of it. On the other hand, the other way to look at the hierarchy is that there are, at any given instant in time, people working simultaneously at several different levels. We still must have our philosophers of science even if their profession is currently in somewhat low regard among the scientific pragmatists. We certainly also must have plenty of the instrument makers at the other end of the hierarchy. The unfortunate thing is that a worker, whose commitment is to one or another level, loses sight of how dependent he is on progress at another level.

We must reiterate, at this point, the notion with which we started. *The approaches to science are manifold.* The sources of the motivations of scientists are neither simple nor single. A very distinguished sensory psychobiologist, Georg von Békésy (1960), has made a somewhat tongue-in-cheek listing of the approaches to science. First, he distinguishes the *theoretical* approach in all its formal majesty. This is usually the format presented to scientific neonates. He then contrasts this theoretical approach with the more realistic *mosaic* approach, in which problems are attacked as they arise with any available tool.

Von Békésy goes on to discuss a number of different types of questions ranging from the "classical questions still unsolved" to the "embarrassing question frequently arising at a meeting and serving no useful purpose." To his list we might also add the "greedy approach" reflecting the motivation of some scientists to pursue their research not for its own intrinsic sake, but for the potential value it might have in helping them achieve some irrelevant ambitions and desires. But even this set of "ulterior motives" must not be completely deprecated. They, like many of the other sources of scientific effort, have been effective in providing incentives for scientific research and have often contributed to our understanding of nature in surprising ways.

B. A Hierarchy of Questions of Sensory Psychobiology

So far we have dealt with a number of very diffuse issues. We have stressed the inherently chaotic and disorganized nature of the true scientific frontier. We have also stressed the great variety of questions that scientists ask about the unknown. Now let us turn our attention to another set of questions based on a far more concrete model. This other hierarchy of questions concerns the sequence of physiological steps occurring in the afferent pathway. The hierarchy is one which is constantly changing as our knowledge of the sensory processes becomes more and more complete. Later in this book we shall very specifically define the nature of the neural coding processes in the afferent chain. We shall point out that some of the most serious problems faced by sensory psychobiologists are inadequately precise definitions of the question that he is asking and the level at which he is asking it. As our knowledge becomes more detailed, it becomes clear that what had once been considered as a single process might later be interpreted as two or more distinguishable subprocesses.

We shall now list some of the more important of these questions concerning the sequence of physiological processes of sensory transduction and transmission. The general guiding sequence will be the afferent one we described earlier, starting from the most peripheral measurements of the physical stimulus and working toward the central nervous system. These are general questions, which seem meaningful to ask today about any sensory modality and which must be answered for each sense in order to complete a description of its function. We shall briefly mention some terms, which will be discussed in great detail later in this book. For the moment, the definitions are unavoidably vague, and the words are only introduced as a necessary means of formulating the questions.

1. What is the nature of the stimulus? Each sense organ is designed to be maximally sensitive to a certain type of physical energy. The description of the range of the physical dimensions of the most effective stimulus is probably the first question that must be asked of any sensory modality. The answer to this question may come either from psychophysical or electrophysiological studies.

2. How is the physical energy transmitted through the accessory sensory structures to the site of transduction? Most sense organs are designed to transmit the physical stimulus to the transduction site by means of accessory and nonneural apparatus, which do not alter, in any substantial way, the nature of the physical energy of the stimulus. For example, the mechanical compression waves, which we call sound, are transmitted to the cochlea by means of a guiding and collecting horn—the external ear, a system of levers and membranes—the middle ear, and finally by a hydraulic medium in the inner ear. The nature of the physical stimulus—mechanical energy—remains, however, the same throughout. There may be some modifications of the pattern of the stimulus by certain selective filtering properties, but it is still mechanical energy with the same physical dimensions that originally arrived at the external ear. Similarly, the optical properties of the eye, while important in defining the visual sensations, do not alter the nature of the photic stimulus—only the relative amounts of each wavelength that ultimately arrive at particular points in the retina.

3. What is the site of the primary sensory action? This question refers to the precise location at which the primary sensory action for each of the sensory modalities occurs. Surprisingly enough, it is not yet clear exactly where incoming stimuli exert their influence when one considers the issue at the level of the microanatomy of individual receptor cells of the various senses. The question has been answered with varying degrees of completeness in the different receptor systems. One of the most important developments in the cutaneous senses has been the observation that there are highly specialized areas of the membrane of the terminal portion of an axon that behave differently than adjacent regions with apparently identical structure. In the auditory sense, the most interesting current hypothesis is that the site of action is the cuticular plate at the base of the cilialike hairs. In the chemical senses, we have only the beginnings of the information needed to conclusively specify where in the cell membrane the critical effects occur. This question is a fundamental one and clearly distinguishable from the others that precede and follow it.

4. *What is the nature of the initial energy absorption process underlying transducer action?* All receptors perform the process of transduction converting one form of energy to another as a result of the primary sensory action. The actual transduction process involves a number of steps, the first of which is the alteration of the chemical equilibrium of the receptor by the physical energy of the stimulus. The nature of the actual process underlying this disequilibriation must be defined and analyzed. As examples, the sequential decomposition of large organic molecules has been identified as the key process for the visual receptor, and the alteration of hair cell membrane permeability by purely mechanical deformation has been implicated in the mechanoreceptor action of touch receptors in the skin.

5. *How does the energy absorption process lead to the generator potential?* One of the most exciting discoveries of recent years in the sensory sciences has been the elucidation of the *generator* or *receptor potential* mechanism of sensory receptors. (See the Introduction to Chapter 4 for a discussion of the differences in receptor and generator potentials.) It is now clear on the basis of a variety of experiments in the various modalities that the propagated spike action potentials conducted in long axons are actually always produced through the medium of some precursor potential of quite different properties. This precursor potential in receptors, which has come to be called the generator or receptor potential, is the first electropotential produced in the transduction process. It turns out that although we know fairly well what the energy absorption process is for most senses, the actual manner in which this absorption leads to the generator potential is, in general, one of the least-well-known stages in the sequence of processes that we have been discussing. The elucidation of the mechanisms responsible for the productions of the generator potentials will be one of the main issues of inquiry during the next decade for sensory neurophysiology.

6. *How are propagated action potentials generated by the generator or receptor potential?* The rapid developments in our understanding of the ionic chemistry of nerve cell membranes and the nature of the regenerative spike action potential, which can be propagated over long distances, has also been accompanied by new insights into the processes underlying the way in which the generator potential produces spike action potentials. The intervention of synaptic effects makes this one of the most interesting and well-known parts of the story.

7. *How are information-bearing electropotentials propagated from peripheral portions of the nervous system to other more central portions?* This question is seemingly too general for the fineness of the sequence we have

been describing. However, we are referring to a more restricted notion. The question of specific interest here concerns the mechanism of spike action potential propagation over the long axons evolved specifically for transmission purposes within the body. We shall only note here that there has been an enormous amount of progress in our understanding of spike action potential propagation throughout the nervous system, and for the purposes of sensory-coding theory, it may even be possible to go so far as to note that a sufficiently detailed answer has been given to this question.

8. How do signals cross from one cell to another at synapses, the points of anatomical discontinuity between neurons in the afferent chain? Synaptic action is, in itself, also a long and exciting story, which is gradually becoming understood. However, it seems as if synaptic action is one of those issues that are in the process of breaking apart into a number of more finely defined subquestions. Of special interest to us is the fact that there appears to be a very strong analogy developing between those portions of the synaptic process that occur on the upstream side of the synapse and the action of the peripheral receptor itself. It is only necessary to substitute a few words like "postsynaptic" potential for "generator" or "receptor" potential for a similar story to be told for each.

The preceding questions are issues of peripheral action and transduction and, in part, represent the subject matter of the first part of this book. There is, of course, also a host of questions which pertain to the central processing of this information once it arrives at the brain. For example, questions of the organization of the cerebral cortex and of the pathways intercommunicating among the various central brain structures are under active scrutiny. Similarly, the large class of psychophysical questions concerning the overall information-processing characteristics of the entire afferent and interpretive systems represents another major grouping of significant issues. Unfortunately, we have not been able to cover all of this and other material of equivalent importance to the depth some would have preferred. Answers to questions 7 and 8, unfortunately represent the main part of an entirely separate text. What we have done is to emphasize another specific question, that of coding or representation, to the maximum possible extent. The archetypical question might be formulated as follows: how are the patterns of information defined by the external stimuli represented at each of the levels of neural processing? And, as a corollary of this general question, what are the neural events that are used as symbols in this representation?

These latter two issues represent the main content of the second part of this book. How we have put this all together can be best introduced by reviewing its general plan.

III. PLAN OF THE BOOK

This book is divided into two major parts. The first part provides what is believed to be a relatively complete foundation of the basic and relevant physical and physiological materials necessary for a complete and indepth understanding of transduction. The second part is devoted to an analysis of the specific coding patterns that have been associated with various attributes of sensory continua.

Now let us consider these two sections in detail, looking at the specific goal of each of the constituent chapters.

The first section of this book is introduced by Chapter 2, an introduction to the basic physics of external stimuli. We classify stimuli in this chapter according to the conventional taxonomies of physics and point out the ways in which stimuli are generated. But most important for later materials we define the metrics used for specifying the amount and kind of each form of physical energy. We emphasize in this chapter the importance of using our well-established physical measures of energy as the starting point in any sensory experiment whether psychological or physiological.

Chapter 3 is dedicated entirely to neuroanatomy with special reference to the structure of the sensory systems. After introducing some of the techniques used by the modern neuroanatomist (with particular attention to modern developments in electron microscopy), the gross anatomy of the nervous system is presented to provide a frame of reference for later discussions. This chapter then collects together, in a single location, what are considered to be some of the finest drawings and photographs of receptor structure. Each modality is presented separately, first at the macroscopic level of organization and then, with increasingly magnified micrographs, in greater detail of fine structure. It is hoped that this brief atlas will not only introduce the various structures in an orderly way, but also emphasize the common anatomical features of this set of remarkable receptor cells. An added feature of the chapter is a set of drawings and discussions of the relay points in the ascending pathways from each modality. So much of the material in later chapters will assume knowledge of their anatomy that it was felt that it would be judicious to present it in a coherent form in this chapter.

The next chapter (Chapter 4) deals specifically with the transduction process or, as some have called it, interenergy transfer. The general problem area is one to which we have already alluded several times. Physical energy is transformed by the receptor organ into electrochemical energy. This chapter is concerned specifically with the processes that are thought to underlie the transformation action up to the stage at which the propagated spike action potential is generated. This chapter treats each of the senses individually for what are believed to be sound biological reasons. It is at the site of transduction that one modality differs more from another than at any later level. We mention the nonneural modification of physical stimuli by the accessory portions of each of the receptor organs. There is a wide variety of processes that tend to alter the physical stimulus before it arrives at the actual transducer tissue. It is important to consider these nonneural processes in terms of their simple physics rather than in the pseudophysical sense implied by a redefinition of the "proximal" and "distal" stimuli.

The material so far presented has been intended to provide an introduction for the second and main part of the book. In this second part, our thesis that there is an orderly relationship between the sensory experiences and the underlying pattern of neural activity is explored and developed in detail. The first chapter of this second section (Chapter 5) presents a statement of what it is that we mean by coding. We distinguish between those discriminable sensory dimensions common to all the modalities and those possible parameters of the neural language that may be associated with them. But the association of a specific neural dimension with a specific parameter of experience is a difficult and sometimes treacherous undertaking. We, therefore, point out some of the hazards faced by the psychophysiological cryptographer as he attempts to unravel the neural code from the multidimensional uproar of activity.

The next six chapters present our view of what is an up-to-date statement of the current views of coding for quantity, time and space, and quality, respectively. Chapter 6 presents the case for the coding of sensory magnitudes. It is initiated by a discussion of the relevant psychological data which must be explained. While it is clear that we cannot completely solve each and every problem or unequivocally define each and every code, enough data have accumulated in the last 20 years to provide at least a tentative statement of the significant coding variables and particularly to emphasize some of the most important consistencies between the psychological and physiological studies of the response dynamic. We then survey the neurophysiological data for as many of the senses for which data have been obtained as a function of variations in stimulus intensity, noting especially the peculiar status of quantity coding in the auditory modality. Stimulus-intensity, response-magnitude relations are considered for the generator potential, peripheral nerve, and central responses in each case. Based on this data, an answer can be proposed to a very important question: at what level does the major nonlinearity of the neural response occur? Finally, to illustrate a general method of inquiry as well for its own substantive sake, we consider whether or not interval irregularity is a "true code" for the representation of sensory magnitudes.

Chapter 7 presents a varied mixture of studies, which illustrate how drastically our attitudes toward the coding of space and time have changed in recent years. We speak, in this chapter, of such phenomena as spatial localization and the interaction of temporally separated stimuli as examples of the loss of fidelity inherent in sensory processing. It is also in this chapter that we discuss the elegant research on the physiological basis of spatial interaction carried out by a large number of physiologists stimulated by the works of H. Keffer Hartline. We then turn to the perception of time, particularly emphasizing some of the newly emerging awareness of the limitations of time as a neural code. We then, in Chapter 8, discuss what has come to be a most important field of modern sensory psychobiology—highly selective neural responses to specific spatio-temporal features of the stimulus pattern. Finally, since so often this type of physiological finding has been misapplied to the explanation of perceptual phenomena, we then discuss, in a critical vein, the relevance of this microscopic neural phenomena to molar behavior.

Chapter 9 presents the various theories of quality coding for vision. It is introduced with a discussion of what it is that we mean by a *quality*. The dictionary definition that quality is that discriminable difference which remains after one accounts for intensive and extensive dimensions in time and space is weak, yet it hardly seems possible to give a more compelling definition. We first consider some of the key psychophysical data and the resulting alternative theories which have been proposed over the years. Not all theories of visual quality coding, which have been proposed over the years, have a neurophysiological basis. Some are merely descriptive and are not therefore germane to the topic of this book. But for those that are relevant, an attempt is made to extract the key neurophysiological elements so that we are really sure what the controversies are all about, at the level of discourse in which we are engaged. Having done so, we then review the neurophysiological data and on that basis describe what is believed to be the best possible contemporary theory of quality coding. Audition is discussed in Chapter 10 in the same way, and the other senses in Chapter 11. In concluding Chapter 11, we seek the generalities common among all of the senses and specifically discuss the ways in which Müller's classic law of specific nerve energies has been modified under the impact of these modern findings.

Clearly, the problems of quality coding are among the most complex to be discussed in this book. While the physics of the stimulus helps us to order our thoughts about visual and auditory quality coding, we do not have appropriate or simple physical dimensions on which we can found our analysis in the somesthetic and the chemical senses. There is no simple analogue in somesthesis, gustation, or olfaction for the roles played by wavelengths of the photic stimulus or the frequency of the acoustic stimulus.

In Chapter 12—The Epilog—we sum up the various facts and theories that we have considered so far in the book. We ask the question: is a unified theory of sensory activity possible in the context of our current state of knowledge of sensory processes? And finally we present a set of emerging "principles" of sensory coding, which help to further sum up current knowledge concerning the neural representation of sensory messages.

The reader should now appreciate that this book covers a wide swath through the sensory psychobiological literature. He should also be made aware of the fact that a single volume can, at best, only do this superficially. To emphasize the point, nothing could be more effective than to note that at about the same time that this book is published, one of the major publishing events of the century will also occur. A many-volumed handbook of sensory physiology will begin to appear from the presses of the Springer-Verlag Publishing Company of Berlin, Heidelberg, and New York. The full extent of this project, which will probably not be fulfilled for some years, is not yet clear, but it is evident at this point that there will be at least 20 volumes, each of approximately the same size as this present text. Obviously, this important handbook will be a virtually inexhaustible and valuable source of information for those who want a much more complete story than this much more modest text can possibly offer. Equally obviously, however, such a handbook is hardly the place to start for the student who is being newly introduced to the psychobiology of sensory coding.

There are, furthermore, a number of important and fundamental areas which we have not covered in detail. For example, if it had not been for the fact that there are numerous good summaries of psychophysical techniques, it would have been necessary for this book to cover that ground too. There are many instances in which we have assumed a knowledge of the procedures and philosophy of psychophysical experimentation, which at least some of the readers of this book may not have. A particularly good discussion, which covers this important material, is to be found in Chapter 7 of Corso (1967). Some readers will also miss a review of the relevant electrochemistry and neurophysiology of transmission in axons and across synapses. Indeed, the draft of this book included chapters on these topics. Limits on the size of the volume as finally published required that they be deleted, and therefore the reader is directed to other sources (for example, Thompson, 1967; Katz, 1966; Stevens, 1966)[2] for modern surveys of the relevant material.

[2] More detailed discussions of this material can be found in D. J. Aidley. *The Physiology of Excitable Cells.* Cambridge, 1971; V. B. Mountcastle (Ed.) *Medical Physiology, VII.* Mosby, 1968; or the distinguished volume by K. S. Cole. *Membranes, Ions and Impulses.* University of California, 1968.

SECTION ONE: FUNDAMENTAL MATERIALS

CHAPTER 2: THE NATURE OF PHYSICAL STIMULI

I. INTRODUCTION

A. What is a Stimulus?

Now that we have set the stage for our discussion by placing the scientific and technical aspects of sensory psychophysiology in their appropriate philosophical context, we can begin our journey up the ascending pathways. We must start, however, with some nonphysiological facts, for it is always some inorganic aspect of the external world of physical energies that is the precursor for each sensory response. Though sense organs in many cases do respond without the presence of some identifiable external physical action, we shall not be concerned with such "spontaneous" or "persistent" activity for the moment. Rather, in this chapter, we shall try to provide the necessary foundation material so that the reader will be able to interpret the metrics used for the specification of stimuli.

The word *stimulus* has a very specific meaning in sensory psychobiology. It is defined as a pattern of physical energy, which produces activity in the sensory pathways. There are a number of restrictions implicit in this definition, which we should discuss explicitly. First of all, note that we have not said that a stimulus is a pattern of physical energy that is merely capable of producing activity. To be a stimulus, the physical energy must actually produce activity. We, therefore, must distinguish between those patterns of physical energy that are *potential* stimuli and those that are *actual* stimuli. Potential stimuli are physical energies that lie within the range of sensitivity of some receptor organ, but that have not yet produced activity in the neural portions of the sensor. Actual stimuli are those potential stimuli that actually have been transduced into forms of neural energy. This chapter, within the scope of these definitions, is concerned with potential stimuli, for we shall be discussing the nature of physical energies as measured with instruments independent of their possible biological effectiveness.

An important point made in the definition of an actual stimulus is that it must produce some subsequent neural response. The organism is constantly exposed to a wide variety of physical energies, not all of which produce electrical activity in the receptors and transmission pathways. Furthermore, not all of these neural responses are either behaviorally or metabolically significant. There appear to be some important neural mechanisms whose function is to *gate* or *allow* only a small number of these signals to actually arrive at the level of consciousness or awareness, or to otherwise affect the function of the organism. Those that are not so allowed are actual stimuli only in a limited physiological way but not psychologically. Electrophysiologists might be unhappy with this definition, but it is necessary for psychobiologists to further restrict the meaning of the term *stimulus* to behaviorally significant ones in order to avoid having it take on such an enormous variety of meanings that it loses all specific meaning.

Another important point to note concerning the definition of a behaviorally significant stimulus is that we have made no specific limitation on the temporal dimension of the term *subsequent*. The response, which is engendered by a stimulus, may be relatively immediate—occurring within a few milliseconds of the time the signal arrives at an appropriate anatomical level—or it may be greatly delayed. Those delays may be as great as several decades. Some of the experiments conducted by Penfield and Roberts (1959) have suggested that when the brain is appropriately stimulated, there may be detailed recall of sensory messages that were recorded many years previously.

Another significant restriction in our definition is that the mere presence of physical energy does not always constitute a behaviorally effective stimulus even if the physical energy is well within the limits of sensitivity of the appropriate sense organ. The physical energy, in most cases, must be patterned or modulated both temporally and spatially to be effective. The notion of pattern is interjected for very specific empirical reasons. Continuous or unchanging modes of physical stimulation seem to lose their efficacy as stimuli very quickly, unless there is some fluctuation of one or another of their dimensions. This fluctuation may be due either to the nature of the stimulus or be introduced by the receptor organ itself. For example, Riggs, Ratliff, Cornsweet, and Cornsweet (1953) have shown that visual patterns, projected into the eye in such a way that they do not move with respect to the retina, tend to disappear very quickly. Their interpretation is that the natural eye movements (saccades) are very important in making a pattern of physical energy effective as a stimulus, because they modulate the energy falling on any given receptor. It is not at all clear why the fading of the stabilized image should take place, but it is clear that in the later stages of fading, the same pattern of physical energy is no longer effective as a stimulus. Furthermore, we shall be discussing instances later in this book in which physical energy patterns that differ only in their shape, speed, or direction of movement may be either vigorously effective or totally ineffective (at least with regard to certain specialized neural elements) purely on the basis of that spatial or temporal difference. These are the sorts of phenomenon that make us restrict and limit the meaning of psychobiologically effective stimuli.

B. The Logical Necessity for Dealing with the Potential Stimulus as an Initial Reference

In any formal logical structure, there is a set of axioms or fundamental beliefs which is used as a starting point for discussion. We do not usually identify all of the axioms upon which we build our formal system. In science this is no less true, even though there is usually at least an illusion of a clearly defined set of definitions and basic measurements which are assumed to be commonly understood by all conversants. We spend a large amount of our collegiate experience learning about the parameters of these basic measures and assumptions. For each of the sciences there may be quite a different set of these axioms. For example, in chemistry many phenomena may be explained even though the unit of discussion is no more detailed than the atomic structures and their associated laws of combination.

In sensory psychobiology it is particularly necessary to have a clearly defined starting point, since the general subject matter is one which, as we pointed out in Chapter 1, is defined in terms of a natural sequence of events which occur in the afferent direction. So where do we begin? What is the set of references to which we can turn when we measure the responses of either some neural step in the chain, or even the most complicated psychophysical judgment? In spite of the fact that we have defined stimuli in terms of their effectiveness in generating a subsequent response, it is only fair to say that in many cases this is not an operational definition. This is so because it is often not possible to specify whether or not a response has actually occurred, or will ultimately occur. Thus, the theoretically pure definition of an actual stimulus cannot provide the concreteness we need in the day-to-day manipulations in the laboratory. The notion of a potential stimulus, however, can be so used. The discussion, which makes up the greater part of this chapter, is therefore a discussion of potential stimuli. It is a discussion of physical energies as they exist, are generated, and are measured in the external world prior to their reception, modification, and transduction by the receptor mechanism.

The class of potential stimuli, of course, enlarges or contracts occasionally as new receptor mechanisms, which are sensitive to unexpected forms of physical energy, are uncovered, or when known receptors are shown to be sensitive to narrower or wider ranges of known potential stimuli. Nevertheless, we feel that it is a better starting point than some confounded measure of actual stimuli. This chapter is, therefore, really a short course in the physics of potential stimuli, independent of their subsequent sensory effects. Nonetheless, the specific subject matter is selected on the basis of known receptor sensitivities.

A precise definition of physical energy patterns is the only meaningful place to start our discussion of sensory systems. It makes little sense, for example, to add the artificial dichotomy of the proximal or distal stimuli in the light of present-day knowledge. The use of these terms was an attempt to emphasize the fact that the physical energy that falls upon the surface of the receptor may be modified in many ways by the time it arrives at the transducer itself. There is, in many cases, a substantial difference in energy content of the stimulus, though usually not in energy type, as a function of passive absorption and modifications performed by the nonneural accessory structures of the various sense organs. We prefer to emphasize the same point in a different way: we shall view the problem as one of a series of energy modifications and transformations, in which the passive properties of the accessory structures are considered in their own right, just as much a biological phenomenon as the neural transduction processes themselves. Throughout this analysis it must be remembered that the actual transduction mechanism has not been definitely identified for all receptors, and many questions remain concerning the specific mode of action of any given stimulus.

For these reasons, and as the reference point from which all other sensory phenomena must be considered, it seems that the only choice is the potential stimulus—the physics of the variety of biologically significant energies.

C. The Notion of the Adequate Stimulus

Having defined a stimulus and distinguished between actual and potential stimuli, it is now necessary to turn to another definition, which has long played an important role in sensory psychobiology—the notion of the *adequate stimulus*. The adequate stimulus is defined, for each sense modality, as the type of physical energy to which the particular receptor is most sensitive. Thus, conventionally, photic energy was considered to be the adequate stimulus for the eye. However, as we have learned more and more about the receptive range of a given receptor, the notion of the adequate stimulus has changed. In vision, for example, it turns out that "photic energy in general" is not a term that has sufficient precision to add very much to our description of the physical process. Rather, it has been found that there are different types of visual receptors, each responsive to a slightly different band of wavelengths of electromagnetic energy. Thus, the adequate stimulus for a long wavelength-sensitive receptor in the eye is, for all practical purposes, a band of wavelengths less than the total visual range, but greater than a single wavelength. The specialized visual receptors may, therefore, be said to be relatively broadly tuned, but yet not sensitive to the full range of visual stimuli. In actual fact, the efficiency of the "quantal catch" for any photopigment is never completely zero for any wavelength of light, visible or not. There is always the possibility of some absorption if the intensity of the photic stimulus is high enough, but the approximation of finite bandwidths for each of the visual pigments is a good one for most of what is known about human vision. Later in this book we shall discuss the important implications of this recurring notion of broadly, yet not infinitely, tuned receptors, but for the moment consider a definition of the most adequate stimulus in terms of a well-specified, moderately broad range of physical energies.

Closely related to this notion of the adequate stimulus is a law of sensory activity, which has been only infrequently challenged since it was put forth by Müller in 1840. This is the famous *law of the specific energies of nerves*. This doctrine states that the sensation resulting from stimulation is a result of the activity of a given set of nerves, rather than the nature of the external stimulus. A modern corollary of this notion is that regardless of the nature of the stimulus, activation of a given nerve produces a sensation characteristic of that nerve. The all-or-none law of nerve spike action potentials, is also closely related to this doctrine. It states that the amplitude and duration of the pulsatile response of an axon are independent of the stimulus characteristics once the threshold of activation is exceeded.

There is reason to suggest, however, that the time has come to modify the connotations, if not the denotations, of the specific nerve energy doctrine at the individual cellular level. The reasons behind such a change arise out of the accumulating mass of data, which indicate that most receptors are broadly, rather than sharply, tuned. Furthermore, there is additional evidence that suggests that it requires a comparison by some decoding mechanism of the relative amount of activity in two or more receptors to establish the quality of a stimulus. Thus, the information conveyed by a single neural element is not sufficient to define a unique stimulus quality. The implications of these developments may profoundly affect the contemporary extrapolation of Müller's law to the idea of single cell specificity. If no single element could carry information adequate to define a sensory quality, then in this sense Müller's law is misleading, for implicit in the modern view of his doctrine is the notion that the particular neuron or the "place in the nervous system" is the critical code for sensory quality. If, on the other hand, this is not the case, but if in addition or instead a comparison of the rate of activity in two or more loci is more important, then we do not really have the pure place coding of quality that is implied by Müller's law. Rather, a mixture of spatial and temporal comparisons is required, which is quite a different concept.

The tale of the particular dimensions of neural activity, which are responsible for coding sensory quality, is one we shall tell in detail in Chapters 9, 10, and 11 but the points we have made in this section are important adjuncts to our appreciation of what is meant by the term *stimulus*.

Now let us consider another aspect of stimulus specification—the dimensions of the physical energy itself. This consideration will be formulated in terms of a brief review of the physics of various forms of energy. For each of the types of physical energy that has been shown to be a potential stimulus for one or another sensory modality, we shall consider the measures that are used to define the kind or quality of the stimulus when applicable, and the typical laboratory sources of the physical energy for experimental purposes. There is no particular order to the discussion other than the one used in the traditional elementary physics course. Table 2.1 is presented as a general preview and summary of much of the material contained in this chapter on stimuli. In addition to listing the various kinds of physical energies in this table, we have also briefly noted the nature of the adequate stimulus, the metric of quantity or amount,

TABLE 2.1. THE DIMENSIONS, SOURCES,
AND UNITS OF POTENTIAL PHYSICAL STIMULI

Sensory Modality		Adequate Stimulus	Metric Associated with Sensory Magnitude
Mechanical	Acoustic	Pneumatic force	Bel and decibel
	Vestibular	Acceleration	g
	Mechanical cutaneous	Mechanical force or gradient of force	Grams, dynes, pounds, etc.
	Proprioceptive	Position & velocity	Degrees & deg/sec or inches & in./sec
Photic		Electromagnetic waves (photons)	Radiometric measures Photometric measures
Chemical		Specific atoms, ions, or molecules	% by weight or volume Mass/volume ratio Molar system Molal system Normal system % saturation
Electrical		Electricity	Voltage — volt Current — ampere Power — watt
Thermal		Temperature or temperature change	°C, °F, °A, etc.

the usual metric of the kind or quality of the energy, and a few possible devices that are conventionally used to generate these energy patterns. The remainder of the chapter is organized in the same fashion as this table with more complete discussions of each of the constituent entries.

II. MECHANICAL STIMULI

A. The Nature of Mechanical Stimuli

Mechanics is that branch of the physical sciences that deals with the action of forces and their relation to the equilibrium, deformation, and motion of

Table 2.1 (*cont.*)

Metric Associated with Sensory Quality	Source
Frequency* (Hz)	Loudspeakers & earphones
Direction	Turntables, linear accelerators
Frequency* (Hz)	Vibrators, hairs, weights, etc.
—	Manipulators
Wavelength (nm)	Incandescent sources Fluorescent sources
Atomic and molecular classification system	Sources of liquids, vapors, and solids
—	Power supplies Waveform generators Coils, etc.
—	Radiant heater Conductive heater Thermoelectric device

solids, liquids, and gases. Mechanical forces are those that tend to deform or accelerate objects possessing mass. This definition is not entirely modern. Modern theoretical physics has made great strides toward unifying the energetics of the various forms of energy (for example, $E = mc^2$). But there is still, at the level at which we shall deal, a system of mechanical language that is quite separate from that used to describe electrical or chemical actions, for example. The language of mechanical actions is based upon the use of the dimensions of mass, length, and time, as well as other functions derived from these three basic dimensions. *Mass* is a property of a material object and is defined in terms of the resistance of the body to changes in its current state of motion. The mass (or inertia) of an object is great for objects that require a great force to change their state of motion, and small for objects that require but a small force to change their state of motion. A change in the state of motion is called an *acceleration*. The term *state of motion* refers, of course, to the velocity (a term that includes direction), or speed (a term that does not include direction), at which an object is moving. An object at rest has a velocity of zero unit of length per second. Objects moving in a direction opposite to some arbitrary positive direction defined by one's current coordinate system are said to have negative velocity. Accelerative forces thus act by adding velocity to an object, or subtracting velocity from it. The fundamental law of physics, which expresses the verbal statements we have just made, in mathematical form is

$$F = m \times a \tag{2.1}$$

In this equation F is the force exerted; m is the mass of the object; and a is the acceleration imposed by the force. The dimension of each unit will depend upon which system of units is being used. The mass of an object is, therefore, measured by applying a force and measuring the acceleration. The larger the force it takes to produce a given acceleration, the larger the mass of the object. The larger the acceleration imposed by a given force, the smaller the mass. The units of force used by physicists are quite varied, but in the metric system they are founded upon a basic unit called a *dyne*. A dyne is defined as a force that will impart a 1 cm/sec additional velocity in 1 sec to a mass of 1 g(gram). 1 cm/sec additional velocity added in 1 sec is also referred to as a 1 cm/sec^2 acceleration.

Within the framework of the sensory sciences, the basic unit of potential mechanical stimuli is also the dyne. For example, all acoustic measurements are defined in terms of this unit. Specifically, the basic reference unit of force for hearing has been defined as an air pressure of 0.0002 dyne applied to 1 cm^2—air pressure being another form of mechanical force. This value has been chosen because this number is very close to the threshold of human hearing at the most effective frequency.

Although forces are defined in terms of their ability to alter the motion of a rigid body, in fact most real bodies are not rigid and do not react at all like the ideal "billiard ball" of the dynamicist's theoretical world. Objects more typically have less than perfect rigidity and considerable spatial extent. Therefore they tend to produce forces that are opposite to any forces that may be acting upon them, just as a compressed spring exerts a force opposite to the force of compression. In this case, the inner elasticity of the object and the external force produce a pair of forces which are equal and opposite. In this manner they ultimately establish an equilibrium state in which no changes occur in the motion of the object. What does occur, instead, is a deformation of the object itself—a deformation that quickly achieves the equilibrium condition and then is static in the sense that no further change in motion or shape may occur. Even in this case, forces measurable in terms of their equivalent ability to accelerate a theoretical rigid object are still operating.

The force applied to a receptor mechanism, however, is not in itself usually the effective stimulus or—in our previously defined terms—the

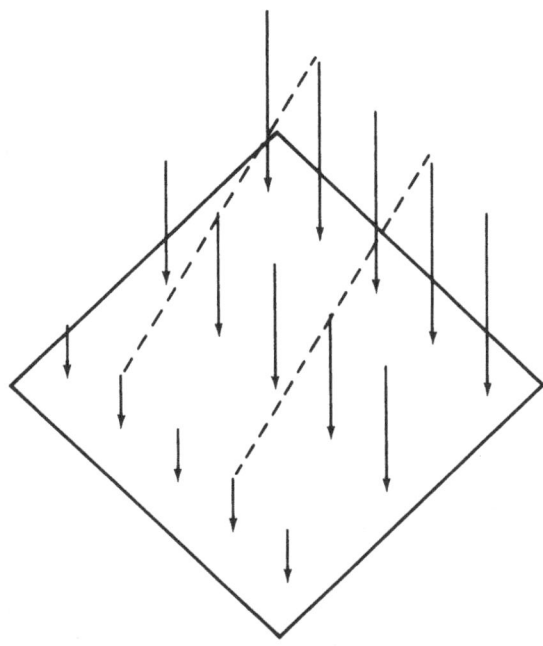

FIGURE 2.1 A field of force with a gradient of intensity varying from one side to the other of the area to which it is applied.

instigator of the primary sensory action. That is, sense organs are in general really not sensitive to forces as such, but rather to the effects produced by the force, such as the deformation or the induced motion imposed on the receptor. This is a subtle point, but it recurs again and again in our analysis of the transducer action of mechanosensitive organs. Driving forces of one kind or another act on tissue to produce effects which themselves are the primary conditions for activation of the mechanoreceptor mechanism. If the same forces had impinged on tissues of different elastic or viscous properties, it is conceivable that they might not even be considered to be potential stimuli. For mechanoreceptors the primary activating effect may be a deformation of some receptor, or the movement of some organ in which receptors are imbedded. It may even be action required to develop a necessary counterforce, which must be generated to produce a state of equilibrium, as described above. In fact, however, we are rarely really able to measure the subtle deformations that occur at the receptor mechanism. In psychophysical experiments particularly, we can usually only state the dimensions of the mechanical forces that are applied, in spite of the fact that they are not usually considered to be the most immediate aspect of a stimulus.

Another concept that we must also note is the gradient. A gradient is a pattern of forces, positions, velocities, or any other physical dimension that is not constant at all places. Figure 2.1 is a plot of a hypothetical force acting on a surface extending from *A* to *B*. Such a force, continuous but varying in amplitude from place to place, is said to possess a gradient over that surface. Gradients can lead to some surprising sensory experiences due to interactive effects among the receptors stimulated by the varying force pattern. We shall consider some of these in detail in Chapter 9.

B. Metrics of Kind

1. *Basic Properties of Sinusoids.* Mechanical stimuli have been defined in simple terms of force. Whether there is a single universal force or several different kinds of forces at the subatomic level is a problem occupying the attention of many physicists today. For the purpose of sensory psychophysiology, however, there is but a single kind of mechanical force. The qualitative differences between the sensations produced by that force are due either to its temporal patterns or to the locus of stimulation. The distinction between two major modalities such as cutaneous touch sensitivity and hearing, for example, depends primarily upon the differential characteristics of the sensitive surfaces. If the force is applied to the skin by means of some appropriate vibrator, the sensation is a cutaneous one. Differences in the magnitude of the stimulus and characteristics of the stimulated site, therefore, bring different sensitivities into play, but the general experience is one dictated by the place on the skin at which the stimulus acts. On the other hand, if the mechanical force of sufficient amplitude is transmitted by means of vibrations in the air, they are very likely to impinge upon the ultrasensitive sensory mechanism of the inner ear and be experienced as sounds at the lowest energy levels. The main requirement for a mechanical stimulus to produce an auditory experience is that the vibrations be within the auditory range of about 20 to 20,000 Hz.

The dimension of physical energy that most strongly affects auditory quality is the frequency of the airborne vibration. This is not the only parameter of the auditory stimulus that will affect quality—the amplitude of the signal is also involved—but in this discussion we are concerned with a description of the nature of the physical energy rather than the correlated perception. In this context and in that of other mechanical stimuli, the best way to describe the different kinds of force is in terms of the differences in temporal patterns of the force. A very useful notation for the time-varying amplitude functions is that general one used in the description of vibratory or sinusoidal motions. Not all stimuli are oscillatory, and not all oscillations are purely sinusoidal, but since it is possible to describe any complex waveform in terms of a superimposition of sinusoids, the convenient and well-developed notation of sinusoidal oscillations has come to be the standard descriptive language for periodically repeating patterns of force. Figure 2.2 is a diagram of a sinusoidal wave pattern. Such a sinusoidal waveform has a number of metrics, which allow us to define it uniquely. This figure is a plot of the changes in the amplitude of an applied force as a function of time. Thus, a simple amplitude measurement at any arbitrary moment is unlikely to give a correct estimate of the maximum or minimum values. There are several ways in which the amplitude of the force can, however, be quantified if the signal has been established to be of a specific waveform such as the sinusoid we are dealing with here. One may specify the peak-to-peak or peak-to-zero level amplitude of the wave.

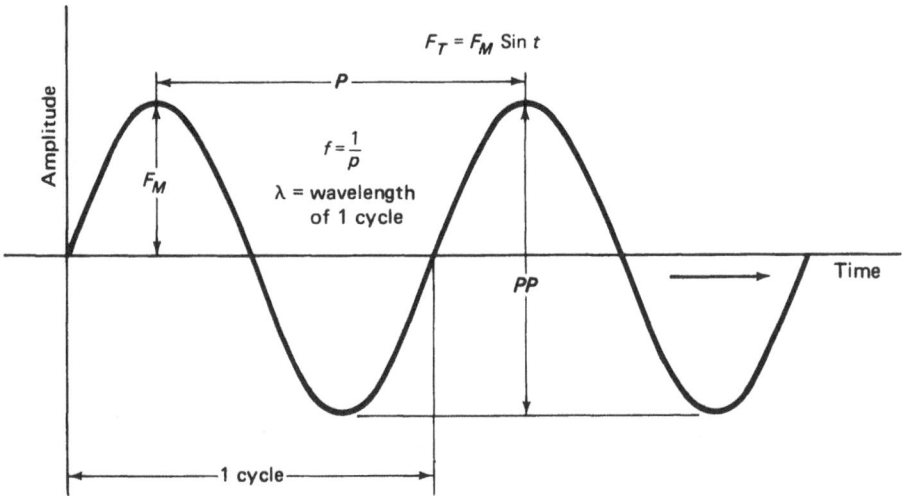

FIGURE 2.2 *A diagram indicating the basic dimensions of a typical sinusoidal wave. F_m is the half-wave amplitude; PP is the peak-to-peak amplitude; P is the period of time (or of space) for one cycle; the frequency f is defined as the reciprocal of the period 1/P.*

The force at any point on the sine wave is precisely defined by the equation

$$F_t = F_m \sin t \tag{2.2}$$

where t is time; F_t is the force at time t; and F_m is the value obtained by the maximum force. Since the wave is precisely defined for each point by means of this equation, and the maximum (either peak to peak or half of that value) force is known, each and every point on the curve is then also defined.

Other measures of amplitude are occasionally used. The root-mean-square value (rms) is obtained by squaring the amplitude of the wave at each and every amplitude, computing the mean of the sum of these squared values, and then taking the square root of that mean value. This procedure is well worth the extra effort, because often the effectiveness of a sinusoidal wave is better specified by this metric than by the simple peak-to-peak measure or an average value. For example, the heating efficiency of an electric sinusoidal voltage is well defined by the rms measure for all waveforms —a feature not shared by the other measures. The rms is, in fact, a measure of the power carried by a varying waveform.

The pattern of a sinusoidal waveform is a repetitive one. After a complete *cycle* (one complete nonrepeating wave), the amplitude of the wave has returned to its starting point. The length of time taken for one complete cycle is defined as the *period* of the vibration. The reciprocal of the period—the number of vibrations per unit time—is defined as the *frequency* of the waveform and is now measured in units of hertz (Hz).

Another set of definitions is required for those waveforms that are not cyclically repetitive. Impulsive forces, for example, are nonrepeated transients, which can be better defined in terms of their wave shape, their amplitude, and their duration, rather than in terms of their frequency.

2. *Frequency Analysis.* There is a very important notion, which occurs repeatedly throughout any discussion of waveform patterns of physical energy. We have spoken of sinusoids and of impulsive forces as if they were, in fact, realistic mechanical stimuli. However, these signals are rarely obtained in natural situations; most potential mechanical stimuli have complex waveforms. Consider, as two examples, the overtones from any musical instrument, or the distortions introduced into cutaneous mechanical stimuli by the various forces and counterforces generated by the elastic and less than perfectly rigid properties of the skin. Even the purest of sinusoidal stimuli can often become unrecognizable after interacting with the various components of the dynamic system involved. However, in each case, almost without regard to the severity of the distortion or the degree of deviation from a pure sinusoid, these signals can be described in terms of a sum of sinusoids.

A powerful analytical mechanism, that has proven itself in many different applications, is the notion of frequency or Fourier Analysis. The basic idea behind this analytical technique is that any waveform can be represented as the superimposition of simpler waveforms. Almost any set of functions can be used as these components in a Fourier Analysis but there are some advantages to using sets that are orthogonal, that is, in which the individual functions are perpendicular to each other in some function space. It turns out that one of the most useful and most commonly used sets of orthogonal functions is the family of sine and cosine functions—$\sin nt$ and $\cos nt$. According to Fourier, the originator of this analytical technique, any function $f(t)$, which is defined as a periodic function, can be analyzed into a specific set of sinusoidal (or other orthogonal) component frequencies. Another way of saying the same thing is that any function $f(t)$ can be approximated to any arbitrarily small degree of error by the summation of a series of sinusoids. The mathematical expression for this relation is:

$$f(t) = \sum_{n=0}^{\infty} (a_n \cos nt + b_n \sin nt) \qquad (2.3)$$

For most mechanical force functions, the variable t is specifically equal to time. The sine functions used in Equation (2.3) are, therefore, functions of time, although in general this need not be so. Standing spatial waves, fixed in time, can also be represented by functions in x, y, or z, rather than t.

Equation (2.3) can be expanded to the following form:

$$f(t) = a_0 + a_1 \cos t + a_2 \cos 2t + \cdots + a_n \cos nt + b_1 \sin t +$$
$$b_2 \sin 2t + \cdots + b_n \sin nt \qquad (2.4)$$

The coefficients a_n and b_n are weighting functions, which determine how much of each of the various sinusoidal components are added to the mixture to form the final waveform. Because it represents the base level around which the resulting function is oscillating, a_0 is particularly significant.

There are a number of conditions that must be fulfilled by functions that are to be analyzed into a Fourier series consisting of a sum of sinusoids. The functions must be defined over at least the range π to $-\pi$ and they must be periodic for multiples of π and $-\pi$. Signals that are nonperiodic can be analyzed by the simple artifact of considering the signal to be only one period of a hypothetical waveform, which is mathematically defined for other periods preceding and following the single real interval. Another condition that the function must fulfill is that both the number of maxima and minima, as well as points of discontinuity, must all be finite. These mathematical restrictions are all adequately satisfied by the continuous stimulus patterns and bioelectric potentials with which we shall deal.

The generation of the coefficients a_n and b_n actually determines the nature of the specific series that will fit a given function. For functions meeting the conditions described above, the coefficients are defined by the following two expressions:

$$a_n = \frac{1}{\pi} \int_{-\pi}^{\pi} f(t) \cos nt \, dt \qquad (2.5)$$

$$b_n = \frac{1}{\pi} \int_{-\pi}^{\pi} f(t) \sin nt \, dt \qquad (2.6)$$

To illustrate the analysis of a given waveform by the Fourier-series technique, consider the function for a straight line with a slope of 45° in time: $f(t) = t$. This function is only defined for one period, which we shall arbitrarily place within the limits $-\pi$ to π. Nevertheless, for the purpose of the analysis, we artificially define it as a periodic function, which repeats itself every two time units. Substituting this function in Equations (2.5) and (2.6), we see that:

$$a_n = \frac{1}{\pi} \int_{-\pi}^{\pi} t \cos nt \, dt = 0 \qquad (2.7)$$

$$b_n = \frac{1}{\pi} \int_{-\pi}^{\pi} t \sin nt \, dt = \frac{-2}{n} \cos n \qquad (2.8)$$

$$\therefore b_n = \frac{2}{n} \qquad \text{for odd } n$$

and

$$b_n = \frac{-2}{n} \qquad \text{for even } n$$

These two expressions tell us that all of the coefficients a_n for the sine functions are equal to zero, and that all of the coefficients b_n for the cosine functions are nonzero. Therefore, the Fourier series for this function is a sum of cosine functions. The Fourier series [Equation (2.2)] for this function can, therefore, be expressed as:

$$f(t) = 2 \sin t - \frac{\sin 2t}{2} + \frac{\sin 3t}{3} - \frac{\sin 4t}{4} + \cdots \pm \frac{\sin nt}{n} \qquad (2.9)$$

For most practical purposes, only a few of the terms in this infinite series are used either in reconstructing or in representing the original function. Figure 2.3 is a diagram of the addition of the first few terms of the Fourier series for the function $f(t) = t$, showing an increasingly good fit as more terms are added together. It should be remembered, however, that the triangular wave is only one half of one period of a mathematical function, which is defined as extending continuously in both directions in time.

This descriptive discussion of frequency analysis is intended to emphasize the uses of the technique. The reader interested in a more rigorous mathematical discussion is directed to any of the standard treatments of time series analysis (for example, Lee, 1960).

Though we have presented the notion of Fourier analysis in this section on mechanical stimuli and although this mathematical procedure is particularly relevant to the hearing process, it should be remembered that any waveform representing oscillations in any form of energy can be equally well represented. Similarly, though this section on the physics of stimuli seemed to be the appropriate place to present the frequency analytical method, it should also be noted that the technique can also be applied to the analysis of repetitive neural or behavioral responses.

The Fourier analysis of any signal results in a set of sinusoidal component waveforms of specified frequencies of specific amplitudes. A very useful way of presenting this same information in an easily interpreted graphic form is a *spectral plot*, an example of which is shown in Figure 2.4. This particular spectral plot happens to be that of the triangular wave we just analyzed.

Spectral plots serve the important purpose of representing many features of complex waveforms, which are not apparent from an inspection of the original signal. For those physical systems that do not pass all frequencies with equal ease (such devices are called filters), a spectral plot allows one to predict the shape of an output signal by subtracting, to the degree necessary, those affected waveforms, and composing the new shape from a summation of the remaining waveforms. Spectral plots can be produced automatically for auditory signals, for example, and are useful guides to the frequency characteristics. In the production of such a plot, however, all information concerning the phase relations of the components and the duration of the signal is lost. Spectral plots of light sources are an important part of the specification of visual stimuli.

Now that we have this very brief introduction to mechanical forces and some of the useful descriptive notations, let us look in greater detail at

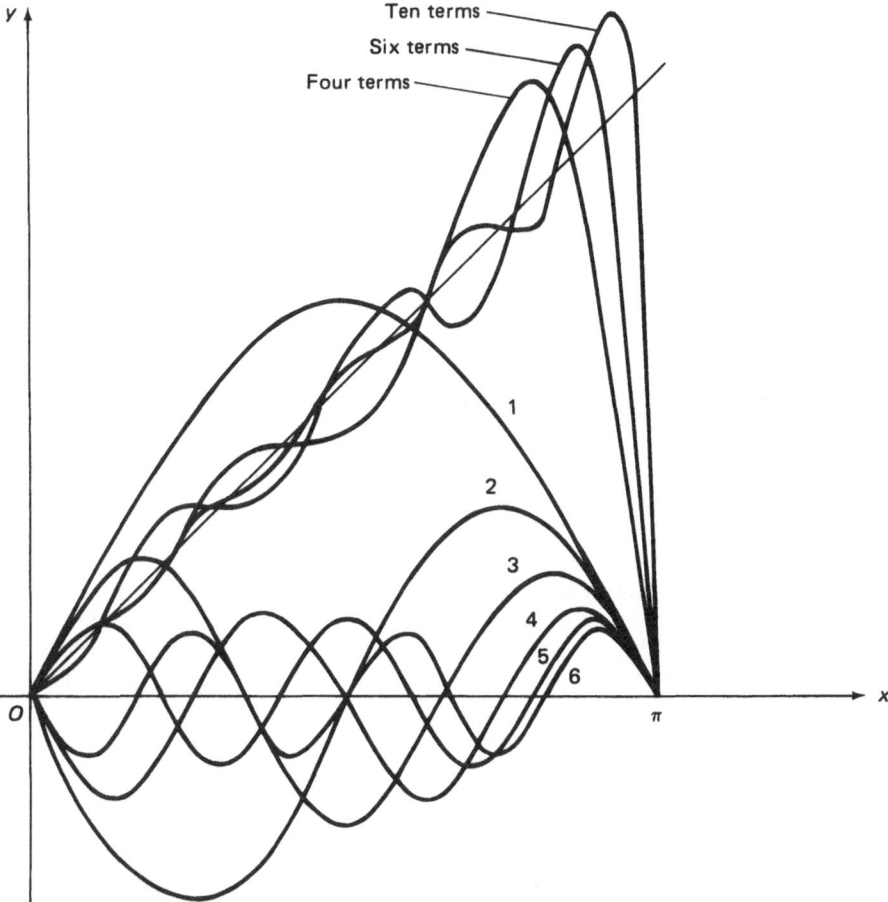

FIGURE 2.3 The synthesis of a triangular wave by the superimposition of several sinusoidal waveforms. Those sinusoids that are initially negative-going are the subtractive terms in Equation (6.7) (from Sokolnikoff and Sokolnikoff, 1941).

the nature of potential mechanical stimuli, with specific reference to each of the major mechanoreceptive sensory modalities.

C. Quantity Measurements of Acoustic Stimuli

The most sensitive mechanoreceptive sense is, of course, the auditory modality. The mechanical energy, which can stimulate the acoustic mechanism, is made up of waves of compression and rarefaction in the air. In addition, vibrations induced directly in the bony tissues of the head can also evoke acoustic sensations.

The waves of compression and rarefaction, which pass through these physical media and which constitute the potential acoustic stimulus, travel at speeds that depend greatly upon the conducting material. This can be

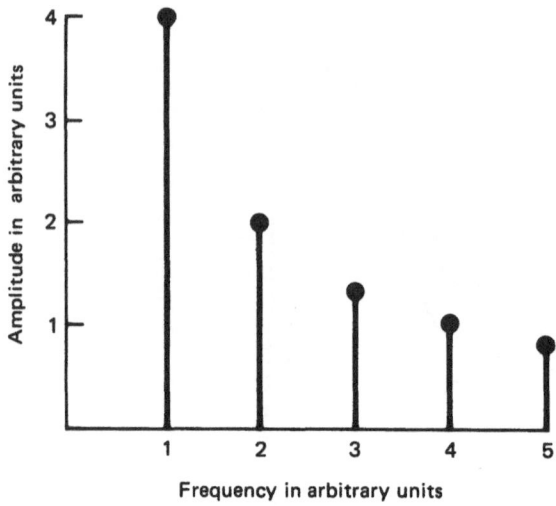

FIGURE 2.4 A power spectrum of the sinusoids used to produce the triangular wave in Figure 2.3.

made intuitively obvious in two ways. If the medium is a loose and elastic material without great rigidity, a mechanical disturbance at one end will be propogated rather slowly to the other, since energy is passed only weakly from one portion of the medium to the next. On the other hand, if the medium is very rigid, a disturbance at one end will quickly emerge at the other end. Thus, the rigidity of a medium is one of the important factors determining the speed of conduction in that medium. Another factor is the density of the material. Density affects the speed of transmission of sound because of the tendency for a material with great mass in each unit volume to be resistant to acceleration imposed by a given driving force. Thus, sounds travel very slowly through dense materials and more quickly through less dense materials. The velocity of sound through a medium is, therefore, inversely proportional to the density of the medium. We may express both this fact and the relationship between the rigidity of the material and the propogation velocity of mechanical vibrations with the following equation:

$$V = C\sqrt{\frac{K}{\rho}} \tag{2.10}$$

where V is the velocity of the mechanical oscillation; C is a constant to adjust the units; K is a modulus reflecting the rigidity of the medium; and rho (ρ) is the density of the medium. C also varies depending upon whether the medium is a solid, a liquid, or a gas. Vibrations travel through air at a speed of 720 mi/hr (1100 ft/sec or 330 m/sec) under normal conditions of sea level pressure and a temperature of 0°C.

We can now consider some metrics, which have been developed especially to describe the amplitude or intensity of the pressure waves used as acoustic stimuli. A general requirement for a nonlinear metric of sound intensity has been generated by the enormously wide range over which the ear responds. Acceptable acoustic stimuli may range in magnitude from physical deflections as small as interatomic distances to the roar of jet engines many billions of times stronger. This fantastic ability to span a great range means that the metric used to describe physical stimuli must, in some way, compress the scale so that when acoustic functions are plotted, the larger values of the stimulus do not hide the smaller values.

Logarithmic units have regularly been used to selectively compress a scale so that both large and small numbers can be meaningfully displayed on a single scale. The logarithmic unit of sound intensity of acoustic stimulus energy is the bel, a measure defined by the following equation:

$$\text{bel} = \log_{10} \frac{P_1}{P_2} \tag{2.11}$$

where P_1 is the power (to be defined below) of the acoustic energy to be measured, and P_2 is the power of a reference sound level. The reference power that is usually used is the value associated with the threshold of normal hearing, 0.0002 dyne/cm^2. Occasionally the alternative 1 dyne/cm^2 is used.

It is important to remember at this point that while the bel as defined above is a direct measure of the intensity of physical energy carried in the transmitting medium, it is only an indirect measure of the psychophysical effect, which will be produced by that stimulus when it falls on the auditory receptor. It is also important to point out that the bel is one of those physical units which, as defined, is too large to appropriately measure the range of real acoustic signal strengths of interest to the biologist. The ability of the human, in particular, to discriminate between two slightly different acoustic energy intensities is so fine that the bel simply represents too gross a measure. To overcome this disadvantage without losing the advantages of the logarithmic scale, the decibel has been simply defined as a unit one-tenth the size of the bel. This means that in 1 bel there are 10 decibels, or:

$$N_{\text{decibels}} = N_{\text{bels}} \times 10 = 10 \log_{10} \frac{P_1}{P_2} \tag{2.12}$$

where N_{decibels} and N_{bels} define the number of decibels and bels, respectively.

This is, however, not the final useful definition of the decibel, for the definition so far is in terms of the power or total energy carried by the acoustic wave. But power measurements are tedious and complicated compared to the simpler measure of the amplitude of the pressure wave we described above. By amplitude we specifically refer to F_m—half of the peak-to-peak value as shown in Figure 2.2. The amplitude in our current context corresponds to either the peak compression in the positive direction, or the peak rarefaction in the negative direction—both values being deviations from the ambient pressure in the medium.

To convert the power definition of the decibel to a definition in terms of amplitude (half peak-to-peak pressure), it is necessary to take advantage of the following formula relating power to amplitude:

$$p = ca^2 \tag{2.13}$$

where p is the power; a is the amplitude; and c is a constant known as the acoustic resistance. We may then substitute Equation (2.13) into Equation (2.12) to get:

$$N_{\text{decibels}} = 10 \log_{10} \frac{ca_1{}^2}{ca_2{}^2} = 20 \log_{10} \frac{a_1}{a_2} \tag{2.14}$$

Or, in other words, the number of decibels that an acoustic signal is above a reference level is 20 times the log (to the base 10) of the ratio of the amplitudes of the sound and the reference.

We now have very precise ways of defining both the quality and the quantity of an acoustic stimulus. We can use the Fourier frequency analysis to define the *kind* of signals making up any speech or musical waveform in terms of its temporal pattern—the parameter most closely associated with sensory quality. We can use the notion of the decibel to define the amplitude of the signal.

Another term, which may be encountered, is called *attenuation*. To attentuate a signal is to reduce its amplitude. The measure of attenuation is also the decibel. Since the decibel is defined as the logarithm of a ratio of two sound amplitudes, we can see that in the case of an attenuation, the ratio would be a number less than 1 and, therefore, the logarithmic decibel measure would be a negative number. The decibel unit still retains its utility, however, with a negative value indicating that the sound pressure level under measurement is less than the reference.

D. Sources of Acoustic Stimuli

To produce practical acoustic stimuli, one must generate waves of compression and rarefaction in the conducting medium of appropriate amplitude and frequency of oscillation. This is accomplished, in general, by transforming the output of electrical oscillators, which produce signals of the proper frequency and amplitude to mechanical oscillations by means of mechanisms that react by converting electrical inputs into mechanical displacements. Such electromechanical transduction devices may be called either loudspeakers or earphones, but the differences between the two are primarily ones of available maximum amplitude, the ability of the device to follow the frequencies of the input electrical signal and different ways in which they may be mounted.

There are three main types of sound producing devices that are used in earphones or in speakers. The first is the *electromagnetic driver*, in which the same principles underlying the action of an electric motor are employed to produce sounds. The electrical energy activates a magnet. This magnet attracts some appropriate material, so mounted that it is free to move. Often the material is a permanent magnet itself. This motion is imparted by levers or directly to the diaphragm which, because of its back-and-forth movement and spatial expanse, is the actual source of the sound waves.

The second most usual type of speaker mechanism is one based on an *electrostatic* system. The mechanical movement, which leads to the production of the sound wave, is produced in this case by the repulsive and attractive forces of like and unlike electrical charges, rather than the attractive interaction of a magnetic field and a susceptible material. Electrostatic speakers are really very large capacitors, in which one of the two electrodes is free to move and the other is fixed. If a voltage difference is developed across the two electrodes, the free one which is, in fact, the diaphragm will move as a function of the amplitude of that voltage. Because electrostatic diaphragms may be very light, it is possible to get a very wide range of frequency responses, but because the amplitude of the movement of the diaphragm is limited for most practical designs, electrostatic speakers cannot produce sounds of great intensity.

The third possible speaker mechanism—the *piezoelectric crystal*—is one which has limited power-producing capacities. Since the amplitude of the mechanical movement is so limited, piezoelectric crystals are primarily used in earphones that do not require high reproduction amplitude. The operation of a piezoelectric earphone depends upon a special property of some crystals to become mechanically deformed when an electric current is passed through them. This is an inverse form of the property of these same crystals to produce an electric current when mechanically deformed. Incidentally, as one might expect, this is one way in which sound waves could be translated back into electrical signals. In that event, the device would be called a microphone rather than a speaker.

The brief description of the three types of converter action given above only begins to suggest the many complications in achieving accurate reproduction of electrical waveforms by loudspeakers. All speakers do not respond with the same output amplitude to signals that are of equal input amplitudes but different frequencies. For these devices, the frequency response curve is said not to be *flat,* and the signals are therefore distorted. The many details of producing high-fidelity sound signals are beyond the scope of this book, but are important factors to remember when setting up an acoustic stimulation situation.

E. The Nature of Vestibular Stimuli

The rarefaction and compression waves in acoustic media represent but one of the ways in which mechanical forces act directly on the body. Anatomically associated with the auditory mechanism is the vestibular mechanism —one of the main sources of information about body position and movement. Though the vestibular system surveys information about position and movement, in fact, it does so only by indirect means. The vestibular mechanism is sensitive to only one type of energy—accelerating forces. The position and the velocity (even though position can be indirectly encoded by gravitational accelerative forces) of the body do not in themselves lead to any stimulation that can lead to either neural activity or a sensation. We do not, for example, experience different sensations solely because we have changed our geographic location, and we certainly are insensitive to the velocity of the earth through space. Accelerating force, therefore, constitutes the single potential stimulus for the vestibular system and for many of the other sensors that help us respond to body position and movement.

The most usual form of accelerative force and the constant level under which most earthly organisms spend their entire lives is, of course, the accelerative force due to the gravitational attraction between their bodies and the earth. This force has been measured very carefully over the years, and it has been well established to have a value of 980 cm/sec^2 or 32 ft/sec^2. In other words, the accelerative force of gravity near the surface of the earth will impart an additional velocity of 980 cm/sec or 32 ft/sec toward the center of the earth every second to an otherwise unimpeded object. Such an acceleration is said to have a magnitude of one gravitational unit or one "g," a convenient unit used for the measurement of artificial gravitational situations. Of course, other factors act in atmospheres to alter the acceleration due to gravity. Friction and air pressure both produce counteracting forces, which reduce the acceleration that would otherwise be imposed by gravity—much to the delight of parachutists.

Though the body is not directly sensitive to position or even orientation, it is easy to understand how we are able to walk upright with our eyes closed. A gravitational force of 1 g always pointing in a specific direction can provide secondary cues. Dense objects immersed in a less dense fluid medium, for example, would tend to drift toward the lowest point in their container, and different locations within that container would, therefore, be stimulated depending upon its orientation. This is apparently the way in which some components of the vestibular mechanism work.

F. Sources of Vestibular Stimuli

The experimental manipulation of accelerative forces has long been a difficult problem. Generally, in order to study the responses to such stimuli, the entire body must be manipulated. One of the simplest and most often used devices for the study of orientation responses is the tilt table. A subject is placed on the table, and the entire body is tilted to the desired orientation. But the use of this device confounds the stimulus presentation, since not only are the vestibular organs stimulated, but there are also other stimuli arising from the press and pull of the body against the restraining mechanisms, which prevent the subject from slipping off the table.

The newest development in the manipulation of normal gravitational attraction is the extraterrestrial compartment. Some experiments of limited duration have been carried out in aircraft descending in precisely defined parabolic paths. During a limited time, "free-falling" subjects within the cabin of an aircraft following such a path appear to have no gravitational forces operating on them relative to the cabin. While such parabolic flights can last for only a short time, zero-gravity flights have, of course, been achieved for virtually unlimited periods of time in capsules orbiting the earth or in trans lunar free falls. This is a technique which, however, is unfortunately not available to the casual experimenter.

On a more down-to-earth level, it is possible to add to the minimum constant gravitational attraction additional g forces directed in various

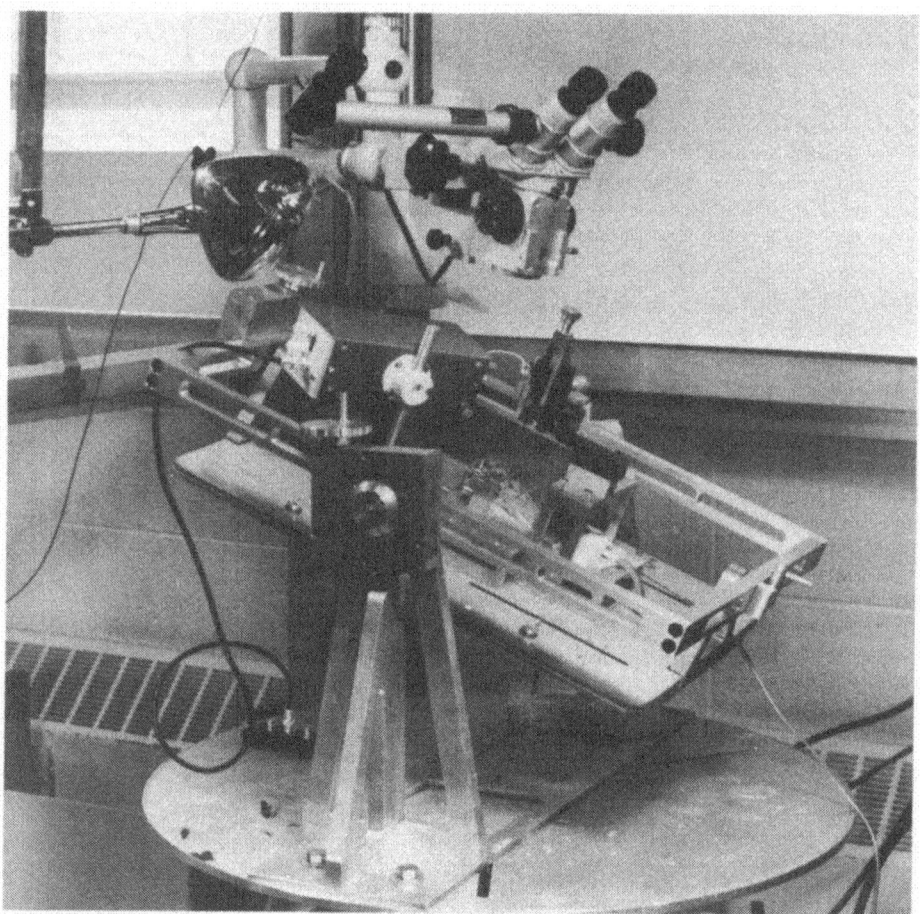

FIGURE 2.5 Photograph of a laboratory turntable, capable of providing vestibular stimulation to small animals (courtesy of Dr. David Anderson, University of Michigan).

directions. The most common form of device is a spinning table, which produces accelerative forces by virtue of its rotary motion. These *centrifuges* may be either very complicated and massive devices, or simpler devices readily constructed from inexpensive components such as that shown in Figure 2.5. Linear accelerations can be imposed on subjects with such devices as the rocket sled shown in Figure 2.6.

In each of these cases, however, it is important to note that the additional accelerative forces are superimposed on the existing gravitational attraction. Vector rules of addition hold for this superimposition. The linear acceleration added to 1 g in an upward-going elevator is an example of this sort. A downward movement in an elevator, however, tends to reduce the force of 1 g in the same way as a falling aircraft. The force intro-

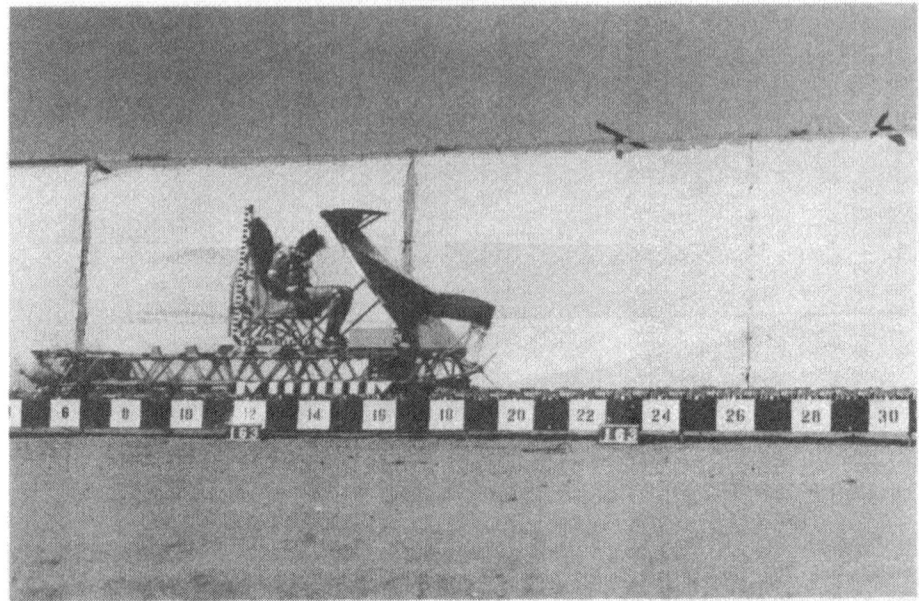

FIGURE 2.6 Photograph of a rocket sled used to provide large linear accelerations to a human subject (courtesy of USAF and Col. John P. Stapp, U. S. Department of Transportation).

duced into the system by a centrifuge or by a linear accelerator, however, need not be solely either in the same or opposite direction as gravity, and thus the addition of these forces leads to forces that must be calculated by the trigonometric rules for vector addition. The interested reader is directed to any elementary physics book for a discussion of the details of vector force addition.

Finally, the vestibular system can be stimulated by other forms of energy that simulate the effects of accelerative forces. For example, both warm water syringed into the outer ear and electrical signals are effective means of nonadequate stimulation of this sense organ.

G. The Nature and Sources of Mechanical Cutaneous Stimuli

Mechanical forces are also potentially capable of stimulating certain receptors in the skin. It is not yet certain how these stimuli effect their action in each case. Equal and evenly distributed forces, even though of high amplitude, are not sufficient to stimulate, but some gradient of mechanical deformation is required. This can be simply demonstrated by inserting one's finger into a pool of mercury. The pressure or touch sensation is felt only at the boundary between the mercury and the air, where the pressure exerted on the skin is not uniformly distributed.

It is eminently adaptive that this should be the case. Some abyssal fish, which are completely blind after thousands of generations of living in the black depths of the ocean, navigate by tactile receptors, which are

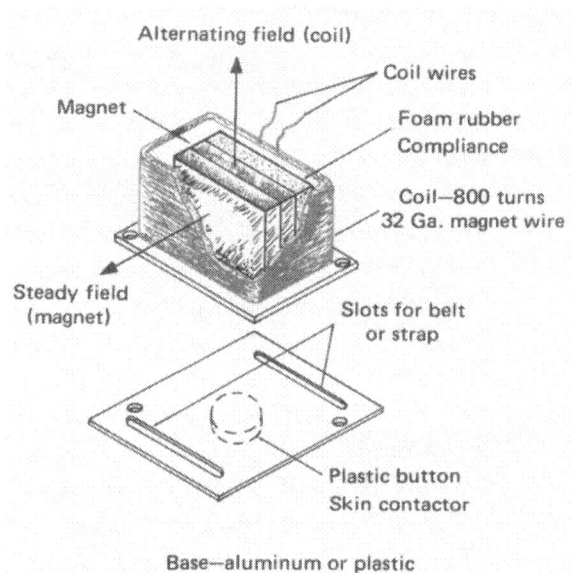

FIGURE 2.7 A simple electro-mechanical vibration transducer that can be used to stimulate cutaneous receptors (from Sherrick, 1965).

dragged along the floor of the sea. The receptors activate neurons, which may be quite long (several inches in the tripod fish, for example). Yet the amazing thing is that the whole transducing and transmitting system, along with the rest of this fish's nervous system, operates effectively at the great pressure under which it lives. Obviously, this sensor is not sensitive to absolute pressures but to some differential factor.

Practically, it can be seen that most mechanical stimuli do tend to produce gradients of pressure due to their restricted size. The classical cutaneous stimulator has been the von Frey hair—a horse hair mounted on some appropriate handle, which is manually applied to the skin. This device is rarely used today, since most work on cutaneous receptors is done with either electrical (to be discussed below) or vibratory stimuli. Vibratory stimulators are generally of the same type as described above for acoustic stimuli, but many special problems have required the development of vibratory contactors. Sherrick (1965) describes one device, whose inertial and frequency characteristics make it unusually suitable for vibratory stimulation of the skin. His device is shown in Figure 2.7. Von Békésy (1960) has also described a variety of mechanical stimulators designed especially for each of several different experiments. His devices are usually driven by conventional electromagnetic vibrators similar to those used for loudspeakers, but by ingenious design of the contactor, the point at which the mechanical energy is conveyed to the skin, he has been able to add greatly to our knowledge of cutaneous as well as acoustic sensory information processing. One of the most interesting of his vibratory stimulators is the one shown in Figure 2.8, which uses a system of levers to impose a controllable gradient of pressure upon the skin.

Specially designed electromagnet or piezoelectric stimulators, which are capable of producing highly controlled micromovements, have been

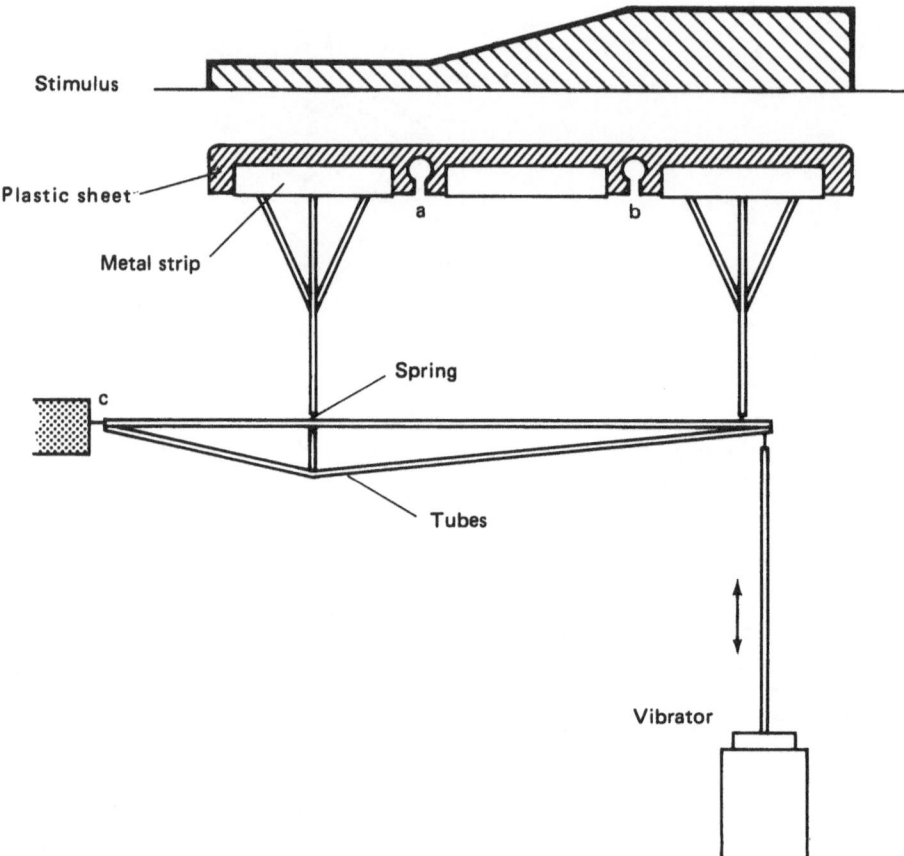

Stimulus

Plastic sheet

Metal strip

a   b

Spring

c

Tubes

Vibrator

FIGURE 2.8 Diagram of an ingenious mechanical lever system capable of providing a gradient of mechanical forces to the skin of the forearm (from von Békésy, 1958).

used by both Loewenstein (1961a) and by Werner and Mountcastle (1965) in their research on the somatosensory system. The details of these devices will be presented in the discussion of the work itself in later chapters because of the special importance the pertinent technique has to the data obtained in their studies.

III. THERMAL STIMULI

A. The Nature of Thermal Stimuli
Heat has been equated by physicists with oscillatory motion of the molecules making up any piece of matter. This oscillation can be conveyed to a group of molecules either by direct mechanical interaction between two solid bodies (conduction), by currents in fluid mediums (convection), or by the absorption of radiant energies of the appropriate wavelength (radiation).

The range of radiant wavelengths capable of inducing those special oscillatory frequencies, which we usually call heat, varies from the upper limits of visible light to the shorter radio waves—from about 7×10^{-7} m to about 3×10^{-4} m. At the shorter end of this range are those wavelengths that have come to be called infrared and that border on the upper edge of the visible wavelengths.

The critical factor for thermal stimulation of the skin receptors appears to be simply the temperature of the skin. Kenshalo, Duncan, and Weymark (1967) have shown that both conducted and radiant thermal energies, if balanced for equal amounts of heat production in the skin, produce equivalent results. Nevertheless, the specific action of thermal energy, which initiates the cutaneous warmth sensation, is unknown. Some investigators believe it operates directly on receptors specifically sensitive to heat and cold in the skin. Other observers have suggested that the expansion and contraction of some of the tissues are the critical factors. This would make the thermal sense merely a special case of the cutaneous mechanical sense. Others have suggested that indirect effects, such as a reduction in the speed of certain metabolic processes as temperature decreases, may mediate the response. Some even have bypassed the question and consider that a reflexive contraction of blood vessels may be the cue for the thermal sensations. But none of the forms of this latter class of theories accounts for the processes that activate these reflexes.

For the moment, let us concern ourselves with the physics of heat and define some of the measures used to quantify its characteristics. Temperature is a very familiar term to all of us, yet its meaning is elusive and generally not well understood. It is insufficient to say simply that the temperature of an object is a measure of its degree of heat or cold. It was this sort of circular definition that led to the notions of phlogiston or caloric heat as a separate form of matter, rather than a property of the material. Current ideas of temperature can all be classified as dynamic theories, since they state that the temperature of an object is a function of the motion of its internal parts. Specifically, these motions have to be within certain limits of size and frequency. The significant point, however, is that heat is not a separate substance, but rather a state of action of the component parts of the material being studied. There is an interesting analogy here between the notion of heat, with an existence separate from the matter that contains it, and the dualistic notions of the mind as something other than a state of action of the nervous system. It seems that both may now be better interpreted in the context of action processes of the underlying mechanism.

B. Quantity Measurements of Thermal Stimuli

Temperature, viewed in this context of molecular motion, is a statistical notion, descriptive of the average kinetic energy of the constituent molecules of some body of matter. Several scales of temperature are commonly in use. The centigrade scale has been designed so that two of the most easily reproducible conditions for calibration are defined as evenly spaced 100° apart. The first of these conditions is the melting point of ice, a temperature which is easily obtained from a container filled with a mixture of ice and water. This temperature has been arbitrarily defined as 0° centigrade. The other calibration condition is the temperature at which water boils at normal atmospheric pressures. This has been equally arbitrarily defined as 100°C.

The other common temperature scale is the Fahrenheit scale. Here the boiling point of water has been arbitrarily defined as 212°F, and the melting point of ice as 32°F. The scale between these two points has been set equal to 180 equal-sized degrees. Translating between the centrigrade and Fahrenheit scales is easily accomplished by using the following equation:

$$C = \frac{5}{9}(F - 32) \qquad (2.15)$$

where C is the number of degrees in the centigrade scale, and F is the number of degrees in the Fahrenheit scale.

The *temperature* of a body, however, is not a measure of the *amount of heat* that is necessary to bring its molecules to a given level of vibratory action. The absorption of a given amount of heat will not have an equal effect on all objects. Other measures, which specify the amount of heat independently of the heating or temperature rise produced in any given material, are therefore required. The *calorie* is the unit of energy used to measure the amount of heat and is defined as the amount of heat necessary to raise the temperature of 1 gram of water by 1°C. This definition of a calorie is further qualified by the fact that this temperature rise must take place when the water temperature is between 14.5°C and 15.5°C. Occasionally, the reader may also encounter the term BTU or British thermal unit. This is a similar but much larger unit—the amount of heat necessary to raise 1 lb of water 1°F at the same temperature.

The property of matter that determines how much the temperature of a given material will be raised by a given amount of heat is called the *specific heat* of the material. Specific heat is defined as the number of calories necessary to raise the temperature of 1 gram of the material 1°C at the standard temperature.

C. Sources of Thermal Stimuli

Controlling thermal energy in such a way that it can be used as a stimulus is also an incompletely solved problem. The thermodynamic properties of the skin do not allow for the rapid impulsive stimulation techniques with flashes or clicks that have been so profitably utilized in vision or audition, for example. Furthermore, the receptors presumed to be activated by thermal stimuli are not usually directly exposed to the stimuli, but are indirectly activated by thermal changes in the tissues in which they are imbedded. The process of thermal stimulation, therefore, is one that is strongly dependent upon the thermal properties of the skin and the resulting efficiency of the different stimulators in raising skin temperature.

Two main thermal stimulation methods have been used. The first is the radiant heating method illustrated by the device developed by Hardy, Wolff, and Goodell (1952), and shown in Figure 2.9. A high-intensity incandescent lamp especially designed to emit a high proportion of infrared rays was aimed at a spot on the skin, which had been blackened with carbon

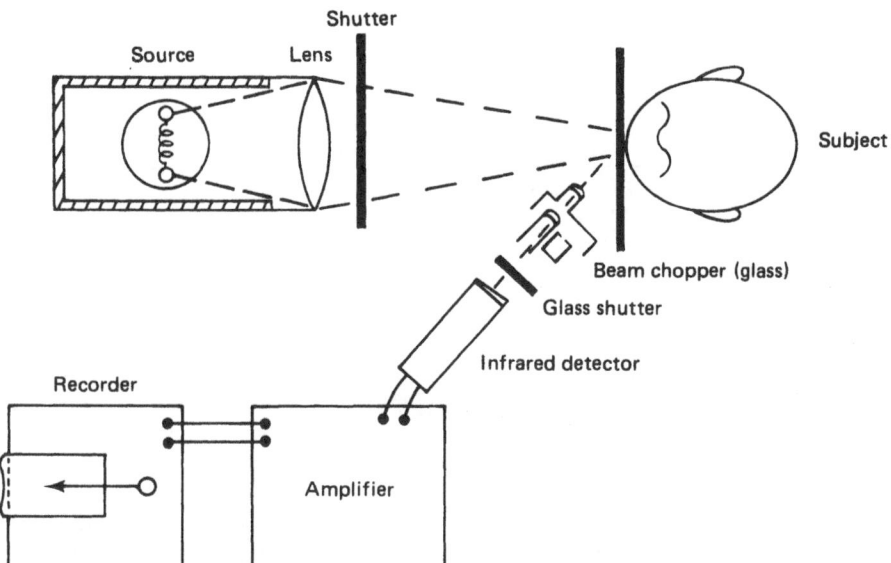

FIGURE 2.9 Diagram of a thermal stimulator created from an incandescent lamp source. This figure also shows how a radiant energy skin thermometer can be used to measure skin temperature without contacting the skin (from Hardy, 1953).

to increase its absorption. A shutter mechanism was interposed between the lamp and the subject to permit the experimenter to control the duration of the stimulus.

The other type of thermal stimulator is one that heats or cools by conduction. Many different devices, which themselves are heated or cooled to the desired temperature before or during contact with the skin, have been used. Typically, large bodies are used. The reason for this is that the heat content of large bodies is sufficiently large to allow heat to be transferred to the skin without appreciably changing the temperature of the stimulator itself.

Recently, single electrical devices capable of both heating and cooling have come into use. One could simply use a resistive heating element of low wattage. Kenshalo (1963), however, has used a device based upon the Peltier thermoelectric effect. The Peltier effect heats one junction and cools the other when a current is passed through two dissimilar metals connected in series with a voltage source. The heating effect is not due to the expenditure of energy as in an ordinary resistive circuit, but depends upon the nature of the two metals. Figure 2.10 shows this type of Peltier element used by Kenshalo for his thermal psychophysical studies.

IV. PHOTIC STIMULI

Measurements of the kind and amount of light have been, for the last 100 years, the most influential empirical influence in furthering our understand-

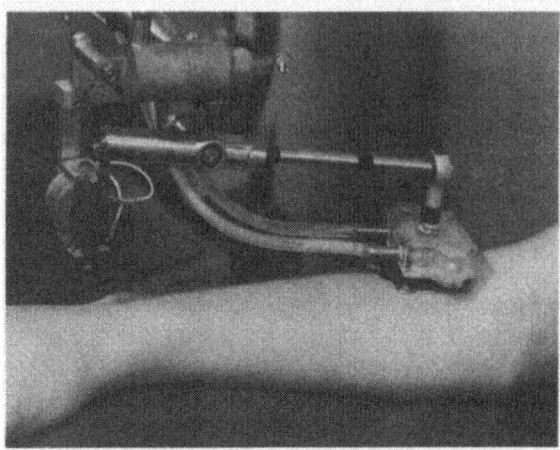

FIGURE 2.10 Photograph of another form of thermal stimulator that uses a Peltier junction as the generator of the desired temperature. Peltier junctions will heat or cool depending upon the direction of the electrical current passing through them and can be extremely accurate—within 0.01 of a degree of desired temperature (from Kenshalo, 1963).

ing of the nature of matter and of our universe. The spectroscopic measurements made at the turn of the twentieth century have led us to a whole new world, for it was a set of intuitions based upon observations of the patterns of light emitted by incandescent bodies that led us to our early theories of the nature of atomic orbital systems. These atomic models subsequently led to the quantum and statistical theories of matter, which still dominate modern physics. Studies of the light emitted or reflected by extraterrestrial bodies have, until very recently, been our sole source of information about the nature of the macrocosm of which our planet is but a very small portion. It appears almost certain, because of fundamental limits on the speed at which mass can move through space, that light and other electromagnetic waves traveling at the speed of light will continue to be the only source of communication with bodies lying outside our solar system for the indefinite future.

It is not, however, with the relationship of light and matter that we are concerned in this book. We must also remember that light has tremendous biological significance. Among other fundamentals, it is responsible for the photosynthetic production of food and the purification of our atmosphere. Our interest in light in the context of this book, however, is specifically in terms of its effectiveness as a means of conveying information about distant events and objects to our sensory nervous system. Visual stimulation requires that light excite the photosensitive cells of a receptive tissue. But, before we can quantitatively discuss the dynamics of the visual process, it is necessary to have a reference set of measures capable of defining the nature, amount, and quality of light. It is with these physical measures of the potential visual stimulus that we shall be concerned in this section.

A. The Nature of Photic Stimuli

The word light, as it is commonly used, is an abbreviation of a more specific notion—visible light. This latter term places this particular kind of electromagnetic vibration more precisely in the context of sensory processes.

Visible light is defined biologically as that range of electromagnetic vibrations having wavelengths varying between about 390 and 760 nanometers (nm). (One nanometer is equal to 1 millimicron which is equal to 10 angstrom units (Å) each of which is equal to 10^{-10} meter.) Electromagnetic oscillations within this range are capable of setting up nervous signals in the optic pathways of man by virtue of their selective absorption by certain photolabile macromolecules. It is this property of specific absorption that defines the bandwidth of visible light, rather than any special discontinuity of the electromagnetic radiation itself.

There has been a classic controversy extending over many centuries concerning the fundamental nature of this light energy. Some scientists, stimulated by the discovery of the photoelectric effect and other related "chunk" phenomena, suggested that light is made up of particles. They championed a theory, which holds that all light is made up of indivisible units or quanta, which can contain only a certain precisely defined amount of energy. The quantum theory was most effective in describing the size of atomic orbits, and explaining the fact that the energies involved in electron jumps between these orbits had to be in precise multiples of certain irreducible energy units. On the other hand, older theories had generally treated light as a continuous wave motion. Though there was a considerable controversy over the nature of the medium in which the waves were propagated, the behavior of light as it was reflected or refracted was well described by models that described light as a continuous wave motion rather than a set of discrete particles.

Modern theorists however, as in so many other similar controversies, have resolved the issue, not by completely accepting one or the other of the two theories, but by acknowledging that both are in part correct. In other words, each theory described different aspects of the same set of phenomena. The first approximation of the wave theory and the early quantum theories were each individually not comprehensive enough to cover all of the experimental results. More limiting, however, was the fact that they could not communicate with each other to allow them to be combined into a single descriptive theory. A compromise of the two theories has been achieved in recent years by means of a remarkable relation linking together the notions of waves and particles. Light is not now considered to be solely particulate, but rather to be composed of "particles with wave properties." Another way of saying this same thing is to say that light is now considered to be "waves of packets."

In any event, both the particle and wave descriptions of light are now transferable into each other by means of the fundamental expression:

$$e = h\nu \tag{2.16}$$

where e is the energy associated with the particle; ν is the frequency of vibration of the electromagnetic waves that make up the light; and h is a fundamental constant of nature known as Planck's constant. Thus we are able, using this simple formula, to convert between the energy content of a particle (which is what we really mean by a quantum of energy) and the vibratory frequency of a light wave.

There is another basic relation, which we also need to complete the transformation from particle energy to the wavelength measure we discussed earlier. This other expression relates frequency of vibration and wavelength of light as follows:

$$c = \nu\lambda \qquad\qquad (2.17)$$

where c is the velocity of light in a vacuum; ν is the frequency of vibration; and λ is the wavelength of the light in the vacuum. It should be noted that this expression also holds when the medium through which the light is being transmitted is not a vacuum. Both the velocity and the wavelength of the light change concurrently in such situations, keeping the equation balanced.

To give the reader a feeling for the magnitude of these units, let us consider a light whose wavelength is about 500 nm. First, using Equation (2.17), we can compute the frequency of oscillation of this electromagnetic wave, which is sensed by the visual system as greenish light. The velocity of light, c, in a vacuum is equal to 3×10^8 m/sec. Therefore:

$$\nu = \frac{c}{\lambda} = \frac{3 \times 10^8}{500 \times 10^{-9}} = \frac{3 \times 10^8}{5 \times 10^{-7}} = 0.6 \times 10^{15} \text{ Hz} \qquad (2.18)$$

Now using Equation (2.16), and with Planck's constant set equal to 6.62×10^{27} erg-sec, we can compute the energy in each quantum of this greenish light.

$$e = h\nu = (6.62 \times 10^{-27}) \times (0.6 \times 10^{15}) = 3.97 \times 10^{-12} \text{ ergs} \qquad (2.19)$$

The particular value of each of these particular numbers is not of critical importance. Different spectral lights (lights of different wavelengths) will have different quantal energies. The important point is that we can transform quantal energies into wavelengths and vice versa in a way that allows us to use whichever model is the most convenient while still maintaining the basic physical notion that light can have both wave and particle characteristics.

Modern theorists have had much more to say about the nature of light. The newer statistical and probabilistic theories tend to avoid the conceptual models of both waves and packets, and speak of light in mathematical terms, which sometimes make it hard for the layman to actually find any concrete model on which to base his understanding. For the purpose of sensory scientists, however, the older models are adequate to provide a basis of discussion even though they may seem somewhat archaic to the new physicists.

B. Metrics of Kind

Light is one of the easiest of the potential stimuli for which to specify quality. The importance of light to our physical sciences over the decades

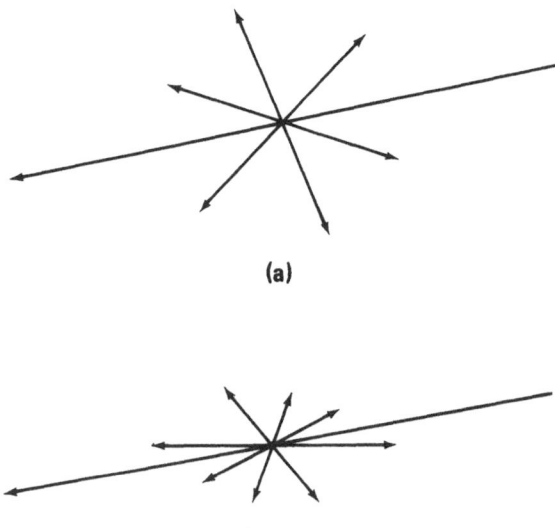

(a)

FIGURE 2.11 Diagram show-
ing the difference between
polarized light and unpolarized light. (a) The ray of
unpolarized light moving in
the direction of the longest
arrow oscillates equally in all
directions perpendicular to
its direction of propagation.
(b) Partially polarized light
oscillates less strongly in one
direction than in the other.

(b)

and the almost unique singularity of the wavelength dimension as a
correlate of psychophysical qualities have led to a very high degree of
sophistication for specifying visual potential stimulus quality. Although
the most commonly used single dimension is wavelength, as we have shown
in the previous section, this may easily be converted to frequency or to the
energy content of single quanta. The latter measure is indeed frequently
used as an alternative to wavelength. It should be noted in passing that
there are some complex interactions among wavelength, amplitude, and
temporal pattern which affect the psychophysical quality of a visual stimulus. But as we shall see later, any mixture of light or different colors can
be represented by a small set of wavelengths (the trichromatic primaries)
in a way that allows us to handle even these complex interactions.

The instruments used to measure the wavelength of light are called
spectroscopes. These devices segregate light of different wavelengths, either
by selective refraction (as in a prism spectroscope) or by selective interference of wave fronts (as in a grating spectroscope). A special spectroscope that has its own internal source of light, any wavelength of which
can be selectively emitted by a simple dial setting, is called a monochromater. Narrow bands of light can also be produced by use of special filters,
which transmit only certain portions of the visible spectrum.

There are other secondary characteristics, which might also be considered as additional ways of specifying the quality of a given visible light.
The degree of polarization, for example, does specify a certain characteristic of light, which has a large number of physical implications. *Polarization* simply refers to the direction of oscillation of electromagnetic waves.
If the light is randomly and equally oscillating in all directions normal to
its direction of travel, as shown in Figure 2.11(a), then it is said to be

TABLE 2.2. THE RADIOMETRIC AND PHOTOMETRIC UNITS USED TO
MEASURE VISUAL STIMULUS QUANTITY (ADAPTED FROM RIGGS, 1965)

		Radiometric		
	Symbol	Name	Unit	Relating Equation
Total Light	P	Radiant flux	Watt (erg/sec)	
Light Through 1 steradian	J	Radiant intensity	W/steradian	$P = 4\pi J$
Light Falling on Extended Surface	H	Irradiance	W/m^2	$H = \dfrac{J \cos \theta}{r_2}$
Light Being Emitted from Extended Surface	N	Radiance	W/steradian/ m^2	$N_{actual} = N_{max} \cos \theta$

unpolarized. If, on the other hand, it has a preferential oscillation as shown in Figure 2.11(b), then it is said to be polarized.

From the point of view of the sensory sciences, there are only a few phenomena in which polarization is important. Some insects seem to be able to utilize the angle of polarization of sunlight as navigational aids. The so-called Haidinger's Brushes—radial bluish and yellowish lines observed when viewing the sky through a polarizing filter—have been cited as effects of polarization sensitivities in human vision, but no other similar effects seem to be of any special significance in man's adaptation to his environment.

C. Quantity Measurements of Photic Stimuli

While a single dimension—wavelength—completely specifies the kind of light for all cases, specification of the amount or quantity of light is not so simple. Not only are there several different units used to specify the amount of light, depending upon special viewing conditions, but there are also two completely different systems for measuring light intensity, in which each of these units is duplicated. The first of these two systems is an absolute and uncorrected energy measurement system, which is used primarily by physical scientists to specify the amount of energy present, irrespective of its ultimate use. These so-called *radiometric* measurements are made with instruments that have been corrected for their own differential sensitivities so that an absolute energy reading is usually given. The second of these two systems for specifying light quantity has a built-in correction factor, which makes its quantity measurements dependent upon the biological effectiveness of the light. The standard correction for effec-

Table 2.2 (*cont.*)

$$(1 \text{ lumen} = 685 \sum_{0}^{\infty} P_\lambda V_\lambda \Delta_\lambda)$$

		Photometric	
Symbol	Name	Unit	Relating Equation
F	Luminous flux	lumen	
I	Luminous intensity	lumen/ steradian (1 candle)	$F = 4\pi I$
E	Illuminance	lumen/m² (1 lux)	$E = \dfrac{I \cos \theta}{r^2}$
L	Luminance	lumen/ steradian/ m²	$L_{\text{actual}} = L_{\text{max}} \cos \theta$

tiveness is the photopic (light adapted) luminosity curve of the human eye. Measurements in this *photometric* system are, therefore, limited to wavelength values between 390 and 760 nm, in agreement with the limits of sensitivity of the human photoreceptor. Thus, light with a wavelength of, say, 1300 nm, even though of very high radiometric intensity, will have zero photometric-intensity. It would simply cook the eye before it could be detected by the human visual system. To repeat this very important point, any light, no matter how intense radiometrically, that has a wavelength outside of the range of visible light, has a photometric intensity of zero.

The devices that are used to obtain radiometric values include such physical instruments as thermocouples and thermopiles, bolometers, and visually uncorrected radiometers and photoelectric cells. The instruments that are used to measure photometric intensities include first and foremost the human eye, and then radiometers and photoelectric cells which have been corrected by filters, whose transmission characteristics are the same as the human eye. Table 2.2 summarizes and previews the entire system of photometric and radiometric units, which will be discussed in detail in the following sections of this chapter. This table and the following discussion are based on Riggs' article in Graham (1965).

1. Radiometric Measures. Now that we have established the critical difference between these two systems of quantity measurements, let us consider in detail the various units that are used to measure light quantity in the various viewing conditions. There are four basic viewing conditions for measuring the amount of light. For each of these "points of view," a separate standard unit has been developed for use in either the radiometric or the photometric system. The four viewing conditions specify units which measure:

1. the total amount of light being emitted from a point source;
2. the amount of light passing through one steradian (defined as the unit solid angle) from a point source. (Since there are 4π steradians making up the sphere around a point source, there are 4π times the amount of light in Condition 1 than in Condition 2 from a source which is radiating equally in all directions.)
3. the amount of light falling on a unit surface at a given distance from a source;
4. the amount of light being emitted from an extended source.

Let us now consider the radiometric or energy-based units that have been developed for these four viewing conditions. In each case we shall also indicate the alphabetic symbol that is usually used to signify the specific measurement.

1. Radiant Flux (P) If we were able to measure the total amount of light being emitted from a point source with some spherical radiometric measuring instruments that completely surrounded that source, we would be able to specify the total *radiant flux* from the source. It would not matter if the source were isotropic (emitting equally in all directions) or very irregular in its directional emission. The measurement of total energy emission would still be accurate, since all emitted energy would intercept the spherical measuring instrument. Such an energy measurement would tell us about the total amount of light being given off by the source. Radiant flux is usually measured in watts (W) or ergs/sec (1 W is equal to 10^7 ergs/sec).

2. Radiant Intensity (J) However, in a practical sense there are no such spherical flux measuring instruments. The receptive area of all practical measuring instruments intercepts only that amount of light passing through a smaller section of the space around the light source. A practical measure of this sort, one that measures the flux through a solid angle of a given size, is called *radiant intensity*. Radiant intensity is measured in units of W/ster where the steradian (ster) is the unit solid angle.

It should be noted that this sort of measurement is independent of both how far the measuring instrument is from the source and the size of the measuring instrument, only if one corrects for the area of the measuring surface and the distance between the source and the instrument. Furthermore, most practical light sources do not emit light equally in all directions and are thus said to be *anisotropic*. For this reason, radiant intensity measurements cannot usually be extrapolated to radiant flux directly by simple multiplication by 4π. It is true only for perfectly isotropic sources that the theoretical relation $P = 4\pi J$ holds true.

3. Irradiance (H) The unit of irradiance has been developed in a further effort to find a practical unit of light intensity. *Irradiance* is defined as the radiometric measurement of the amount of light energy falling on a surface. This measurement is, of course, dependent on the distance and magnitude of the source of the light. But since it is measured at the

destination rather than at the source, it is usually a better measure than radiant intensity for evaluating the amount of energy that is really involved in some stimulus situation. Irradiance has basic units of W/m^2. Since the solid angle cut by a given surface is dependent upon its deviation from perpendicularity, and the proportion of a steradian which is cut is also inversely dependent upon the square of the distance of the surface from the source, it is possible to calculate the radiant intensity from an irradiance value by use of the following equation:

$$J = H \frac{\cos \theta}{r^2} \tag{2.20}$$

where r is the distance of the surface from the source, and θ is the angle of deviation from the perpendicular. It must be emphasized that, in this case, this equation is precisely accurate, given a good value for H. However, it cannot, in general, be extrapolated to a total estimate of the flux for the same reasons that radiant intensity cannot—the possibility of anisotropy in the emission.

4. Radiance (N) All of the three preceding measurements have been specified in terms of an idealized point source of light. However, most light-emitting sources are extended surfaces rather than points. Such distributed light sources also require a unit that takes into account the fact that the light is coming from an extended source. Radiance is such a unit having the physical dimensions of $W/ster/m^2$. The amount of light being emitted by such a surface also must be corrected for the angle of view. This is intuitively obvious when one considers that at an angle of 90 deg, the area is but a horizontal line, which theoretically has no surface area. Thus:

$$N_{actual} = N_{max} \cos \theta \tag{2.21}$$

where N_{actual} is the amount of light measured; N_{max} is the amount that would have been measured by an instrument situated perpendicularly to the radiant plane; and θ is the actual angle of incidence of the line of sight of the measuring instrument.

2. *Photometric Measures.* These then are the radiometric measures. An exactly equivalent set of photometric measures exists. The only difference between these photometric measurements and the radiometric measurements just described is that all photometric measures are corrected by the average sensory effectiveness of each wavelength of light. The sensory effectiveness of light is defined by the scotopic and photopic luminosity curves of human rod and cone vision and will be discussed in detail later in this book. For the present, let us simply consider the luminosity curve shown in Figure 2.12 as a set of measures of the effectiveness of light of different wavelengths for a relatively light adapted eye. This curve tells us, for example, that it takes a much more energetic source of red light to produce a given subjective brightness (complicated, of course, by a difference in hue) than to produce a yellowish sensation of the same brightness.

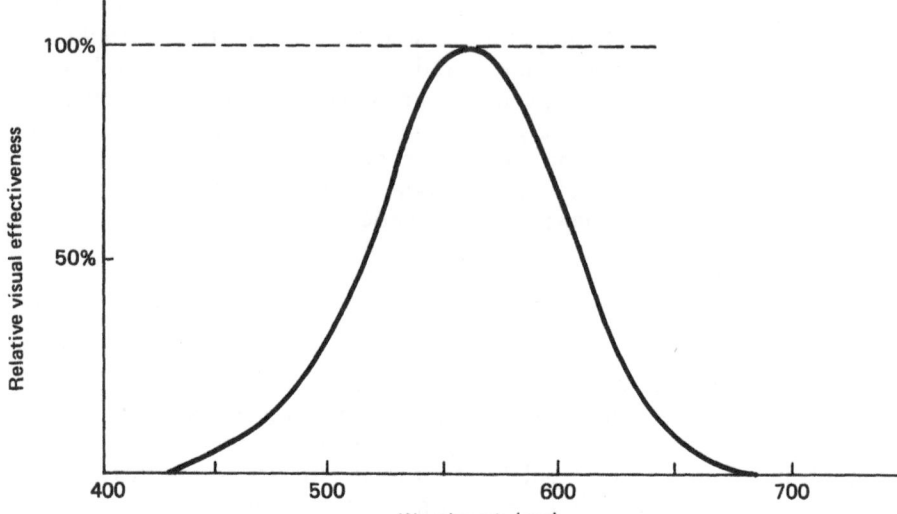

FIGURE 2.12 *A simple photopic luminosity curve showing the difference in relative visual effectiveness of light of varying wavelengths. It is this curve that is used to convert radiometric energies to the photometric units, but compare with Figure 9.2.*

The formal relation tying the radiometric and photometric systems together is a transformation based on the two units of flux. With this relation, we are able to calculate the luminous flux, which is produced by a given amount of radiant flux. Since the correction is the photopic luminosity curve, which is really a set of constants rather than a single constant, and since light brightnesses sum as the colors are mixed, the total luminous flux is a sum of all the corrected component wavelengths. Thus, the calculation is not a direct multiplicative correction, but a more complex summation. The formal relation transforming watts to lumens (the lumen being the basic unit of luminous flux) is:

$$\text{number of lumens} = 685 \sum_{0}^{N} P_\lambda V_\lambda \Delta_\lambda \tag{2.22}$$

where 685 is the number of lumens per watt of the most effective stimulus, that is, light with a wavelength of about 555 nm; P_λ is the radiant flux at each wavelength component λ; V_λ is the photopic luminosity coefficient (the proportional height of the luminosity curve at λ) for each component; and Δ_λ is the width of each of N wavelength bands. Such a corrective equation has the effect of inserting the eye into the quantitative measurements mathematically. Other instruments, which actually involve the visual process or which correct radiometric measures by appropriate filters, can also be used. In either case, the units of the photometric system that de-

application, but it is used frequently by investigators as a more convenient way of specifying the actual significant amplitude of the stimulus. The troland is particularly useful when used in conjunction with an artificial pupil, a small aperture place in the optic pathway close to the natural pupil. The size of an artificial pupil is usually chosen to be slightly less than the minimum size attainable by a highly constricted pupil. For humans, this minimum size is about 2 mm. When the artificial pupil is used, a stimulus is unaffected by the continuous fluctuations in the natural pupil and thus, retinal stimulation remains more constant than it otherwise would. This is particularly important in situations in which adaptive or situational variations in pupil diameter might be present.

D. Sources of Photic Stimuli

There are two principal physical means of producing light. The first involves the thermal agitation of molecules. This process, called *incandescence,* can be accomplished by any device capable of heating a material to a point at which it can give off light. Since the thermal agitation of molecules is a random process, all frequencies are emitted by an incandescent source. The spectrum (a plot of the component wavelengths of the light) is, therefore, said to be continuous. Although the spectrum may shift its peak as the temperature rises, it does remain continuous over the entire wavelength range in which the source is emitting light. The shift in the peak of the distribution is the reason that most materials as they are heated to higher and higher temperatures tend to shift through a precisely defined series of colors from red to yellow to bluish white, as well as increasing the total amount of energy emitted, in accord with the Stefan-Boltzmann law.

The second means of producing light is by a process called *luminescence.* Luminescent sources emit light as electrons in the atomic orbits drop from an excited state to a state with lower energy content. The surplus energy so released can be given off, in large part, in the form of visible light. It should be remembered that the initial energy required to excite a luminescent light has to come from some external energy source. It may come from a chemical reaction, such as that used by luminescent insects and fungi, or from ultraviolet or electron bombardment. Luminescence is better illustrated, however, by the operation of the cathode-ray tube (CRT). Within a CRT a stream of electrons is produced by running a current through a resistive filament. These negatively charged electrons are accelerated by a positive voltage, which also directs them in the general direction of a luminescent material on the face of the CRT. After the electrons are properly focused and positioned, they impinge upon a particular point on the luminescent screen. There, accelerated electrons, arriving at relatively high velocities, are able to "kick" other electrons out of the atomic orbits of the salts composing the screen. The vacancies so created are filled by free electrons dropping into the empty orbital positions under the attractive force of the newly positively ionized atoms. In so doing, these replacement electrons must give up the excess energy that allowed them to at least temporarily remain outside of the atomic orbits. This excess is in substantial part, if the salts are correctly chosen, in the form of those quantum values that constitute visible light, and it is this visible light that emerges as the trace on the CRT display.

Since only certain energy values, in accord with quantum principles, are possible as the electrons fill the empty orbital positions, the light from a luminescent source, if analyzed with a spectroscope, will be found to be a series of lines rather than the continuous spectrum produced by an incandescent source. The particular lines that are present will be a function of the materials that make up the luminescent material or, as it is more generally known, the phosphor. The deposition of different materials can result in different colors and such delights as color television.

Because of the low-level light intensities generally available from luminescent sources, incandescent sources have, in the past, been more often used in psychophysical experiments. But the use of incandescent sources has a number of inherent disadvantages primarily associated with their temporal characteristics. Incandescent sources must be heated to do their work, and due to the thermal inertia of the constituent parts, this often requires turn-on and turn-off periods, which are quite long in comparison with the visual processes under investigation. The timing of incandescent light patterns is, therefore, generally done with shutters of one sort or another, which mechanically obscure the light. On the other hand, some flourescent sources, which have rapid ignition times of the order of a few microseconds, have now been developed, and such sources are regularly used in tachistoscopes to expose an image for a brief period of time. Even this sort of device, however, suffers from certain problems. Often these sources have an initial ultrabright transient which, although lasting for only a millisecond or so, may interfere with the requirements of many visual threshold experiments. Oscilloscope screens themselves are often used as stimulators. Phosphors, which have ignition times as short as a microsecond and extinction times of a few tens of microseconds, can be chosen, but luminous intensity is usually low.

Some researchers have attempted to utilize (but unfortunately, it must be admitted, generally without success) electronically controlled light sources such as the Kerr cell or certain electrooptical crystals. These devices regulate light transmission by electrooptical rotation of the plane of polarization of a beam of light. But the complexities and the finite light-dark ratios of these devices limit their utility, and the reader is advised to avoid this oft-attempted dead end.

As mentioned above, another problem with light sources has been the difficulty of controlling intensity variations, which are introduced by fluctuations in the subject's pupil size. There are two main ways in which this control has been achieved. The first is the artificial pupil described above. The second way to guarantee that the pupil fluctuations do not inadvertently affect the light intensity is to bring all of the light to a focus exactly at the center of the pupil. Since in an ideal situation all of the light would then pass through this focal point, pupil contractions have no effect on the available amount of light. Such an optical arrangement is called a Maxwellian view and is diagrammed in Figure 2.13.

The experimental control of the intensity of light is not only a problem of guarding against artifactual intensity variations such as those re-

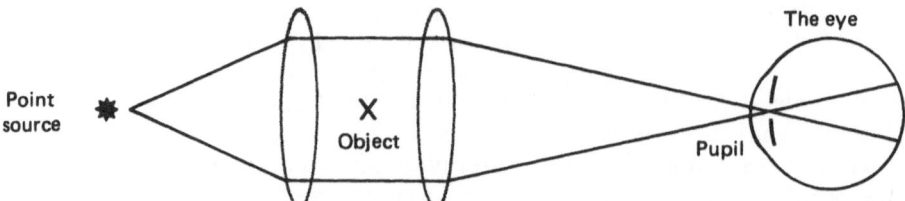

FIGURE 2.13 A Maxwellian view optical system. The incident light is focused at the entrance pupil so that fluctuations in the pupil size have no effect on stimulus intensity. Objects to be imaged on the retina must be placed between the two converging lenses to be seen in sharp focus.

---

sulting from the pupilary response, but also one of controlling light intensities as an independent variable. This may be done most easily by means of neutral density filters of one sort or another. Neutral density filters do not change the color of the light, but decrease the amount of light equally for all colors. These filters may be in the form of thin sheets of plastic, or of optical "wedges," which allow continuous and automatic control of intensity by simply positioning the appropriate part of the wedge in the optical pathway. Even though originally optical wedges were exactly that—wedge-shaped pieces of glass—it is now possible to obtain a flat film, which is an optical wedge by virtue of an increasingly dense optical quality, rather than an actual change in physical thickness. In general, direct control of the intensity of luminous sources is difficult, unless neutral density filters are used.

V. CHEMICAL STIMULI

A. The Nature of Chemical Stimuli

In later chapters of this book, we shall describe how nervous cells are made up of semipermeable membranes, which separate solutions of slightly different chemical composition from each other. These slight ionic concentration differences are thought to represent the fundamental process that underlies all of the behavioral and neurological phenomena, which distinguish the sensate from the inanimate. It is not surprising, therefore, that there should be some sense organs that are especially sensitive to chemical compounds. In fact, as we shall see, the primary receptor action of all sense organs is probably an alteration of some such ionic balance. In this section, however, we shall concern ourselves with the nature of those chemicals that can affect those receptors that are almost uniquely sensitive to chemicals. Receptors found in the nose, the tongue, and possibly, in a general way, in many other body cells seem to be very primitive mechanisms in which the stimulus acts without an elaborate transduction and conversion mechanism like those so elaborately evolved in the ear, the eye, or the skin.

Substances that are effective as stimuli for the chemical senses must have a number of properties. First, they must possess the ability to dissolve in water. Dissolution of salts, in particular, involves a breaking of the bonds, which bind the constituent elemental atoms into molecular systems. When these bonds are broken, the charged atomic fragments, or ions, are available for chemical interaction. In some instances, this chemical interaction may be direct. The available ions may simply add to the existing concentrations and thus alter the potential gradients across the cell membrane in ways that lead immediately to the elaborate membrane responses we shall discuss later. For other species of ions, however, there often are intermediate reactions. Thus, for example, a given species of ion, which does not in itself contribute to the important transmembrane potential gradient, may act as a carrier to remove another ion, which is a part of the concentration system. Binding reactions of one sort or another may also alter the semipermeable properties of the nerve cell membrane and allow passive flow of the ions that define transmembrane potential.

Another important property of chemical stimuli, which is especially relevant in the olfactory process, is the necessity for volatility. Gaseous or airborne vapors are, of course, a physical necessity for stimulating the olfactory epithelium. Furthermore, once these vapors have arrived, they must also be water soluble if they are to have any effect. As we shall see in a later section of this book, some minor theories of olfactory reception, which supposed that the electromagnetic properties of certain large molecules was a significant factor in their biological effectiveness, have not stood the test of time.

With this general introduction, we can now consider somewhat more specifically what is meant by a chemical stimulus. We shall assume that the reader is familiar with the basics of chemical structure and that the terms atom and molecule are known to him. The notion of the ionization process deserves a somewhat more elaborate discussion because of its critical importance in our subsequent discussion. Chemical molecules are formed by the binding together of atoms. Sometimes the number of atoms involved may be very large. Consider, for example, the very complex macromolecules involved in the genetic materials. One kind of DNA (deoxyribonucleic acid) has a molecular weight of about 15×10^6. This number is roughly equal to a count of the protons and neutrons that compose a single molecule of DNA. Since the atomic weights (also defined as the number of protons and neutrons) of most atoms vary from 1 (for helium) to only about 300, the number of atoms involved in one large biological molecule can be very large indeed.

On the other hand, some molecules are very small. The very important molecule NaCl (common salt) has an atomic weight of only 58.45[1] and is composed of only two atoms. After ionization, the charge on the ions—the resulting charged particles—is not dependent on the molecular weight of the atom, but only upon the nature of the bond that was disrupted. The NaCl molecule ionized to Na^+ and Cl^- ions, indicating the transfer of one electron from the sodium atom to the chlorine atom. Some

---

[1] Atomic weights may differ from whole numbers, depending upon what atom is taken as the reference, the mixture of various isotopes, and slight mass losses due to the energetics of nuclear combination.

ions with very large molecular weights may also have an ionic valence of ± 1.

There are two main binding processes, which hold molecules together, of significance to our present discussion. The first kind of binding—electrostatic binding—results from the fact that the orbital electrons around an atom have a strong tendency to form complete sets of eight electrons (octets) in the outermost electron shell. This tendency is known as the octet law. Thus when an atom of sodium (Na), which has but one very loosely bound electron in its outer orbit, comes close to an atom of chlorine (Cl) with seven electrons in its outer orbit, the octet completing tendency is so strong that the sodium atom actually loses an electron to the chlorine atom. In this manner, both the sodium and chlorine atoms end up with an ultrastable octet of electrons in their outermost shells. However, in giving up the electron, the previously neutrally charged atom of sodium now has a deficiency of one negatively charged electron, and this results in that sodium atom now being effectively positively charged. In the same way the chlorine, which has picked up an extra electron, is now effectively negatively charged. The attraction of these unlike charges on the two ions draws them toward each other, and they form a relatively stable molecular structure. When the molecule dissolves in water, however, the two component atoms can overcome this attractive force and separate. In doing so, however, they are not able to overcome the strong octet force, and thus they remain in the form of charged ions with either one extra or a deficiency of one electron. Dissolution, therefore, results in a population of charged ions, which are especially able to participate in other chemical reactions.

The second kind of binding is found predominantly in organic compounds and is called *covalent binding*. In covalent binding, the strong tendency to create a stable octet of electrons is accomplished by sharing electrons. Thus, an atom with four electrons in its outermost orbit can share four other electrons with another similar atom in such a way that each seems to have a full octet, even though only half as many electrons as are really needed are present. Covalent bonds are especially powerful and cannot be broken in a way that leads to ionized (charged) particles. The sharing process itself, rather than electrostatic attraction, is the source of the binding force within covalently bound molecules.

How do we specify the kind of chemical stimulus involved in a given experiment? There is no single dimension that serves the same role that frequency does for vision or hearing. On the other hand, the whole elaborate chemical classification and taxonomy system, which has evolved over the years, is a highly specific means of defining the chemical constituents of an olfactory or gustatory stimulus. It is, of course, completely beyond the scope of this short section to describe the complete chemical nomenclature system.

B. Quantity Measurements of Chemical Stimuli

The actual effective amount of a chemical, which is presented as a psychophysical or neurophysiological test stimulus, is sometimes difficult to specify exactly. Although there are relatively specific measures which can be used for concentration and volume, for example, it is not at all certain in most cases just how much of the stimulating material actually comes into close enough proximity to the receptive tissue to be considered a part of the effective stimulus. A drop of water pipetted onto the tongue or a blast of scented air may represent a far larger potential stimulus than the effective volume of the actual stimulus material. It is not as easy to correct such a measure as it is to correct for absorption of the ocular media. In addition, neither the tongue nor the olfactory chamber, nor for that matter most experimental equipment, can be completely scourged of all possible contaminants, and thus the possibility that a very pure material may be contaminated by the residue from an earlier trial is very, very large. If there are complicated interactions among different chemicals, the possibility of distortions from the true sensory properties is also, therefore, very large. Perhaps it is for this reason—inadequate stimulus control—that our knowledge of the chemical senses is more limited, and our theories are generally less sophisticated than for the other senses.

Forewarned of these difficulties, let us first consider the metrics of quantity, which are used to describe the concentrations of solutions. True solutions differ from other mixtures of chemicals in that there is a complete molecular intermingling of the solute (the material present in the lesser amount) and the solvent (the material present in the larger amount). Considering the difficulty in specifying the effective quantities of the materials that are really involved, these relative amounts of the solute and the solvent, therefore, can be even more important than the absolute volume of material presented to the subject or experimental animal. The following list describing the ways in which concentrations of chemicals in solutions can be measured is modified from a discussion in West and Todd (1961).

1. Percent by weight: the number of grams of solute divided by the number of grams of solvent.
2. The mass-volume ratio: the number of grams of solute divided by the number of milliliters of solvent.
3. The molar system: If the atomic weight or molecular weight of any substance is expressed in grams, that *gram molecular* or *gram atomic weight* of the material contains 6.02×10^{23} atoms or molecules. This is known as Avogadro's number. There is considerable advantage in comparing the number of atoms or molecules rather than the weight of the material, and the *molar system* allows one to do exactly that. Thus 1 gram molecular weight of hydrogen (atomic number $+1$) weighs 1 gram and contains the Avogadro number of hydrogen atoms. The same number of atoms is contained in 1 gram molecular weight of glucose, but because of the higher molecular weight, 1 gram molecular weight is equal to 180 grams of that sugar. The specific measure for the molar system is the number of gram molecular weights of a given solute in 1 liter of solvent. The unit of the molar system is the mol. Therefore, a 1.0 molar solution contains 1 gram molecular weight of the solute per liter of the solvent.

4. The molal system: Another often used measure is similar to the molar system, but instead of using a standard solvent volume of 1 liter, a standard weight of solvent is used. This standard weight is usually 1000 grams. Thus, for different solvents, a 1.0 molal solution may vary considerably in the volume of the solvent. However, all 1.0 molal solutions consist of 1000 grams plus the gram molecular weight of the solute. In this manner, it can be seen that for a given solvent equal molal concentrations of two different substances would also have equal numbers of atoms of the solute. These equal numbers, however, would be contained in differing volumes of solvent, if solvents of different gram molecular weights were used.

5. The normal system: Another system for indicating the concentration of a solution is based upon the fact that different chemicals are effective to differing degrees in their ability to release chemical ions. Specifically, the *normal system* is used in situations where acids, bases, and oxidizing solutions release and extract different amounts of H^+, O^-, and OH^- ions into and from the solvent. Normal solutions do not contain a specific weight of the solute, but rather contain an amount of solute which is capable of releasing a specific gram molecular weight of the particular ion desired. For example, a 1 normal acid solution contains a weight of the acid sufficient to release into the solution 1 gram molecular weight of H^+ ion. Further, a 1 normal basic solution contains a weight of the base sufficient to release into the solution 1 gram molecular weight of the OH^- ion. In each case, different amounts of given acids and bases will have to be added to release a 1 gram molecular weight of the H^+ and OH^- ions. In addition, it should be remembered that the actual weight of 1 gram molecular weight of H^+ is different from the actual weight of 1 gram molecular weight of OH^-

This brief outline has described a number of alternative systems for measuring the concentration of any given chemical in a solution. These measures are the appropriate means for specifying the quantity of a stimulus for those sense organs that can accept solutions. On the other hand, the olfactory system must have its stimulus presented to it in a vaporous form, and means for specifying the mixture concentrations of various volatile materials are required. There are immense problems, however, in the specification of the amounts of an odorous material that are necessary for a threshold sensation even after an appropriate metric has been defined. Some difficulties result from the fact, as we have noted, that the threshold amounts of many chemicals are so small that minor contaminants, leakages, and indeed even temperature changes all contribute to great variance in the measured values. It must not be forgotten that some chemicals can be sensed when only a few molecules are present. Another more serious problem is that some volatile solvents, even though they themselves may have no odor, can affect the biological effectiveness of the stimulus solute by altering its chemical activity. This may depend upon the density and molecular weight of the solvent in extremely complex ways (Jellinek, 1964).

Now with these constraints in mind, let us consider some of the measures used as metrics of amount of odorous stimuli.

1. Milligrams or micrograms per cubic meter: One of the most often used measures of olfactory stimulus strength is a simple measure of the weight of material that is present in a given volume of the carrier gas. As we have said, this measure can at best be only approximate. Injection procedures create local eddies and local pressure conditions, which can compress or rarify the carrier and thus alter the weight per unit volume considerably. This sort of distortion is in addition to the always present question concerning what portion of an injected stimulus actually arrives at the receptor.

2. Parts per million/trillion/and so on: A measure that partially overcomes the difficulties of the volumetric measure of milligrams or micrograms per cubic meter is one based upon parts per million or trillion. This measure indicates the relative proportions of the molecules of the odorous material in relation to the number of molecules of the carrier gas. This ratio remains constant as the pressure varies. Since the "parts" in parts per million is considered to be the number of molecules of the stimulant, Avogadro's number can also be used to make this calculation from the measured weight of the material and its known molecular weight.

3. Degree of saturation: Another measure, which is often used in olfactory experiments, is the percentage or degree of saturation. A given solute is allowed to completely saturate a given gaseous solvent by being present in the original mixing container in a superabundant supply. For a given set of temperature pressure and vapor pressure conditions, a maximum amount of the stimulant will mix with the carrier. This mixture is then further mixed with a known volume of the carrier gas to give a new gaseous solution, which is said to be saturated in proportion to the quantities of the two.

C. Sources of Chemical Stimuli

Stimulation techniques for eliciting gustatory responses are, for a number of reasons, usually very simple. The technique that is still predominantly used is to pipette a measured amount of a chemical onto the tongue. In some slightly more elaborate procedures, a running stream of the test solution is washed across the area of tongue in which the investigator is interested. The only really significant recent innovation in taste stimulation techniques seems to have been von Békésy's (1966) utilization of a vacuum to raise a single taste bud up out of the pit in which it is usually buried. The solutions can then be more directly applied to what is presumably the taste sensitive structure.

Stimulation of the olfactory system, on the other hand, has become almost an engineering specialty in itself. Technical *olfactometry* is a systematic effort to adequately specify the amount of the chemicals involved in stimulation of the sense of smell.

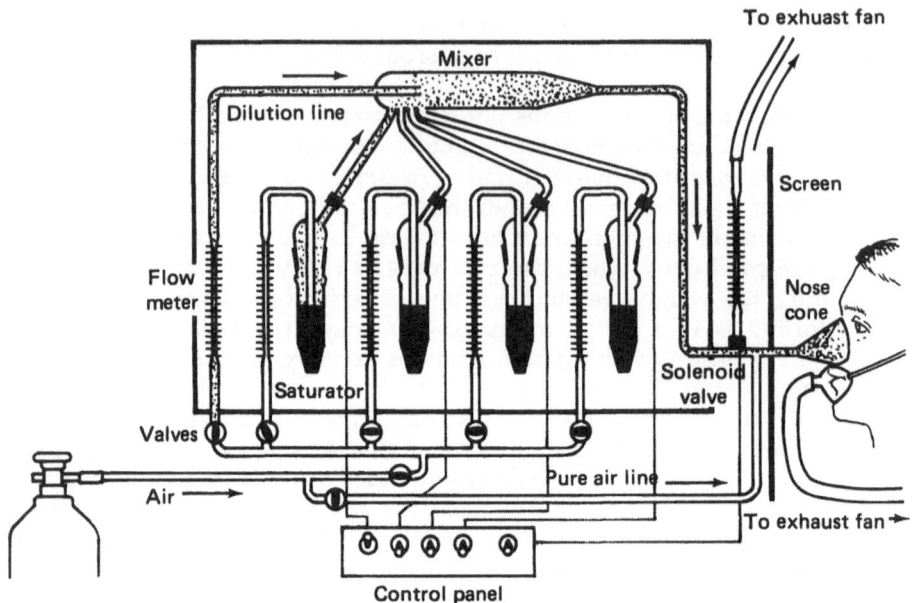

FIGURE 2.14 *An elaborate modern olfactometer showing the mixer that combines pure compressed air with any one of four test substances under the control of electrically operated solenoids (from Amoore, Johnston, and Rubin, 1964).*

The original olfactory stimulating devices used by some of the earlier investigators included measured blasts of air from bottles or streams of air regulated by the subject's own inspiration. But these early devices have evolved into complex and elaborate systems such as that shown in Figure 2.14. In this drawing, a common source of a pressurized carrier gas is filtered through charcoal to remove organic substances and through silica gel to remove water. This dried and filtered gas is then divided, so that portions of it can pass over several chambers containing odorous stimulants. In addition, a separate passageway is provided for the filtered gas itself. A mixing system is then used to mix together the appropriate proportions of the odorant required for any given experimental trial. Great care must be taken to use materials for the various containers, passageways, and connectors that do not appreciably absorb any of the odorous materials used in the experiments. Otherwise, contamination of current experimental trials by earlier ones is a distinct possibility, particularly in light of the extraordinary sensitivity of the olfactory system to trace amounts of stimulants.

This same problem of contamination is also a factor even when the olfactometer itself is not subject to trace absorption. The other parts of the body, the subject's clothes, and the room in which the subject is sitting all can contribute to the special difficulties of controlling olfactory stimuli. To overcome further many of the problems, Foster, Scofield, and Dallenbach (1950), among others, have developed "odor noise"-free rooms, which they call "olfactoria." In this sort of chamber, all parts of the subject's body, scribe the same four basic viewing conditions used in radiometry are as follows:

1. Luminous Flux (F) Luminous flux is defined as the total amount of visually effective light being emitted in all directions by a point source. The standard candle is the basic reference of the photometric system and it, by definition, emits 4π lumens.

2. Luminous Intensity (I) Luminous intensity is defined as the amount of visually effective light being emitted through 1 steradian (ster)—the unit solid angle. It is measured in lumens/ster. One standard candle emits 1 lumen through each steradian.

3. Illuminance (E) Illuminance is defined as the amount of visually effective light falling on a surface. The unit of illuminance is the *lux*, which is defined to be equal to 1 lumen/m². As in the definition of irradiance, the angle θ of deviation from the perpendicular and the distance r from the light source determine the illuminance according to the following rule:

$$E = I\frac{\cos \theta}{r^2} \tag{2.23}$$

4. Luminance (L) Luminance is defined as the amount of visually effective light that is being emitted by an extended source. The units are, therefore, measures of luminous flux per square meter or lumens[8]/steradian/m². Other units of luminance are commonly used. For example, 1 lumen/steradian/m² is equivalent to 3.14 millilamberts (mL). As in the definition of radiance, the angle of view of the source is critical in defining the amount of light that can be seen according to the following rule:

$$L_{\text{actual}} = L_{\text{max}} \cos \theta \tag{2.24}$$

where L_{actual} is the amount of visually effective light, which can be seen at an angle θ from a source whose emission is equal to L_{max} when viewed perpendicularly to its surface.

Both photometric units and radiometric units are measures of the amount of light being emitted by light sources either in terms of physical energy or visual effect and do not include in their formulation any information about the optical characteristics of the eye. From time to time various investigators have attempted to define units that include the necessary corrections and, thus, more precisely specify the light that actually falls on the retina. The absorption characteristics of the ocular media and the size of the pupil are two additional factors, which one would ideally also like to have included in the definition of the visual stimulus amplitude. Photometric measures do, implicitly, include estimates of the passive absorption of the visual system because of their correction by the luminosity curve, but fluctuations in the size of the pupil add a parameter of uncertainty about luminous measurements if total stimuli energy is important.

As an approach to such a measure of retinal rather than corneal stimulation, L. T. Troland proposed a unit, which was the product of the luminance of a light source multiplied by the area of the pupil. This unit, now known in his honor as the *troland*, has a number of limitations in its with the exception of his nose, may be topologically outside of the stimulating chamber, and thus most contaminants can be excluded.

VI. ELECTRICITY—THE UNIVERSAL STIMULUS

In defining the adequate stimulus, we pointed out that each of the sensory modalities was especially sensitive to one or another form of energy. With the exception of possible electroreceptors in some electric fish, there are no known receptors for which electricity is the primary adequate stimulus. Yet electrical signals are almost unique in their ability to stimulate any and all of the sense organs as well as neurons directly.

A. The Nature of Electricity[2]

1. Charge and Voltage. Electricity is a fundamental property of matter. The atomic model that we now accept as the best description of matter tells us of a world in which the basic building blocks of the elements are made up of a set of fundamental particles, some of which carry an electrical charge. We shall consider this notion of a charged body as the starting point for our present discussion. Charge is divided into two kinds: "negative" and "positive." This definition is based on the physical forces that are created when two or more charges are brought into proximity to each other. Charged objects have been found to either repel or attract each other, and the familiar laws that unlike charges attract and like charges repel are well known. It is not so well appreciated, though, that all electrical units are defined on this same basis.

At the most primitive level, the unit charge found on the basic atomic particles has a value that appears to be remarkably constant and has, therefore, become the basic unit of electrical quantity measurement. Specifically, we use as our basic measure the amount of electricity associated with the negatively charged electron. However, even though the charge on an electron is a convenient laboratory unit, it is much too small for practical charge measurements, which almost always involve many billions of electrons. The *coulomb* has, therefore, been defined as the total charge of 6.28×10^{18} free electrons and is the practical unit of charge.

Charge in itself is not, of course, a useful stimulus and does not even exert an effective physical force until it interacts with other charges. When charges interact, either repelling or attracting each other, they produce forces. These forces tend to put charge in motion and thus are able to do useful work or create other effects that are of special significance in our particular biological field of interest.

First, let us consider the nature of the force that occurs when two charged bodies interact. The magnitude of force that is produced is defined by the following inverse square law:

$$F = k \frac{q_1 q_2}{r^2} \tag{2.25}$$

[2] Much of this material has been adapted from my more detailed discussion in an earlier work (Uttal, 1968).

where F is the force; k is a constant characteristic of the medium surrounding the charged objects called the permitivity ($k = 1$ for a vacuum); q_1 is the charge on the first object; q_2 is the charge on the second object; and r is the distance between the two. The force produced is defined as 1 absolute volt if an erg of work is done, moving a charge of 10 coulombs from the more negative to the more positive point. The absolute volt is, once again, much too small a unit for most practical purposes and a larger unit—the volt—has been defined as 10^8 absolute volts, to accommodate the levels practically found. It is very important to remember that the volt is defined in terms of the force existing between two charged bodies. In practice, this means that no electrical work can be done, or voltage measured, unless a comparison between two points is made. Generally, one of these points is assumed to be common to many voltage measurements. The most common reference used is the earth or ground, although many electrical circuits are referenced to some common voltage level within the circuit, which is not itself referenced to the ground.

The effect of a voltage on free charges produced by a difference in charge distributions is to move them from one place to another. This movement of charge—called *current*—is measured in units called amperes (A). One ampere is defined as the movement of 1 coulomb (Q) of charge past a given point in 1 sec. The practical unit for most electronic circuits is the milliampere (mA), or one-thousandth of an ampere, or the microampere (μA), one-millionth of an ampere. Some instruments are sensitive enough to accurately measure micro-microamperes, or even micro-micro-micro-amperes. Only power lines and supplies usually deal in full amperes.

Voltage sources and the currents produced by them may be constant in time (direct current), or they may vary in time (alternating current or other more complex waveforms) as a function of the mechanics of the original voltage source. The most usual present source of electrical voltage is generation by rotating machinery, which generally produces sinusoidally shaped voltage waveforms. These signals can be described in exactly the same way (in terms of frequency and amplitude) that we describe the sinusoidal waveforms of acoustic stimuli. Voltages produced by chemical cells, on the other hand, are dc.

Voltage sources may be combined in two different manners to enhance their capacity to perform a given task. Some tasks require higher voltages than that available from a single voltage source. For example, batteries produce a voltage that is dependent upon the basic electrochemical reaction of the substances of which they are composed. The only way to get a voltage higher than this chemically defined case is to combine batteries into *series* circuits such as that shown in Figure 2.15(a). The total voltage of such a series circuit is defined by the following equation:

$$E_{\text{total}} = E_1 + E_2 + E_3 \tag{2.26}$$

Automobile batteries, for example, are made up of several independent cells, each of which puts out about 1.1 volts (V)—the basic voltage of a lead-acid battery unit. The 6- and 12-V batteries required for ignition and

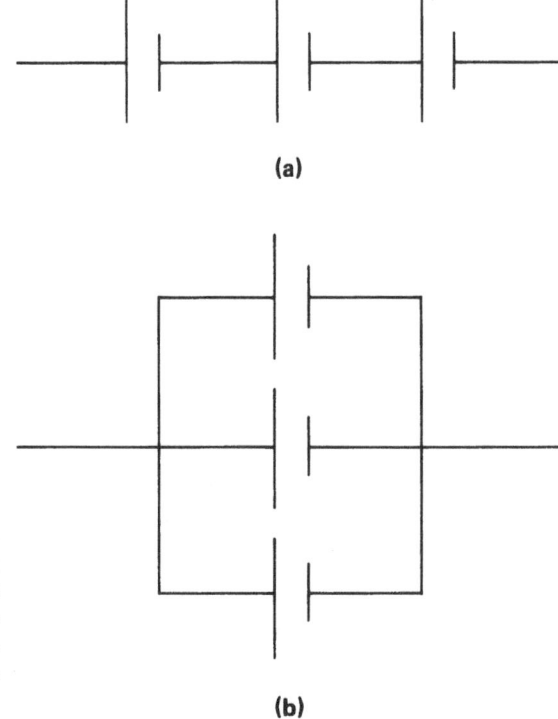

(a)

(b)

FIGURE 2.15 Electrical batteries connected in series (a) and in parallel (b). Series connection provides higher voltages, while parallel connection provides higher current.

the other electrical functions of an automobile are produced by series grouping of these cells.

On the other hand, it is often necessary that additional current capacity, rather than driving voltage, be available. This can be accomplished by means of the arrangements shown in Figure 2.15(b). Voltage sources wired in this manner are said to be arranged in *parallel*. It is intuitively obvious, as well as formally demonstrable, that voltage sources so connected result in a combined voltage equal to the voltage of the individual units. The voltage of the individual units must, however, be equal to each other, or currents will flow uselessly between the units. The advantage of the arrangement is that it can produce a greater current than that available from a single battery.

In practice, electrical energies are generally transmitted from place to place as ac signals because of the simplicity with which voltage levels can be altered by transformers and the lower power loss in ac transmission lines. However, electronic equipment requires dc voltages for stable operation. Special converters changing ac to dc are usually built into any special purpose equipment that receives its main source of energy from the ac main lines. Of course, battery-powered equipment does not require this additional conversion equipment.

2. *Impedance and Current.* Voltage, however, is not the only factor that specifies the magnitude of a current through a conducting circuit. The characteristics of the circuit itself are also important, and particularly the characteristics of the circuit known as *impedance.* Impedance is the property of an electrical component, which tends to inhibit the flow of charge through the circuit of which it is a part. There are many different kinds of physical implementations of devices that exhibit impedance of one kind or another, but in fact, the situation is not as complex as it first appears. All impedances can be classified into three different subtypes—resistive, capacitive, and inductive impedance. It is, furthermore, true that all three types operate by virtue of their tendency to develop a countervoltage in opposite polarity to the applied voltage. With these general notions in mind, we can now consider each of the three different types of impedance separately.

The first kind of impedance is *resistive impedance* or, more simply, *resistance.* Resistance is exclusively a property of the material from which the resistor is made and the shape into which it is formed. Specifically, each atomic element has a *resistivity coefficient* associated with it that is primarily a reflection of the number of electrons in its outermost or valence orbit. If this orbit is filled with a complete set of eight electrons, then these electrons are tightly bound, and the material is a very poor conductor; its resistivity coefficient is very high. Such a material is said to be an *insulator.* If the outermost orbit, on the other hand, contains only one, two, or three electrons, these electrons are easily detached and can act as "carriers." In this case, the material conducts electricity very easily. Such materials have very low resistivity coefficients and are said to be good *conductors.* If the outermost orbit contains four, five, or six electrons, then the material is of some intermediate level of resistivity and is said to be a *semiconductor.* All of the critical factors influencing the resistance of a conductor are contained in Equation (2.27):

$$R = \rho \frac{L}{A} \tag{2.27}$$

in which R is the resistance in ohms; ρ is the elemental resistivity coefficient; A is the cross-sectional area; and L is the length of the conductor.

For a given applied voltage, the impedance of the conductor will determine the current that flows. For purely resistive circuits, the well-known Ohm's law holds:

$$I = \frac{E}{R} \tag{2.28}$$

where I is the current in amperes; E is the voltage in volts; and R is the resistance in ohms.

A large portion, but not all, of the impedance exhibited by biological tissue to electrical currents is resistive. A second kind of impedance is that produced by circuit devices called *capacitors.* The capacitance (C, measured in farads) of a capacitor is defined as the amount of charge (Q, measured in coulombs) per applied volt (V), or:

$$C = \frac{Q}{V} \qquad (2.29)$$

The instantaneous voltage across a charged capacitor is obtained by solving this equation for V:

$$V = \frac{Q}{C} \qquad (2.30)$$

This voltage on the capacitor is the inverse voltage impeding the applied voltage once the capacitor has charged.

It must be remembered, however, that the capacitance of a capacitor is not the same as the impedance (measured in ohms) of the capacitor. Capacitive impedance is very sensitive to the frequency of the applied voltage as defined by the following equation:

$$X_c = \frac{1}{2\pi f C} \qquad (2.31)$$

where X_c is the capacitive impedance in ohms; f is the frequency of applied voltage; and C is the capacitance in farads. Thus, for signals equal or very close to dc (where f is vanishingly small), the impedance of a given capacitor is very large. For very-high-frequency signals, the same capacitance will result in a very small capacitive impedance.

The skin exhibits capacitive characteristics that alter its impedance to different kinds and frequencies of applied stimuli. It is for this reason that the constant current devices described below are necessary for electrostimulation through electrodes applied to the skin. Careful preparation of the skin by sanding and scrubbing with cleansing agents can tend to reduce, but not eliminate, these capacitive effects.

The third kind of impedance, *inductive impedance,* is not often a matter of concern when one is stimulating biological tissue, since it is usually a function of electromagnetic effects found in coils of wire. Some of the electronic circuits used for generating stimuli may, however, exhibit inductive impedance. We shall merely say that coils exhibit a reverse potential due to the buildup of a magnetic field that tends to oppose current flow, just as the inverse voltages of a capacitor or a resistor impede current flow. Biological tissues can, in some instances, exhibit an impedance dependent on the rate of change of ionic current, but it is rare.

B. Sources of Electrical Stimuli

As we have said, electrical stimuli are remarkably efficient in their almost universal ability to activate receptors and other neural tissues. There is a continuing debate over whether the critical feature of the electrical stimulus is the voltage applied across the sensitive tissue, or the current through it.

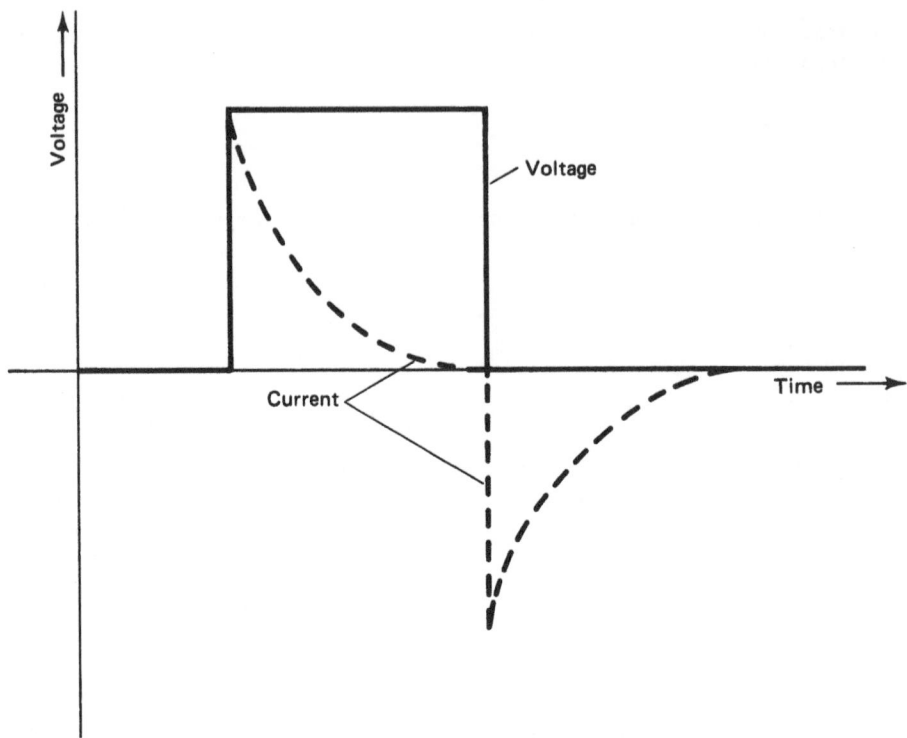

FIGURE 2.16 Diagram showing the shape of the current produced in a circuit that has both resistive and capacitive components (like the skin) by the application of a perfectly square voltage pulse. This differentiation of the current waveform is the reason that constant current stimulators must be used in electrostimulation experiments.

Probably, as so often happens, this argument is spurious, since voltage and current are directly related by an impedance coefficient. What is important is that the stimulus be adequately defined and controlled so that experimental conditions are repeatable. For these reasons, rather than any subtle special property of current or voltage, most experimenters have chosen to define their electrical stimuli in terms of current. Applied voltage pulses are extremely susceptible to distortion due to the impedance characteristic of the tissue or electrodes. Therefore, while applied voltages may be constant, the current through the tissue and, therefore, the voltage across some interior portion of the tissue may vary considerably. The difference between the waveform of an applied voltage pulse and the current produced in a capacitive load is shown in Figure 2.16. The most desirable electrical stimulus is, therefore, a constant current applied through some appropriate electrodes. Thus, even if the impedance of the skin or of the electrodes does vary, the current flowing through the underlying tissue will still be adequately defined.

The timing and shaping of electrical signals is a subject within the realm of electronic instrumentation and is a long and detailed story in itself. Assuming the availability of a given waveform, the key issue for sensory psychophysiology is how one goes about connecting these waveforms to the receptor tissue.

There are several further technical issues with which the experimenter must be concerned when he specifies electricity as the experimental stimulus. First of all, very often electrical stimulation is used in conjunction with very-high-gain preamplifiers, whose purpose is to detect and amplify the resulting neural signals. The signals from biologically active tissue may be, at the very largest, a few millivolts, and are more likely to be of the order of a few tens of microvolts. The stimulus voltages associated with the typical impedance conditions of the electrode-tissue interface may, however, be as large as a couple of hundred volts. This means that the very sensitive amplifier tuned for extreme sensitivity to those low-level bio-potentials would suddenly be exposed to these enormous stimulus amplitudes. In most cases, high-gain amplifiers simply "block" or are saturated with such high signal levels for periods that may last up to several seconds. The best way to protect the detecting amplifier and prevent this blockade is to isolate the electrical stimulus from the amplifier electrically. This can be accomplished by being sure that the voltages of the stimulators are not referenced to the same ground used by the preamplifier. This process is called *voltage isolation*. Thus, the amplifier will be unable to sense the stimulus voltage except for the small amount due to capacitive leakage to the common ground. Electrical stimulus isolation can be accomplished with special transformers, or by radio-frequency isolation units, various kinds of which are now commercially available. This latter type of unit, originally developed by Schmitt and Dubbert (1949), is actually a very small radio transmitting and receiving station built into a common circuit. The Schmitt isolator accomplishes the same function that the transformer does, isolating the stimulus from ground by transmitting a ground referenced signal across an air gap, but differs from the transformer in that it actively generates the high-frequency carrier signal.

With constant current regulation and stimulus isolation both present, the electrical stimulus is now ready to be presented to the subject. The final task is the selection of appropriate electrode or contact materials. It is at the interface between this electrode and the biological tissue that many of the most serious obstacles to efficient and controlled electrical stimulation occur. Stimulating electrodes may be classified into one of two types. The first category includes metallic electrodes, and the second category includes electrolytic solutions. The latter group is most commonly made of a solution of some salt, while metallic electrodes of zinc, copper, stainless steel, silver, platinum and, among others, tungsten have been used. But even metallic electrodes are often used in conjunction with some sort of a salt solution or jelly to decrease the contact resistance.

Silver, tungsten, and stainless steel are the most often used metal stimulation electrodes. Figure 2.17(a) is a photograph of an elegant set of stainless steel stimulating electrodes developed by Gibson (1968) for electrocutaneous stimulation.

Electrolytic electrodes can be very simple. Figure 2.17(b) is a photo-

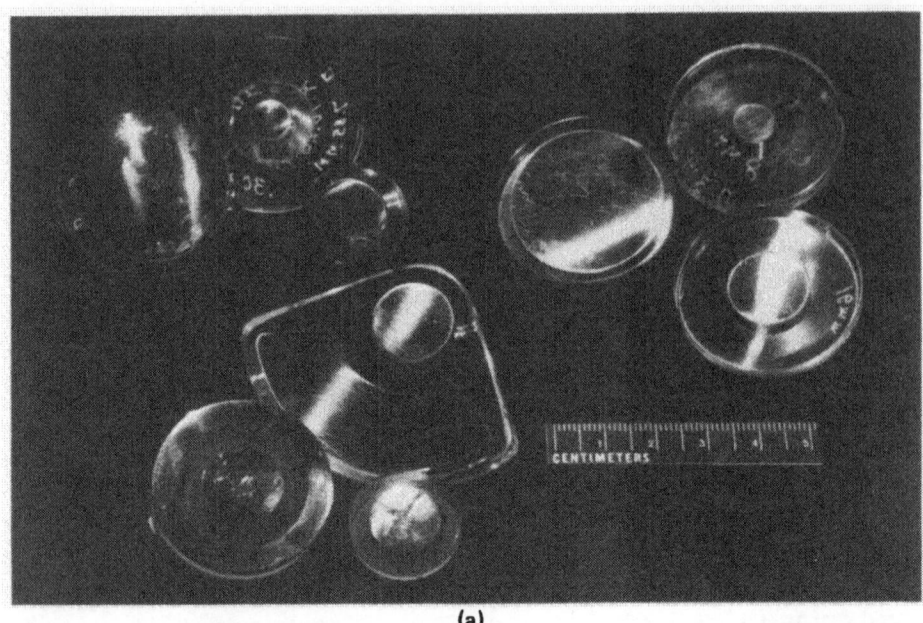

(a)

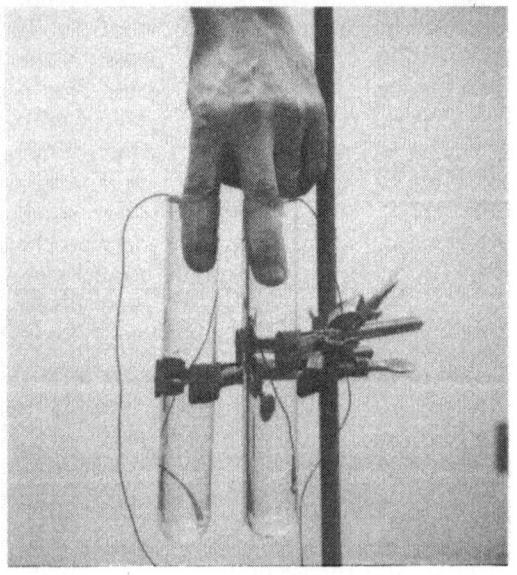

(b)

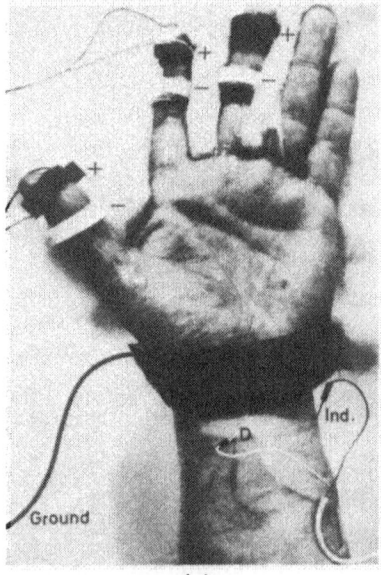

(c)

FIGURE 2.17 (a) An elegant set of electrodes used for electrostimulation of the skin (courtesy of Dr. Robert Gibson). (b) A simple electrical stimulator consisting of two test tubes of body normal NaCl solution into which the fingers are inserted. Note the insulated electrical wires terminating in metallic electrodes (from the author's laboratory). (c) Electrostimulators made up of cloth bags soaked in saline solution and held to the hand by lead bands. Note also the electrodes used for the recording of the induced nerve action potentials (from Buchthal and Rosenfalck, 1966).

graph of a stimulator used by the author to stimulate nerves in the fingers. The subject inserts his fingers into two test tubes of a salt solution. Contact is made with the electronic apparatus by simply immersing a metallic contact into the solution. No electrode jelly or any other special preparation is required by this type of electrode, since there is a very large involvement of the immersed skin resulting in a very low interface impedance.

Figure 2.17(c) is a picture of an alternative form of electrolytic electrode, used by Buchthal and Rosenfalck (1966). Flannel bags surrounding a soft lead electrode were soaked with a salt solution and then bent around the finger. The lead acted both as the contactor and as the support for the salt-soaked flannel electrode. The electrode could be easily kept wet by application of the salt solution to the flannel.

We have now discussed the essential elements of an electrical stimulator capable of providing constant current and isolated electrical stimuli. The waveform of the signal applied to the electrodes is dependent upon the particular experimental design. In the large number of situations in which the purpose of the experiment is to excite nerve action potentials, the waveform of choice is a brief pulse lasting for less than the duration of the action potential. This type of signal has a number of advantages, not the least of which is that a single pulse electrical stimulus, if brief enough, results in only a single nerve action potential. It is, therefore, possible to control the temporal sequence of the nervous response by patterning the external stimulus. This is a special condition quite unobtainable in those situations in which the usual adequate stimuli are activating the usual receptors. The broad implications of this technique will be discussed later in this book (in Chapter 6) when we discuss the neural coding of sensory intensity.

Other workers have used ac voltages as their stimuli for studies of cutaneous amplitude and frequency discrimination. But in general, the skin has been shown to be insensitive to frequency changes using this technique, and it seems to some that ac voltages are inappropriate stimuli in light of the pulse coded mechanisms of the transmitting neurons. Primarily for these reasons, ac stimuli have been used less and less in recent years.

VII. THE SPECIFICATION OF PATTERN

In previous sections of this chapter, we concentrated on the quantification of the quality and quantity of the physical energy of the stimulus. However, it has repeatedly been shown to be the case that a simple statement of only the physical energetics of the stimulus is often grossly insufficient to account for the complexity of a response. Very often two stimuli with identical average physical energies can produce extraordinarily different responses due to other organizational properties. The patterning of equal amounts of photic energy into different geometrical patterns can strongly affect such diverse responses as our attitudes toward a painting or the evoked brain potential. Figure 2.18, for example, shows a set of stimulus patterns from an experiment (Beatty and Uttal, 1968) in which an attempt was made to specifically test the hypothesis that pattern itself was a significant determinant of the amplitude of the evoked brain potential. The patterns shown all contain the same amount of physical energy. The only

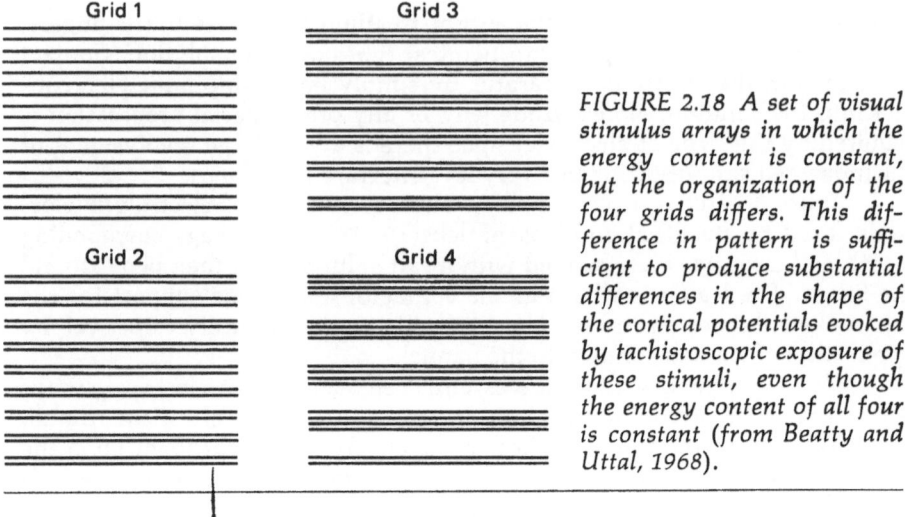

FIGURE 2.18 A set of visual stimulus arrays in which the energy content is constant, but the organization of the four grids differs. This difference in pattern is sufficient to produce substantial differences in the shape of the cortical potentials evoked by tachistoscopic exposure of these stimuli, even though the energy content of all four is constant (from Beatty and Uttal, 1968).

difference among them is in the overall organization (in this case, grouping) of the stimulus lines. Yet the results of the experiment showed that there was a very strong effect on the evoked potential as a function of the grouping, namely, that the larger the number of lines in a group, the smaller the evoked potential. Indeed, this effect was considerably stronger and more reliable than the effect produced by varying the intensity of a visual stimulus.

Equally certainly, the patterning of a musical composition is a far more significant determiner of our response than the absolute frequencies and amplitudes of its constituent sounds. The difference between the Appassionata and the same set of sounds presented in another order or pattern is so profound as to be almost unnecessary to mention. Neurophysiologists and psychologists, working with the senses of many different animals, have found what seem to be specific sensitivities to pattern (Lettvin, Maturana, McCulloch, and Pitts, 1959; Roeder and Treat, 1961; Segundo, Moore, Stensaas, and Bullock, 1963; Uttal and Krissoff, 1968) that transcend even at the receptor level the sensitivity to the simpler metrics of physical energy. The result of these and other related observations over the last few years has led to a very much increased interest in the use of stimuli with complex patterns and a decrease in interest in the use of impulsive unitary stimuli. In Chapter 8 we shall discuss this problem in very great detail.

The experimental specification of stimulus pattern, however, is often difficult and is, in some cases, an underdeveloped technology in spite of its demonstrated importance. In other realms, it is almost overdeveloped, but unfortunately underused in psychological experimentation. Consider, for example, the musical notation system. A musical scale is one precise statement of a sequence of sound stimuli. As more and more experimenters begin to use patterns of musical tones as their stimuli, we shall probably see more precise means of stimulus specification.

The frequency analytical techniques, which are used to characterize signals as sums of sinusoid components, and the related correlational techniques, which extract general periodic tendencies, must also be considered as representational systems for pattern. They do, however, eliminate a large amount of the critical detail information of a given temporal pattern. Nevertheless, they do emphasize the pattern aspects in an important way and ought not to be overlooked in our present discussion.

The specification of temporal acoustic patterns, as we have said, has the rich background of musical notation systems to depend upon. Spatial patterns, however, have no equivalent artistic notational schema. The spatial arts, sculpture, painting, and architecture have never used anything other than their own pictographic representation. Sketches or starkly diagrammatic blueprints are about all that has classically been available as a spatial shorthand. Recently, however, some of the automatic machine tool techniques have required that geometric forms be represented by a sequence of coded instructions. This technique may have the germ of a future notational system for geometrical forms implicit in it. Presently, however, the representation of two and three dimensional objects in space is usually done by a direct analogue—a map—which pictures the form in almost its complete detail. But it is often as difficult to deal with a map as it is to deal with the multidimensional object itself. Consider the small differences between an original painting and a reproduction. About the only advantages that are forthcoming from maps are reductions or enlargements of the scale of the original object, or the removal of an extraneous dimension. This latter notion is exemplified by a map of a geographical area in which the height of various items is ignored. The map is smaller, and it can be carried in one's pocket, but for the purpose of this discussion, it is still very much a pictographic representation of the original object. Maps, of course, are used frequently to specify visual stimuli for psychological experiments. A collection of slides of different geometrical forms is essentially a set of maps in which no information reduction or coding scheme is used.

Many investigators, on the other hand, have searched for algorithms, that is, computation rules or formulas that generate sets of geometrical forms according to certain generative rules. In many of the procedures, there is a random element inserted so that a general algorithm can produce a large number of similar but unpredictable geometrical forms. In this case, the algorithm itself cannot be used to uniquely define any given character, a priori, since the specific figure generated will depend, to a great extent, upon the specific random numbers that are produced during the generation process. The final output of such a routine, however, may represent a geometrical form in a reduced fashion in the sense we use when we refer to a notational or coding system.

Some of the more interesting figure generation routines are described in the following paragraphs:

1. The "quasi-random histogram." Fitts and his colleagues (Fitts, Weinstein, Rappaport, Anderson, and Leonard, 1956) suggested a system for making random forms that has a number of advantages for psychological research. All shapes generated by this system are similar, yet differ enough to provide a sufficiently variable dimension for experimental manipulation. Figure 2.19 shows two of these patterns. The rule for generating

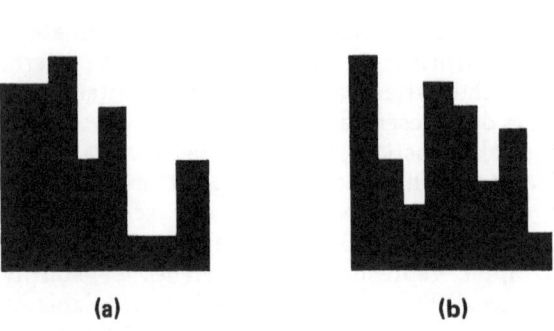

FIGURE 2.19 Two stimulus patterns formed by random selection of the height of columns in an 8 × 8 matrix. The pattern in (a) has been formed by true random sampling with replacement, while the one in (b) was formed by constrained random sampling without replacement (from Fitts, Weinstein, Rappaport, Anderson, and Leonard, 1956).

this type of pattern is that a number between 0 and the maximum allowable height of a bar is randomly selected for each of the bar positions. This results in a pattern like that in Figure 2.19(a). If the random selection process is constrained so that a given height can be chosen only once (random selection without replacement), then a form like that in Figure 2.19(b) results. It is interesting to note, in passing, that the figures formed by the latter procedure are much more difficult to identify in a group of similar patterns than are those that are generated by the first fully random rule. Considering that the information content of the constrained random group is less because of the introduced redundancy, this is not too surprising a result.

2. The random polygon. Attneave and Arnoult (1956) developed an algorithmic technique for generating a variety of polygonal visual stimulus patterns. Random locations were selected on a sheet of graph paper. These locations were then connected, forming an exterior limit on the size of the polygon. Then any remaining interior points were used to make indentations in the otherwise relatively regular polygon. Figure 2.20 shows one of the shapes and the generation process. Attneave and Arnoult in their publications have been especially adamant in their appeal for precise metrics of geometrical form, for they, like the author of this book, feel that without an adequate specification of the nature of the stimulus, little formal progress is possible in our understanding of sensory processes.

3. The "random" dot pattern. The problem of form can also be approached in a three-dimensional context as well as a two-dimensional one. Julesz (1960, 1971) has been interested in the study of depth perception, specifically in the cues that are introduced by retinal disparity independent of the other stereoscopic cues. To provide stimulus materials that had no other cue present but retinal disparity, he chose to use a novel and ingenious display composed of what appeared, when seen monocularly, to be an absolutely random dot pattern. Figure 2.21 shows a pair of these patterns. However, when the objects are viewed dichoptically, certain regions of the dot pattern can, under the proper convergence conditions, fall on corresponding points of the retina. Because certain regions of the dual pictures are not really completely random, but rather are identical in both pictures except for uniform lateral shifts in plotted position, they can be

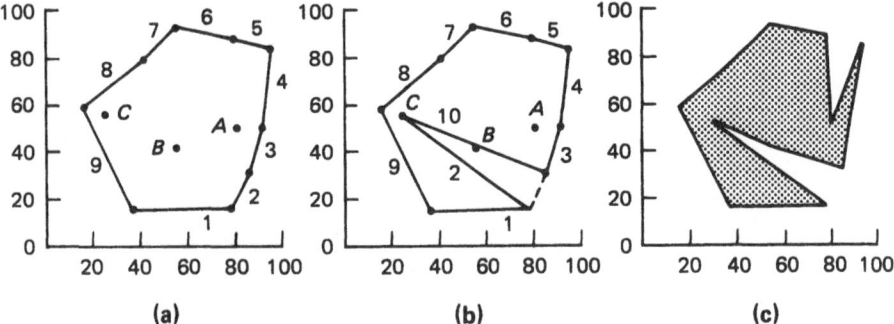

FIGURE 2.20 Steps in the construction of a random polygon, using the procedure invented by Attneave and Arnoult (1956). Random points are first plotted, and then the exterior points are connected. Then slices are taken out of the external polygon to connect the internal points, thus forming irregular polygons with both convexities and concavities.

interpreted by the visual system in exactly the same way as the slightly shifted aspects of a more conventional stereoscopic pair produced by differences in the position of the two eyes or two camera lenses. Images that had not been obvious to any degree in the original pattern suddenly emerge in sometimes awesome complexity.

It is obvious that the very powerful responses elicited by these random dot patterns have little to do with the simple physical energetics of the stimulus and that the "pattern" of dots is the all-important variable. Julesz has done some work in quantifying these patterns in terms of the introduced disparity, but the best models of all, of course, are the computer generation routines, which plot out the pictures.

There is no question that these algorithmic generation routines do play an important and useful role in defining stimuli for psychological experiments. However, they do not completely define a metric that can be used to specify the exact configuration of the generated characters because of the random factors that appear throughout all of the methods. Thus, while a given routine might generate the members of a particular class of patterns, it is not known which particular item will occur with any given evaluation of the algorithm. This limitation may, indeed, not be a handicap if one is interested in the problem of a general theory of form perception, but it does not help us in the specification of the critical differences in the perception of forms like the alphabetic characters, which are already predetermined. This same problem occurs in an analogous form in the study of speech, where, of course, the same generalization holds; namely, the energetics of the speech sound are secondary and almost incidental compared to the pattern of sound and meanings involved in an utterance. Stochastic procedures and analytical techniques are commonly used in speech analysis to help describe the sequential dependencies and general statistical structure of speech sounds, but again statistical models fall short of the desired goal—a specific and full metric for the representation of pattern and form.

FIGURE 2.21 A dicoptic stimulus pattern in which no figure is apparent when viewed monocularly. When viewed in a stereoscope, however, the single cue of retinal disparity generated by systematic variation of dot position gives rise to a strong impression of a center square rising above the background (from Julesz, 1971).

Perhaps the next closer approximation to a complete map is a computer program. Unfortunately the problems of communicating this particular longhand description of a geometrical form have still not been solved, and few psychological experiments report the construction of the computer program defining the stimulus, in the methods section.

In this chapter we have attempted to gather together the basic measures and fundamental principles of physics that are necessary for a full understanding of the sensory process. We have stressed the point that the physical stimulus must be the starting place for all discussions of neural coding of sensory messages. We have distinguished between a potential stimulus and a realized actual one and have, in conclusion, stressed the point that the gross energetics of the physical stimulus may often play a secondary role to those distributions of energy in time or space which we call patterns, but for which we have not yet developed an adequate descriptive notation. With this introduction to physical stimuli, we can now proceed to the biological aspects of sensory processing and consider the anatomy and physiology of the information input mechanisms in the remainder of the first section of this book.

CHAPTER 3: THE ANATOMY OF RECEPTORS AND THE SENSORY PATHWAYS

I. INTRODUCTION

The discussion in the preceding chapter has provided a foundation of the necessary physics, which must serve as a reference point to which we shall anchor all studies of sensory communication. The energetics and organization of the physical stimulus are, as has been pointed out, the only meaningful referrents for all of the stages of transduction and coding that follow. However, before we can meaningfully discuss transduction and the coding neural signals, it is necessary that we make some further preparatory steps. In this chapter, we shall concern ourselves with the structure of those highly specialized receptor structures in which these transduction actions occur and the neural pathways which convey information from them to the central nervous system.

There are three levels of anatomical information concerning the receptors with which we must deal: the macroscopic, the microscopic, and the ultra or electron microscopic. In recent years there has been great progress in our understanding of these cells, highly specialized as they are for the conversion of almost unimaginably slight amounts of energy into transmittable neural signals, particularly at the ultramicroscopic level. This is primarily the result of some extraordinary progress in the field of electron microscopy. In addition, there has also been considerable progress made, at a grosser level, in tracking the ascending sensory pathways. The emphasis in this latter case is on the location of the synaptic interconnections and the tracing of the sensory nerves and tracts from the receptor organs to the areas of the upper reaches of the central nervous system at which, presumably, the communicated information becomes, in some unknown manner, the stuff of which experience is made. In presenting this information, we shall deal with the anatomy of the receptors and the associated pathways of a single modality as units, rather than adopt the alternative strategy of describing all of the receptors and then, separately, all of the pathways. As far as possible, the anatomy of ascending pathways and of receptor structures presented will be that of man himself. Occasionally infrahuman data will be used where human findings are not available for one reason or another or to make a particular point.

To fully understand the nature of modern neuroanatomical knowledge, there are three pieces of preparatory material that must first be discussed. We must first consider the need for, and the operation of, the electron microscope itself, the tool, par excellence, of the microanatomist. Second, we must consider some of the techniques that are routinely used for the elucidation of neuroanatomical structure. Finally, we must also consider some grosser features of the general organization of the central nervous system, without which our subsequent discussion of the ascending pathways would be very difficult to fully understand.

II. THE ELECTRON MICROSCOPE

In the rest of this chapter, we shall be dealing with the sensory organs at several different levels of magnification. Gross structural analyses and the application of optical microscopy have both contributed much and will continue to contribute substantial amounts to our knowledge. The continued fertility of optical microscopic techniques is well illustrated by Johnsson and Hawkins' (1967) recent work using phase contrast microscopy to elucidate the structure of the cochlea. Nevertheless, the real cutting edge of ultrastructural research in the last decade has certainly been the application of the electron microscope to the study of receptor and neural anatomy. It is for this reason that we shall pause for a moment to consider exactly why one has to use an electron microscope, and then how this incredibly effective machine actually operates. To understand the operation of the electron microscope, we must first understand something about the wave properties of electromagnetic energy and the limitations of the optical microscope. We must consider the nature of the concept of resolving power and its relation to the wavelength of the radiation being used in the magnification process.

It is not possible to review completely the principles of optics that underly the optical microscope; however, a few reminders of the basic mechanism of the refraction of light by lenses might help the reader to understand some of the material that will follow. We have already discussed, in the previous chapter, some of the ways in which the quantal characteristics of light are exhibited (for example, in the line spectrum of a luminescent light source) and have mentioned how it is possible to convert from quantal energy measures to the wavelength or frequency measures. Discussion of the optical properties of lenses is one that is always framed

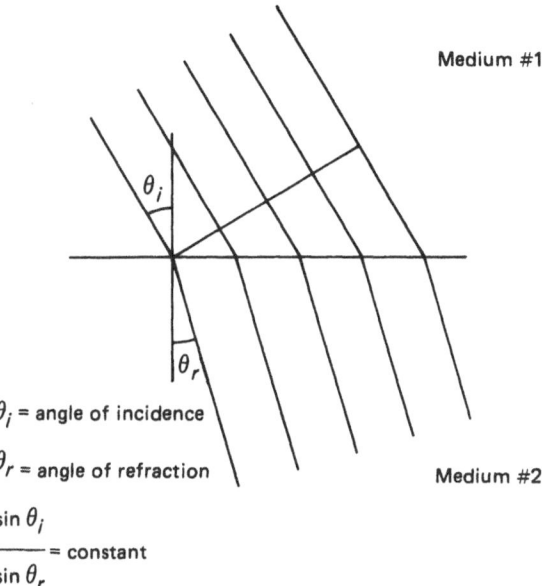

FIGURE 3.1 Diagram show-
ing the change in the direction (refraction) of a beam
of light as it enters a medium
of a different index of refraction than that of the one in
which it had been traveling.
Refraction is the basis of all
optical lens effects including
magnification and is analogous to the refraction of electron beams by magnetic
fields.

Medium #1

θ_i

θ_r

θ_i = angle of incidence

θ_r = angle of refraction

Medium #2

$$\frac{\sin \theta_i}{\sin \theta_r} = \text{constant}$$

in terms of the wave properties of light and constitutes the science that is
usually called geometrical optics.

The basic premise of geometrical optics is that light is diverted in
direction as it enters *at an angle* a medium with a different index of refraction than that in which it had been traveling. Since the velocity of the
light changes with the index of refraction, the effect is to alter the direction
of the wave front by retarding one portion earlier than the others (see
Figure 3.1).

A lens will divert or refract rays of light, an amount which depends
upon not only the index of refraction of the component glass but also upon
the curvature of the lens. Thus, each lens has a characteristic "focal length,"
which is defined in terms of the distance from the lens at which parallel
rays (coming from infinitely far away) are brought to a focus. For light
sources (the object) that are not infinitely far away, the distance Q at
which an image is formed depends upon the distance P to the object and
the focal length F of the lens in accord with the following relation:

$$\frac{1}{P} + \frac{1}{Q} = \frac{1}{F} \tag{3.1}$$

These notions are summarized by Figure 3.2 for a simple thin lens.

The degree of magnification M of a lens can be defined as the ratio
of the image size to the object size, and it can be shown that this is
simply equal to the ratio of P and Q. Therefore:

$$M = \frac{P}{Q} \tag{3.2}$$

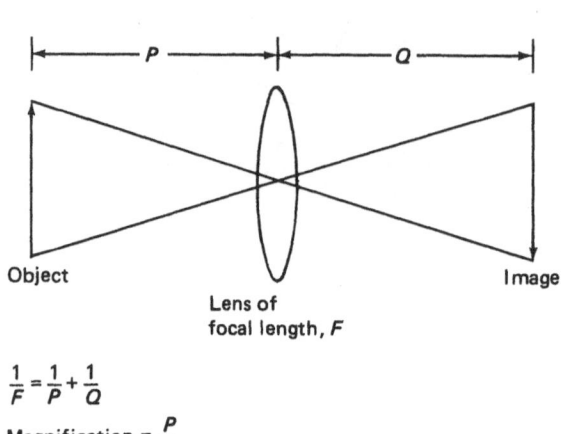

FIGURE 3.2 Diagram of the action of a simple thin lens. Light will be imaged at a distance Q from the lens, which is a function both of the distance of the object from the lens P and the focal length F of the lens. The magnification will be exactly equal to P/Q. Several lenses of this sort can be used to gain additional magnification according to a multiplicative rule (magnification total * = magnification₁ × magnification₂ × . . . magnification_n), but only up to the resolving power limit which, for an optical microscope, is approximately equivalent to a magnification of 2000.*

Since the relation between P and Q is a function only of F, it is clear that the degree of magnification of a glass lens will be solely a function of its focal length and where the object is located. The magnification of a lens or lens system (the magnification of one lens can be concatenated with that of another to give even larger magnifications than those possible with a single lens), however, is unrelated to the so-called resolving power of a microscope. Magnification can, for all practical purposes, be increased without limit, but a limit is imposed upon any microscope by the fact that the light being used is also being magnified as much as the object under study. Thus, there comes a time at which the individual wavelengths of the light begin to be large enough to interfere with the imaging of the object. This limit is the basis of the idea of the "resolving power" of any microscope.

Because of diffraction effects produced by the interaction of wave fronts from the much magnified individual light waves,'there is no realizable way of improving the optical properties of any microscope to distinguish between two adjacent points that are closer than a certain minimum amount. That is to say, even with perfect optical elements the wavelength of the utilized radiation specifies a minimum separable distance (resolving power) for any magnifying system. An expression, which can be used to estimate the maximum possible resolving power of any given magnifier, can be derived and shown to be a function of both the wavelength of the radiation and the geometry of the magnifying system:

$$r = \frac{0.5\lambda}{\text{NA}} \tag{3.3}$$

where r is the resolving power (the minimal separable distance achievable by the magnifier); λ is the wavelength of the utilized radiation; and NA is the "numerical aperture" of the magnifying system. For optical microscopes, the numerical aperture is defined by:

$$NA = \mu \sin \theta \tag{3.4}$$

where μ is the index of refraction of the medium through which the light passes, and θ is half the angle subtended by the lens. Under optimum conditions of viewing, using an appropriate fluid immersion system and appropriately slanted light pathways, the numerical aperture of a microscope using visible light can only be as great as 1.5. Therefore, the resolving power of the best quality optical microscope is limited to about a third of the wavelength of the magnifying light. The shortest visible blue light that can be seen under normal conditions is about 380 or 400 nm. Resolving power is thus limited to separations of about 130 or 140 nm. By use of even shorter invisible lights, such as ultraviolet radiation, and special photographic or electronic detection systems, resolving power can be extended even further. Finally, however, the problems of lens transparency and of lens aberrations begin to take over, and the limits of the optical microscopes cannot be extended by any means. Unfortunately, this technological limit is not identical to the limit of the sizes of many of the elements of biological concern. As one important example, the lamellar layers of the outer segment of a retinal rod are only 50 Å thick (see Porter and Bonneville, 1968, p. 181), and it is at this ultramicroscopic level that most significant transductive phenomena occur. Alternative means of increased magnification are, therefore, necessary if one is to have fuller information about the details of microstructure.

Equation (3.3) leaves two different routes open in the search for a means to improve the resolving power of a magnifying system; the wavelength of the radiation may be decreased, or the numerical aperture of the system may be increased. For many practical reasons, it has generally not been possible to greatly increase the numerical aperture of any magnifier. The optical or electrical properties of lenses and magnets seem to be recalcitrant to much improvement in this direction. Therefore, it has been necessary to work on the other factor in the equation, the wavelength of the radiation used in the magnifying process. This strategy is facilitated by the fact that visible light is but one small region of the continuum of electromagnetic energies and wavelengths, which spans the energy spectrum from long, low-frequency radio waves to the ultrahigh-frequency equivalents of some of the basic particles of matter when they are accelerated to high velocities.

It is not germane to the present discussion to detail further the relationship between the particle and wave properties of the basic building blocks of matter. Let us simply reiterate that modern physical theory treats electrons, along with all other elementary particles, as packets of waves, which exist in only a certain statistical sense in any place at any given time, the limit on their precise localization being a function of the Heisenberg uncertainty principle. The critical fact in the context of the present discussion is that a beam of electrons, just like a light ray, has associated with it wave properties which result in the fact that it can be refracted, reflected, and focused by appropriate "lenses" just as can visible light. The lenses that can accomplish this for the electron beam, however, are not made of glass or quartz, but must be either electrostatic plates or electromagnetic coils of exactly the same nature one would find in an oscilloscope or a commercial television set.

By applying electrostatic or magnetic fields to a beam of electrons, the path of the particles can be altered in a selective manner, depending upon their course and the shape and magnitude of the deflecting field. Electrons from a point source, spherically divergent in their initial paths, can be collimated into a nearly parallel stream or focused by the action of, say, an appropriate magnetic field. The amount of deflecting force exerted on each electron is proportional to the component of its velocity, which is at right angles to the local magnetic field. This is, of course, the famous right-hand rule of motors.

Deflection control by magnetic force is exactly analogous to the focusing action of a glass lens in the optical microscope and can be used in the same way to magnify an image. Magnetic lenses also have "focal lengths" and refractive properties analogous to glass lenses. But in the case of the electron beam, we are dealing with an electromagnetic wavelength that is far shorter than that of visible light, and thus the resolving power of the electron micrographic system can be much greater. In practical fact, assuming a relatively constant numerical aperture (and, as we have said, there is relatively little that can be done in modifying the numerical aperture of magnifying systems), rather than 150 nm resolution ability, typical of a good optical microscope, a good electron microscope will have an ability to resolve two objects only 1 nm apart. This separability can be even further improved to a few angstrom units as the energy of the electron beam is increased beyond a million volts as it is in some modern machines. The associated decrease in equivalent wavelength as a function of electron energy is the basic reason that the more highly resolving electron microscopes are also much larger physical instruments. They simply require higher accelerating voltages and the correspondingly more complex and massive instrumentation to achieve and maintain these higher-energy electron beams.

It is also a practical result that electron microscopes do not operate as near their theoretical limit on resolving power as does the optical microscope. The art of designing the deflecting coils for an electron microscope simply has not achieved the same relative level of freedom from aberrations of one sort or another that the equivalent optical arts have.

A focused and magnified beam of electrons from the electron microscope, after passing through or being reflected from a specimen, of course, is still invisible to the human eye. The information contained in such a beam must be converted to a visible image or a photographic record by projection of the beam of electrons onto a luminescent screen capable of emitting light within the visible spectrum. Additional amplification is often achieved by image intensifiers, closed-circuit television, or other electrooptical methods of light enhancement.

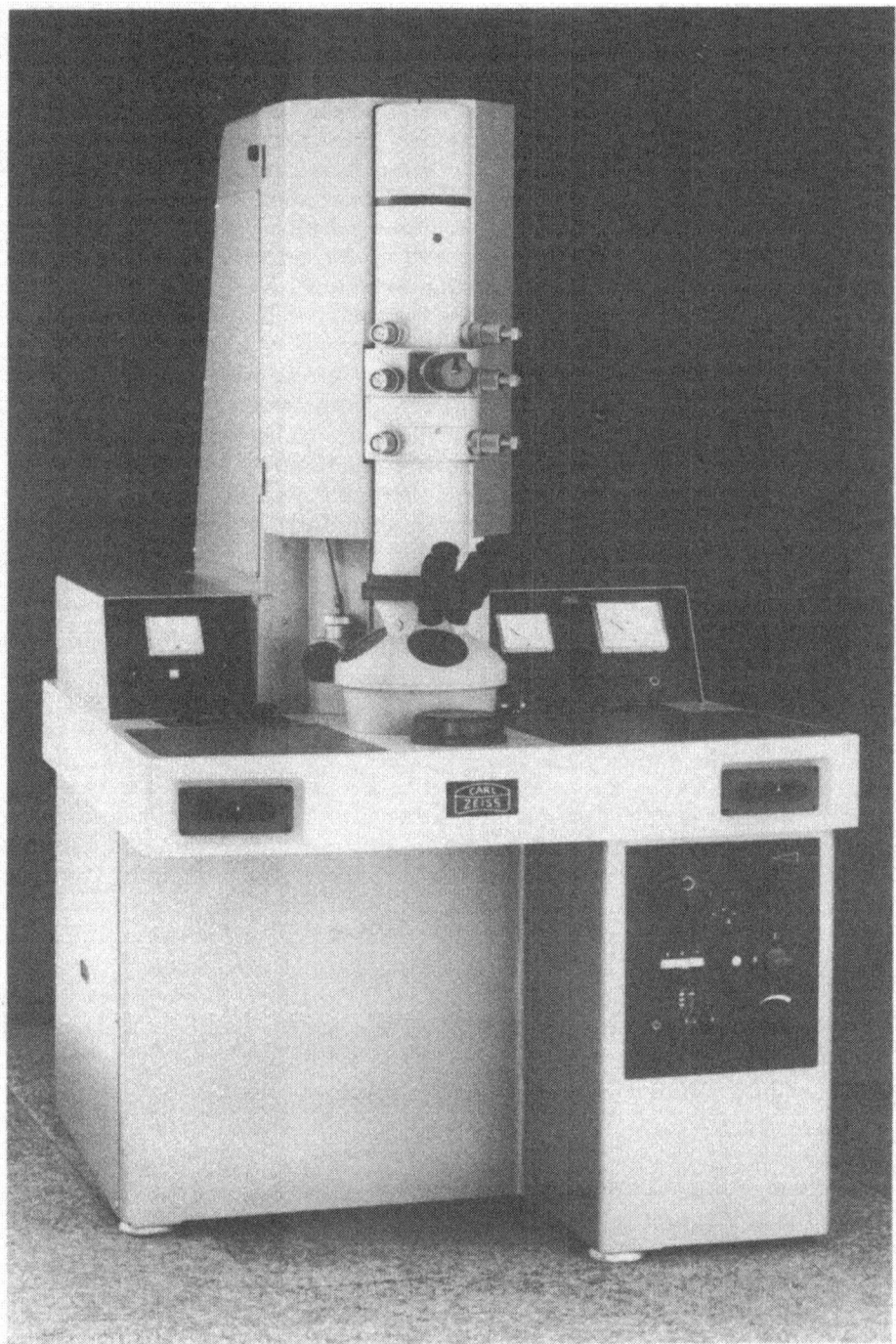

FIGURE 3.3 A photograph of the outside of a modern electronmicroscope (courtesy of Carl Zeiss, Inc.).

Electron microscopes, like optical ones, may be either reflection or transmission types. In either case, a special and appropriate technology of speciment preparation has developed. To minimize the absorption and thus the associated heating of the electron beam in the transmission electron microscope, specimen tissues of extremely thin cross section must be prepared. Ultramicrotomes capable of slicing a section of a fraction of a micron in thickness are routinely used. These ultramicrotomes may require blades made from specially fractured pieces of glass. For reflection electron microscopy, a process specialized for the examination of the surface detail of a specimen, special metallizing techniques have been invented. In this process a thin coating of a metal, especially selected for its ability to reflect electrons, is sputtered onto the surface of the specimen. The reflected electrons are then guided to the fluorescent screen or photograph film. Figure 3.3 shows a photograph of a modern electron microscope.

An important new development in electron microscopy has been the recent availability of the scanning electron microscope. This device has the advantage of enormous depth of field—so great, in fact, that in many instances objects appear to be in focus over their entire volume. Figure 3.4(a), for example, is an example of what would have been an impossible micrographic task prior to the development of this instrument. An entire receptor organ is seen at a relatively low level of magnification. This same sort of three-dimensional accuracy is also available, furthermore, at magnifications of many thousands as shown in Figures 3.4(b) and (c).

The scanning electron microscope operates on the basis of the secondary ejection of electrons from the specimen after the surface is bombarded with the primary electrons produced by the electron gun of the microscope. The key point is that not all loci on the surface of the specimen are bombarded simultaneously, but rather a highly focused beam of electrons "scans" each point in sequence and in synchrony with the painting of an image on a cathode-ray oscilloscope. It is this sequential scanning procedure similar to that used on an ordinary television that is the basis of the name of this form of the electron microscope, as well as of the great depth of focus.

Figure 3.5 is a cut away diagram of the main features of a scanning electron microscope, showing the electronic synchronization and control circuitry, the specialized detector capable of selectively sensing the number of secondary electrons ejected from the specimen and the display oscilloscope. Very often, the specimen is coated with some material to increase the number of secondary electrons. This material is usually some metal capable of being vaporized and deposited in a coating only a few angstrom units thick. As we shall see later in this chapter, some important insights into receptor anatomy have emerged through judicious application of scanning techniques.

The technical details of the construction of an electron microscope are, however, only secondary in interest to the astonishing pictures these elegant machines have provided for students of many of the biological sciences and particularly for those of us interested in the senses. There is no better way to make this point than to present in later sections of this chap-

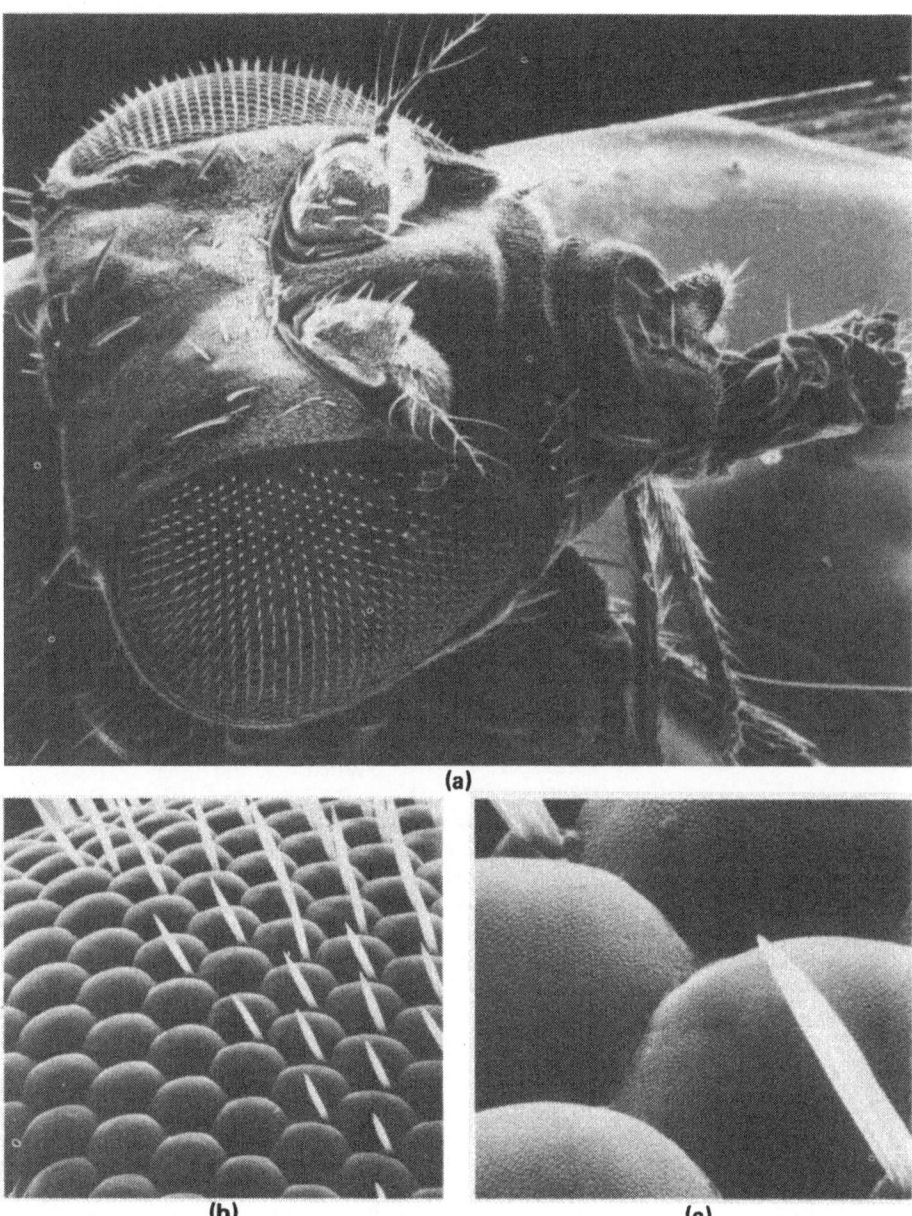

FIGURE 3.4 A series (a), (b), and (c) of scanning electronmicrographs of the visual organ of a fruit fly in increasing order of magnification showing the astounding three-dimensional effects produced with this instrument. (a) The whole head (× 108). (b) Several ommatidia (× 302). (c) A single ommatidum (× 11,200) (courtesy of Dr. Lloyd Beidler, Florida State University).

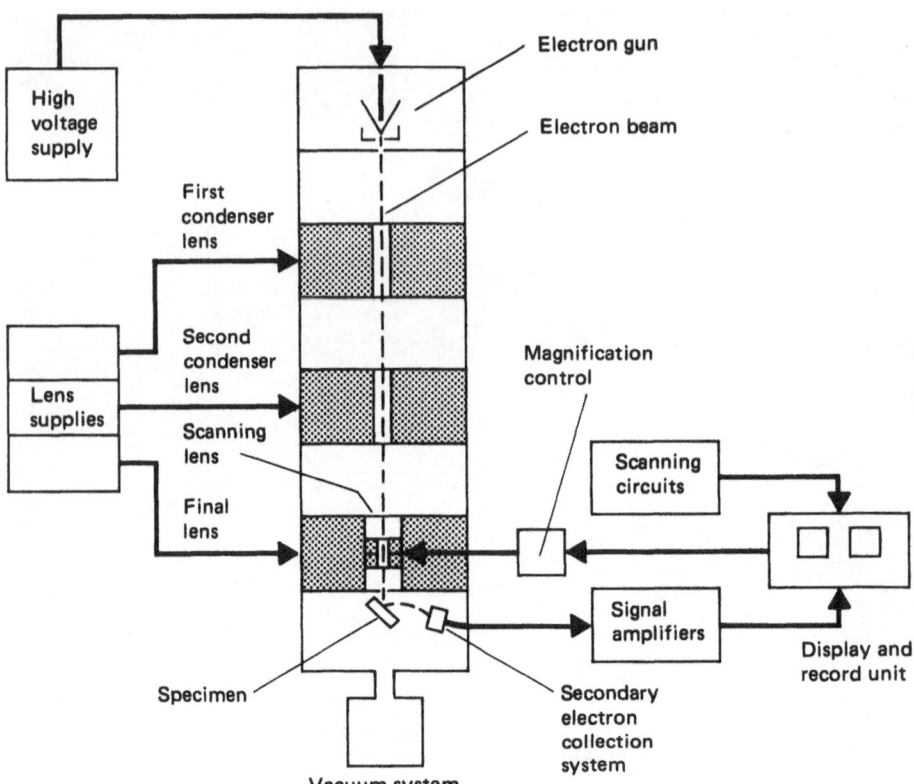

FIGURE 3.5 *A cutaway drawing of a modern scanning electronmicroscope show-ing the additional scanning and display circuitry necessary to scan the matrix of points on the specimen in sequential order. The bottom electromagnetic lens controls the scanning of the electron beam. The serial information emitted from the specimen in the form of a stream of secondary electrons of varying intensity is then measured and used to plot out a picture on an oscilloscope for photo-graphic purposes (courtesy of Kent Cambridge Scientific, Inc., Morton Grove, Illinois).*

ter a sampling of some of the better ones and some of the interpretive drawings made from them. The general scheme we shall follow in this chapter will be to proceed from the gross to the ultramicroscopic anatomy. In a very true sense we shall thus be saving the best for the last. But all of the levels of structural complexity at which we shall look in this chapter will appeal to the esthetic senses of the reader in a way quite distinct from the impact of some of the later chapters. However, before we can look at sensory anatomy in particular, we must consider central neural anatomy in general. The next two sections accomplish this function. We first con-sider some of the general techniques used for neuroanatomical research and then the gross structure of the central nervous system as it is presently known.

III. SOME BASIC RESEARCH TECHNIQUES IN NEUROANATOMY

A. Additional Optical Microanatomical Techniques

The optical microscope, as we have said, has played and will continue to play an important role in mapping the central nervous system. To use a microscope to observe what are normally transparent tissues, special techniques must be employed to make the cells visible. The classic technique has been to use some sort of a dye or stain, which is relatively specific to a particular kind of tissue. Thus, there are stains like toluidine blue, which are highly specific for cell bodies alone, and others like the silver based stains, which act in little understood ways to selectively stain some parts of some cells including the axons and dendrites. Many pictures of whole neurons have been processed with a technique known as the Golgi impregnation method. In this procedure, crystals of silver chromate fill the cell completely, and thus it is really not so much a membrane "staining" technique as it is a sort of "fossilization" procedure. In other silver staining techniques like the Holmes and Bodian procedures, the silver atoms combine with neurofibrillar elements, and a true stain is thus achieved.

More recently, new techniques, that allow unstained nervous tissue to be observed, have been developed. Phase contrast optical techniques take advantage of the minute differences in the refractive index of the different parts of individual cells, so that the microscopist can observe almost completely unprepared tissue. In fact, it is possible in some instances to actually see a living cell going through its normal metabolic activities with this type of microscope.

Fluorescence techniques, which allow examination of tissues in a form very close to their natural states, have also been developed. The fluorescence technique usually involves some specialized preparation of the tissue including the injection of special fluorescent dyes, however, and living cells cannot usually be observed in this manner. Typically the tissue is frozen and then dried in a vacuum. The prepared tissue is then placed in a special microscope, in which the light source is rich in ultraviolet rays. Different tissues pick up different amounts of dyes and thus fluoresce in different colors when they are exposed to ultraviolet light. It is this secondary emission of light that is seen by the observer, rather than transmitted light filtered by a stained slice of tissue, as is the case in a conventional optical microscope. (The particular color of the cell can thus indicate which cells are histochemically alike and perhaps, even more important, functionally similar.)

A very recent development (Stretton and Kravitz, 1968) in fluorescence microscopy takes advantage of a special dye known as Procion yellow. This dye has a number of important advantages. One of the most significant is the fact that it is relatively harmless to a living neuron. It is, therefore, possible to inject this material into a physiologically responsive cell through a micropipette and, for a short time, observe the anatomy of the living cell while simultaneously recording its electrophysiological signals. Another important advantage is that the neuronal membrane seems to be very impermeable to the Procion yellow dye. Thus, all of the dye remains within the single cell into which it is injected, yet it is also capable of diffusing to most of the branches of the neuron. A cell can, therefore, be anatomically studied as if it were perfectly isolated from its neighbors if the injection is appropriately done.

Procion yellow fluoresces in the yellow portion of the spectrum when irradiated by a bluish light, while most cells that do not contain dye will fluoresce with a greenish color. The injected cell will stand out clearly, therefore, including most of its smaller ramifications. The dye is also stable during normal fixation procedures and remains in serial sections so that it is still useful for postmortem microscopic examination.

The microanatomical techniques, which we have so briefly mentioned here, help to directly distinguish one anatomical structure from another. Some fiber bundles and nuclei are separated from their neighbors in sharp and distinct patterns when observed through the microscope. The constituent cells of each region may be quite different from one area to another. In other cases, however, the microanatomical difference may be quite small, and no obvious line of demarcation may exist between two adjacent regions. Furthermore, microanatomical techniques also may show greater differences in sequential portions of the same pathway than in adjacent portions of different pathways. Since so much of our neuroanatomical interest at this microscopic level is based upon our interest in the functional rather than the structural properties, neuroanatomists often turn to the following procedures to define the limits of a tract even when it shows very little visible anatomical differentiation from its neighbor.

B. Evoked Potential Techniques

Stimulating and recording procedures and electronic instrumentation are often used to trace out the anatomy of the nervous system. The procedure typically involves the activation of one portion of the nervous system with some stimulus and the probing for electrical responses in other locations. The stimulation may be accomplished in a number of ways. Adequate stimuli may be applied to the normal receptor channels; electrical stimuli may be used to activate almost any region of the nervous system; or chemicals such as strychnine may be applied to a portion of the brain. A relatively large electrode may then be used to determine the regions of the brain or spinal cord that are activated by the stimulus.

One of the major problems with this technique is that the number of remote regions that may be activated by any stimulus may be very large due to abundant interconnectivity. In the cat, for example, it seems as if stimulating any one part of the brain activates a large number of other regions of the brain. For this reason, the most powerful application of this evoked potential technique has been to the analysis of sensory systems that are sufficiently simple so that afferent conduction can be very well traced. Much of what we know of sensory localization in the cortex has come about through this sort of approach.

C. Degeneration Techniques

We mentioned earlier that if an axon is disconnected from its cell body, the axon will die. This is due to the fact that the metabolically important structures of a cell are located in the cell body; peripheral structures, like axons,

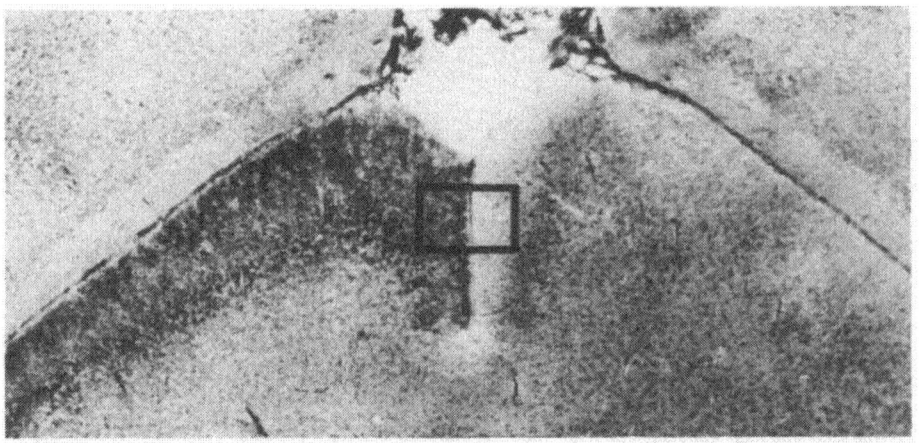

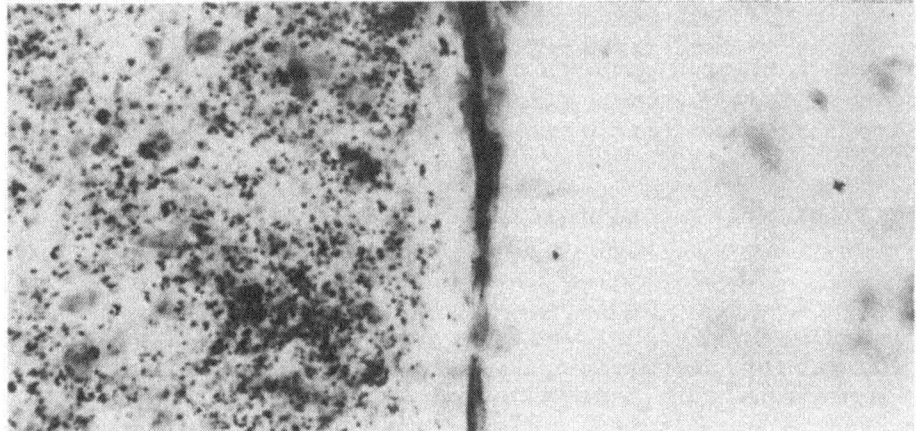

FIGURE 3.6 Micrograph of a degenerating tract in the superior colliculus of a hamster. This degeneration was produced by removing the controlateral eye of the animal a week prior to the time it was sacrificed and the histological sample taken. The evidence of degeneration is the accumulation of the dense granular material, a phenomenon which is shown in more detail in the more highly magnified lower photograph. (A photograph of a sample collected by Dr. G. Schneider, reproduced with the courtesy of Dr. L. Heimer, 1970.)

cannot survive alone. This fact has been used as a useful adjunct to the stimulation and recording and microanatomic techniques to trace sensory pathways. If a cut is made between the originating cell bodies and the axons of a major pathway, there will appear, over the next few days and weeks, a neurological lesion along the entire pathway, ending only at the next synaptic junction. The degeneration of the myelin sheath is the microscopically observable result of axonal degeneration. In some of the ascending pathways of the spinal cord that are quite long, this provides an exact means of mapping the course of the tract. Figure 3.6 shows a prepared slice of the superior colliculus of a hamster showing the granulated appearance of a sharply circumscribed degenerated region produced by removing the contralateral eye.

Axonal degeneration of this sort is known as prograde degeneration. Degeneration of a cell body can also occur when the axon is cut loose. This is known as retrograde degeneration and is exhibited as a systematic change in the intracellular structure of the cell body or perikaryon. In the peripheral nervous system, retrograde degeneration is often reversible, and the perikaryon may return to normal after regeneration of the axon. In the primate central nervous system, however, the process is not reversible, and once the axon is disconnected, the entire cell usually dies.

Transynaptic degeneration has also been reported, adding a further complication to some of the obvious difficulties encountered when one depends too much upon degeneration techniques as a source of anatomical information.

These, then, are some of the basic techniques that are used to trace out the functional anatomy of the nervous system. Before we consider the current state of our knowledge of the specific anatomy of the individual sensory pathways, we must digress to a discussion of the general organization of the central nervous system.

IV. THE GROSS STRUCTURE OF THE CENTRAL NERVOUS SYSTEM

Later in this chapter, when we discuss the anatomy of the various sensory channels, we shall refer to various relay stations or nuclei along the ascending pathways where, for example, synaptic associations between sequential neurons may occur. In many previous instances in which this sort of material was presented, the discussions were sometimes obscured by the fact that no accompanying presentation was made of the general gross anatomy of the central nervous system. In this section, we shall present a brief gross anatomy of the central nervous system, introducing the various centers in a way which, it is hoped, will make the subsequential detailed discussion of the ascending tracts more intelligible.

The central nervous system is made up of three main portions: the brain, the spinal cord, and the retinae. The retinae are associated for embryological reasons with the other two portions, but will be considered separately in our discussion of receptor anatomy. In this section, we shall concentrate only on the brain and spinal cord. Figure 3.7 is a drawing of the central nervous system as it would appear after an initial gross dissection. Because of the evolutionary growth of the cerebral hemispheres in particular, this drawing obscures the overall structure and important relationships among many of the various parts that are going to be referred to later.

When the brain and spinal cord are dissected and observed without any special preparation, there is little to indicate the rich and orderly array of pathways that convey sensory information from the periphery to the highest portions of the brain or among the constituent parts of the brain. Some regions of the central nervous system are particularly rich in myelin sheaths and display a whitish cast. These regions are predominantly

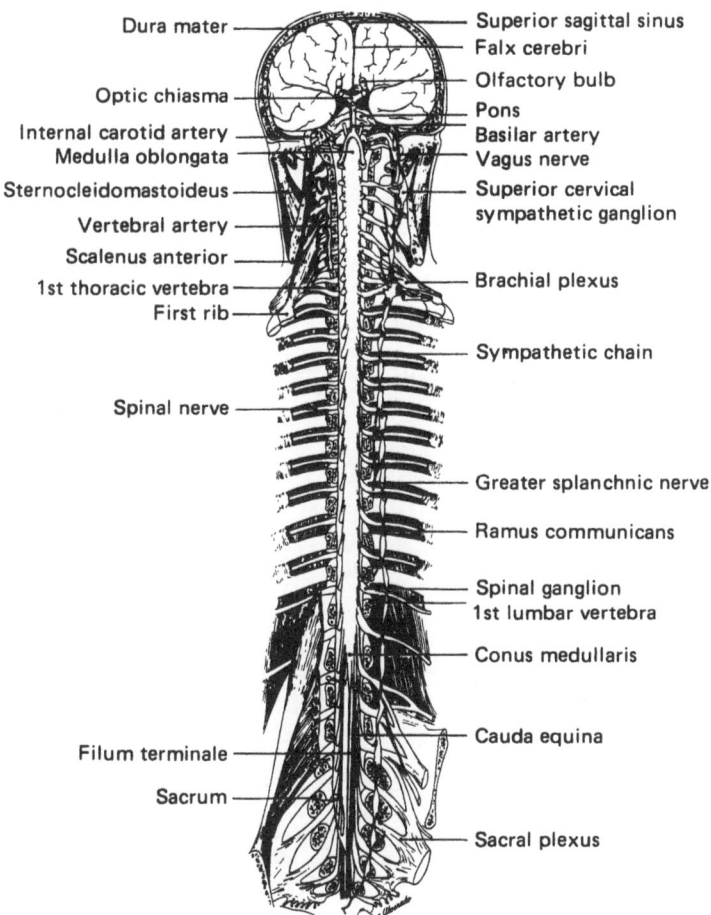

Dura mater — Superior sagittal sinus
Falx cerebri
Optic chiasma — Olfactory bulb
Pons
Internal carotid artery — Basilar artery
Medulla oblongata — Vagus nerve
Sternocleidomastoideus — Superior cervical sympathetic ganglion
Vertebral artery —
Scalenus anterior —
1st thoracic vertebra — Brachial plexus
First rib —
Sympathetic chain
Spinal nerve —
Greater splanchnic nerve
Ramus communicans
Spinal ganglion
1st lumbar vertebra
Conus medullaris
Cauda equina
Filum terminale —
Sacrum —
Sacral plexus

FIGURE 3.7 Drawing of the central nervous system as it would appear in a gross dissection approached from the back (from Goss, 1973, after Hirschfeld and Leveille).

axonal bundles and thus mainly serve the function of transmitting information from one portion of the brain to another. Other regions are pinkish grey and are made up mostly of neuronal cell bodies and other unmyelinated processes. But the boundaries between these two regions are often not obvious in the gross dissection. Yet when one looks at a chart of a slice of the central nervous system in a conventional anatomy text, a complex pattern of ganglia and tracts is usually seen. To emphasize this difference, we have presented in Figure 3.8 both an unretouched photograph of a lightly stained slice of the rat's brain and a more detailed stereotaxic grid and anatomy indicating some of the many known centers involved in the same region.

The discrepancy, between the two parts of the figure of course, is due

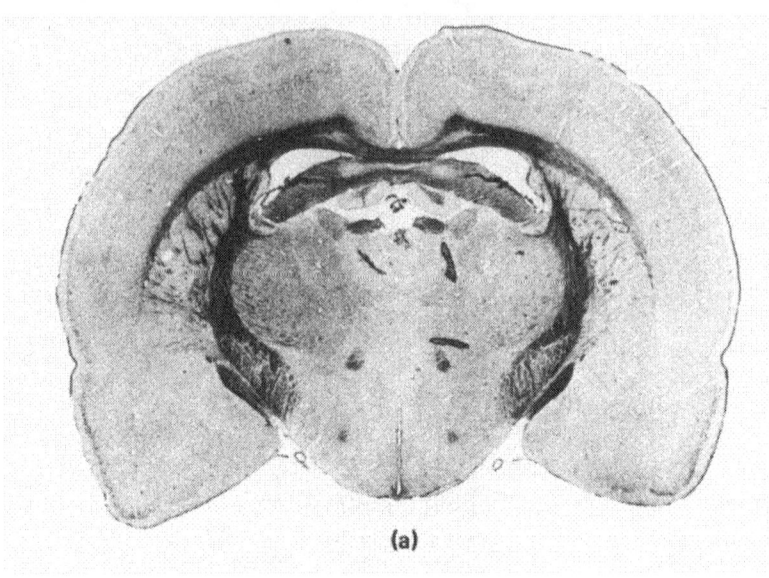

(a)

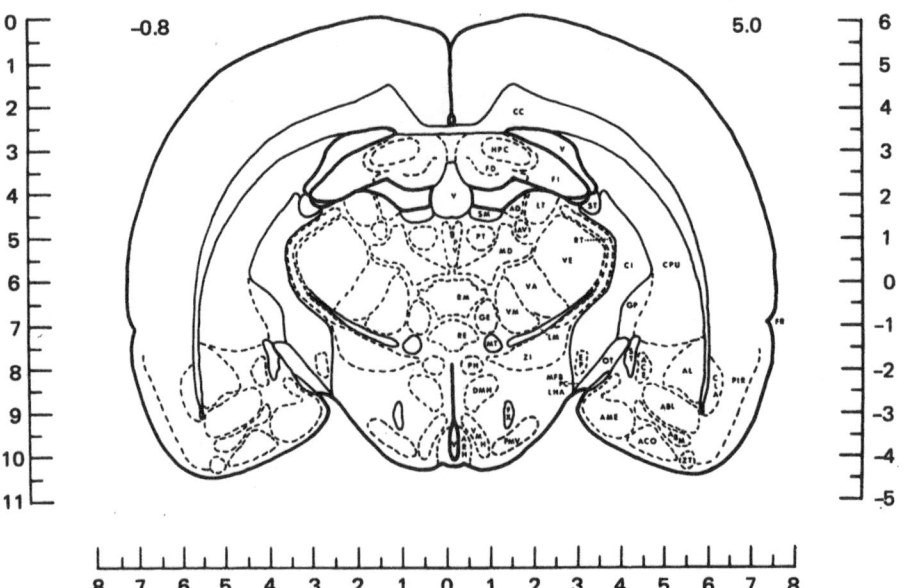

FIGURE 3.8 Photograph (a) showing the appearance of a lightly stained section of the brain of a rat and a stereotaxic map (b) with abbreviations of some of the many known centers and nuclei of the same section. Since most of these centers and nuclei cannot be seen in the original photograph, it is clear that they have had to be tediously traced by degeneration, evoked potential, and other anatomic locating procedures (from Pellegrino and Cushman, 1967).

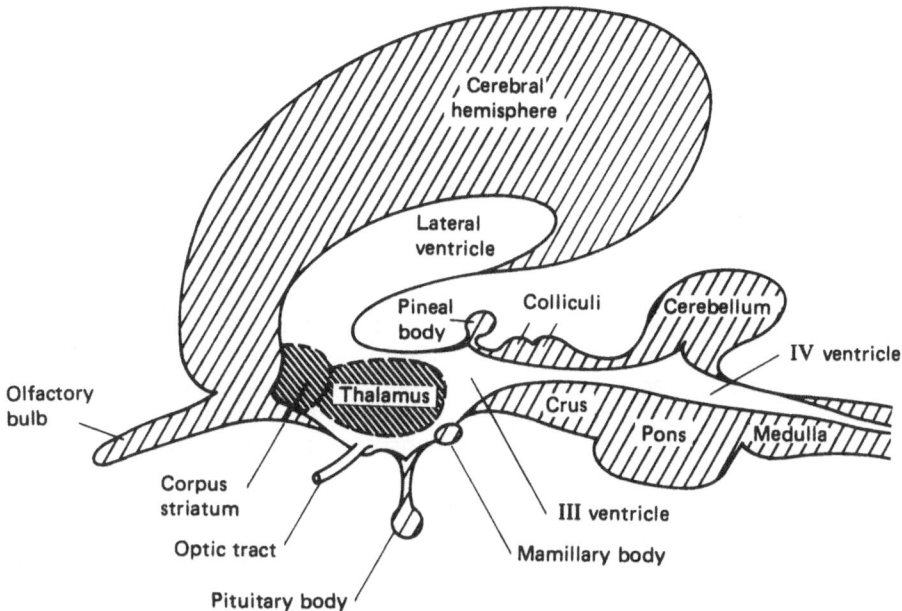

FIGURE 3.9 Diagrammatic sketch that maintains the topological relation of the central nervous system, but distorts the actual physical dimensions. The central nervous system is seen to be organized as a tube with various hypertrophied centers (from Morgan and Stellar, 1950, after Lickley, 1919).

to the enormous amount of work that has been done to plot the structure of the central nervous system by anatomists using some of the techniques described above.

Another useful pictorial display of the central nervous system is shown in Figure 3.9. In this figure, a plan proposed and first used by Lickley (1919) and later adapted by Morgan and Stellar (1950), the topological relationships of the central nervous system have been maintained, but in so doing the actual physical dimensions have been distorted to emphasize the tubelike structure and the relatively linear order in which the various major centers are organized.

The original neural tube, the primitive and simple precursor of the nervous system seen in the first few weeks of embryological development, has had an extraordinary growth by the time a vertebrate is an adult. The structure has swollen at several places and is, in the adult animal, represented by a series of major relay and integrative centers at various levels along the course of the brain or spinal cord. The grandest development from the original neural tube is certainly the great cerebral hemispheres, which now physically overlay almost all portions of the rest of the brain, completely hiding some of the lower centers. Not only do the cerebral hemispheres physically overshadow the lower centers, but it is, of course, also thought that it is in these giant cerebral ganglia that the mechanisms underlying the highest accomplishment of organic evolution—cognitive behavior—reside.

Neural connections between the hemispheres are conveyed through the cerebral commissures—the anterior and posterior commissures and the corpus callosum. Signals into the hemispheres come via a variety of ganglia and tracts conveying information upward mainly from the thalamus and the ascending reticular formation. The thalamus is the great sensory relay station of the brain, passing messages from the lower centers to the cortex. Below these more anterior portions of the brain, a region which is often collectively referred to as the forebrain (composed mainly of the cerebral hemispheres, the thalamus, and the hypothalamus), lies the anterior portion of the brain stem, which is also known as the midbrain. The midbrain is primarily made up of a series of relay stations for both ascending sensory and descending motor information. On the dorsal (or back side) of the human midbrain lie the two pairs of inferior and superior colliculi, which together make up a general region known as the tectum or roof. The colliculi are especially important relay stations for sensory information, and we shall find many synapses here of especial importance to the auditory and visual pathways. Ventral to these structures, or on the front of the human midbrain, lies the crus, a region through which many sensory and motor tracts pass up and down the central nervous system.

In the hindbrain, the pons contains a number of important nuclei and also has many important tracts passing through it without synapsing. The cerebellum of the hindbrain is primarily a center for motor control, and while it does receive some sensory information, notably from the proprioceptive and vestibular receptors, we shall not give it any extensive coverage in this book. The medulla, on the other hand, is richly endowed with a wide variety of sensory ganglia and tracts and will appear as one of the important relay stations in many of the discussions of the ascending pathways. The spinal cord is mainly a collection of giant tracts, but some cell bodies and synaptic connections, of which we shall speak in detail later, are also present there.

Table 3.1 summarizes the anatomy of the central nervous system as discussed in the preceding paragraphs. It also does two other things. This table introduces certain additional terminology used to describe the various structures and also acts as a locator for certain of the major centers of interest in our later discussions. I am glad to acknowledge that Table 3.1, and much of this present discussion, are based upon the presentation in Morgan and Stellar's (1950) textbook on physiological psychology.

Another major feature of the central nervous system is the complex net of nerves that enter and leave it. Neuroanatomists distinguish two different classes of these nerves—the spinal nerves and the cranial nerves—depending upon where the nerves enter or leave the nervous system. Table 3.2 lists the various cranial nerves, many of which are mainly sensory. The main distinction of importance to our present discussion is that the spinal nerves, unlike the cranial nerves, travel at least a portion of their course in the spinal cord, and all are related to bodily sensory or motor functions. Depending upon the level of their entry into the spinal cord, the spinal nerves are classified as cervical, thoracic, lumbar, sacral or coccygeal.

We now should have a general notion of the organization of the central nervous system, including the sequence of centers and tracts to be

TABLE 3.1 THE VARIOUS NULCEI AND CENTERS OF THE CENTRAL NERVOUS SYSTEM

			MAJOR CENTERS	FURTHER SUBDIVISIONS OF SENSORY IMPORTANCE
The Brain	Forebrain	Telencephalon	Cerebral Hemisphere	Sensory Regions of Cerebral Cortex Association Regions of Cerebral Cortex
			Olfactory bulb Corpus straitum Basal ganglion	
		Diencephalon	Thalamus Optic tract and retina Hypothalamus	Lateral geniculate body Lateral nucleus Medial geniculate body Hypothalamus Arcuate nucleus Ventrolateral nucleus
	Midbrain	Mesencephalon	Superior colliculus* Inferior colliculus* Crus (the floor)*	Red nucleus Substantia nigra Mesencephalic nucleus Basis pedunculi Oculomotor nucleus Trochlear nucleus
	Hindbrain	Metencephalon	Cerebellum Pons*	Trigeminal nerve nucleus Parabrachial nucleus
		Myelencephalon	Medulla*	Gracile nucleus Cuneate nucleus Dorsal, ventral, and cochlear nuclei Solitary nucleus Superior, medial, and lateral vestibular nuclei Superior olive Inferior olive Trapezoid body
The Spinal Cord				

(Reticular Formation — spanning vertically through Mesencephalon and Metencephalon/Myelencephalon rows, marked with arrow)

TABLE 3.2 THE CRANIAL NERVES (ADAPTED FROM THOMPSON, 1967)

Number	Name	Functions
I	Olfactory	Smell
II	Optic	Vision
III	Oculomotor	Eye movement
IV	Trochlear	Eye movement
V	Trigeminal	Masticatory movements Sensitivity of face and tongue
VI	Abducens	Eye movement
VII	Facial	Facial movement
VIII	Auditory vestibular	Hearing Balance
IX	Glossopharyngeal	Tongue and pharynx
X	Vagus	Heart, blood vessels, viscera
XI	Spinal accessory	Neck muscles and viscera
XII	Hypoglossal	Tongue muscles

found. Once again, we repeat that while our emphasis will be heavily on the communication properties of the brain, most of the centers to be described have other functions besides. The thalamus, for example, which has been referred to as the great sensory transmission center, contains several different nuclei, which do not directly receive afferents from the sensory pathways. The distinction that we make here is slightly artificial, because even the process of integration, for example, is based upon the communication of information from place to place. Nevertheless, we feel it is necessary in the context of modern neurophysiology to separate out those processes that represent stages in the transmission of information from the peripheral receptors to the cerebral cortices, from purely internal communication links.

The sensory tracts through the brain and spinal cord, which we shall discuss, are the most direct access routes to the specific upper portions of the brain associated with each of the senses. We must also take note of an additional common pathway through the *reticular system*, which also plays an important role in sensory functions.

The reticular system has been known anatomically for many years, but only recently has been shown to have important functional properties associated with arousal and wakefulness (Moruzzi and Magoun, 1949). It is a central tube of poorly defined anatomy lying within the direct ascending pathways, which we shall discuss in detail in the following section. Anatomically it has been described as an almost structureless "reticulum" of cells with relatively short fibers and lacking the linear ordering of the usual afferent pathways. In addition to the specific sensory nerve tracts that pass to the sensory cortical areas, there are collateral sensory inputs from all of the sense organs to the reticular formation which have been physiologically, if not structurally, defined. The reticular formation has, as its output, a general and nonspecific pattern of signals, which are conveyed almost universally to almost all parts of the forebrain. These nonspecific outputs can produce a state of activation or excitement in these cortical regions, which many researchers believe may correspond in some way to the psychological states of attention, awareness, and consciousness. The many complex properties and functions of the reticular system are fully discussed in another volume of this series (Thompson, 1967).

This then completes our discussion of the preliminary anatomic material. We shall now consider the specific material of importance to an understanding of the anatomy of sensory receptors and the ascending sensory pathways.

V. THE VISUAL SYSTEM

A. The Anatomy of the Visual Receptor

From some points of view, the paired photoreceptors of the vertebrate visual system may be considered to represent the highest evolutionary development of any sensory system. Certainly if one used some arbitrary comparative measure of, say, the possible amount of information transmitted, the visual system would stand at the top of the list. Yet, in some curious way, people are often able to cope with blindness more easily than loss of some of the other less rich senses. Total deafness, for example, cuts one off from human communication in ways that some would consider even more profound than blindness. Loss of the proprioceptive system, which has a very low information-processing rate, on the other hand, is probably lethal, as is a total loss in cutaneous sensitivity. The point is—it is not always possible to use information-processing capacity as the single measure of sensory importance; rather, the adaptive utility of a sensory system may be more important to the organism in ways that go beyond richness of information flow.

Our plan for this chapter, as noted above, is to go from the macroscopic to the increasingly microscopic for each sense organ. Therefore, let us first consider the structure of the eye as it might be observed by another naked eye or with a low-power hand magnifying glass. Figure 3.10 is a cross section of the eye observed from the top. The most anterior portion of the eye is the transparent cornea, the interface between the external and internal worlds. The cornea performs a passive information-transmission function in addition to the protective and supportive functions it shares with the two other layers of the eye, the sclera and the choroid. Behind the cornea lies the anterior chamber of the eye filled with a clear watery fluid known as the aqueous humor. Behind this anterior fluid-filled

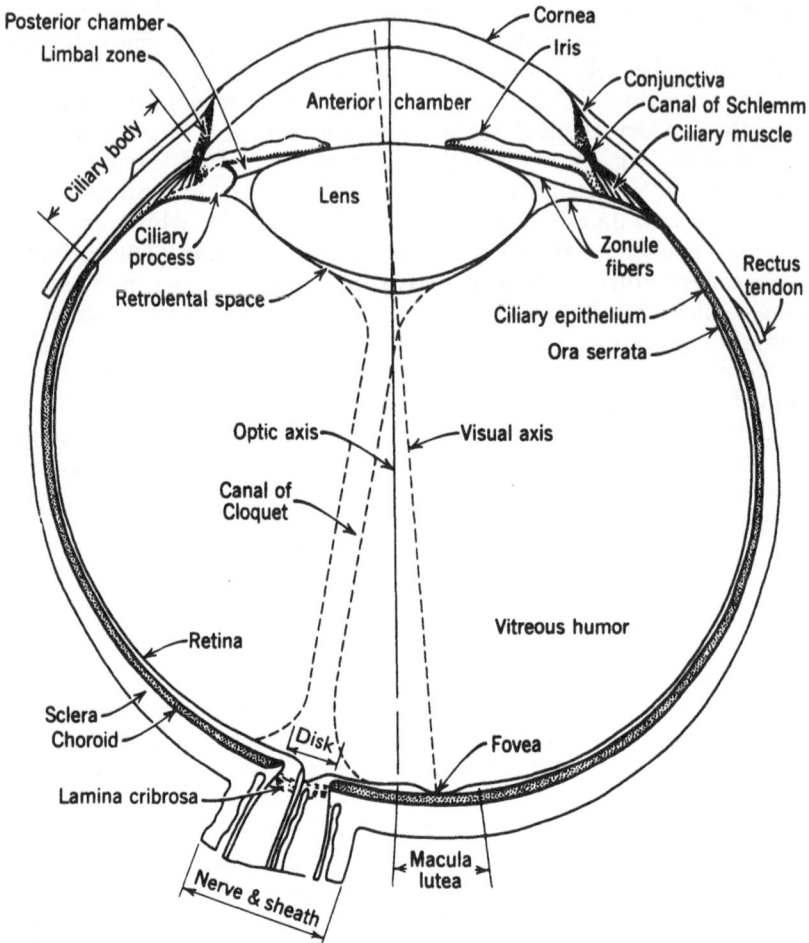

FIGURE 3.10. A cross section of the eye from the top, showing many of the important structures involved in the visual process. See text for full details (from Brown, 1965, after Walls, 1942, as modified from Salzmann, 1912).

chamber lie two mechanically active units of extraordinary capability—the iris and the crystalline lens.

The iris, colored by the deposition of various pigments, is a diaphragm composed of two counteracting muscular bands, the sphincter and the dilator. The sphincter is an anterior layer composed of muscle fibers running parallel to the perimeter of the circular iris. It is capable, upon contraction, of reducing the diameter of the pupil—the aperture in the iris—to less than 25 percent of its relaxed dimensions. The dilator, on the other hand, is composed of radial muscle fibers which, when contracted, tend to pull the pupil to its maximum opening.

Pupil diameter is a function of many different variables. The amount of incident light can directly affect pupillary diameter, but the internal emotional state of the animal can also have dramatic effects. Hess (1965), for example, has shown that the "attractiveness" of a male or female portrait correlates highly with pupil dilation. Kahneman and Beatty (1966) have also shown that such intellectual activities as mental arithmetic affect the pupil diameter. It is not too surprising then to realize that the muscles of the iris are smooth muscles controlled involuntarily by the autonomic nervous system. Dilation is stimulated by sympathetic signals, and the constrictor action of the sphincter muscle by parasympathetic nerve action.

The action of the iris, like any other mechanical diaphragm in an optical system, reduces the amount of light entering the eye. However, pupil area can vary only over a range of about 16 times the minimum size. Other neural and photochemical factors must be invoked to explain the full range of light level adaptation. Reducing the size of the pupil, furthermore, can also increase the depth of field of clear vision and the overall sharpness of the retinal image by cutting off the rays coming from the periphery. These peripheral, oblique rays contribute more to the spherical, cylindrical, and astigmatic aberrations of the visual image than the central direct rays. Their absence, therefore, greatly decreases the amount of blur, and in a crisis situation, this may be a truly useful advantage for an animal.

Another mechanically active tissue behind the anterior chamber is the crystalline lens. Its actions are equally as remarkable as those of the pupil, but are mainly associated with retinal focussing rather than the control of stimulus intensity. The lens, as it necessarily must be, is also a transparent object in the normal eye and is made up of a series of lamina very much like those of an onion. The lens is suspended by a series of "zonule" fibers from another muscular ring, the ciliary muscle, which lies just under the sclera below and to the outside of the iris. The action of this ciliary muscle is to automatically adjust the shape of the lens to provide the appropriate focusing action for objects at differing objective distances. The lens must be flattened to provide increased focal length for objects that are far away. This is achieved by a relaxation of the ciliary muscle, producing an increased tautness of the zonule fibers overcoming the natural elasticity of the lens and thus flattening its shape. For near objects, the focal length of the lens must be shortened by making the lens less flat. This is achieved when the ciliary muscle contracts with a resulting decrease in the strain on the zonule fibers. Then the lens' natural elasticity tends to make it more spherical.

The ciliary muscle is, like the iris, also a smooth muscle controlled by the autonomic nervous system. Accommodation is, therefore, not under voluntary control. Rather, information about the degree of retinal blur is conducted from the central nervous systems to the autonomic nervous efferents and then to the muscles that control the lens' shape. The exact nature of this communication link is not fully known.

Behind the lens lies the great posterior cavity of the eye, which is filled with the gelatinous vitreous humor. The canal of Cloquet, the dim structure shown running through the posterior chamber from the lens to the retina in Figure 3.10, is a vestige of the pathway of the hyaloid artery, which actually connects the lens to the blood supply during the embryonic development of the eye. It degenerates during childhood.

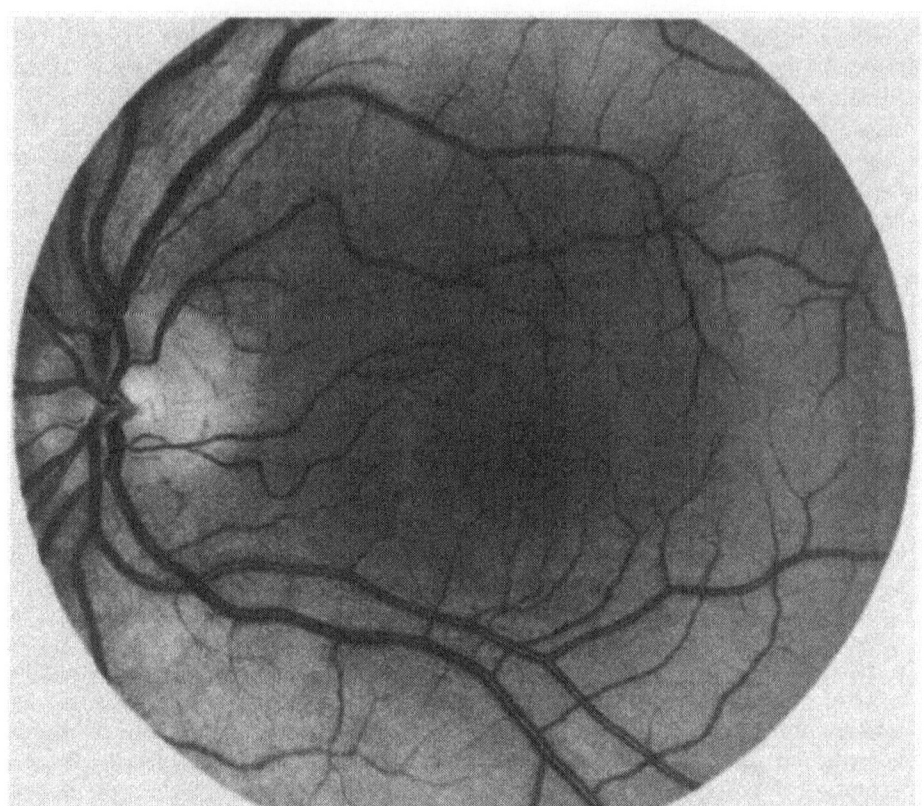

FIGURE 3.11 *A photograph of the fundus of a human eye as it might be seen through an ophthalmoscope. The fovea is at the center of the macula—the dark area at the center of the picture (courtesy of Mr. C. L. Martonyi of the University of Michigan).*

Other gross features are also visible without magnification to an observer when he views the retina through an opthalmoscope. One of these features, which can be seen in Figure 3.11, is the optic disk or, as it is better known, the "blind spot." It is in this region that the retinal blood vessels and the optic nerve both enter or leave the eye through a region in which there are no photoreceptors present. Another easily seen feature is the tiny bright spot, which indicates the position of the fovea. The fovea is a highly specialized region of the retina, mediating the most spatially and chromatically acute visual processes due mainly to the fact that it is here that the maximal density of cones occur. It is also interesting to note that the arborization of the blood vessels can actually be observed in one's own eye by shining a small light into its corner in a darkened room.

Most important of all ocular structures and the *raison d'être* for the presence of all of the other accessory structures is the retina. This tissue, visible only as a slight discoloration at the gross level at which we are

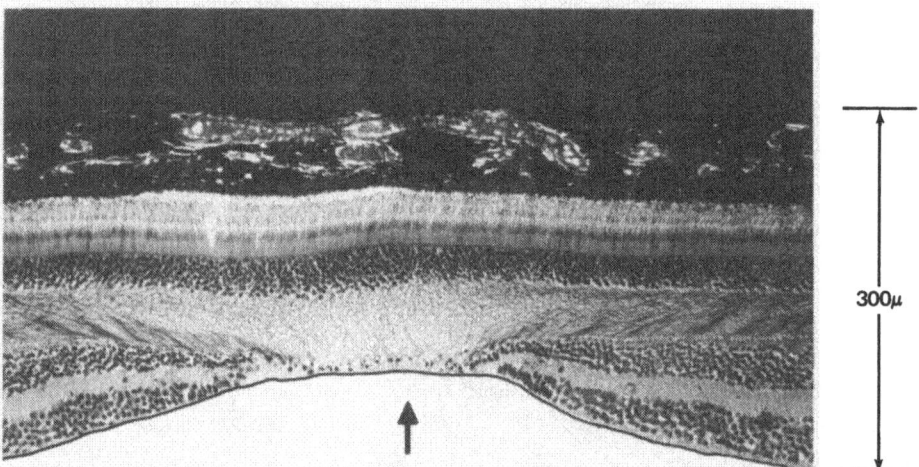

FIGURE 3.12 A photograph of a cross section of the monkey retina at the fovea. The arrow indicates the direction from which light enters the eye (× 40) (courtesy of Dr. M. Glickstein of Brown University).

examining the eye, contains the critically important receptor cells and the neural plexus, which mediate the transductive and initial neural processes of vision. To appreciate the structure and the significance of this astonishing receptor tissue, we must take our first step down into the microscopic world. Our guide in this exploration initially will be the two volumes that sum up the monumental work of Steven Polyak (1941 and 1957). Polyak dedicated his entire life to the study of the optical micrography of the primate retina, and recent progress had added little to the story he told until the application of the electron microscope to the problem of retinal anatomy.

Figure 3.12 is a microscopic cross section of the human retina taken from a region near the fovea. First, the reader should consider the thickness of this tissue. The retina is exceedingly delicate, varying in thickness from 125 μ at the fovea to about 300 μ at the periphery, and this of course includes ten distinguishable structural layers. Even more surprising than the delicacy of the tissue, however, is the fact that the retina seems to be inverted. The broad arrow in this figure shows the direction of light coming in from the outer world after having passed through the ocular media. Before the light arrives at the photoreceptors themselves, it must traverse the entire thickness of the other neural and supporting cell layers of the retina. The absorption of visible light by these initial layers is relatively slight, fortunately, for they are nearly all completely transparent. Nevertheless, it is measureable and, therefore, it is especially important that the absorption spectrum of this tissue, as well as that of the lens and vitreous, be understood and corrected for in any calculations that attempt to distinguish absorption spectra of the retinal receptors from that of the whole eye.

Looking at Figure 3.12 once again, we see that there are three main

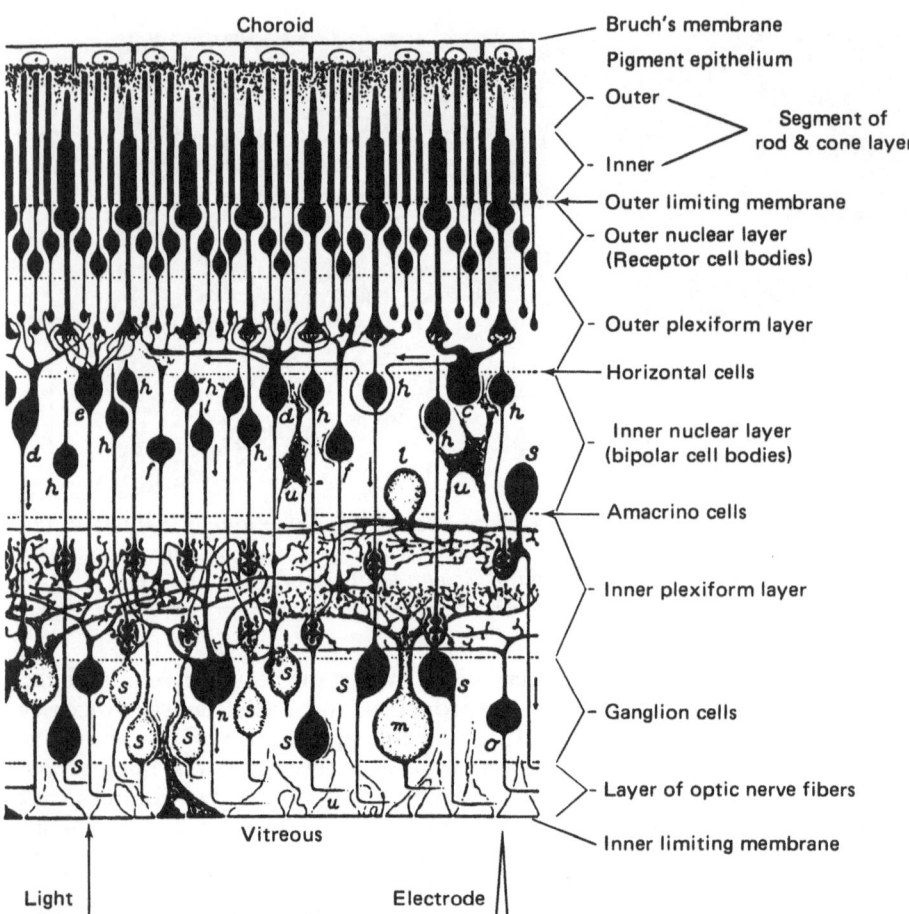

Choroid — Bruch's membrane

Pigment epithelium

Outer — ⎫ Segment of
Inner — ⎭ rod & cone layer

Outer limiting membrane

Outer nuclear layer
(Receptor cell bodies)

Outer plexiform layer

Horizontal cells

Inner nuclear layer
(bipolar cell bodies)

Amacrine cells

Inner plexiform layer

Ganglion cells

Layer of optic nerve fibers

Vitreous   Inner limiting membrane

Light   Electrode

FIGURE 3.13 Diagrammatic rendition of a cross section of the retina at a region
that has both rods and cones present. The normal direction of incident light and
of an electrode penetration are shown. (This diagram, from Ruch and Patton
[1965] has been modified from an earlier drawing by Polyak [1941] and is used
through the courtesy of Mrs. Stephen Polyak.)

cellular layers in the vertebrate retina. The initial layer, defined functionally
in terms of the photic action, if not anatomically, is the photoreceptor layer.
The second layer is composed of short bipolar cells which convey information from the receptors to the third layer, the ganglion cells, whose
axons make up the optic nerve and pass without a synapse to the thalamus.
Figure 3.13 is a much more diagrammatic sketch, from Ruch's (1965) modification of a Polyak drawing, which defines the 10 different regions of the
retina to which we have referred. This division is based upon the cellular
anatomy and also indicates some other structures we have not described
in any detail. In addition, both of these figures show the presence of various kinds of horizontally connecting cells.

The photoreceptor layer in all vertebrate eyes is made up of one or both of two highly specialized types of neurons. On the basis of their shape, these cells have been distinguished and named rods and cones. However, it is clear from surveying the anatomical literature that this dichotomy refers to what is actually a continuously graded series of cells of varying shape. There are both rodlike cones and conelike rods to be found in the primate retina. Nevertheless, the two groups also differ in their function, and the duplicity theory of retinal function is one of the basic tenets of retinal psychophysiology.

The rods and cones themselves have only minimum axons, if their terminal axonal brushes can be dignified at all with that nomenclature. They synapse almost immediately with the layer of bipolar cells and other horizontally interconnecting cells.

Horizontal cells are found in the second layer of the retina and interconnect among rods and cones, often synapsing at several different points in a horizontal plane. Amacrine cells are also horizontally conducting units, but interconnect at the level of the junction of the bipolar and ganglion cells.

This, briefly, was the anatomical story as it was known up to about the early 1950s. In the last 10 or 20 years, the electron microscope has begun to contribute much more to our knowledge. This is particularly so in regard to the ultramicroanatomy of the rods and cones and the synaptic interconnections in the retina.

Our current knowledge of the anatomy of the rods and cones has been summarized in some recent contributions of Young (1967, 1969). He describes not only what appears to be a major anatomical distinction between rods and cones, but also presents a description of how these delicate photoreceptive cells repair themselves after damage. Figure 3.14 shows the structure of a typical rod and cone from the retina of a frog. The obvious difference in the shape of the outer segment is the primary feature, which had led to the original dichotomy of retinal receptors into these two categories; however, it can also be seen that there are a number of other differences between the two types of cell. Most notably, the outer segment of the rod is considerably longer. There is also an oil droplet typically found in the frog cone's inner segment, which may also have some optical properties associated with color vision.

A major structural aspect in Young's drawing is the fact that the outer segments of both the rod and the cone are connected to the rest of the cell by a very thin stalk. The presence of this stalk was first reported by De Robertis (1956). It is presumably through this connecting cilium that the metabolic necessities and newly formed protein must be transported. An important related fact is illustrated in Figure 3.15. While the outer segments of both rods and cones had long been known to be composed of flat lamella or disks, Young's electron-micrographic studies showed that there was a major difference in the construction of the rod's disks as compared to those of the cone. The disks in the rod are free-floating toward the terminal end of the outer segment, and their outer membranes are apparently quite separate from the outer cell membrane. Near the base of the rod's outer segment, however, the outer membrane of the disk is

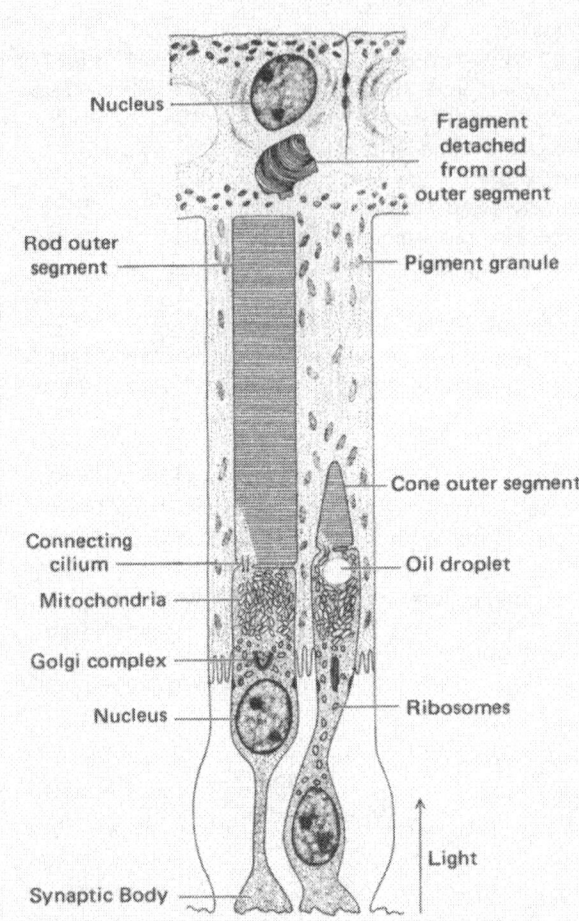

Nucleus

Fragment
detached
from rod
outer segment

Rod outer
segment

Pigment granule

Cone outer segment

Connecting
cilium

Oil droplet

Mitochondria

Golgi complex

Ribosomes

Nucleus

Light

Synaptic Body

*FIGURE 3.14 Drawing of a
single rod and a single cone
from a frog, showing the
characteristic difference in
shape. This figure also shows
the connecting cilium, a feature not visible until electronmicrographs were taken of
this cell (from Young, 1970).*

apparently continuous with the outer membrane of the cell. The arrangement of the membrane of the disks in the cone, however, is solely like that
of the rod disks near the base; the outer membrane of the cone disks always retains physical continuity with the membrane of the outer cell wall.

Careful further microscopic examination of the region beyond rod
outer segments showed debris, which was apparently made up of fragments of cast-off, free-floating rod disks. Radiographic tracer techniques,
which tracked the course of newly formed rod disks, also showed that
new protein was first incorporated into disks near the bottom of the outer
segment, and then this new disk gradually migrated to the end of the
outer segment, where it disappeared. The ultimate disappearance of the
labeled disk at the terminus of the outer segment was apparently associated
with its "casting off" at the end of its useful lifetime.

Such a renewal process in the rod is one way in which the outer
segments of photoreceptors can be maintained and rejuvenated over the
lifetime of the animal. Young found, however, that the cone, quite to the
contrary, does not incorporate new protein in the same way. In the cone,

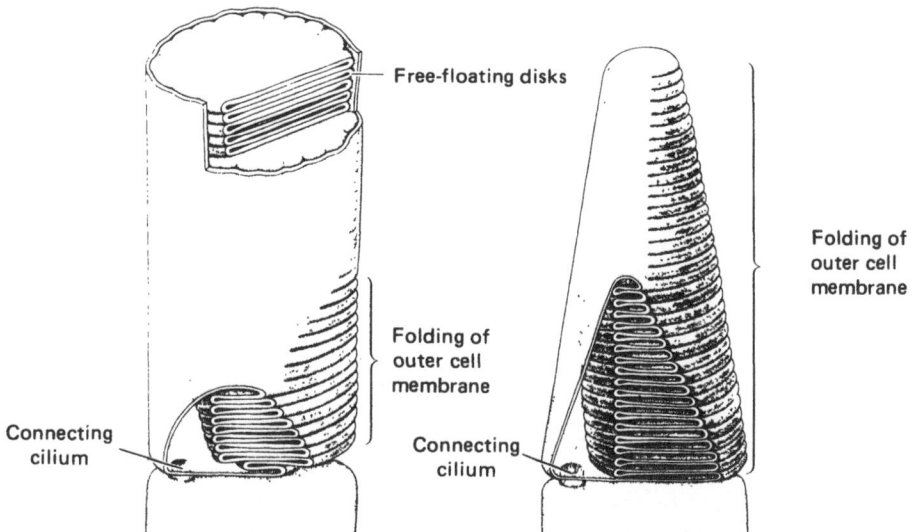

FIGURE 3.15 *Drawing of an even further magnification of the outer segments of a rod and of a cone. There is a characteristic difference between the two in the manner the disks are formed. In a rod the disks are formed from invaginations of the cell membrane, but gradually become detached from it as they migrate toward the terminal end. In the cone there is no such disk migration, and the disks remain fused to the outer cell membrane throughout the life of the cell (from Young, 1970).*

there is apparently no regeneration of disks and no migration. In fact, he believes that the cones are cone shaped primarily because the outermost segments were created early in the life of the animal and the more proximal larger ones later in its development. No further development of new disks occurs after the animal has matured. New protein is formed and introduced into the disk structure, but rather than being entirely incorporated into a newly generated disk, at the base of the cone outer segment, which then migrates outward, the new protein diffuses outward and is uniformly incorporated into all of the cone's permanent disks throughout the outer segment simultaneously.

Dowling and Werblin (1969) have taken advantage of the electron microscope and the very large cells of the retina of the mud puppy (Necturus) to demonstrate some of the details of the interconnections between the various cells. Figure 3.16 is one of their electron micrographs showing a number of important features. One of the most notable details is that there are several different kinds of synaptic contacts present on the receptors. Synapses may be invaginated, with protrusions of one cell actually extending into the body of another cell. The synapses may, on the other hand, only be superficial, merely "denting" the surface of the recipient cell.

Dowling and Werblin believe, on the basis of their anatomical studies, that rods often have to make synaptic contact with bipolar and horizontal cells, whose perikaryon lie in positions laterally displaced from the rod

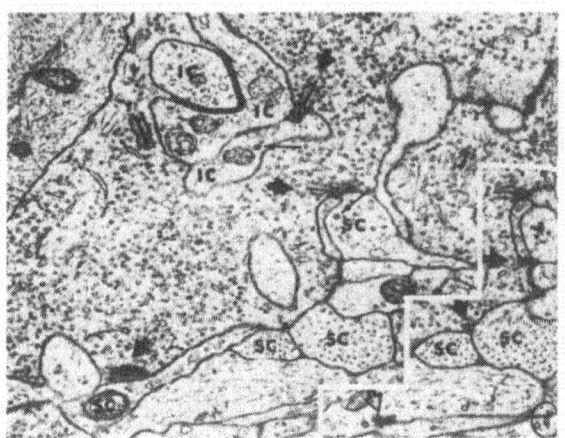

FIGURE 3.16 Electronmicrograph of the synaptic region at the bases of a cone of the mud puppy retina. Two different kinds of synapses have been observed. One makes only a superficial contact (SC), while the other makes contact within an invagination of the cell wall (IC). The arrows indicate synaptic vesicles in what may be a chemical synapse from a horizontal cell to a cone (from Dowling and Werblin, 1969).

itself. In fact, they believe that many rods terminate in the region under a cone, while the cone typically has its synapse directly beneath itself in this animal. The two types of ganglion cell, which are believed to occur in the mud puppy, differ in that one type is mainly connected to bipolar cells, while the other is mainly connected to Amacrine cells, which are themselves directly activated by bipolar conducted information.

Dowling and Boycott (1966) have also used electromicrographic techniques to study the primate retina, and their findings are of special interest in the context of this book. Their summary sketch is displayed in Figure 3.17. Some of the important features of this drawing are:

1. The primate rods and cones each have specifically shaped terminal arborizations.
2. The rods and cones in the primate retina connect to three differently shaped classes of bipolar cells. The rods connect only to "rod mop" bipolars, while the cones connect to either "midget" or "flat" bipolars.
3. Each synaptic invagination of a primate rod usually contains between four and seven synaptic filaments, while each synaptic invagination into a cone contains no more than three filaments.
4. The horizontal connections at the base of the primate receptors (mediated by the horizontal cells) are far less complex than those at the bases of bipolars (mediated by Amacrine cells). Presumably this could allow substantially greater integrative information processing in the latter than in the former.

B. The Ascending Visual Pathway

Figure 3.18 is a diagrammatic presentation of the anatomy of the primary visual pathway. For all its awesome information-processing capacity, the ascending visual pathway is among the easiest of the sensory tracts to describe. We have already discussed the triple-layered retina with its two synaptic layers. Beyond the retina there are at least three different path-

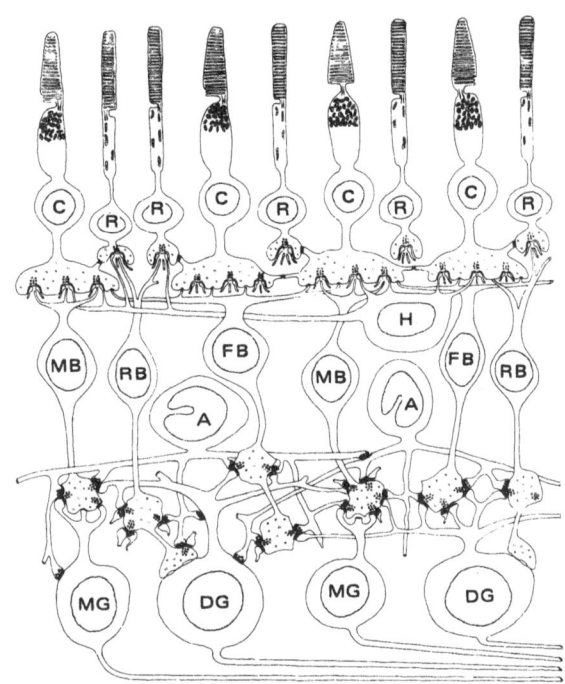

FIGURE 3.17 A schematic drawing showing the organization of the primate retina. Note particularly that Dowling and Werblin have distinguished among midget bipolars (MB), flat bipolars (FB), rod bipolars (RB), midget ganglion (MG), and diffuse ganglion (DG) cells. Note also the several different varieties of synaptic contact that are evident in this figure (from Dowling and Boycott, 1966).

ways through which signals can get to the cortex. The classical pathway is through the optic nerves and tracts to a single synaptic contact in the lateral geniculate bodies. From there, the signals project to at least three visual areas in the occipital cortex—the areas known as 17, 18, and 19. An additional pathway passes through the reticular system, which is thought to be associated with nonspecific activation of widely distributed portions of the cortex.

A third major pathway carrying relatively specific information to the cortex, although less well known, has recently received additional attention. Schneider (1969) and Travarthen (1968) have emphasized the importance of a pathway from the retina through the superior colliculus with somewhat different properties than those of the geniculate pathway. This collicular pathway is characterized by very large receptive fields and seems to be more involved in gross spatial localization than in fine form perception. Kaplan (1970) has suggested that it serves a number of functions, which are quite important and observable in human psychophysical processes such as walking or texture sensitivity.

Superficially, this is all that seems necessary to be said about the neuronal pathways of the visual system. However, there are a number of other extremely interesting points of anatomy, which are vital to our understanding of visual perception. For example, though the ganglion cell axons pass without synapse to the lateral geniculate body, there is a most important and significant sorting out of these axons at the optic chiasma, the junction point that separates the part of the visual pathway known as the

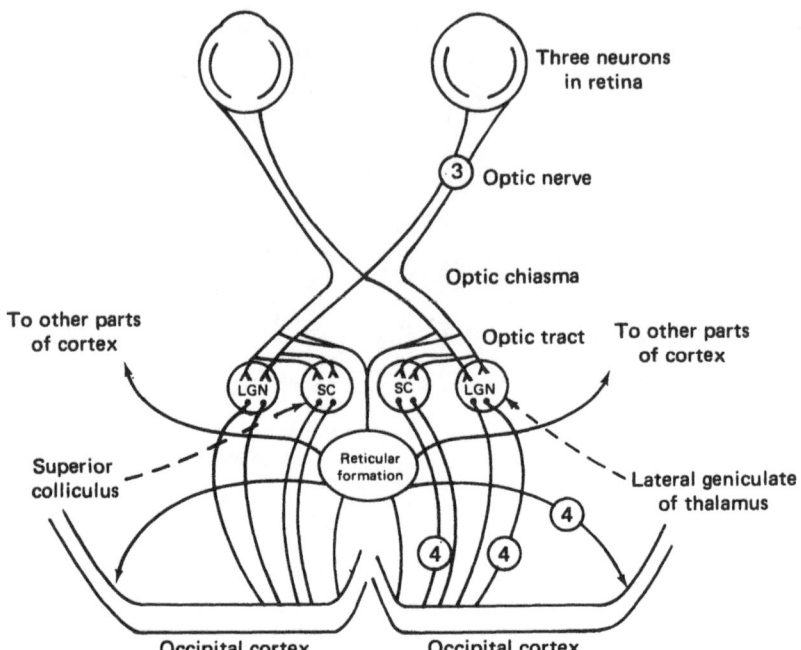

FIGURE 3.18. A schematic drawing of the entire ascending visual pathway. Small circled numbers indicate the order of the neuron in the chain from the receptor to the cortex.

optic nerve from that known as the optic tract. Each retina is functionally divided into two regions, which gather visual information from the left and right visual field respectively. In the right eye, the right field of view is mediated by the nasal hemiretina. In the left eye, the same right view is mediated by the temporal hemiretina. On the other hand, the left-hand view for the right eye is mediated by the temporal hemiretina and in the left eye by the nasal hemiretina. So many different perceptual phenomena are mediated by fusion of the corresponding images from the two left or the two right viewing hemiretina that it is not surprising to discover that the evolutionary forces operating have produced a system in which the necessary crossovers provide exactly this sort of image conjunction. As shown in Figure 3.18, ganglion cell axons from the left temporal and the right nasal hemiretina project to the left cerebral hemispheres, and ganglion cell axons from the right temporal and left nasal hemiretina project to the right cerebral hemisphere. Interhemispheric connection almost certainly exists through the corpus callosum, but such processes as steroscopic depth perception can presumably be handled from each field of view within a single hemisphere. As we shall see later, there is no known interaction between the two eyes at any level more peripheral than the geniculates of the thalamus.

As we have said, visual signals project primarily to the visual centers in the occipital lobe through the lateral (and perhaps also through the medial) geniculate bodies, as well as through the colliculi. In addition, it is probably also true that there are other cortical destinations of visual signals. Visual information is also capable of producing generalized brain activation by virtue of its connections to the nonspecific reticular system as noted above. Furthermore, there have been many reports indicating that many regions of association cortex contain "polysensory" cells, which can be activated by stimuli of several different modalities. Thus, vision, audition, and somatosensation may all be acceptable inputs to a single cell of this type.

VI. THE AUDITORY SYSTEM

A. The Anatomy of the Auditory Receptor

The visual system excels at making fine spatial discriminations. The auditory mechanism, on the other hand, has evolved into the system *par excellence* for the interpretation of very fine temporal patterns. However, a very curious and important fact is that the ears' ability to deal with temporal patterns is, in fact, also mediated by spatial encoding processes. Later in this book, we shall emphasize in greater detail that the sensory systems generally seem to operate in this manner; that is, they do well with spatial discriminations, but badly with temporal ones. In those instances in which fine temporal discriminations are made by a sensory system, one generally finds that such performance is achieved by converting temporal codes into spatial ones. To understand how such conversions can come about in the ear, we must understand the structure and the ultrastructure of the acoustic mechanism and, in particular, the anatomy of the elegantly organized array of receptor cells within the coiled cochlea.

Surprisingly, even many of the relatively macroscopic features of the anatomy of the auditory mechanism were not known until the last few hundred years. This is probably due to the fact that some of the most important parts of the auditory mechanism are embedded within the bony structure of the skull. Initial attempts at dissection often obliterated the delicate inner structures, which we now know are critical to auditory transduction. The massive destruction of bony tissue required to observe the middle and inner ear requires special care so that the delicate inner structures could be salvaged. It was not until the sixteenth century, therefore, that the three ossicles, the three tiny bones of the middle ear, were discovered, and the general spiral arrangement of the cochlea and the orthogonal arrangement of the tubes of the bony vestibular labyrinth described. Even then, however, no one understood the significance of the tiny droplets of water that emerged when the cochlea was opened. It was not until 200 years later that it was confirmed that the inner ear was entirely filled with fluid in its normal state. This discovery was the key fact in the development of the several theories of auditory quality coding, which were subsequently to emerge.

The major technological development, which was to so significantly affect knowledge of auditory anatomy, of course, was the invention of the

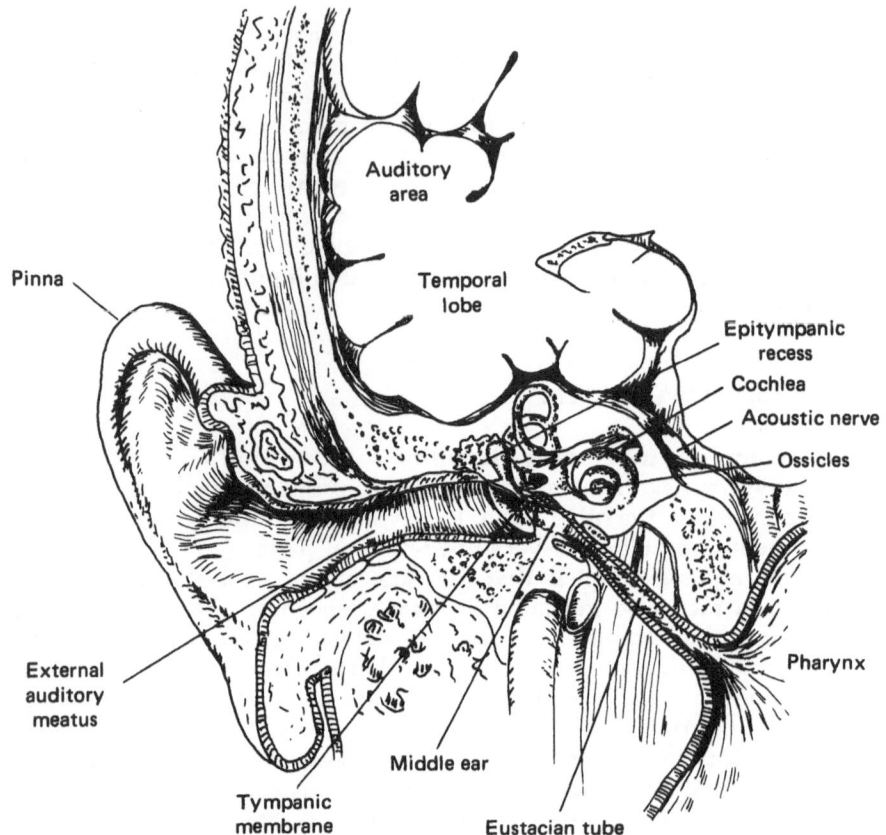

FIGURE 3.19 Gross anatomy of the auditory system showing the external, middle, and inner ears and the associated vestibular mechanism (courtesy of B. J. Melloni and Abbott Laboratories, N. Chicago, Illinois).

compound microscope by Jannsen in 1590. But it was not until the beginning of the nineteenth century that it was being regularly applied to auditory structure analysis, and those years were filled with one startling discovery after another concerning cochlear microanatomy. In 1851 Reissner discovered the delicate membrane now known by his name. That same year Corti made the extraordinary contributions to an understanding of the auditory receptor tissue itself. His findings resulted in his name being associated with several parts of the cochlear apparatus, as well as the inclusive term describing the actual sensitive tissue itself—the organ of Corti.

We shall consider the history of some of the theories of auditory pitch encoding that have appeared over the years in Chapter 10 of this book. But for the moment, let us turn our attention to some diagrams of the auditory apparatus that are currently accepted as examples of the anatomists' best work on the auditory system.

Figure 3.19 is a drawing of the gross anatomy of the human auditory mechanism as it might be seen with the unaided eye or with a hand magnifying glass. The pinna of man is a vestigial organ, no longer capable of any substantial amount of directional movement, but still serving effectively as a hearing horn. The pinna collects signals from a wide area and feeds them in a concentrated form into the external ear passage—the external auditory meatus. It also may aid in directional hearing by selectively attenuating signals coming from behind or from one side of the head. The eardrum or, as it is otherwise known, the tympanic membrane, separates the outer ear cavity from that of the air-filled middle ear. In the middle ear is found the chain of three tiny bones, the auditory ossicles, which convey mechanical perturbations from the tympanic membrane to the oval window. The ossicles not only transit the mechanical deformations of the tympanic membrane, but they also considerably amplify the forces applied to it. This occurs because the three ossicles are arranged as a series of levers. Thus, while the amplitude of motion is greatly reduced, the applied force can be proportionately increased. The reduction in acoustic signal amplitude, coupled with the exquisite nervous sensitivity of the auditory system, allows displacements of the oval window as small as one-tenth the diameter of a hydrogen atom to be detected in psychophysical experiments.

The air of the middle ear is continuous with that of the outside environment. This continuity is normally achieved through a most unusual pathway. If the tympanic membrane is not perforated, the continuity of the air in the middle ear with the outside air is solely through the eustachian tube, which connects the middle ear to the throat. The existence of this tube explains why swallowing can equalize or relieve the pressure in the ears and why sore throats sometimes lead to middle ear pain or, indeed, infection.

Both the external and the middle ear are nonneural processors and are capable only of modifying the amplitude of the mechanical action of the acoustic stimulus. There is no energy transduction in these outer regions. It is only in the fluid-filled inner ear that the actual neurologically active elements reside. The inner ear is made up of two regions, which are functionally quite distinct: one, the cochlear mechanism, transduces acoustic signals, whereas the other, the vestibular mechanism, is associated only with the sense of balance. However, the spiral cochlea can be seen in Figure 3.19 to be continuous with the vestibular apparatus—the three semicircular canals and the two oval chambers. Therefore, both systems are filled with the same fluid. For the moment we shall concentrate only on the anatomy of the cochlea—the auditory receptor structure.

As noted previously, the optical microscope is still a profoundly useful instrument, contributing important information to our knowledge of cochlear anatomy, even though the newer electron-microscope techniques are becoming increasingly important. Foremost, among the optical microscopists working on the auditory mechanism today are Joseph Hawkins and Lars Johnsson of the University of Michigan's Kresge Hearing Research Institute. Their new methods allow very fresh tissue from cadavers to be studied before the inevitable deterioration allowed by prolonged staining preparation procedures occurs. To introduce us to this level of magnification of the cochlear microanatomy, let us consider Figure 3.20(a), which is a slightly enlarged photograph of a dissection of the human coch-

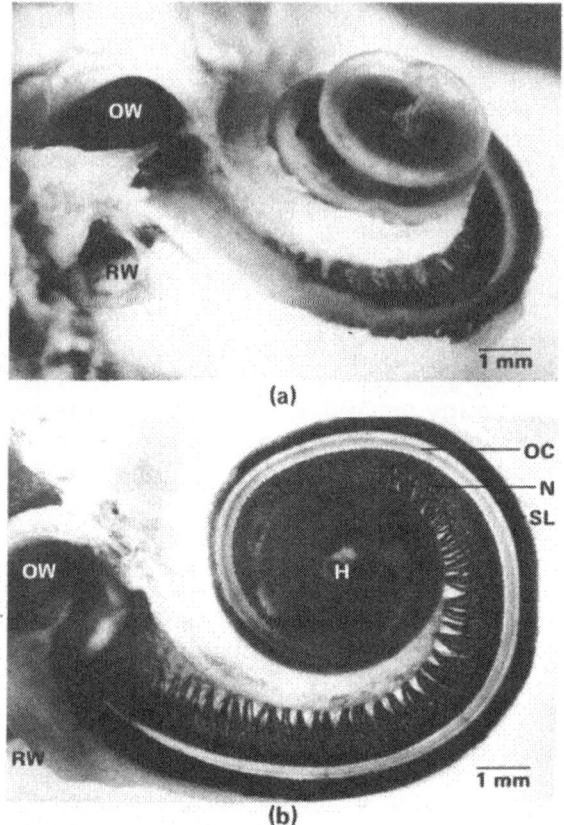

FIGURE 3.20 (a) Photograph of a slightly enlarged dissection of a human cochlea showing the spiral structure, the oval window (OW), and the round window (RW) (from Johnsson and Hawkins, 1967). (b) A more detailed view showing the heliocotrema (H), the organ of Corti (OC), the spiral ligament (SL), and the auditory nerve fibers (N) from Johnsson and Hawkins, 1972).

lea carried out and photographed by Johnsson and Hawkins (1967). The two and a half turns of the human spiral cochlear structure can be clearly seen. It is also possible to see dark traces, which are the bands of fibers of the cochlear nerve, somewhat better in Figure 3.20(b). A plane view of a cochlea at a slightly increased magnification is shown in Figure 3.21. In this figure we begin to see the structure of the mechanically sensitive tissue on the basilar membrane itself. The dark structures indicated by N are auditory neurons lying within the bony shelf or osseus lamina. The lighter band is the basilar membrane, while the slightly darker band indicated SL is the spiral ligament. IHC and OHC indicate the inner and outer hair cells, respectively. Figure 3.22(a) shows, at an even further degree of magnification, the general arrangement and the surprising regularity of the four rows of hair cells as observed with a scanning electron microscope. Unlike the previous three figures, this is of a cat. Figure 3.22(b) completes the series by showing a scanning electron micrograph of a tuft of stereocilia on a single hair cell.

Johnsson and Hawkins point out that these views from the top are somewhat unusual, yet most instructive in their presentation of the orderly

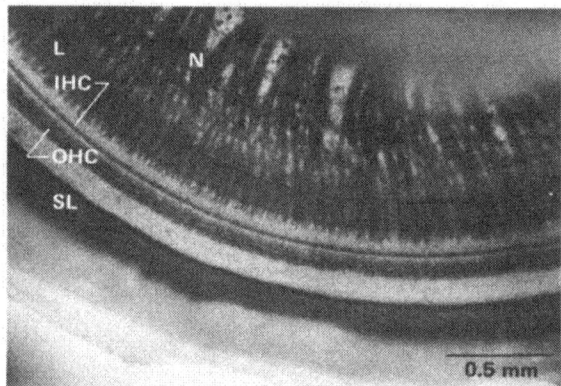

FIGURE 3.21 A more highly magnified microphotograph of a top view of the interior of a human cochlea, showing the auditory nerve fibers (N), the limbus (L), and the spiral ligament (SL), as well as the rows of inner (IHC) and outer (OHC) hair cells (courtesy of Dr. Lars Johnsson, University of Michigan).

array of receptor cells. Most students, they say, are indoctrinated into the anatomy of the inner ear from a different perspective, that of the cross section of the cochlea. The cross section is indeed better suited for helping to explain the next smallest level of microscopic reduction to which we now turn. Figure 3.23 is a very up-to-date cross-sectional drawing, showing in detail what the dark and light surface bands of Figure 3.21 can only suggest. It can be seen in this figure (which, incidentally, was also prepared by Hawkins) that the cochlea is really a tube within a tube. The scale vestibuli and the scala tympani are really two parts of a single continuous outer cavity, which interconnect through a small hole called the heliocotrema at the apical end of the cochlear coil. This continuity means that the perilymph, the fluid that fills these two scalae, is virtually identical throughout both, although small potential differences indicating some ionic concentration differences have been reported by some investigators.

The scala media, however, is separated from the other two scalae by two barriers. The superior wall of the scala media is made up of a very thin tissue known as Reissner's membrane. Reissner's membrane is believed to be only a single cell in thickness and has virtually no mechanical properties. However, it does act as an ionic barrier and thus helps to maintain substantial ionic concentration differences between the perilymph filling the scala vestibuli and tympani and the endolymph filling the scala media.

Also preventing perilymphatic-endolymphatic mixing is the tripartite inferior wall of the scala media, a group of tissues which we observed from the top in Figure 3.21. One major portion of the scala media's inferior wall is the bony shelf, the osseous lamina, through which the fibers of the cochlear nerve pass. From the terminus of the bony shelf, the basilar membrane, the structure supporting the other tissues of the acoustic receptive mecha-

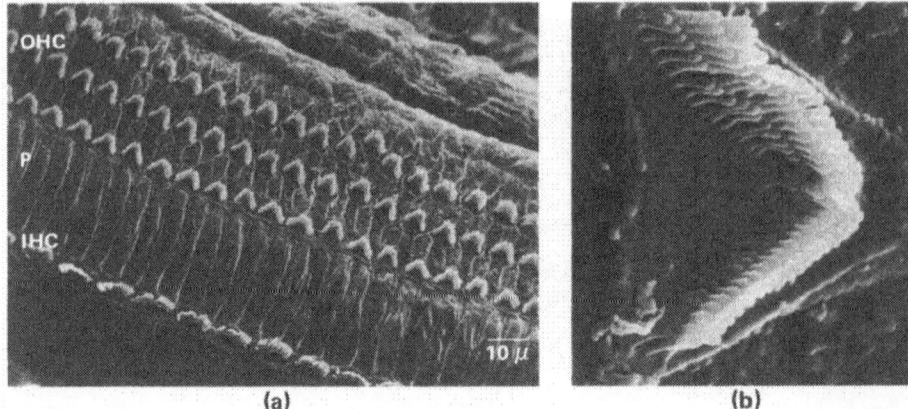

(a)   (b)

FIGURE 3.22 (a) A scanning electronmicrograph at an even greater magnification, showing the highly ordered arrangement of the three rows of outer hair
cells (OHC) and the one row of inner hair cells (IHC) as well as indicating the
Pillar cells (P) in the cat's basilar membrane (× 1000). Note the V-shaped tufts
of stereocilia on the outer hair cells, which are visible only because the tectorial
membrane has been removed (courtesy of Mr. Robert E. Preston of the University of Michigan) (b) A scanning electronmicrograph at an even higher magnification (× 15,000), showing the stereocilia of a single outer hair cell from a
baboon (courtesy of Dr. Hans Engström of the University of Göteborg).

nism itself, constitutes the next portion of this inferior wall. Finally, when
the basilar membrane terminates, the spiral ligament, attached to the outer
bony wall of the skull, completes the barrier. The receptor cells and the
associated supporting cells that make up the organ of Corti, a major portion of the basilar membrane, are of the greatest importance for us, and we
shall now consider them in some detail.

In addition to the specific nervous tissues, the receptor cells, and the
axons of the cochlear nerve, various kinds of supporting cells are also
found within the organ of Corti. Deiter's cells, Jansen's cells, and the cells
of Claudius have all been identified in Figure 3.23. While these cells perform important functions, they are not thought to be involved in the
auditory transductive process. Another important accessory structure, the
triangular and cartilagenous arches of Corti, at one time was thought to be
tuned resonators primarily responsible for acoustic quality encoding (see
Chapter 10). It is now thought, however, that they merely are supportive
structures.

The elements that are thought to be of the greatest significance in the
transductive process are the tectorial membrane and the hair cells. The
tectorial membrane is a flap of tissue growing from the spiral limbus. What
is now known to be its outer edge, the reticular lamina, was once thought
to be an outer sheaf on the layer of Hensen's cells, but most acoustic anatomists now believe this to be an error due to artifacts in the older microscopic techniques. The tectorial membrane is loosely attached to the limbus
and is able to move in relation to the hair cells, which are more rigidly

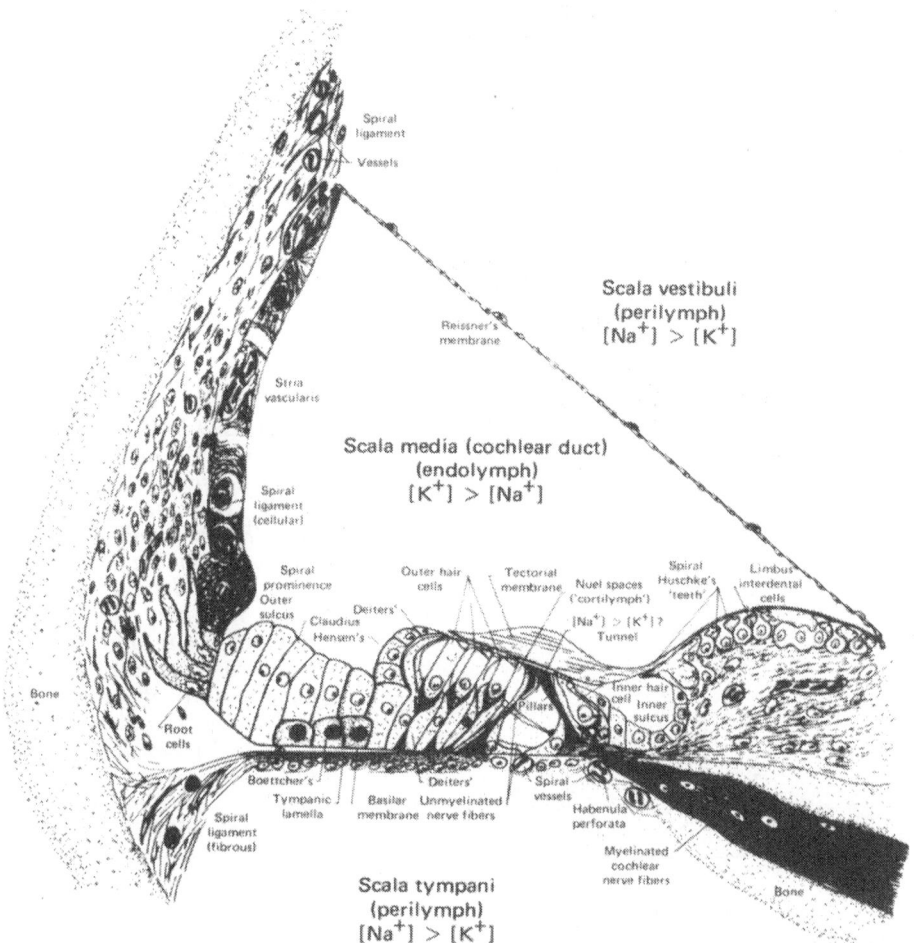

FIGURE 3.23 Cross section of one coil of the cochlea, showing the elaborate structure of the organ of Corti (courtesy of Dr. Joseph Hawkins, University of Michigan from Best and Taylor, 1966).

supported by the basilar membrane. This relative movement of the tectorial membrane with regard to the hair cells results in a shearing action, in which the tiny cilia (the hairs) of the hair cells are bent or otherwise displaced. It is this action that is considered to be the primary sensory action in acoustic transduction.

Hair cells lie in four parallel rows as shown in both Figure 3.21 and Figure 3.22. Three of the rows are outside (away from the center of the spiral) of the arches of Corti and are known as the outer or external hair cells. There is but a single row of inner or internal hair cells located inside (toward the center of the spiral) the arches. To understand the structure of these hair cells and the significance of their structure in developing an ex-

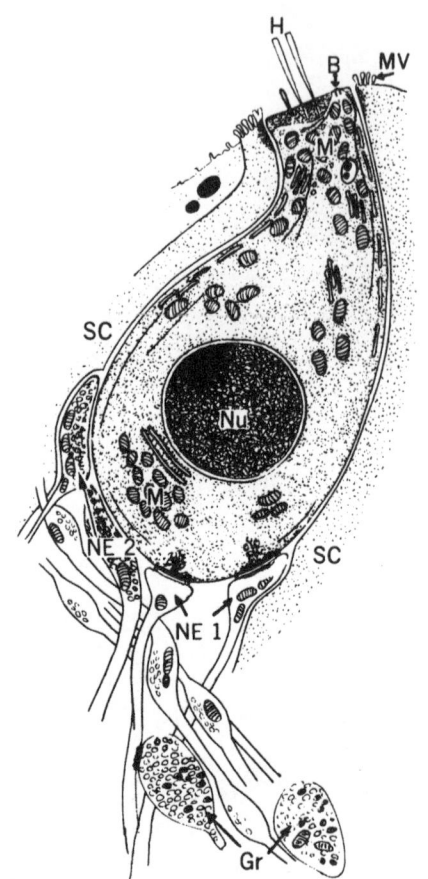

FIGURE 3.24 Drawing of a guinea pig's auditory inner hair cell, showing the cilia or hairs (H), the basal body (B), the microvilli (MV) on the surrounding supporting cells (SC), the cell's nucleus (Nu), two kinds of synaptic terminals, one of which appears to be afferent (NE 1) and the other efferent (NE 2), and some granulated structures (GR) which are possibly axo-axonal junctions (from Engström, Ades, and Hawkins, 1965).

planation of the transductive process, we must increase our magnification and descend to the even more microscopic level of cellular ultrastructure. It is at this level of magnification that the electron microscope is the only instrument capable of providing the necessary degree of resolution.

Figure 3.24 (taken from the works of Engstrom, Ades, and Hawkins [1965]—the basis of much of the rest of our discussion on acoustic hair-cell microanatomy) is a drawing made from electron micrographs of an inner hair cell. An important feature of the acoustic receptor cell is that it has no elongated axonal process. It is unquestionably a true neuron, but like the rods and cones of the eye, it synapses almost immediately. Another extremely interesting anatomical observation made by Engstrom and his colleagues, which could be of special significance in our interpretations of receptor interaction (see Chapter 7), is that there are two different classes of synapse among the several that are usually observed to make connection at the base of each inner hair cell. The first type is a heavily granulated structure, while the second exhibits much less of this granular intracellular material. It has been suggested that this anatomical difference

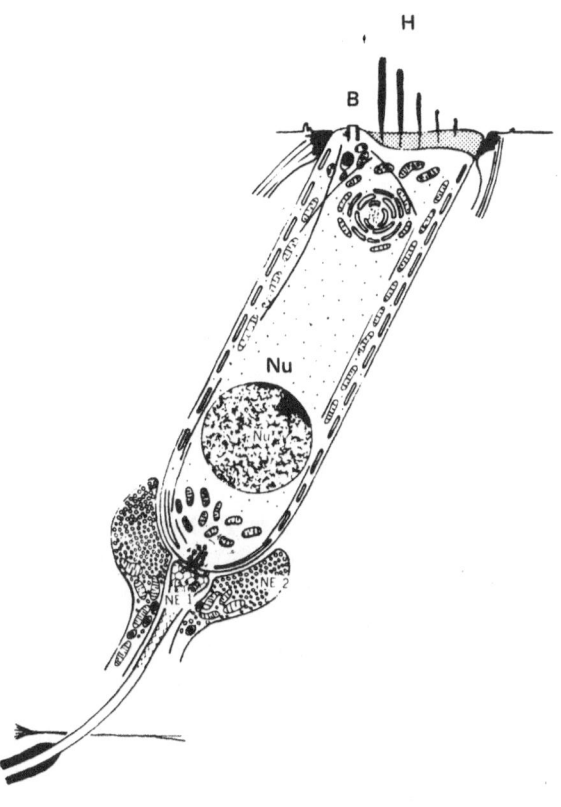

FIGURE 3.25 Drawing of a guinea pig's auditory outer hair cell. Abbreviated captions are the same as in Figure 3.24 (courtesy of Dr. Hans Engström of the University of Göteborg).

reflects the fact that both afferent and efferent neurons synapse with the hair cell, since the granules may be synaptic transmitter substance. If this suposition is correct, it would be a most important fact, for it would mean that central nervous activity or activity from adjacent receptors would both be potentially capable of modulating the sensitivity of the receptor cell itself. The complications that such feedback mechanisms would introduce into the stimulus-response relationships even at the receptor level are profound, indeed.

Perhaps the most important portion of the hair cell is the almost invisible body that lies under the basal end of the hairs or, as they are more correctly known, the stereocilia. Whatever the mechanism of the auditory transduction, which is ultimately accepted as the actual one, there is not much doubt that the basal body will be found to play a very significant role. It is almost certain that it is the junction at which the mechanical action is finally converted into a neural signal.

Figure 3.25 (also from Engstrom, Ades, and Hawkins, 1965) depicts a typical outer hair cell. The cilia of the outer hair cell, more numerous than on the inner hair cell, lie atop a similar basal body, which once again is thought by many of the workers in this field to play the key role in auditory transduction. The synaptic arrangements at the base of the outer hair cell are somewhat more regular than those found at the base of inner hair cells, but both the afferent and efferent types of synapse also appear to be present. The efferent cells, if that is indeed what they are, appear to envelop the afferent ones, the latter being connected more centrally to the base of the outer hair cell. Such an arrangement would allow considerable interaction. It should also be noted that the very intimate relationship of the possible candidate afferent and efferent cells at the base of the hair cell raises another possibility. The two may actually be communicating with each other directly rather than indirectly via the altered properties of the receptor.

This, then, is a structural analysis of auditory receptor cells. As with any other sensory system, this sort of transductive structure would be irrelevant unless information could be conveyed to the central nervous system. We shall now consider the anatomy of the ascending auditory pathway, which serves this communication function.

B. The Ascending Auditory Pathway

Figure 3.26 diagrams the ascending auditory pathway. As we have seen, cochlear hair cells, the primary auditory receptors, do not have any axons of their own. Nevertheless, they certainly must be considered to be the first neuron in the auditory chain. Synaptic connections at their base connect the hair cells to the dendrites of the bipolar cells of the auditory or cochlear nerve. The cell bodies of the fibers in the cochlear nerve collectively make up the spiral ganglion, which is embedded in the bone of the skull adjacent to the cochlea. The cochlear nerve, itself, bifurcates in the ventral cochlear nucleus immediately upon entering the medulla. At this branching point, one of the resulting bands of fibers immediately synapses with other neurons, which then pass horizontally across the medulla, sending some fibers to the ipsilateral and some to the contralateral superior olivary nuclei. The other branch of the cochlear nerve goes directly to the dorsal cochlear nucleus and, after an additional synapse, crosses over to the superior olive. Ascending fibers from the superior olives pass begin their ascent through the midbrain along the great tracts known as the lateral lemnisci. Once again, however, these tracts bifurcate, and as can be seen in Figure 3.26, some portion of the fibers synapses again at the mesencephalic nucleus of the inferior colliculus. Again the band of fibers bifurcates. Some fibers go directly to the medial geniculate body of the thalamus, while others cross over to the opposite inferior colliculus before ascending to the contralateral medial geniculate body. From the geniculates, the final neuron, the fifth or sixth in the chain, projects directly to the auditory cortex, which is buried within the lateral fissure of the cerebral hemisphere.

VII. THE VESTIBULAR SYSTEM

A. The Anatomy of the Vestibular Receptors

Figure 3.19, in addition to depicting the gross structure of the cochlea, also showed the macrostructure of the rest of the fluid-filled inner ear. The ad-

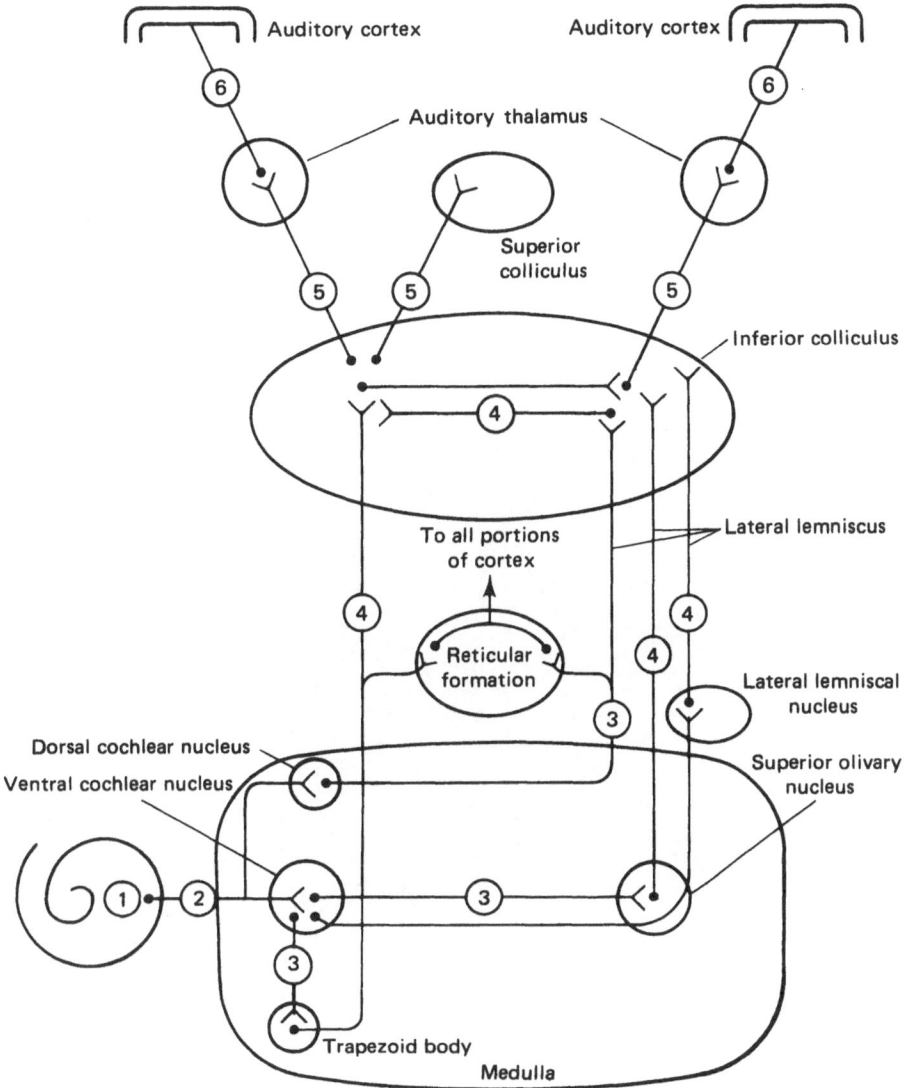

FIGURE 3.26 A schematic drawing of the entire ascending auditory pathway. Small circled numbers indicate the order of the neuron in the chain from the receptor hair cells to the auditory cortex.

ditional structures, of course, do not serve an auditory function, even though they share a common fluid medium and a common embryological history with the cochlea. Rather, the canals and bulbs of the vestibular system are the basic receptors of a sensory system responsible for the maintenance of balance and of our spatial relations to accelerative fields. The vestibular receptors are made up of five cavities: two nearly perfectly oval bulbs, and the three semicircular canals.

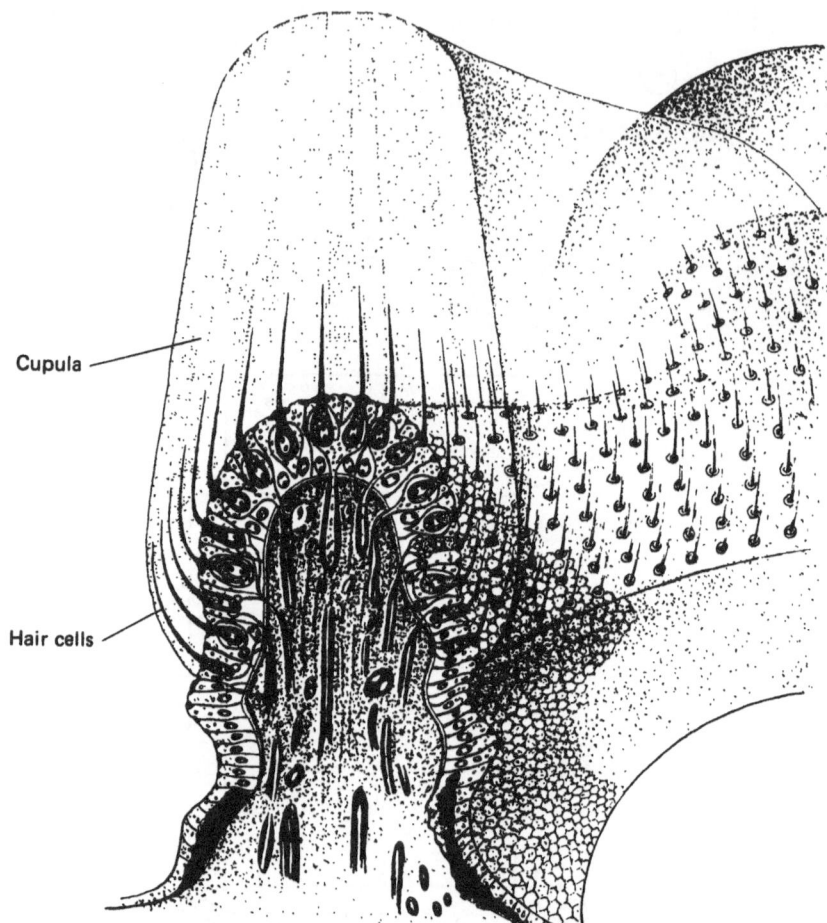

Cupula

Hair cells

FIGURE 3.27 Drawing of the crista ampullaris of the vestibular system's semi-circular canals. The gelatinous cupula transmits mechanical energy to the hair cells (from Flock, 1971, after Wersäll).

The two oval structures, the sacculus and the utriculus, are immediately adjacent to the basal end of the cochlea. The sacculus is actually connected to the cochlear inner ear by a tiny duct—the canal of reuniens, thus providing continuity of the endolymphatic fluid throughout the inner-ear structure. The utriculus, in turn, is connected to the sacculus through another tiny duct.

The three semicircular canals all terminate on the surface of the utriculus in enlarged bulblike regions known as ampullae. The inner surface epithelium of these ampullae and of the utriculus and the sacculus contain the vestibular receptor structures, which are capable of being activated by the accelerative forces operating on the fluid medium.

Figure 3.27 is an interpretive drawing of a micrograph of a cross section of the ridgelike crista ampullaris, the receptor structure found in the

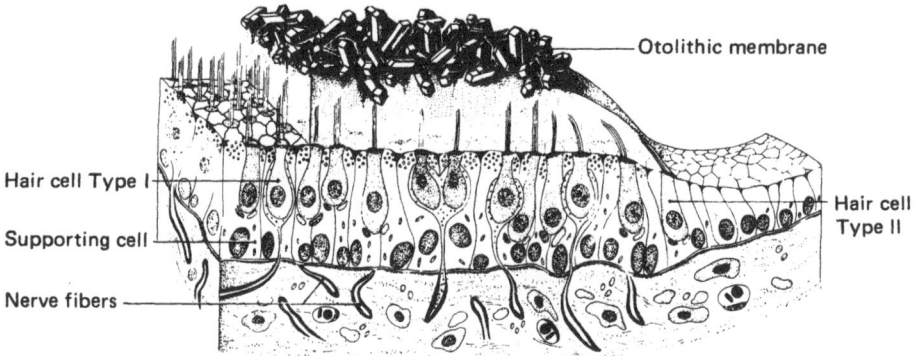

FIGURE 3.28 Drawing of the receptor area of the utricle and saccule, showing the gelatinous membrane (analogous to the cupula of the crista ampullaris) supporting calcium carbonate crystals or otoconia (from Iurato, 1967).

ampulla of the semicircular canals. (This figure is taken from Flock, 1971, but originally had been drawn by Wersäll, 1956.) The gelatinous cupula acts as an intermediary mechanical linkage to convey the forces imposed on the semicircular canal fluid to the epithelium of the crista and, thus, to the receptor cells. In this figure can also be seen the epithelium containing the receptor cells on the surface of the crista.

In the utricular and saccular regions, a different sort of receptor structure exists. Their surfaces are also covered with a specialized epithelium containing receptor hair cells, but the epithelium is arranged more in a flat sheet, and the gelatinous material is organized differently. Figure 3.28 (from Iurato, 1967) is a greatly enlarged drawing of a large region of the sensory epithelium from the utricule. This figure shows that the gelatinous mass, which covers the sensory epithelium, is in turn covered by a fine layer of calcium salts known as otoconia. The difference in the structure of this otoconial layer and the cupula is the basis of a major difference in the function of the vestibular receptors of the saccule and utricule on the one hand and the ampullar cristae on the other. The ampulla cristae are activated entirely by velocity changes resulting from rotary or linear motion of the head. The three semicircular canals, therefore, are primarily sources of information about changes in the velocity dv/dt of the head, and thus can be thought of as being the transducers for discontinuous accelerations. The receptors of the utricule and saccule on the other hand, because of the overlying layer of otoconia, are continuously activated by constant accelerative fields like gravity. As such, they constantly provide information about the orientation of the head rather than discontinuous accelerations as do the semicular canals.

Thus, armed with the general anatomy of the vestibular macrostructure, we are now prepared to descend to a more highly magnified level of microscopic examination. This particular body of knowledge results from the electron-microscopic investigations of Ades and Engstrom (1965) and Wersäll (1956). As in the cochlea, there are two distinguishable varieties

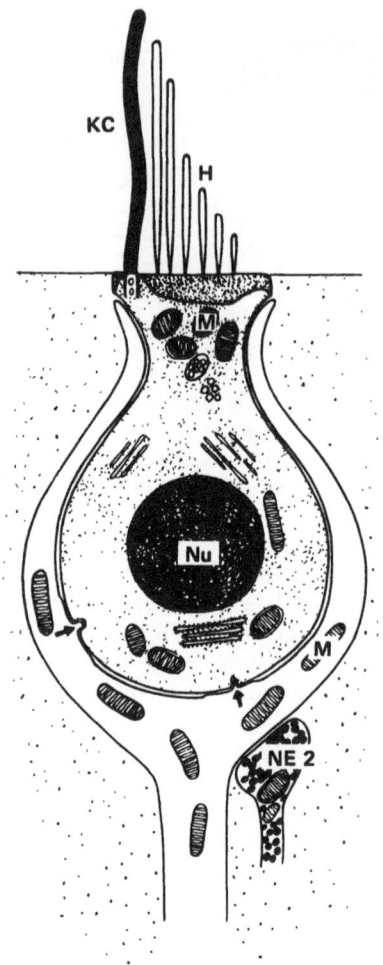

FIGURE 3.29 A Type 1 vestibular hair cell, showing the kinocilium (KC), the stereocilia (H), some mitochondria (M), the cell's nucleus (Nu), and, as with the auditory hair cell, two kinds of synaptic connections. One afferent type occurs in several locations (arrows) on the interface between the hair cell and a surrounding "calyx" (NC), while the other appears to be efferent (NE 2) (from Ades and Engström, 1965).

of vestibular hair cells. The two types are distinguished on the basis of their shape as well as the nature of the synaptic connections between the vestibular hair cell and its connecting axons. As Engstrom and Ades point out, however, these two categories may be but two extremes of a continuum, which actually includes many different intermediate varieties.

Figure 3.29 is a typical Type 1 vestibular receptor cell. It is seen to be flask shaped and to contain all of the usual cellular metabolic apparatus necessary for the maintenance of any cell, such as mitochondria and the nucleus. Like so many other of the receptor cells we have seen so far, it is a hair or ciliated cell. Each cell possesses a single kinocilium and as many as 70 smaller stereocilia arranged in an orderly array. While the kinocilium appears to contain an extension of the cytoplasm of the receptor cell, the stereocilia appear to be extensions of the cuticular base plate overlaying almost all of the distal end of the cell. Just as with the auditory hair cell, it is possible that this cuticular plate is, in fact, the critical organ of transduction for vestibular sensitivity. Thus, it is suspected that this is the point at which the primary sensory action occurs, but this is not certain and extremely difficult to establish one way or the other with our current technology.

Type 1 cells have two very distinct kinds of synaptic connections. The first, according to Ades and Engstrom, is a "calyx," which almost completely encloses the proximal end of the receptor cell body itself. This structure is indicated by the label NE1 in Figure 3.29. Synaptic contact is believed to be made at the slight indentations where the membrane of the calyx seems to enter invaginations of the membrane of the receptor cell. In electron micrographs little, if any, granular structure can be observed in the calyx and, thus it is presumed to be afferent. However, the second type of axonal connection—the smaller synaptic knob indicated by NE2 in Figure 3.29—has rich granulation. Ades and Engstrom infer from this structural difference that this second type of synapse is an efferent one and may provide a means of modulating receptor sensitivity by central mechanisms in a way similar to that hypothesized in the auditory system.

Figure 3.30 shows the structure of a Type 2 vestibular epithelial hair cell. The terminal end of the Type 2 cell is also covered with a microforest of cilia. They appear to be organized almost identically to the array found on the Type 1 cell. The major differences between the Type 1 and the Type 2 cells are found in the overall shape of the cell and the nature of the synaptic junctions. Type 2 cells are much more regular cylinders with little evidence of the bulbous or flask shape of the Type 1 cell. Similarly, the synaptic calyx typically enclosing the Type 1 cell is a feature completely absent from the Type 2 cell. Synaptic connections for the latter type are, in general, far simpler in structure. The tiny invaginations, where the synaptic junction is thought to occur, can still be seen, however. These synapses also seem to be divided into two different categories, on the basis of the amount of granular structure seen in electron micrographs, and, therefore, both afferent and efferent communications are also indicated for in Type 2 vestibular hair cells.

An interesting feature of both types of vestibular hair cells emphasized by Ades and Engstrom is that the second smaller type of hair, the stereocilia, are very regularly graded in length. The further a stereocilium is from the kinocilium, the shorter it tends to be. This arrangement, Ades and Engstrom speculate, may serve an important function by "polarizing" the hair cell, so that forces applied in one direction are more effective than in another. In such a manner, directionality might be introduced into vestibular sensation. Other investigators (Wersäll and Flock, 1965) have suggested that the polarization is effective enough to entirely reverse the neural effect of displacements in opposite directions. According to them, displacement of the hairs in one direction will inhibit the cell's activity, while displacements in the other direction will lead to excitation. Considering the possible direct relation between the mechanical distortion of the base plate by the hairs and the permeability to ion flow, such a possibility seems eminently feasible.

Another interesting and slightly different point of view has been expressed by Hillman and Lewis (1971), based on scanning electron micro-

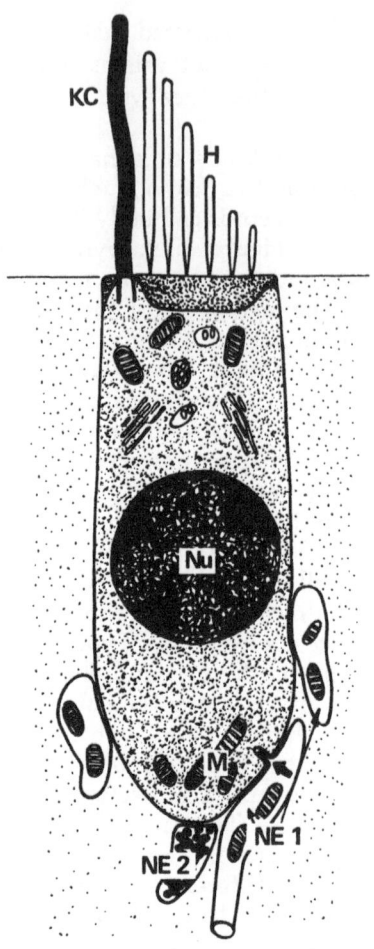

FIGURE 3.30 A Type 2 vestibular hair cell; nomenclature as in Figure 3.29 (from Ades and Engström, 1965).

graphs of the vestibular hair cells. They have observed that the many stereocilia are attached to a bulblike growth on the end of the single kinocilium. This arrangement is clearly seen in Figure 3.31, a reproduction of one of their scanning electron micrographs of the hairs of a single vestibular receptor cell. As we saw earlier, the stereocilia all emerge from the cuticular base plate, while the kinocilium is simply attached to a portion of the cell membrane. Hillman and Lewis' suggestion is that the mechanical linkage of the stereocilia and kinocilia acts to produce a "plungerlike" motion, maximizing the conversion of the mainly transverse motion of the stimulus into the up-and-down motion at the base of the kinostereocilium. From Hillman and Lewis' point of view then, the base plate may not be the key factor in the transduction, but may merely serve a mechanical role assisting the nearby cell membrane of the cell to do that important job.

There are also a number of other anatomical curiosities that may be

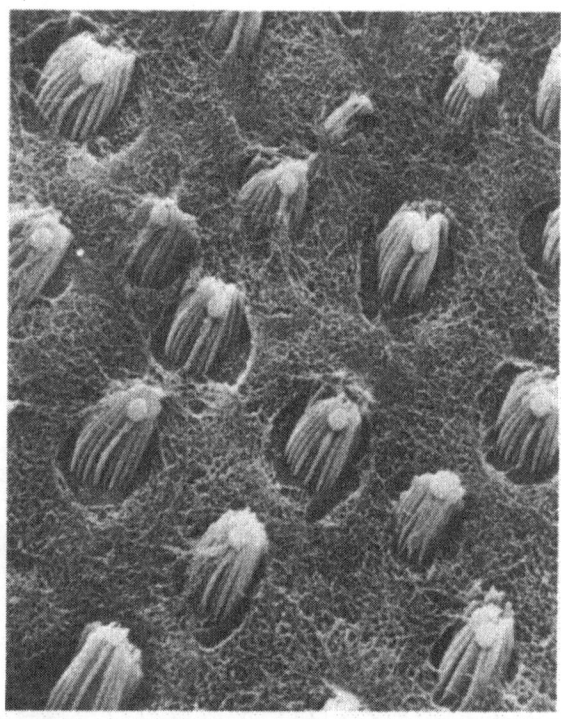

FIGURE 3.31 A scanning
electronmicrograph of the
cilia of vestibular hair cells,
showing the bulbous ending
on the end of the kinocilium
and the arrangement whereby
back-and-forth motion is converted into a plungerlike
up-and-down motion (from
Hillman and Lewis, 1971).

important in enhancing the interaction among the vestibular receptor cells.
Figure 3.32, again from Ades and Engstrom (1965), shows a complex relationship between the calyx surrounding a Type 1 cell and two Type 2 cells.
In addition to what may be a functional bridge connecting two cells, there
also appears to be an efferent synapse impinging upon the bridge. If this
efferent synapse were inhibitory, it might be able to modulate the interaction mediated by the bridge.

B. The Ascending Vestibular Pathway
It may be somewhat inappropriate to refer to the vestibular pathway pic-
tured in Figure 3.33 solely as an "ascending" system, for it also has descending and direct motor outputs. At the base of the vestibular receptor
hair cells, as we have seen, there is a synapse with a set of second-order
axons. These axons are the fibers of cells, whose perikarya lie in the
vestibular (Scarpa's) ganglion near the head of the medulla. After the
fibers enter the medulla, the vestibular nerve branches into four parts.
Branches are sent to the superior, medial, lateral, and spinal vestibular
nuclei. The course of each of the four branches is different for the fibers
that emerge, after another synaptic relay, from each of these nuclei.
    The fibers emerging from the superior vestibular nucleus ascend,
without crossing over, to the ipsilateral oculomotor and trochlear nuclei,
where afferent nerves conduct motor information directly to the muscles
controlling eye position. Here, also, the pathways synapse again and pro-

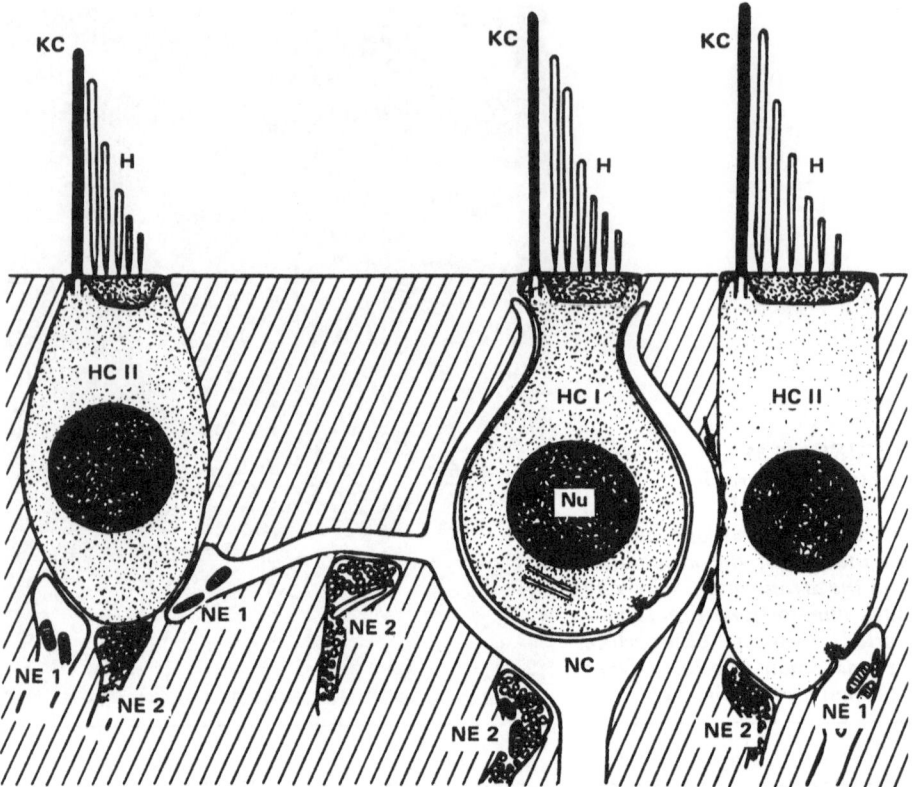

FIGURE 3.32 Drawing of some possible synaptic interconnections of vestibular hair cells, suggesting that there may be some sort of lateral interaction even at this most peripheral level. Nomenclature as in figure 3.29 (from Ades and Engström, 1965).

ject to unknown regions of the cerebral cortex. Postsynaptic fibers from the medial vestibular nucleus, on the other hand, send ascending fibers, which cross over immediately to the contralateral oculomotor and trochlear nuclei. In addition, crossed fibers are projected through both the ipsilateral and contralateral medial longitudinal fasculi, a pair of spinal pathways, to ventral motor nerve roots for direct control of skeletal muscles. An auxiliary pathway branches off to the spinal accessory nucleus, which is responsible for the control of some of the muscles of the head and the neck.

The lateral vestibular nucleus, which receives fibers from the third branch of the vestibular nerve, projects fibers that descend ipsilaterally along the lateral vestibulo-spinal tract into the spinal cord. Finally, the fourth branch of the vestibular nerve synapses in the spinal vestibular nucleus and then sends both crossed and uncrossed fibers descending through the two medial longitudinal fasciculi to various muscles. The several direct pathways to the skeletal musculature are important to many

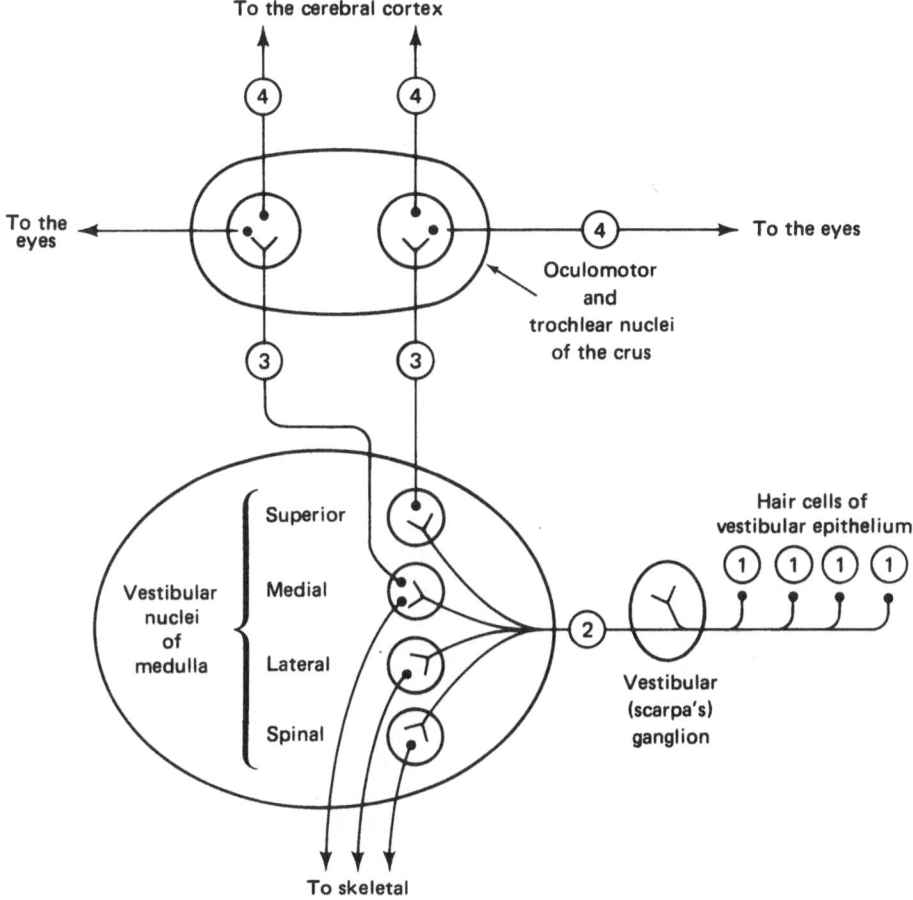

FIGURE 3.33 A schematic drawing of part of the ascending vestibular pathway. Beyond the crus little is known of the details of the pathway.

of the motor skills exercised by animals. The ability to respond without the involvement of cortical reaction times makes possible the splendid co-ordination of a diver, an acrobat, or a cat.

VIII. THE SOMESTHETIC SYSTEM

A. The Anatomy of the Somesthetic Receptors
The psychophysical discovery that the skin displayed punctate patterns of sensitivity to touch, heat, cold, and pressure was made at about the same time as the anatomical discovery that the nerve plexus ended in the skin in similar pointlike end organs. Therefore, some physiologists and psychologists were led to correlate end organ anatomy with the individual cutaneous submodality. In fact, however, a century of continued research along

several different lines has failed to show any specific correspondence between the varied end organs of the skin and the cutaneous sensory functions.

Kenshalo and Nafe (1960) have summarized this century of failure in a review, which has been adapted and reproduced in Table 3.3 below. They distinguish among three different types of experiments that strive to associate specific receptors with specific sensations. The first category included direct microscopic investigations of the tissue excised below psychophysically identified sensory "spots." The first part of the table shows that this approach led to virtually nothing that could be even remotely considered to be a correlation between any specific receptor of the skin and any given sensory modality.

The second category of investigation included statistical studies. Larger areas of the skin were examined for the general distribution of the sensory spots, as well as for the general histological distribution of various kinds of receptors. Even with regard to general distributions, it is difficult to see any pattern emerging in the studies listed in this second part of Kenshalo and Nafe's table.

The third category of investigation included simple histological examinations of the skin. It was found that, in general, hairy skin has few, if any, of the specialized end organs found so plentifully elsewhere on glabrous (smooth) skin. Yet hairy skin does have sensitivity to pain, cold, pressure, and warmth, just as do the glabrous areas.

All three categories of investigation leave the reader with the feeling that little evidence exists for what is probably one of the most persistent misstatements of fact in the sensory literature, namely, that specific receptor structures are associated with specific modalities and underly specific sensory spots. We shall speak more of the general problem of cutaneous sensory end organs and their relation to theories of quality coding later in Chapter 11 of this book. For the moment, we shall only briefly point out that other difficult-to-explain facts (for example, the mobility of sensory spots) also seem to mitigate against the association of specific end organ structures with specific sensations. A more enlightened future theory will probably look upon sensory spots as functions of the organization of the neural plexus and of interactions between nearby neural units at several different levels of the nervous system rather than as perceptual analogues of specifically sensitive punctate end organs.

The encapsulations and end organs we shall discuss may be no more than consequences of the fact that cutaneous end organs are very much exposed to the ravages of the external environments. Coupled with this environmental barrage, as a possible source of structural diversity, is the fact that cutaneous neural end organs are also highly unusual portions of the neuron—remote terminal structures where bizarre metabolic and membrane states may obtain even under the best of conditions.

The important fact is that, in some manner, cutaneous and proprioceptive nerve end organs have become generally specialized in ways that allow them to act as transducers of physical energies. By some evolutionary process, the terminal ends of the nerve have become exquisitely sensitive to mechanical, thermal, and noxious stimulation. The notion, which it is

TABLE 3.3 A HISTORY OF THE VARIOUS EXPERIMENTS
ATTEMPTED TO SHOW CORRELATIONS BETWEEN ENCAPSULATED
NERVE ENDINGS AND THE PUNCTATE SKIN SENSATIONS*

Investigator	Skin Area Glabrous	Skin Area Hairy	Sensations Tested	Encapsulated Endings Reported
TYPE I INVESTIGATIONS				
Donaldson (1885)		Forearm	Cold	None
Goldscheider (1886)		Forearm	Cold, warm, touch, pain	None
Haggqvist (1913)		Forearm	Cold, warm	None
Dallenbach (1927)		Upper arm	Cold, warm	None
Pendleton (1928)		Forearm	Cold	None
Woolard (1935)		Thigh	Cold, pain, touch	None
Bazett (1941)		Forearm	Cold	None
Weddell (1941)		Forearm	Cold	Krause endbulbs
Belonoschkin (1933)	Nipple		Cold	Complicated plexuses without capsules
TYPE II INVESTIGATIONS				
von Frey (1895)	Conjunctiva		Cold	Krause endbulb
	Cornea		Cold, pain, touch, warm	None
		Forearm		Krause endbulb
Strughold (1925)	Mouth mucosa		Cold	Krause endbulb
Strughold & Karbe (1925)	Conjunctiva		Cold	Krause endbulb
Bazett et al. (1932)	Prepuce		Cold, warm, touch	Krause endbulb Ruffini cylinders
Sinclair et al. (1952)	Finger		Cold, warm, touch	Meissner corpuscle Merkel's Disks Krause & Ruffini endings
		Forearm		None
		Auricle		None
TYPE III INVESTIGATIONS				
Gilbert (1929)		Thigh		None
		Epigastrium		None
		Chest		None
		Breast		None
Gilmer (1941)		Back		None
Hagen et al. (1953)		Abdomen		None
		Finger dorsum		
Dastur (1955)		"232 specimens from hairy skin"		
Winkilmann (1955)		"Hairy skin"		None
Woolard (1936)		Thigh		Meissner corpuscle Merkel's disk
Gilbert (1929)	Foot sole Nipple			Meissner corpuscles Golgi-Mazzoni capsules
Williams et al. (1929)	Prepuce			Krause endbulb Ruffini cylinders Meissner corpuscles 4 unnamed types
Cathcart et al. (1948)	Nipple			Krause endbulb (rare) Unnamed smaller capsules
Gairns (1951 & 1955)	Palate Gum			Meissner corpuscles Krause endbulb Unnamed varieties
Gairns (1953)	Tongue			Krause endbulb Meissner corpuscles

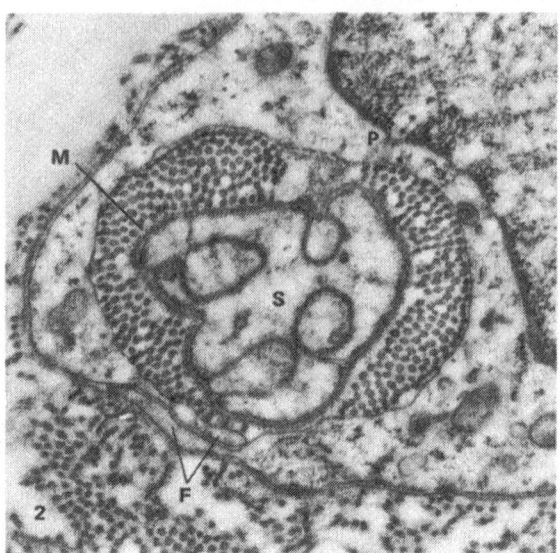

FIGURE 3.34 An electron-micrographic cross section, showing some of the structures that can surround even supposedly "free" nerve endings. In this case, a Schwann cell (S), the source of myelin, as well as another membrane (M), surrounds four "free" nerve endings. Furthermore, the whole cluster is surrounded by collagen fibers (F) overlapping folds of even another encapsulation layer formed from a perineural cell (P). Are free nerve endings truly "free"? (from Cauna, 1968).

desired to stress here, is that there is at best only minimum evidence to support the notion that the encapsulations and other external structure of the end organs play any but an indirect role in determining which of the several different kinds of physical energy is going to stimulate a given fiber. It is the suspicion of the author that in the long run we shall find that it is more important *where* a cutaneous fiber is located than *what* its structure is like in the definition of the stimulus energy to which it will be most sensitive. We shall deal with this further in Chapter 11.

Having noted the lack of a clear correlation between receptor structure and sensory specificity, we are in a better position to critically consider the simple anatomical facts, which are shown to us by the optical and electron microscopes. Cauna (1968) emphasizes that the categorization of cutaneous receptors is best made as a simple dichotomy: free nerve endings and encapsulated end organs. However, he also points out that the "free nerve endings" are almost never completely free, for the Schwann cells of the myelin sheath extend in almost all fibers down to the very tip of all fibers, even those that appear under relative low degrees of magnification to be covered by only naked nerve membranes. Figure 3.34, for example, is an electron micrograph of the cross section of some free nerve endings from the human skin taken by Cauna. The neuron still shows the partial Schwann cell sheath, which is a vestige of the more elaborate myelin coating of the more central portions of the cell.

It is also probably true that the encapsulated endings of the skin represent a much more highly diverse set of corpuscular endings than is usually appreciated. Not only is there a much larger anatomic variety of cells present than is usually discussed in elementary textbooks, but there is also a far greater diversity of shape and form within a given receptor type. The standard types usually listed probably represent only the distinguish-

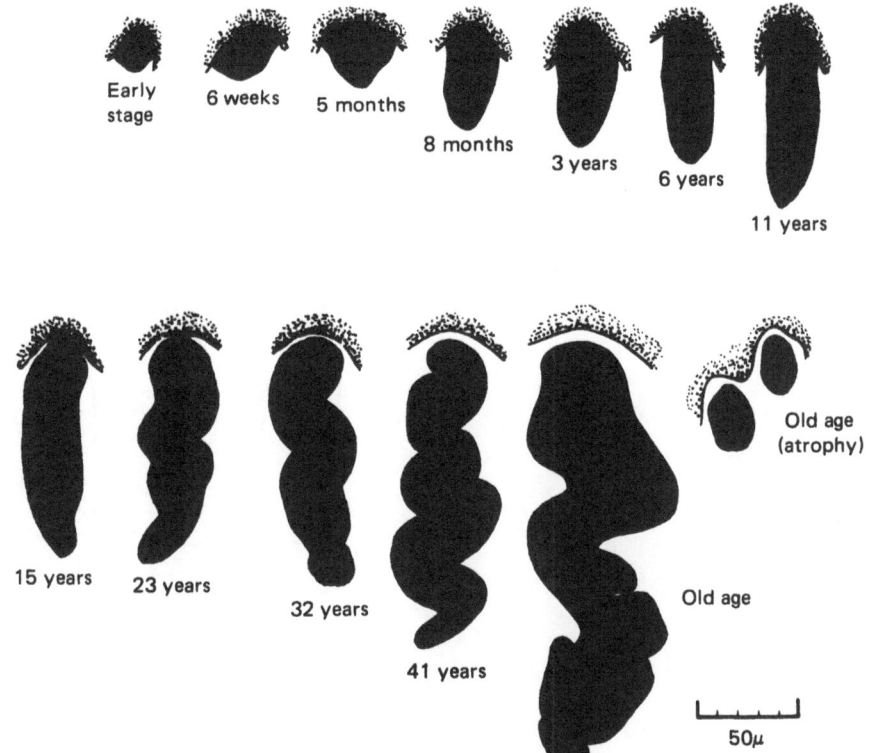

FIGURE 3.35 Drawings of a series of Meissner's corpuscles taken from humans of different ages. What is the typical shape of a Meissner corpuscle? (from Cauna, 1965).

able nodes of a continuum of varying shapes. Meisner corpuscles, Merkel disks, Pacinian corpuscles, and Golgi corpuscles all exist, but the full range of forms is widely divergent even within each type. Even the age of the animal can be very important in defining the shape of a given kind of corpuscle. For example, Figure 3.35 is a set of drawings showing the gradual change in shape of the Meisner corpuscle from animals of different ages. Figure 3.36 (a) and (b) show two related corpuscular endings—a mammalian Pacinian corpuscle and an avian Herbst corpuscle.

Iggo and Muir (1969) have recently described the structure of a "touch corpuscle" found in the skin, which seems to have a number of important properties in mediating cutaneous experiences. The Iggo corpuscle is not a single cell, but rather a cluster of about 50 Merkel cells gathered together under a dome of epidermis. Figure 3.37 shows the general arrangement as deduced from electron micrographs.

These drawings emphasize the very great diversity of type that can be observed in cutaneous end organs. As we shall see in a later chapter, the transductive process in the case of the Pacinian corpuscle, however, is almost completely independent of the integrity of the extra neural

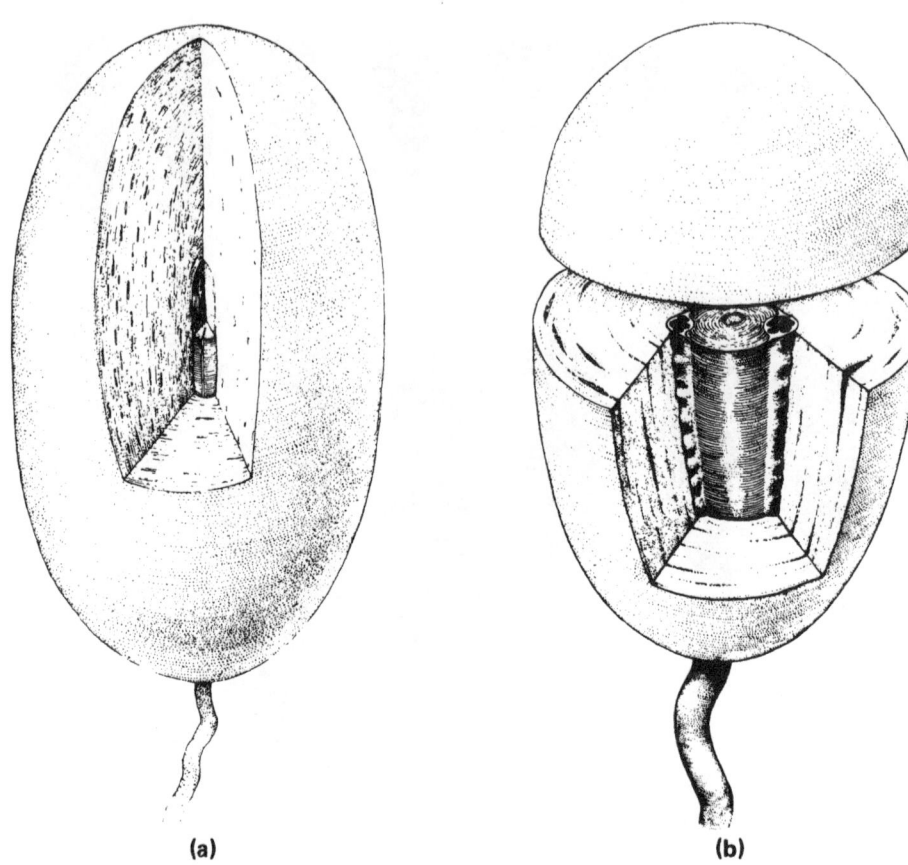

FIGURE 3.36 (a) Drawing of a mammalian Pacinian corpuscle (from Munger, 1971). (b) Drawing of an avian Herbst corpuscle (from Munger, 1971).

corpuscle itself. Presumably, the Pacinian corpuscle and most of the other accessory structures serve only secondary nonneural functions. It is to the terminal portions of the cutaneous neuron itself, rather, that we shall probably have to look for the locus of the primary sensory action.

The receptor cells of the proprioceptive system are similar, though somewhat different and specialized compared to those found in the skin. These cells signal information about the position and movement of the portions of the body. Several different types have been identified, but the best known are the Golgi tendon organs (see Figure 3.38) and the several different types of muscle spindles. These latter structures are extremely interesting in that they make intimate contact with muscle fibers in either a "flower spray" or "spiral" arrangement, both of which are illustrated in Figure 3.39. Other receptor types of various kinds are found throughout the animal kingdom in various joint, muscle, tendon, and even mesentary structures.

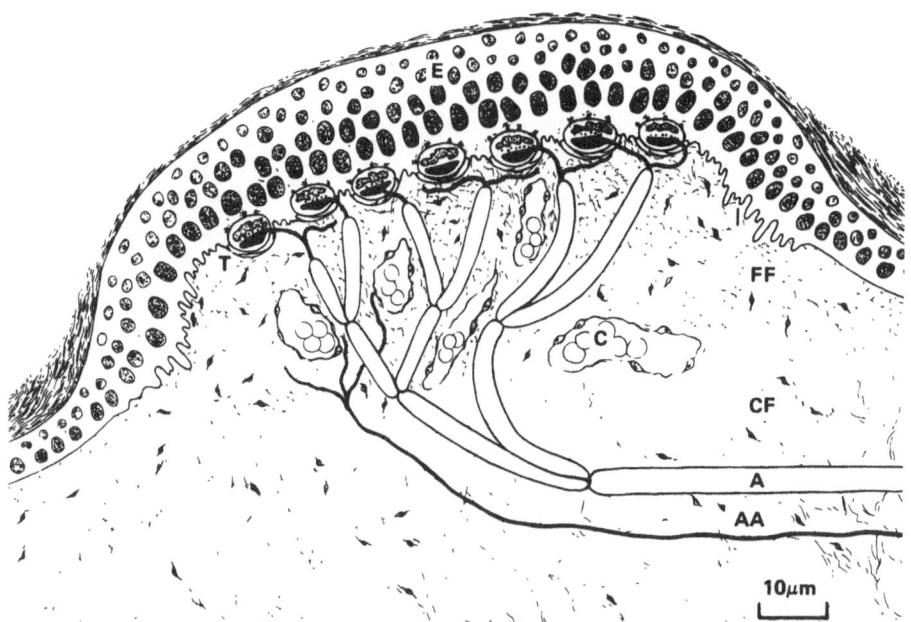

FIGURE 3.37 Drawing of an Iggo cutaneous receptor corpuscle, showing the myelinated axons (A), the unmyelinated axons (AA), collagen fibers (FF and CF), the epidermis (E) and the tactile cells (T) (from Iggo and Muir, 1969).

B. The Ascending Cutaneous and Proprioceptive Pathways

1. *The cutaneous pathways.* It is important to note that the peripheral somatosensory nerve net, though it initially appears to be very complex, is organized in an eminently simple fashion. There are no synapses and no important interactions of any other sort among the parallel fibers in any peripheral nerves. The individual neural fibers are simply bundled together. In spite of the great numbers of the nerve fibers, they all can be considered functionally as independent pathways. Figure 3.40 is a famous dissection of the peripheral nervous system of a human preserved in the Johns Hopkins Medical School. The nervous system shown here could be dissected free in some idealized *in vivo* experiment and spread out in a great sheet with little change in the function of each component part.

In recent years several investigators, most notably Wall (1961) and Rose and Mountcastle (1959), have concluded that there are two separate and relatively independent pathways for the cutaneous senses. The first, primarily concerned with the communication of high definition, high information content messages and the rapid signaling of touch and pressure, is characterized by passage through a brain stem tract known as the medial lemniscus. The other pathway, primarily concerned with the slower acting and less localized cutaneous spatial experiences as well as with pain and temperature senses, passes through the spinothalamic tract of the spinal cord and brain stem.

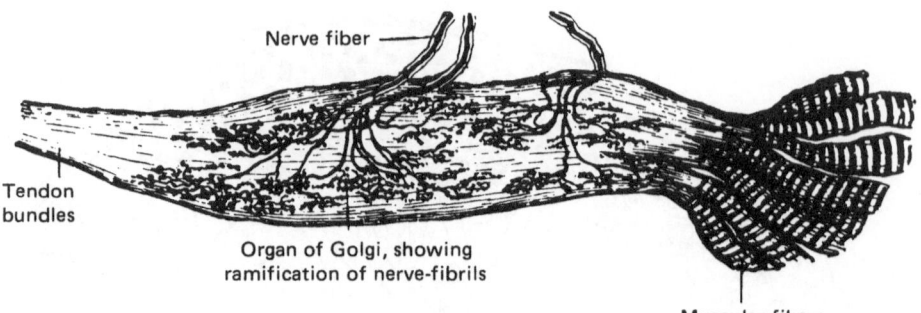

Nerve fiber

Tendon
bundles

Organ of Golgi, showing
ramification of nerve-fibrils

Muscular fibers

FIGURE 3.38 Drawing of a Golgi tendon organ (from Goss, 1973).

We shall first consider the medial lemniscal system for fast touch and pressure signals from the skin of the trunk and limbs. The initial action, as we have said, is the transduction of the physical energy of the external stimulus into neural activity at one of the cutaneous receptors just discussed. It should be remembered, however, that in contrast to the visual, auditory, and vestibular systems we have just discussed, the sensitive transductive membrane for the somatosensory system is on the terminal of a long axon rather than a separate receptor cell. Touch and pressure signals so generated are then transmitted through the peripheral nerves in the limbs and trunk toward the spinal cord along the axons of cells, which have their cell bodies located in the dorsal spinal roots. Most lemniscal fibers than ascend, without crossing over or synapsing, to the brain stem via the dorsal columns and the spinocervical tracts of the spinal cord. When they reach the level of the medulla, they then cross over to the contralateral side of the brain. The entire group of fibers now makes up the great brain stem pathway known as the medial lemniscus.

The next synaptic junction (the second for the medial lemniscal pathway) does not occur until the axons have passed into the thalamus where, in the lateral nucleus, they synapse to the final neuron in the pathway and ascend to the cortex. This final neuron then extends into the somatosensory regions of the post central cortex. Figure 3.41 illustrates, in a schematic manner, the major details of the anatomy of this medial lemniscal portion of the somesthetic system.

Now let us consider the other major cutaneous system—the one passing through the brain stem spinothalamic pathway. As noted, it conveys the slower and less well localized signals associated with pain and temperature reception. The anatomy of this pathway is shown schematically in Figure 3.42. Fibers from the pain and temperature receptors enter the spinal cord through the same dorsal roots that convey the medial lemniscal signals and synapse for the first time in the dorsal horns. All of the spinothalamic fibers are then thought to cross over immediately and ascend up the spinal cord through the lateral spinothalamic or the spinotectal tracts. At the level of the mesencephalon, these fibers join with other fibers from

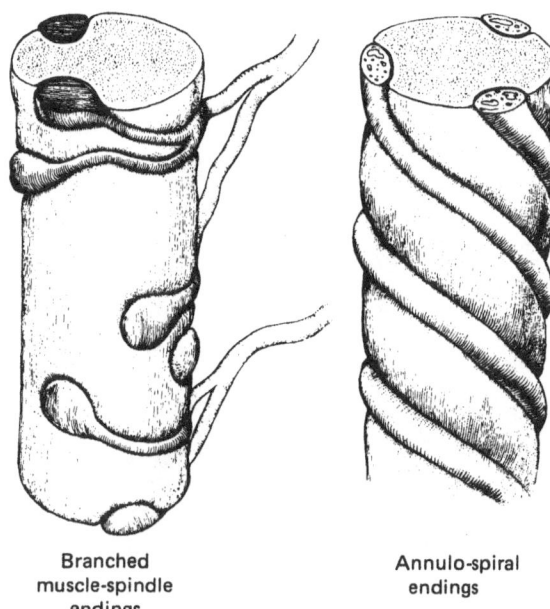

FIGURE 3.39 Drawing of two different kinds of muscle spindles. One has branched endings, while the other forms a concentric spiral around the muscle fibers (from Munger, 1971).

Branched muscle-spindle endings

Annulo-spiral endings

the head and neck to form the brain stem spinothalamic tract itself. The second synaptic interconnection occurs when these fibers arrive at the lateral nucleus of the thalamus. The final and third neuron in the chain then projects directly to the somatosensory cortex.

2. *The proprioceptive pathways.* The proprioceptive pathways of the somatosensory system convey information from the muscle, tendon, and joint receptors. Both an important similarity and an important difference emerge when we compare the proprioceptive and the somatosensory pathways. The similarity shared by the two systems is that fibers from proprioceptive receptors are merged into the medial lemniscal pathway with cutaneous signals and project to the same somatosensory area of the cerebral cortex. The difference is that in addition to projecting to the cerebral cortices, proprioceptive signals also project to the cerebellar cortices, where they play an important role in regulating involuntary muscle tonus, body position, and general motor synchronization.

Since the general anatomy of the medial lemniscal projection of proprioceptors to the cortex is so similar to that of the cutaneous pathways, we shall only briefly mention in addition the cerebellar proprioceptive pathway. Information from the proprioceptive receptors enters the spinal cord, as does all sensory information from the body, through the spinal roots. Some of the fibers cross over to the other side of the spinal cord and ascend to the cerebellum through the medulla and pons. Others ascend directly without crossing over through various tracts of the medulla to the various parts of the cerebellum.

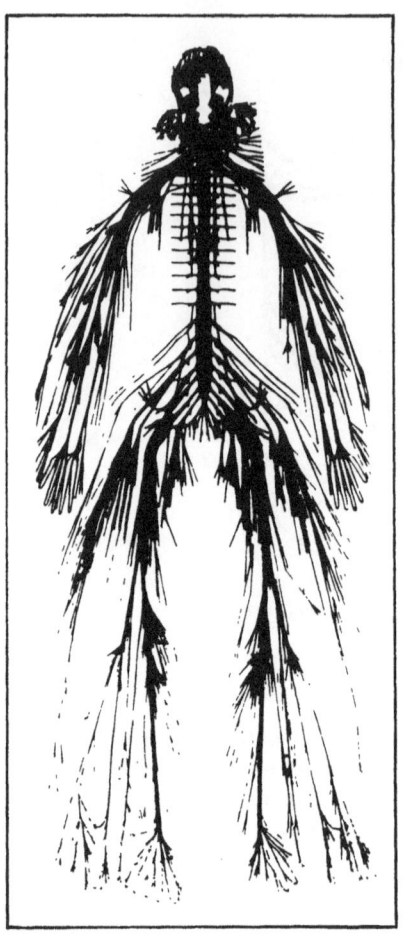

FIGURE 3.40 Photograph of a dissection of the entire nervous system now in the Johns Hopkins University Medical School (courtesy of Time-Life, Inc.).

Though our interest at this moment is entirely directed toward the proprioceptive inputs of the cerebellum, it should also be pointed out that the cerebellum also receives inputs from other sensory pathways. It is certainly obvious that an organ like the cerebellum, which is involved in the maintenance of posture, should also receive afferent signals from the vestibular organs. But, furthermore, recent studies have shown that visual, auditory, and even cutaneous inputs also project to the cerebellum. Thus, it is now clear that this organ is more like the cerebral hemispheres in terms of its inputs than previously had been suspected.

IX. THE OLFACTORY SYSTEM

A. The Anatomy of the Olfactory Receptor
We now turn from senses that are tuned to be most responsive to slight amounts of photic or mechanical energy to two that are able to respond to

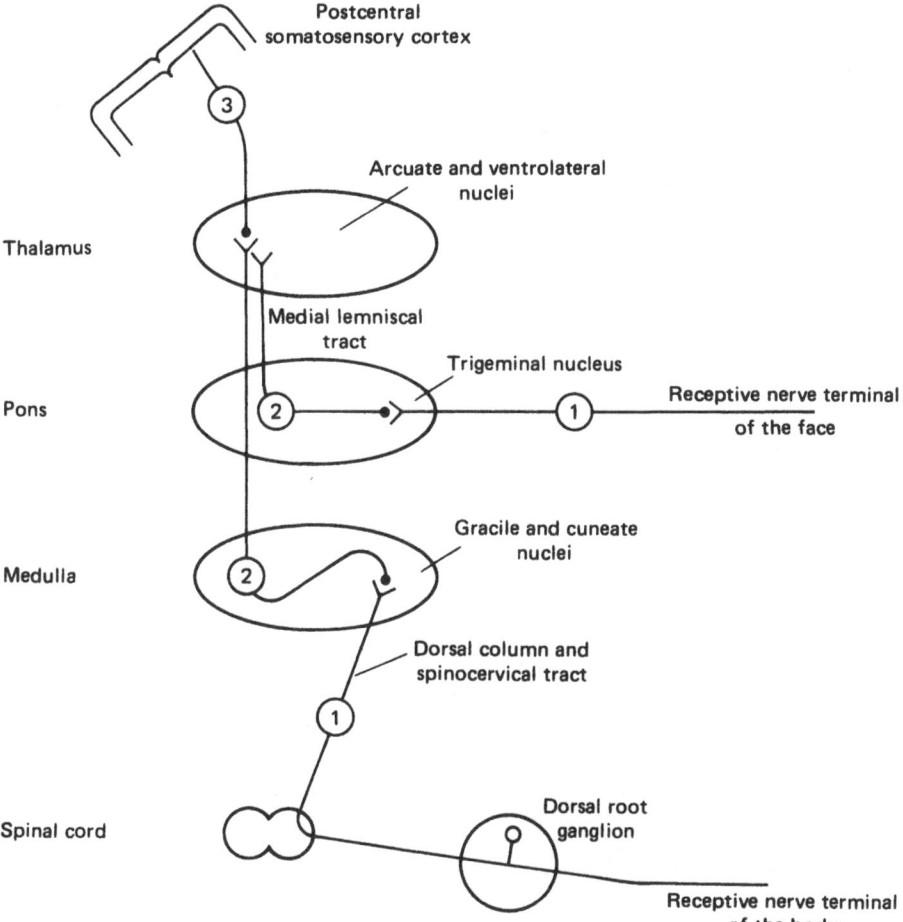

FIGURE 3.41 A schematic drawing of the entire lateral lemniscal ascending pathway of the somatosensory system. Small circled numbers indicate the order of the individual neuron.

almost infinitesimal amounts of chemicals. The olfactory and the gustatory senses have evolved into microscopic chemical laboratories with an exquisite sensitivity far beyond that of the best man-made chemodetectors. It is thought that the olfactory system, for example, is able to respond to concentrations as low as 1 part in a billion for certain chemicals.

The olfactory receptor structure is buried within the nasal cavaties of the skull. The external nose is, needless to say, plain on your face and needs little further description; but within the nares, or nostrils, the structure becomes a little less familiar. Figure 3.43 is a dissection of the nose, showing the bony septum dividing the two nostrils and the cavity within which lie the two patches of yellowish tissue, which have long been thought to be the sole olfactory receptor areas.

A possible contradiction to the statement that these yellowish patches

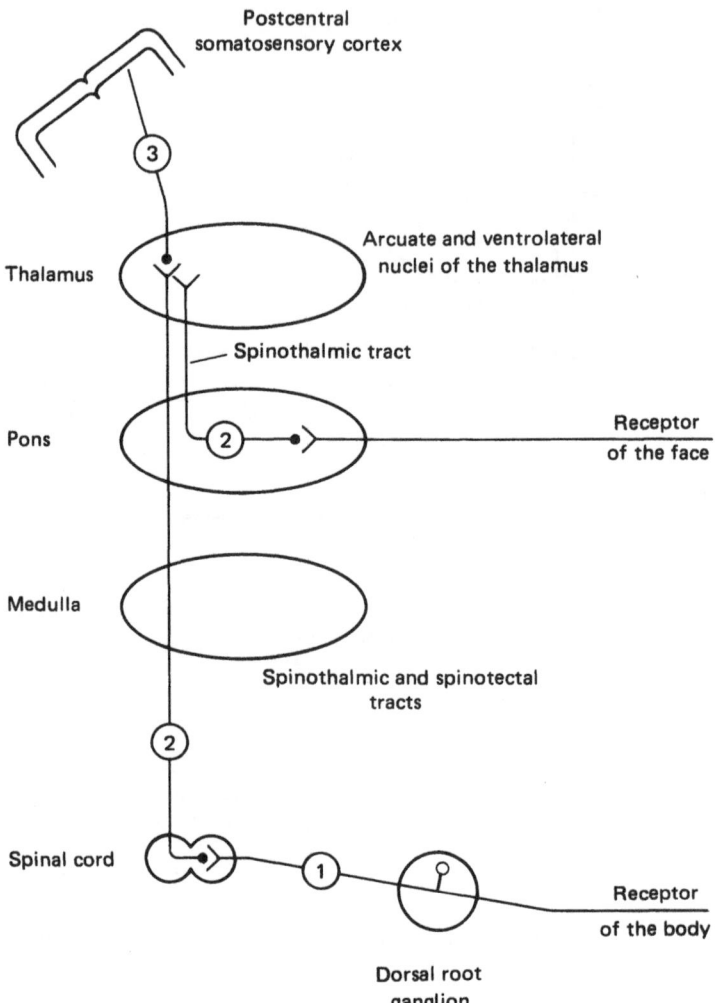

FIGURE 3.42 *A schematic drawing of the entire spinothalamic ascending pathway of the somatosensory system.*

are the sole olfactory receptors has recently emerged. Henkin (1967) has noted that some patients, operated upon for cancer of the bony shelf that underlies the brain, leading to the destruction of the yellowish olfactory patches, can still maintain odorous sensitivity. Thus, it is possible that there is either a population of olfactory receptors outside of the yellowish patch or that olfaction may be mediated by a more generalized sensitivity of other less complex receptors in the upper nasal cavity. Figure 3.44 is an optical micrograph of a cross section of the olfactory epithelium showing the general arrangement of the receptor cells and the neurons that emerge from this receptive area.

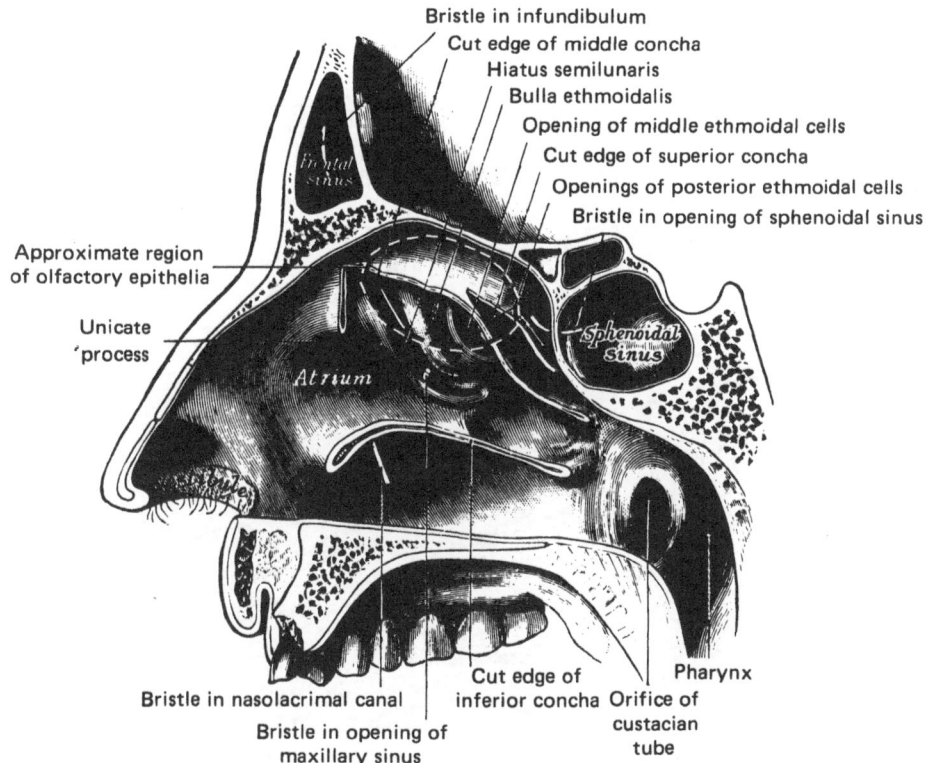

Bristle in infundibulum
Cut edge of middle concha
Hiatus semilunaris
Bulla ethmoidalis
Opening of middle ethmoidal cells
Cut edge of superior concha
Openings of posterior ethmoidal cells
Bristle in opening of sphenoidal sinus

Approximate region
of olfactory epithelia

Unicate
'process

Frontal
sinus

Sphenoidal
sinus

Atrium

Bristle in nasolacrimal canal

Bristle in opening of
maxillary sinus

Cut edge of
inferior concha

Pharynx
Orifice of
custacian
tube

FIGURE 3.43 *A drawing of the interior of the nasal cavity, showing the approximate location of the olfactory epithelium (from Goss, 1973).*

The discussion that follows describing the ultrastructure of olfactory receptors is based upon the contributions of de Lorenzo (1963). His inquiries into the structure of the olfactory epithelium have produced the diagram shown in Figure 3.45. This drawing is a cross section taken through the plate of cells, which are arranged perpendicularly to the plane of the olfactory epithelium. The tissue can be seen to be composed of an array of receptor and sustentacular (supporting) cells, all of which are columnar in shape. The sustentacular cells are of only secondary interest, and we shall say no more of them other than to point out that they are, in some cases, quite similar in shape to the receptor cells even to the extent of having the same sort of cilia at their terminal end. Whether this is a functional similarity and whether these cells are, in some way, involved in receptor action is not known.

The olfactory receptor cells are composed of two major portions: the cell body and the axon. The cell body terminates in a crownlike projection, on which are supported a group of from 6 to 12 cilia. The cilia presumably contain the actual chemosensitive sites. The axon of the olfactory receptor

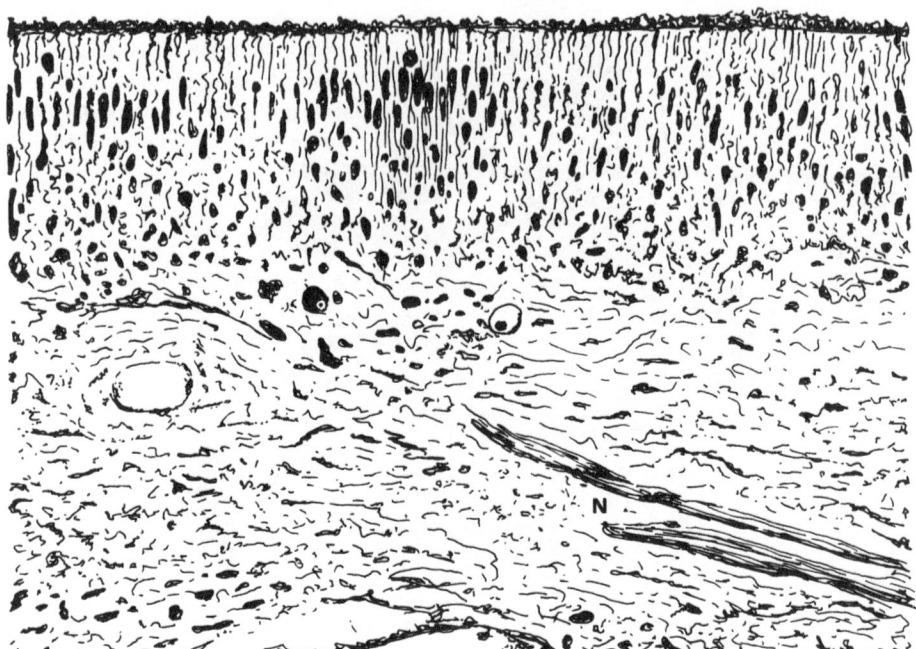

FIGURE 3.44 An optical micrograph of a cross section of the olfactory epithelium (from de Lorenzo, 1963).

cell is a long, but very fine fiber projecting upward toward the olfactory bulbs. These axons, which average only 0.2 μ in diameter, are bunched together in a surprising way. They form a cable of cells not superficially unlike any other sensory nerve, but differing in the fact that the axons are all embedded within the invaginations of a small number of relatively large Schwann cells. Figure 3.46, also reproduced from de Lorenzo's work, displays this curious pattern of organization.

The nature of the receptor sites on the cilia is unknown. As we shall see later in Chapter 10, theories of olfactory transduction are currently quite speculative and, while several have been presented over the years, none has received general acceptance.

B. The Ascending Olfactory Pathway

Figure 3.47 depicts the olfactory pathway. We see here that the olfactory receptor cells send their axons without synapsing up through perforations in the ethmoid bone at the base of the skull. After passing through this bony plate, the axons enter the olfactory bulbs, which lie under the anterior portion of the cerebral hemispheres. In the olfactory bulb, these axons

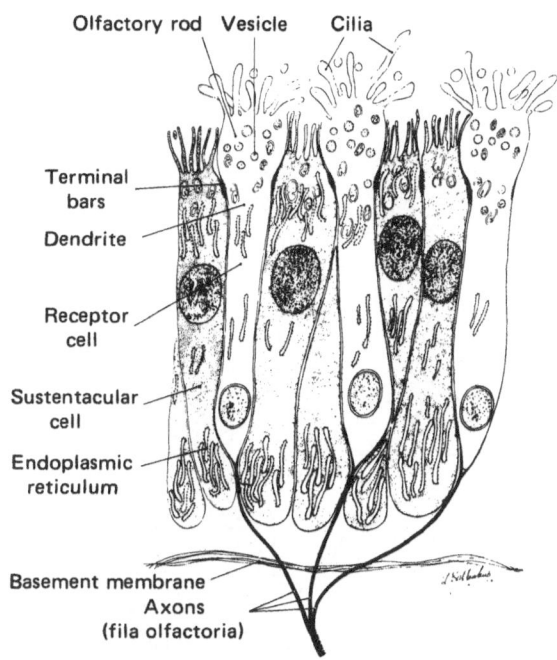

FIGURE 3.45 *Drawing of some receptor cells and sustentacular cells of the olfactory epithelium. Note particularly that there is no synapse at the base of the olfactory receptor. The axon is its own (from de Lorenzo, 1963).*

which collectively make up the stranded fila olfactoria—the primary olfactory nerve—synapse for the first time, but in highly delicate and complex structures known as the olfactory glomeruli. Fibers in each strand of the fila olfactoria seem to branch only after they have entered the glomerulus and then spread over wide areas. Each glomerulus, according to Allison and Warwick (1949), receives inputs from 26,000 receptor cells in the region of a given perforation in the ethmoid bone. The precise nature of the complicated synaptic tangle in the glomeruli is not well understood. The very fine size of the fibers and the complexities of the interconnections have made it difficult to discern exactly what structural or regional specificity may be maintained there.

However, in recent years some progress has been made in understanding olfactory bulb structure and ultrastructure. Andres (1970) has summarized much of the material stressing the comparative constancy of the olfactory bulb anatomy as one ascends the phylogenetic tree. Both fish and primates have very similar olfactory bulbs. A sketch as interpreted from electron micrographs of the microstructure of the bulb is reproduced from Andres' article in Figure 3.48. The large mitral cells can be seen to send axons centrally directly, but there are also other interneurons that convey information from the mitral cells to other afferent neurons indirectly. Inserted in this figure are also other sketches based on electron-micrographic data showing the types of synapses that have been observed in the connections between the filia olfactoria and the mitral cells of the bulb and other bulbar synapses.

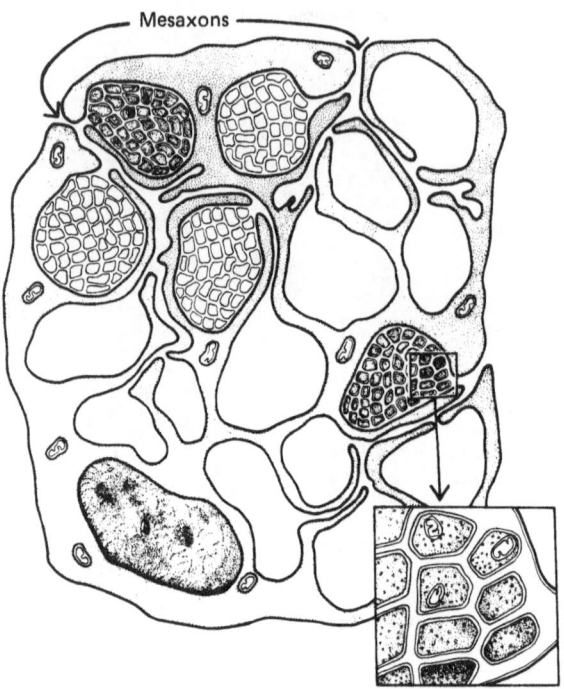

Mesaxons

FIGURE 3.46 Drawing of the manner in which the axons of the olfactory receptor cells are clustered together within the invaginations of a Schwann cell on their way to the olfactory bulb (from de Lorenzo, 1963).

Little information is available about the projections of the second- or third-order fibers from the olfactory bulbs. It is these axons that make up the olfactory tract. The next synapse of the ascending pathway is either in the amygdala or in the subcallosal gyrus of the cerebral hemisphere, depending upon which of a pair of branches of the olfactory tract one follows. From either of these centers further projections course to olfactory areas on the hippocampal and dentate gyri as well as to other lower brain centers, where olfactory information may be involved in more primitive regulatory functions than those mediating conscious experience.

X. THE GUSTATORY SYSTEM

A. The Anatomy of the Gustatory Receptor

The gross structure of the tongue is shown in Figure 3.49. It is seen to be covered with numerous bumps, hills, and ridges which are called papillae, each of which is easily seen under low magnification. Figures 3.50, 3.51, and 3.52, for example, show foliate, circumvallate, fungiform, and filliform varieties of papillae. It must be remembered that these papillae are not the receptor structures, but are more comparable to the ridges of the skin. The taste buds, which are the actual receptor structures, are smaller and are generally found in the groves between the papillae; but the fungiform

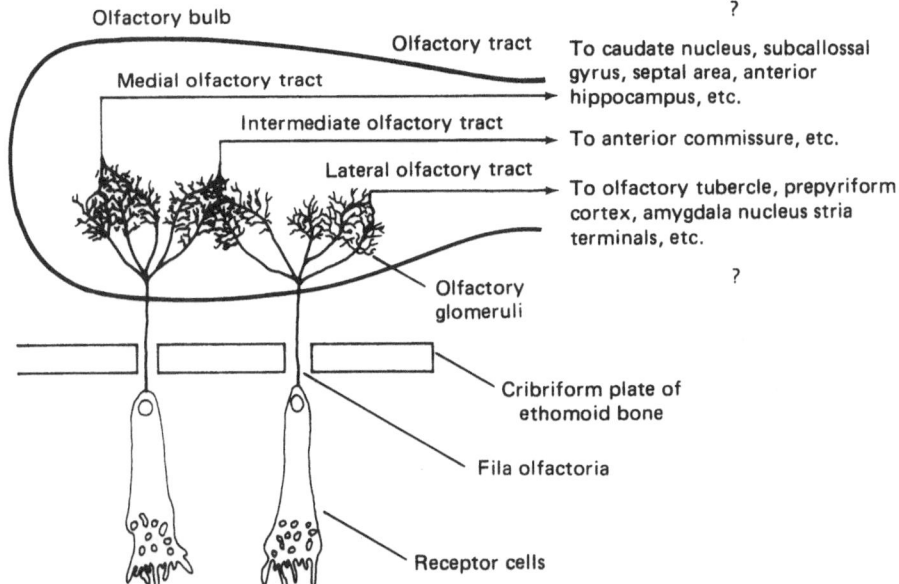

FIGURE 3.47 *A schematic drawing of part of the olfactory ascending pathway. Beyond the olfactory bulb, little is known of the specific details of the pathway.*

papilla, for one divergent example, usually has the taste bud centered in its surface. Note, in particular, the porelike opening to the receptor taste bud itself in the photograph of the fungiform papilla. The arrangement of a typical taste bud is more specifically illustrated in Figure 3.53, showing that each bud is in fact a cluster of cells.

Originally, optical studies had tended to support the notion that the cells in a taste bud were also of two distinct kinds—sustentacular and sensory—and the assumption was that the organization was very much the same as the receptor tissue of the olfactory system. Several different lines of investigation have clearly shown, however, that the story is not at all similar.

The first indication that this story was too simple arose as a result of the optical micrographic techniques themselves. What had originally appeared to be a simple dichotomy between sensory and sustentacular cells turned out to be, once again, two extremes on a continuum. Many cells, transitional in form between the sustentacular cells and the receptor cells, were frequently observed. A second line of evidence, also derived from optical micrographic technique, was the appearance of a very large number of receptor cells, which seemed to be in an advanced state of disintegration.

Beidler, Nejad, Smallman, and Tateda (1960) and de Lorenzo (1960) all realized that both of these pieces of information hinted at the existence of an extraordinary mechanism, namely, that the sustentacular cells and the receptor cells are one and the same, and that the observed structural

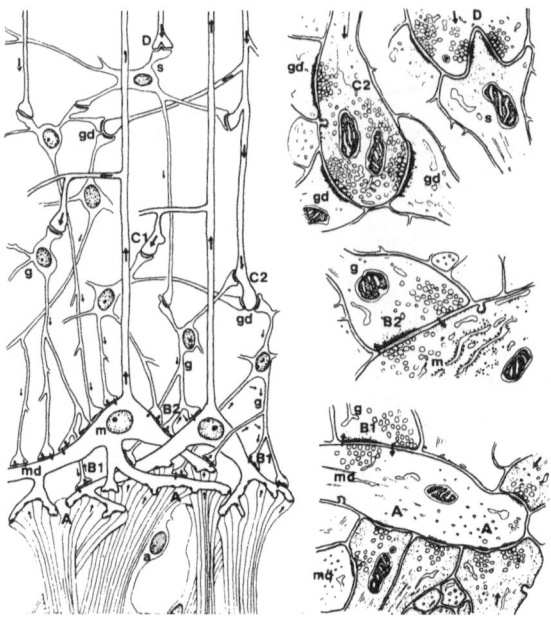

FIGURE 3.48 A drawing based on electronmicrographic studies of the fish's olfactory bulb, showing the variety of synaptic interconnections. Small arrows indicate the afferent direction, and all letters refer to different classes of synaptic connections. Insert figures show some of the synaptic contacts in more detail (from Andres, 1970).

differences reflect different stages in the life cycle of a single kind of cell. Such a cellular metamorphosis has the advantage of making practical sense in another way. Of all of the sense modalities, the gustatory receptors are the ones that are the most vigorously insulted by their environment. The visual and auditory senses deal with the most delicate stimulus energies and are protected in a number of ways. (Yet even so we have already discussed regenerative mechanisms for rods and cones.) The olfactory receptor is only exposed to the delicate vapors of gaseous stimuli. The skin is the only receptor system in which energy levels approach those falling on the tongue, and even then its receptors are protected by various means. But, consider the gustatory environment. Corrosive juices of all kinds, wide temperature differences, and mechanical abuse are all the lot of the gustatory receptors. Furthermore, the receptor tissue is not even continuously bathed in a protective fluid or buried deep in an inaccessible inner chamber. The delicate membrane of this neuron, perhaps more than any other neural tissue, might be expected to deteriorate as a result of this onslaught of energetic and destructive stimuli.

An adaptive solution to this problem of environmental insult is to have a replaceable sort of receptor. Two problems, then, must be solved. The first, of course, is where would the new receptor come from? The second concerns how the receptor can be disengaged from its afferent axons so that they, too, will not have to be replaced.

The answer to the first question regarding the source of new receptor cells has been answered by Beidler, Nejad, Smallman, and Tateda's (1960) experiments using radioactive isotopes. (See also Beidler and Smallman,

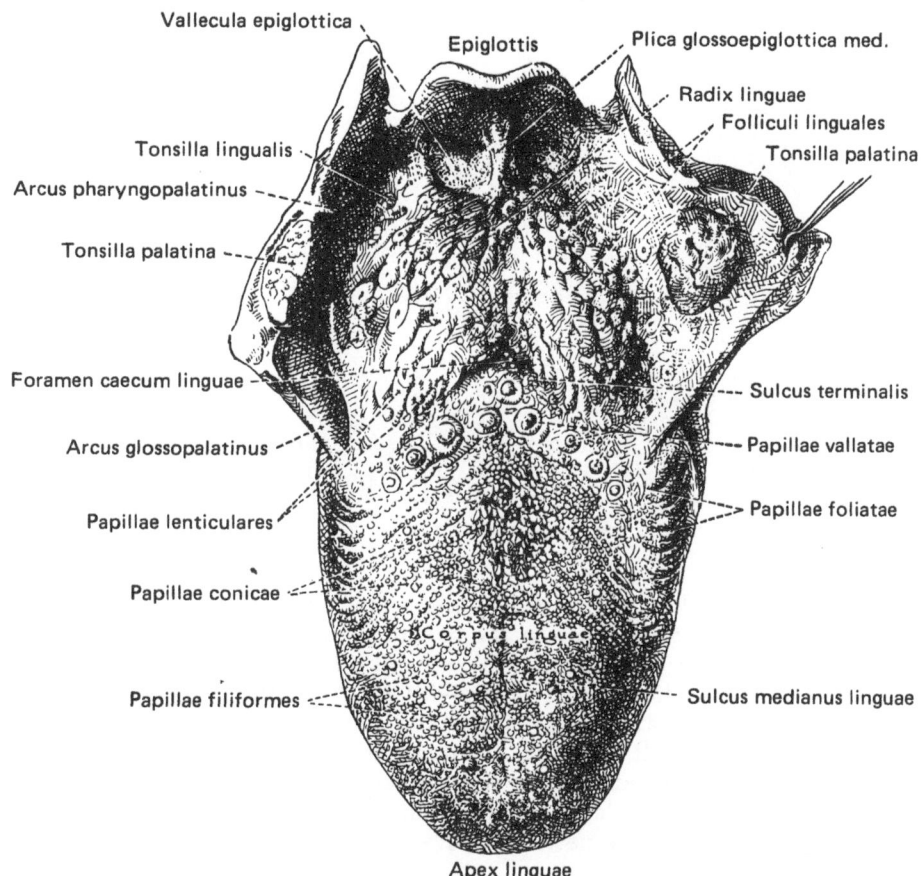

Vallecula epiglottica

Epiglottis

Plica glossoepiglottica med.

Radix linguae

Folliculi linguales

Tonsilla lingualis

Tonsilla palatina

Arcus pharyngopalatinus

Tonsilla palatina

Foramen caecum linguae

Sulcus terminalis

Arcus glossopalatinus

Papillae vallatae

Papillae foliatae

Papillae lenticulares

Papillae conicae

Corpus linguae

Papillae filiformes

Sulcus medianus linguae

Apex linguae

FIGURE 3.49 A drawing of the gross anatomy of the tongue (from Goss, 1973, after Eycleshymer and Jones).

1965.) Assuming that during metamorphosis, receptor cells would be exhibiting a very high degree of growth and change, Beidler and his colleagues decided to briefly irrigate the tongue of a rat with a solution that contained radioactive thymidine, one of the amino acids required in protein synthesis. Figure 3.54 is a graph showing the amount of radioactive material present at any given time after the irrigation. The amount of radioactive material is measured by a photographic technique (autoradiography), in which slices of the tissue taken at different times following irrigation are placed on a sensitive plate. The emitted radioactivity from the radio-thymidine exposes the silver grains in the plate in proportion to the amount of activity still held within the cell. Cells that were in an active stage of division and growth tended to acquire the radioactive thymidine and incorporate it into their structure. During the period in which a cell is

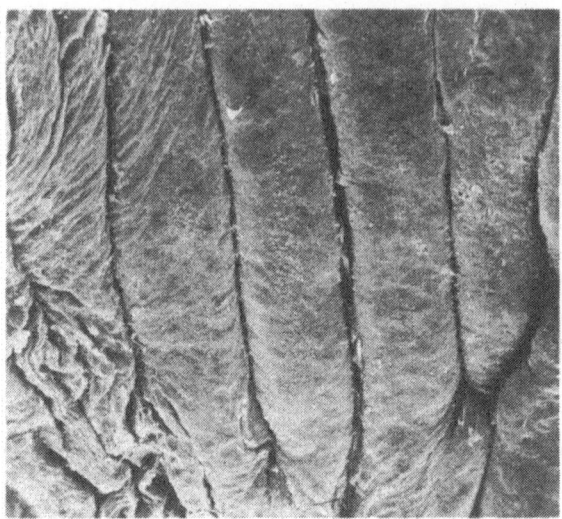

FIGURE 3.50 Foliate papillae of the rabbit's tongue (from Beidler, 1969).

rapidly metamorphizing, it absorbs increasing amounts of the thymidine, and this increase is reflected in the gradually increasing amount of radioactivity during the early hours following the irrigation. After the cell has completed its division and is stable—that is, no further mitotic division or growth is occurring—the amount of radioactivity remains relatively constant. Then the cell begins to disintegrate, and the radioactive thymidine is released to be washed away in the animal's mouth. The autoradiographic density then begins to decline until finally all of the activity is gone. This suggests that at this time new cells have replaced the radioactive older ones

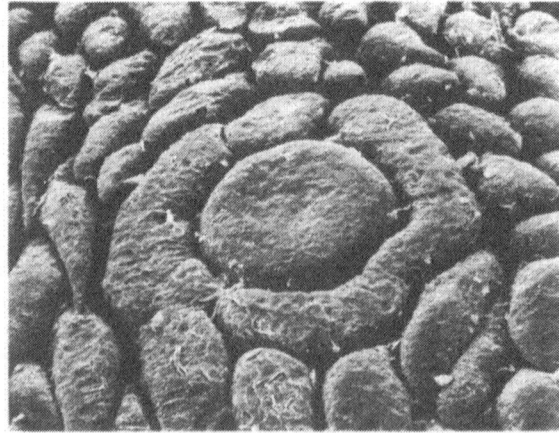

FIGURE 3.51 Circumvallate papilla of the dog's tongue (from Beidler, 1969).

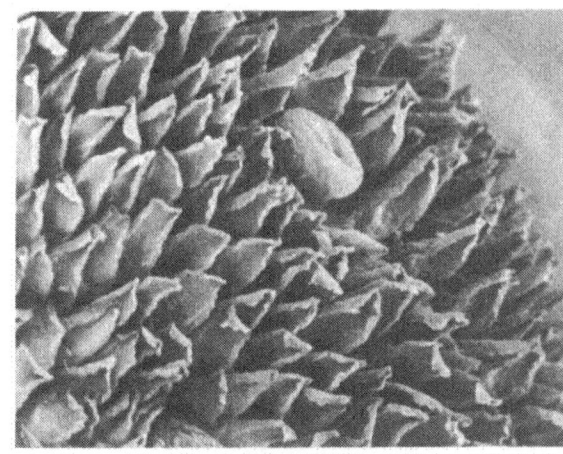

FIGURE 3.52 Filliform (leaf-like) and one fungiform papillae of the rabbit's tongue (from Beidler, 1969).

that have died. Since the radioactive material was not present during their metamorphosis, it is not available to be incorporated into their structure, and they do not display any activity beyond that of the normal background. The answer to the question of where the new receptor cells come from is, therefore, that they metamorphize from sustentacular cells.

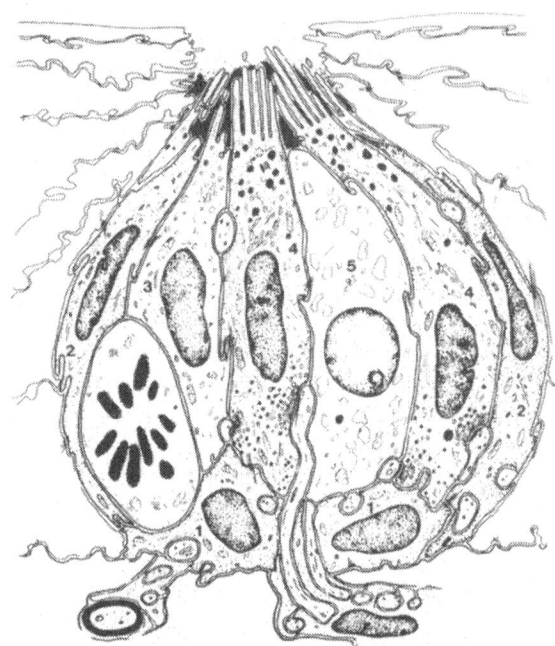

FIGURE 3.53 Cross-sectional drawing of a taste bud in a rabbit, showing a basal cell (1), an epithelial cell (2), a metamorphising epithelial cell (3), a fully matured receptor cell (4), and a degenerating receptor cell (5) (courtesy of K. H. Andres of Ruhr-University Bochum).

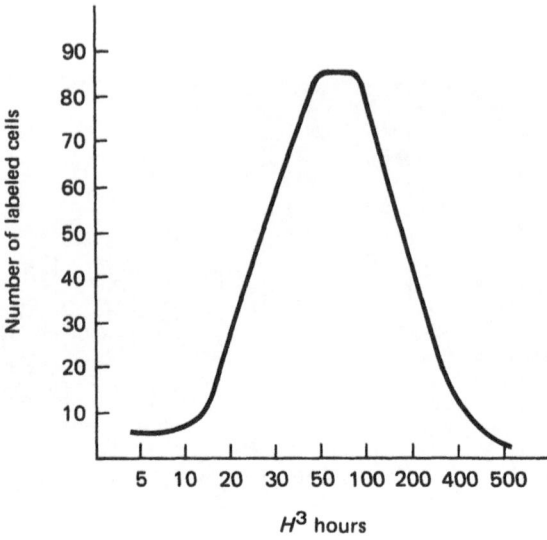

FIGURE 3.54 A graph show-
ing the number of radioac-
tively labeled cells present in
the taste bud of a rat as a
function of the number of
hours following the injection
of radioactive thymidine.
This sort of data is the basis
of the suggestion that there
is a gradual replacement of
the receptor cells in taste
buds over a period of several
weeks (from de Lorenzo,
1963).

This migration and renewal of gustatory receptor cells has also been
shown to occur in other mammals. De Lorenzo (1963) demonstrated the
phenomenon in the rabbit, and Conger and Wells (1969) have shown it
to occur in the mouse's tongue.

The second problem, which now has to be dealt with, is how these
cells are connected with their afferent axons. If the receptors were connected in the same way as the olfactory cells, that is, their axons were continuous extensions of the receptor itself, the disintegration of the receptor
would be expected to destroy the gustatory axon as in any cell that has lost
its nucleus. From de Lorenzo's pictures it can be seen, however, that the
gustatory axon and receptor are, quite to the contrary, not parts of the
same cell, but that there is a synapse between the two. Figure 3.55 suggests
the nature of this synapse. De Lorenzo has observed two different kinds
of terminals near the base of the gustatory receptor cells. They may be
distinguished on the basis of size. The larger neuronal endings always seem
to be squeezed between two receptors in a way that suggests that they
have only superficial functional contact with either one. In fact, de Lorenzo
has also considered the possibility that they do not synapse at all with the
receptor cells, but that these "free" nerve endings may represent an alternative possible receptor mechanism. He also points out that if these large
axons are synaptically connected with receptors, then it is also clear that
they always innervate more than a single one.

The smaller axons, however, have a far more intimate interconnection
with receptors cells. Each small axon terminates in an invagination in the
body of the receptor, where the synaptic connection is presumably made
and the tiny axon connects, without branching, to one and only one cell.

The most important point to remember about these gustatory receptor
synapses is that they are all transient. As the receptor cells metamorphisize,
migrate, and degenerate, the nerve fibers must be passed along from one

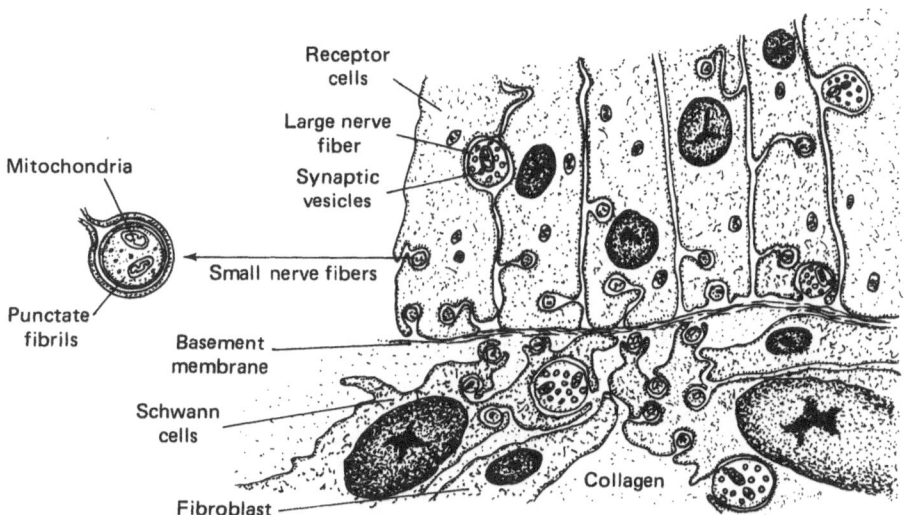

FIGURE 3.55 A drawing based on electronmicrographic data of the synaptic arrangements at the base of a gustatory receptor cell, showing the temporary arrangement whereby a neuron can be passed from a degenerating cell to a newly metamorphising receptor (from de Lorenzo, 1963).

cell to the next. That is, neurons, which presumably remain almost stationary, must disconnect themselves from a dying receptor and reconnect themselves to the new cell moving in to replace it. Thus, a certain constancy of localization is maintained in spite of the movement and death of gustatory receptors. Cells, at a particular stage of their development, may be located at a specific place and possibly even have a specific sensitivity or, more properly, a specific range of sensitivities. The neurons with which they interconnect then would be capable of maintaining whatever spatial information is characteristic of that place or stage of development. Whatever the exact details of the gustatory transduction process, it is quite clear that this transient synaptic interconnection and the migrating receptor cell represent parts of a remarkable adaptive mechanism of great interest to the student of sensory coding.

B. The Ascending Gustatory Pathway

Because of the difficulty of applying impulsive gustatory stimuli, perhaps less is known of the anatomy of the ascending pathway for taste than for any of the other senses. The axons that synapse with the taste receptors themselves are the fibers of cells that have their cell bodies in the dorsal root ganglia of the seventh, ninth, and tenth cranial nerves. Figure 3.56 traces a possible pathway, but ignores other complications of the path from the tongue to the solitary nucleus of the medulla. From there, however, the route of the gustatory pathway is almost completely unknown until the fibers arrive at the contralateral arcuate nucleus of the thalamus. Only very recently has a relay in the parabrachial nuclei of the pons been dis-

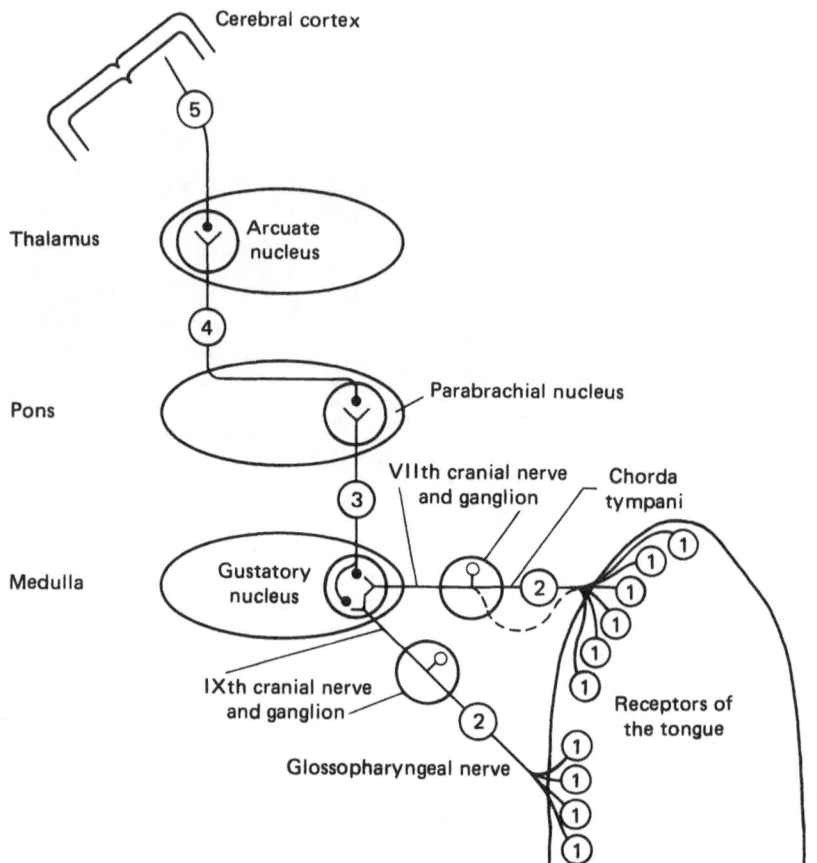

FIGURE 3.56 A schematic drawing of the gustatory pathway. This figure omits much of the complexity of the course of the nerves parallel to the chorda tympani.

covered by Norgren and Leonard (1971) in rats. From the thalamus the fibers presumably project to the precentral region of the cortex, which is supposed to be associated with taste sensory experience. It is also probably true, however, that this is a gross oversimplification of a pathway, which most certainly has other projections in the brain stem and the cortex.

XI. AN INTERIM SUMMARY

So far we have considered the anatomy of each of the sensory systems in a more or less independent manner. Yet it is clear that there are many common features that all share with the others. For example, it is interesting to note that many of the sensory structures have some sort of ciliated projection or are themselves ciliary derivatives. A consideration of the general function of receptors suggests why such a process would be an adaptive one. Receptors must necessarily come into contact with the outside world, and an elongated ciliary structure not only provides a convenient means of protruding the sensitive surface toward the stimulus energy, but also increases the receptive area at very little expense in cellular volume. The outer segment of the rod or cone in this context compares with the hairs of the auditory or vestibular receptor as well as the more obviously ciliated structures of the olfactory and gustatory receptor cells. Even those receptor endings that are nothing more than nerve endings (with or without encapsulations) also fall into the general range of this rubric. Whether this anatomic similarity reflects some sort of biochemical similiarity is probably not a question that can be answered at the present time.

Another important general consideration concerning receptor structure is that there appear to be two different kinds of receptor cell organizations present. In the first case, the cell has no real axon of its own —only a brief terminal arborization, which is not capable of producing spike action potentials. In the alternative case, the cell does have an axon, and this conducting fiber may not synapse until some more central portion of the nervous system. The meaning of this dichotomy of structure may lie in any one of several possible explanations. Clearly those cells that disintegrate and are replaced (like the gustatory ones) do well to have no axon of their own to drag along in this replacement process. Clearly also, additional opportunities for information processing occur when the synaptic connections are more peripheral.

Furthermore, it has become increasingly clear in recent years, particularly as a result of some of the extraordinary electron micrographs, that many more receptor structures than had previously been thought to do so receive control information from the central nervous system. The appearance of so many of what are apparently efferent synapses on the auditory and vestibular receptor cells and second- or third-order olfactory and visual cells suggest possibilities of centrifugal control of sensitivity at the most peripheral levels. Few electrophysiological studies have yet examined this potentially important process (indeed, we are just beginning to read of studies in which stimulus-produced electropotentials are recorded from receptors), yet it is certain that systematic studies of the feedback properties of peripheral neural structures will play an important role in the research of the decades ahead.

This, then, brings our discussion of the anatomy of receptor systems to a close. This material is important in providing a basis for further discussions of the processes of sensory action, as well as in the interest intrinsic in the structures themselves. We shall now turn to a discussion of the molecular and membrane properties of these structures, which underly transducer action in the receptors.

CHAPTER 4: SENSORY TRANSDUCTION

I. INTRODUCTION

Sensory transduction has been defined as the combination of processes that converts the physical energy of a potential stimulus into neuroelectric energy. Within this broad rubric, we shall try to emphasize that there are several distinct and sequential processes involved in sensory energy conversions. It must be understood that reference is not being made to the separate fact that the several different receptors use several different energy conversion mechanisms, but rather that within each of the sensory modalities, transduction cannot be considered a unitary process. Quite to the contrary, it must be considered to be a train of distinguishable stages, each of which must be explained in turn before we can claim to have full knowledge of the transduction process of any given modality.

The anatomical units of prime importance in the transductive process are, of course, the receptor cells, those specialized neurons in which, typically, the most distal elements have evolved remarkable abilities to convert incredibly small amounts of one or another kind of physical energy into nerve cell membrane potential changes. We have already described the anatomy of a wide variety of receptor cell types in Chapter 3. The infinitesimal quantities of potential stimulus energy required to activate any of these receptor cells is emphasized by the fact that the thresholds of some of these cells are at or near the minimum theoretical limit. For example, a single quantum of light is thought to be able to activate a single photoreceptor in the human eye. As another example, it has been calculated that if the hair cells of the cochlea were tuned to any finer degree of sensitivity, we would constantly be aware of the rush of blood through the vessels of the ear or even of the Brownian motion of molecules in the air.

Though we are knowledgeable about many of the details of transduction in some sense modalities, it is also important, on the other hand, for the reader to remember that there are great lacunae in our knowledge of the various neuroelectric steps and membrane properties of some others. While we have a remarkably detailed picture of the primary photochemical process in the eye, very little is known about the mechanism of the next stage—how the photochemical breakdown products are able to produce the generator potential. In the ear we can conceptualize a plausible mechanism for the production of the generator potential, but it is not so clear what particular mechanical mechanism can be identified as the primary sensory action. To understand the incompleteness of our knowledge as well as to emphasize the multilevel nature of the transduction process, it will be useful to pose a hierarchy of questions. Each of these questions emphasizes one of the several different intermediate stages of the total transduction process at which any given discussion is being carried on.

1. What pretransductive modification of the adequate stimulus is produced by the nonneural sensory apparatus of each sense organ?
2. What is the site and nature of the primary sensory action?
3. How does the energy absorbing process of the primary sensory action lead to the generator or receptor potential?
4. How does the generator or receptor potential lead to the production of the propagated spike action potential?

Figure 4.1 is another way of considering this same idea—that there is a series of sequential steps involved in the transductive process for any receptor modality. This figure depicts several current notions. First, it symbolically emphasizes the multilevel nature of the transductive process. Second, it also reminds us of the fact that though our attention is focused in this book on the information processing in the ascending or afferent direction, there are also demonstrable modifications of even the most peripheral stages of the transductive mechanism by efferent feedback information from the central nervous system. The accommodation of the lens of the eye, pupil contraction, stapedial muscle reflex action in the middle ear, and complex synaptic effects in all of the receptor systems are all examples of how the sensory process can be altered by signals from central nervous structures.

Another important new general notion, which is introduced by Figure 4.1, is that there really are two distinguishable pathways by which spike action potentials may be produced. Receptor cells may produce either receptor or generator potentials. These graded, summatable, and nonpropagated potentials are both presumed to be alternative first steps in the neural encoding of a physical stimulus, and both act as pre-

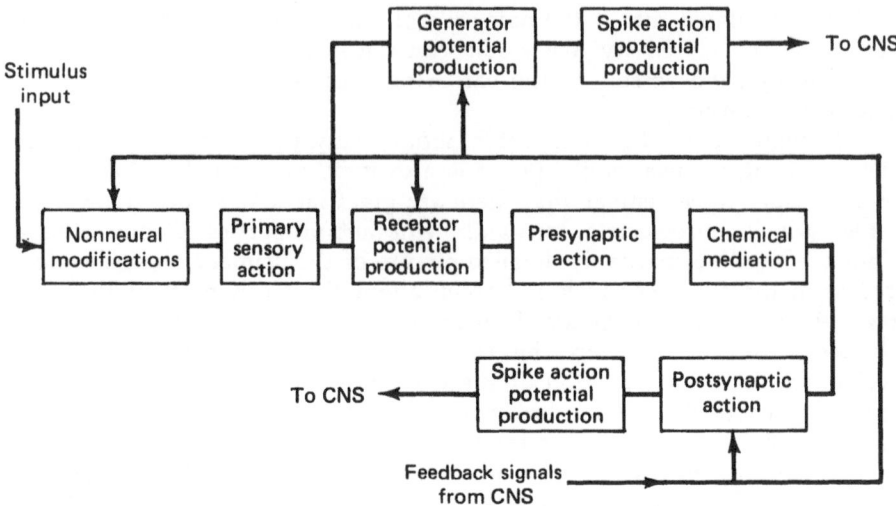

FIGURE 4.1 *A schematic drawing emphasizing the steps in the transduction process and the two alternative pathways (one involving synaptic transmission and one direct) possible in the process converting physical energy to pulse coded spike action potentials.*

cursors of propagated signals. But a distinction must be drawn between a receptor and a generator potential based on an anatomical difference between the two different receptor cell types. We shall define a receptor potential as one that does not lead to a spike action potential within the same cell. Its effect is felt through the mediation of a synaptic action, and thus a variety of different kinds of other forms of encoding occur prior to the production of the propagated spike action potential. A generator potential, on the other hand, is a graded potential produced in a receptor cell that has its own axon. The generator potential, therefore, is the direct precursor of a spike action potential. The distinction, obviously, is one based on whether or not the receptor itself is but a specialized terminal portion of a neuron with its own elongated axon, or whether it is only an axonless unit, which synapses almost immediately, and which has no membrane capable of supporting a spike. In either case, generator and receptor potentials appear to be universal intermediate mechanisms in receptor function even if they have not been unequivocally identified in all modalities.

The problem of the criterion for accepting some candidate graded potential as the true receptor or generator potential deserves some brief mention here. In almost all of the sense modalities, there is some sort of a potential recordable, which could possibly be that potential. Proof that a given potential plays that role is not always easy to find. But there are certain criteria that can be applied to limit the range of possible candidates. For example, the candidate receptor potential must be related to the stimulus in a way that makes it clear that it is a direct result of the application of the stimulus. Second, it must be independently shown to be necessary for the elicitation of the spike action potential train. If a graded potential can be reduced without substantially reducing the spike frequency, it is unlikely that it is a receptor potential no matter how closely it follows the stimulus. Furthermore, it should also be appreciated that there is always the possibility that these graded potentials are, in fact, signals reflecting some other more fundamental (perhaps chemical) process, which really is the direct intermediary between the stimulus and the spike train. Thus, the electrical potential itself may not be the immediate stimulus for a spike train—only a concomitant of the more or less graded chemical processes, which are produced by the stimulus, but which we have no way yet to directly observe. If this latter alternative is true, and if the generator potential is closely associated with the more direct process, everything we shall have to say will still hold, but the words "generator or receptor potential" will become something of an allegory for the more basic process, which we do not yet know how to measure.

In general, receptor potentials are excitatory, that is, increase subsequent neural activity, but this is not a universal. Arvanitaki, Takeuchi, and Chalazonitis (1967) report that both excitatory and inhibitory generator potentials can be produced in the same large and general-purpose receptor cells of the subesophageal ganglion of certain molluscs as a function of the kind of olfactory stimulus. Boeckh (1967) also discusses some olfactory receptors in the carrion beetle, which can produce either inhibitory or excitatory potentials depending upon the nature of the stimulating chemical. It is not at all clear whether an inhibitory potential produced by a sensory stimulus ultimately leading to a reduction in the amount of subsequent activity should be termed a generator potential, but there is no generally agreed-upon term to describe such actions. Nevertheless, we must accept the general notion that both excitatory and inhibitory generator potentials can be produced by receptors. It is obvious that inhibitory generator potentials may play an important role in establishing patterns of sensory coding even though their primary action is to reduce the amount of information flowing through the receptor.

It should be clearly appreciated that there is no direct relation between excitatory and inhibitory on the one hand, and depolarizing and hyperpolarizing (respectively) on the other. Excitatory receptor potentials are hyperpolarizing in the vertebrate retina, but depolarizing in the invertebrate eye, for example. In general, it seems that if the spikes are produced in the second-order cell, then excitation is associated with depolarization. On the other hand, if the second-order cells (like the bipolars of the retina) do not propagate spikes, then the direction of polarization is not associated uniquely with either excitation or inhibition.

In general, inhibitory signals are as good candidates for the receptor potential as excitatory ones. Some systems operate on a basis in which any deviation from some spontaneous level is considered a signal. Others operate through integrative circuits, which can actually enhance signal output at one point by inhibitory inputs at another. Furthermore, sometimes inhibitory effects can establish neural patterns more sharply by increasing the contrast between inhibited and excited regions.

Finally, it should be noted that inhibitory effects can be produced by locking the membrane permeability, as well as by a heightening of the potential difference that has to be overcome by any stimulus whose effects are depolarizing.

We can sum up this brief introduction to the transduction process by emphasizing the specific functions of receptor cells. They have all evolved specific abilities as energy transformation systems capable of interfacing the organism with the events in his environment. These mechanisms evolved out of and are specializations of more primitive generalized forms of organic sensitivity to chemical, thermal, or photic and mechanical stimuli, which can still be observed in simple animals and single cells. Of course, in the sense organ these primitive excitabilities have been so refined that the individual receptor cell displays a very much heightened sensitivity (lowered threshold) to one particular stimulus energy form, thus providing the initial means of differential encoding of the different kinds of stimulus energies. In more primitive cells, these organic excitabilities were, and are, combined with effector capabilities: the same cell would both sense and respond. But it is a general property of higher organisms that the extreme increase in sensitivity to one kind of energy is coupled with specialization in function and few, if any, sensory cells retain any effector capability in the higher animals.

In the rest of this chapter, we shall try to answer each of the questions in the hierarchy outlined above for those sensory modalities for which some reasonably complete story exists. For some of the receptors, we can paint a rather complete picture of one stage of the transductive process, while for others we know more about some other stage. Although we shall emphasize, in later parts of this book, the uniformity and common features of neural coding, it is not possible to do so in this section. The individual receptor cells have evolved in unique ways to increase their sensitivity to a particular adequate stimulus.

II. TRANSDUCER ACTION IN THE EYE

A. Nonneural Stimulus Modifications

Before light can participate in the primary sensory action, it must pass through a large amount of intermediate tissue. In fact, as we saw in our chapter on anatomy, incident light must even pass through the several retinal layers before impinging upon the receptors.

One possible explanation for the inverted retina is based upon the fact that the photoreceptors (in particular, rods) are critically dependent upon intimate contact with the pigment epithelium. Since the pigment epithelium is so opaque, a formidable barrier to light transmission would exist if the photoreceptors faced the outside world. Other explanations of the inverted retina have also been based on the fact of its origins from the ectoderm of the primitive embryo.

Thus, among other changes, light passes through tissues, which selectively absorb certain wavelengths of the incident light; it is modulated in intensity by an iris diaphragm, whose opening is dependent upon the amount of light; it is focused by a lens with centrally controllable accomodation; and it is scattered by imperfect optics of all of the components. The important generality to remember, however, is that all of these changes do not involve, in any way, any kind of an energy transformation. The light may be redirected or reduced in intensity, but it is always the same sort of electromagnetic energy as when it initially entered the eye. It is not until the light falls on the highly specialized photochemicals in the outer segments of the rods and cones that a chemical action, which initiates the conversion of the electromagnetic energy to electroneural activity, takes place.

B. The Primary Sensory Action in Vision

On the basis of the work of a number of distinguished biochemists, but most notably that of George Wald and his colleagues, the story we have to tell about the primary sensory action in vision is one of the most complete of any we shall discuss in this chapter.

To summarize very briefly, the picture of the primary sensory action of vision, which Wald and others have developed over the years, asserts that the outer segments of the rods and cones contain large molecules that break into two parts under the influence of incident light. The breakdown products resulting from the photodecomposition of these molecules in some unknown way induces a change in the membrane polarization, which can be considered to be the receptor potential. Wald's most important contributions lie in his elucidation of the mechanisms of the breakdown of the photochemical and the sequential series of intermediary substances, which are produced by spontaneous decomposition following the initial configurational change in the original photosensitive macromolecule. In other words, he was mainly responsible for establishing the various steps in the photochemical "cycle" underlying the primary visual action.

Now let us consider the story in a little greater detail. For a number of years, it had been known that a curious violet chemical was involved in the visual process. Boll in 1877 had discovered this substance and had named it rhodopsin. The general idea that there was a cycle, which involved rhodopsin and its breakdown products, had been suggested by Selig Hecht in the 1930s. Wald (1968) states (in his Nobel acceptance speech) that it was under the influence of Hecht that he began a search for the chemical constituents, which had appeared as only hypothetical structures in Hecht's theories. In 1933 Wald made an initial, though not unexpected discovery; vitamin A was present in large amounts in the retina, and in the next year he followed this up with another important discovery. Wald (1933) detected the presence of an organic substance he at that time was to call retinene. Retinene ultimately turned out to be an aldehyde of vitamin A—a substance long known to play an important role in night vision. We shall consider this issue in more detail later, but first let us skip ahead a few years and alter our terminology to the more modern one. Wald and others have now agreed that vitamin A should be called retinol and retinene, its aldehyde, retinal, to emphasize their very important role in the visual process. (An aldehyde is a chemical product produced by the oxidation of a precursor such as retinol.)

The picture was now set for the formalization of the original notion of the photochemical breakdown that Hecht had proposed and the identification of some of the specific chemicals, which had only been algebraic expressions in his mathematical model. Wald defined the steps in what is now known as the "Rhodopsin Cycle." He and his students and colleagues have identified the specific molecules and the nature of the reactions that occur under the influence of incident light. In doing so, they have provided us with a very specific statement of the primary visual action.

The essence of the now generally accepted Wald model is that the visual pigment found in each of the receptor cells of the eyes of a wide variety of animals always consists of a typical kind of photosensitive molecule composed of two essential parts or moieties. The one part—a carotenoid (so named because pure suspensions often have a typical orange-red color)—is a relatively simple structure. In fact, the carotenoid is a special isomeric form of retinal. The other part of the visual pigment is a much larger organic structure—a protein with a molecular weight of 30,000 to 40,000. Though we now appreciate that there are many different kinds of this large proteinaceous portion, Wald has coined the generic name opsin for all of these complex structures regardless of the animal or photoreceptor in which they might be found.

Opsins differ in two ways. Details of the organic structure vary from species to species and are, therefore, said to be species specific. But even within one animal, there are frequently several different kinds of opsins. In vertebrates one opsin is responsible for the compound visual pigment found in the rods, while the trio of photochemicals observed in cones suggests three different kinds of cone opsins. In some other animals, the anatomical separation may be quite a bit more unusual than simply different cells in the same sense organ. For example, two photopigments each containing a different kind of opsin are found at opposite ends of the body in the crayfish. One is found in the anterior eye, while the other is found in a simple photoreceptor cell in the tail.

Nevertheless, the model of a composite molecule composed of a large proteinaceous moiety bonded to a smaller structure is probably the standard configuration of all visual photopigments and the key notion of the present Wald theory. We shall now consider some of the details of the smaller part—the carotenoid—as an initial step in elucidating the full details of this most important theory.

Retinol exists within the body in a balanced equilibrium between itself and its aldehyde—retinal. The structure formula of one kind of retinol—retinol$_1$—and one kind of retinal—retinal$_1$—are shown in Figure 4.2 (a) and (b). It can be seen that the two differ very litle. Only the bonding of the terminal OH or O group differs. Retinol$_1$, however, is not an active participant in the visual process. Its main importance is in the role it plays as a precursor of retinal. The quantities of retinol$_1$, therefore,

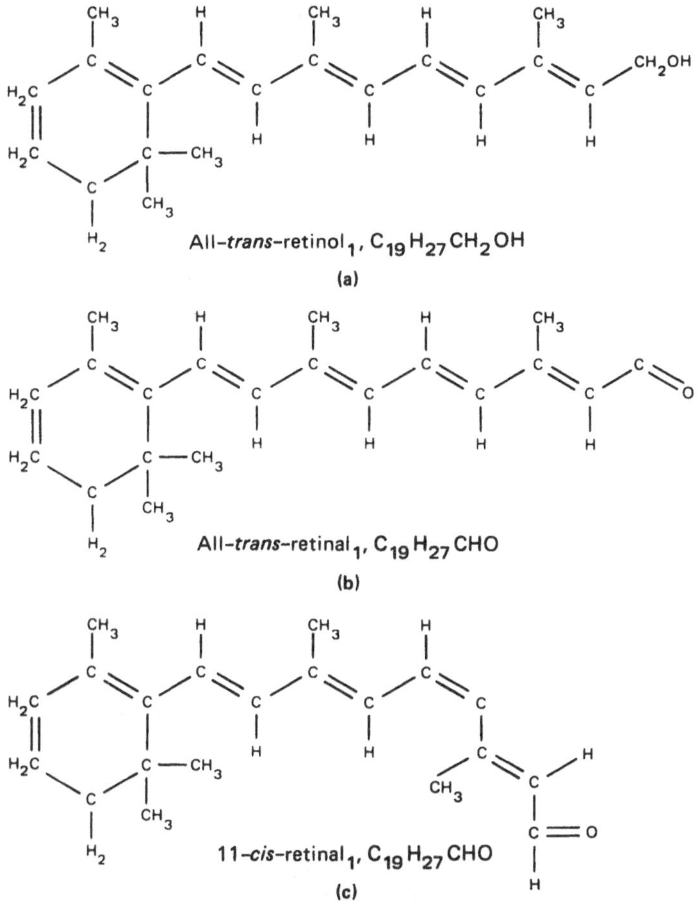

FIGURE 4.2 The structural formulas of three of the important molecules involved in the photochemical cycle. See text for details (adapted from Wald, 1968).

determine directly the availability of retinal₁, and thus retinol₁ deficiencies in the diet lead only indirectly to visual inadequacies. The equilibrium between retinol₁ and retinal₁ is balanced such that the oxidation process producing retinal₁ has the lesser rate constant of the two reactions; thus retinal₁ is produced and maintained only as it is used in the visual cycle and only, it is thought, in the retina.

A structure analysis of retinal₁ is further complicated by the fact that it can exist in several different stereoisomeric forms. All of the isomers of retinal₁, of course, have the same chemical formula $C_{19}H_{27}CHO$, but they differ in the three-dimensional pattern into which the molecules are arranged. The physical shape of the molecule is a function of the angles assumed at bonding points between adjacent molecules. The various stereoisomers of retinal₁ differ principally because of differences in bonding angles at carbon-to-carbon junctions. An important fact, upon which visual photochemistry is based, is that the chemistry of stereoisomers can differ even though their formulas are identical.

The two most important of the several stereoisomeric forms in which retinal$_1$ can exist are the *all-trans* and the *11-cis* shapes. The all-trans form was illustrated by the drawing in Figure 4.2 (b) above. The shape of its tail is essentially straight, because all of the carbon-to-carbon bonds in that tail are in the same direction.

The 11-cis stereoisomer of retinal$_1$ is illustrated in Figure 4.2 (c). In this case there is a bend at the 11th carbon atom, which puts a kink in the tail. As Wald points out in a recent discussion of his model (Wald, 1968), the 11-cis configuration should not be expected to exist at all, since molecular dynamics suggest that it is intrinsically unstable. The extraordinary fact, however, is that 11-*cis*-retinal$_1$ exists and does maintain this stable stereoisomeric form, *but only as long as it is kept in the dark*. This deceptively simple statement is, in fact, the key to the whole story of the primary visual process. There are two very important reasons for the key role. First, 11-*cis*-retinal$_1$ is the only stereoisomer of retinal$_1$ that is capable of forming a stable bond with the organic macromolecule, opsin. Second, the action of light on the rhodopsin molecule serves only to stereoisomerize 11-*cis*-retinal$_1$ into its all-trans form, thus forming an unstable substance which goes through the various stages of the visual cycle spontaneously without the necessity for any other external force.

The net effect of these very special characteristics of retinal$_1$ is that the primary sensory action in vision can be specifically identified as the straightening or stereoisomerizing of the 11-cis to the all-trans form of retinal$_1$. No other action of light is necessary once this trigger process occurs.

When 11-*cis*-retinal$_1$ is stereoisomerized by light and the combined photomolecule breaks down, a complex series of spontaneous further decompositions occur. The rhodopsin molecule, for example, does not immediately degenerate into all-*trans*-retinal$_1$ and rhodopsin, but rather goes through a number of intermediate states, each of which has its own specific properties. These intermediate states occur very rapidly, and it had been extremely difficult to determine their characteristics by the ordinary spectral absorption techniques used for the stable final breakdown products. A remarkable innovation introduced by Wald's group, however, has made it possible to take "temporal snap shots" of the intermediaries. The technique, which might be called "freeze chemistry," took advantage of the fact that the sequence of intermediary photochemicals are produced by reactions with different temperature thresholds. That is, each of the processes can occur only at a successively higher temperature. Thus, the initial breakdown of rhodopsin into an intermediary called prelumirhodopsin will lead to a stable mixture of rhodopsin and prelumirhodopsin if the experiments are carried out at $-195°C$. If the temperature is allowed to rise to $-140°C$, then prelumirhodopsin will spontaneously decay further into another intermediary called lumirhodopsin.

FIGURE 4.3 A schematic drawing of the complete rhodopsin cycle. Those portions of the cycle that are connected by wavy lines are driven by light, but those connected by straight lines occur in the dark. The wavelengths indicated in parentheses are the peaks of the absorption spectra of the particular intermediate breakdown product. The temperatures are thresholds for the next step in the reaction. Cooling the mixture below any of the thresholds can stop the reaction at any intermediate stage desired (adapted from Wald, 1968).

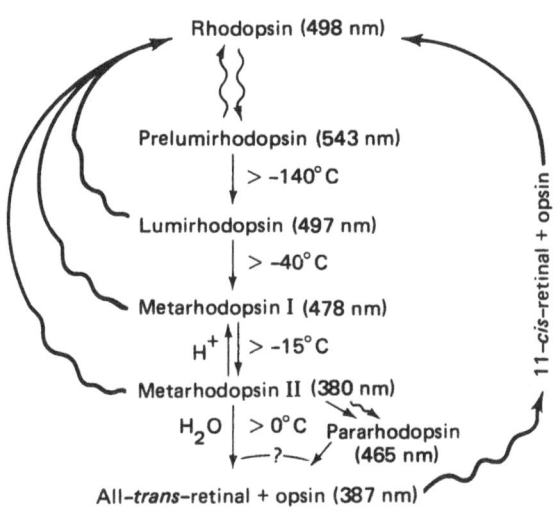

At −40°C, lumirhodopsin further decays spontaneously into a substance called metarhodopsin I which, when in the presence of H^+ ions, is converted into another substance known as metarhodopsin II. Metarhodopsin II is further decomposed into the final breakdown products, retinal$_1$ and opsin, through two alternative routes. Wald has shown that as the temperature rises to O°C, in the presence of water, metarhodopsin II will spontaneously decompose into the final breakdown products, but it may also go through an auxiliary pathway involving another intermediary called pararhodopsin.

The whole process is diagrammed in Figure 4.3, which is adapted from Wald's 1968 paper. In addition to showing the sequence of breakdown products, this figure also shows the key temperature at which each sequential step is "unfrozen," as well as two other very interesting and important sets of data.

First, the peak wavelength of the absorption curve of each of the intermediates is indicated. We can see that each of these chemicals absorbs maximally at a different part of the visual spectrum. This placement of the absorption peak is a key measure in the identification of each breakdown product and the only present way of showing that they are really separate and distinct chemicals.

Second, the figure also indicates by the shape of the arrow in each reaction—which reactions are spontaneous and will occur in the dark (straight lines) and which are reactions that must be driven by light (wavy lines). It is important to note that there is only one light-driven breakdown reaction, and this means that the visual response only requires light to trigger the string of dark reactions that lead to the free final breakdown products—retinal$_1$ and the protein opsin. The other light reactions, interestingly enough, are all in the opposite direction and contribute to the regeneration of rhodopsin from the various intermediaries and thus to the final equilibrium mixture of the various substances.

The main advantage of the technique of freezing the chemical reactions is that processes that last for only a few microseconds and that are, therefore, too brief to be examined at body temperature can be isolated in time for a sufficiently long period so that measurement of their optical and chemical properties can be made. It is, of course, not at all certain that each of the processes isolated in this manner is not really itself a combination of several subprocesses with the same or similar threshold temperature. Indeed, current investigations have suggested that, in fact, lumirhodopsin may be two substances (now known tentatively as lumirhodopsin A and B), but the details are at present not completely established.

The complete story of the biochemistry of the visual photopigments is complicated further by the fact that just as there are many different types of opsins found in different species and two different kinds of opsins (rod and cone types) found in many animals, there are also known to be two different types of retinol and thus two different retinals. The two different kinds of retinal are usually found in different species of animals, but some animals seem to be able to change from a retinal$_1$ system to a retinal$_2$ system (or vice versa) as they mature. The structural formulas of retinol$_2$ and retinal$_2$ are shown in Figure 4.4 (a) and (b), respectively.

Retinal$_1$ and retinal$_2$ and their respective retinols are not simple stereoisomers of each other, but are distinct chemical structures with differing formulas. Retinal$_1$ has a formula of $C_{19}H_{27}CHO$, as we have seen, while retinal$_2$ has a formula of $C_{19}H_{25}CHO$. The critical structural differences can be observed in the benzene ring body of the molecule, where a double bond between two carbons in retinal$_2$ replaces a pair of auxiliary hydrogen atoms in retinal$_2$.

Retinal$_1$ has classically been assumed to be found in land vertebrates and marine fish and adult frogs. Retinal$_2$ was assumed to be found in vertebrates who spend at least the early part of their lives in fresh water. This group of animals includes freshwater fish and lampreys and some other amphibia. Recently, however, Schwanzara (1967) surveyed the pigments of a large number of freshwater fishes and found that both retinal$_1$ and retinal$_2$ systems were to be found in this group. He attributed the presence of both systems to the fact that different freshwater fishes live in different conditions of ambient lighting, and somehow this led to a natural selection of what was an optimum pigment for each environment.

Let us review and summarize the situation as we have described it so far. There are two different kinds of retinal. Usually only one of the two is found in any given animal species that possesses this kind of photochemistry. There are, however, many opsins that differ in minor details from species to species. This explains the slight differences in the absorption spectra obtained as one compares different animals. But within a given species, it is also possible for at least two distinct kinds of opsin to be present. In some animals the two opsins may be located in com-

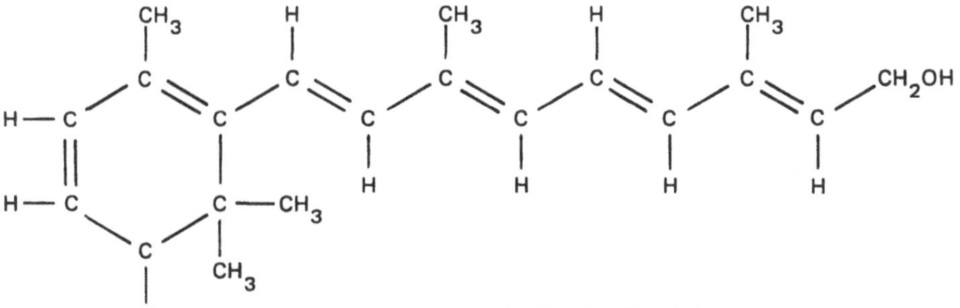

All–*trans*–retinol$_2$, $C_{19}H_{25}CH_2OH$

(a)

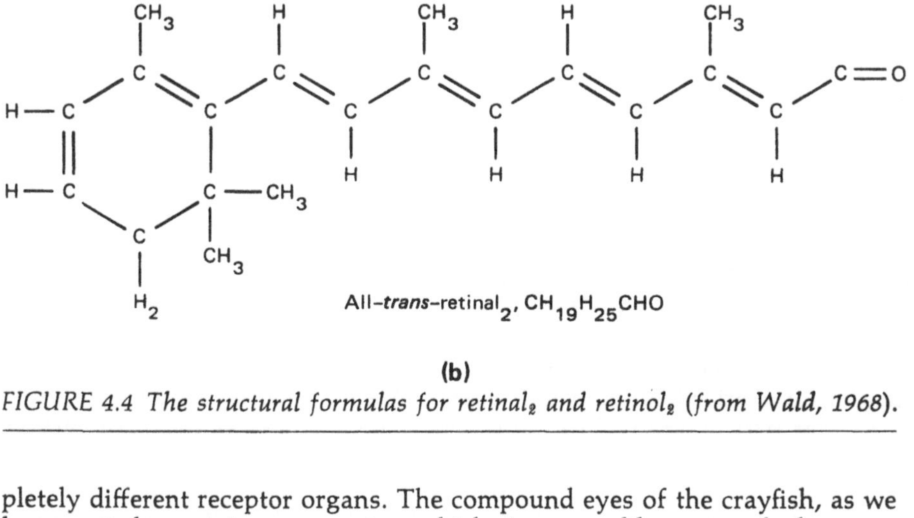

All–*trans*–retinal$_2$, $CH_{19}H_{25}CHO$

(b)

FIGURE 4.4 *The structural formulas for retinal$_2$ and retinol$_2$ (from Wald, 1968).*

pletely different receptor organs. The compound eyes of the crayfish, as we have noted, contains an opsin, which is more like one of the cone opsins of vertebrates, while the caudal photoreceptor in the animal's tail has a spectral sensitivity very much like rhodopsin, and this presumably has an opsin more akin to the vertebrate rod component. In other animals, like man, the two kinds of opsins may exist in adjacent cells in the same receptor structure. The rods and cones of the human eye are examples of this latter type.

As we have suggested, a further and very important complication relating to color vision is that there appears, in some animals, several different kinds of cone opsin. Based on direct spectrophotometric measurements by Brown and Wald (1964) and Marks, Dobelle, and MacNichol (1964), we now know that there are probably three different kinds of cone pigments in the human eye. Since the retinal in each of these cone pigments would presumably be the same, the observed differences in absorption spectra must be due to the fact that there are three different kinds of cone opsin present. Each cone has one, and only one, of each of these chromatically distinct photopigments, which Rushton (1962) has named

TABLE 4.1 THE TYPES OF PHOTOPIGMENTS THAT CAN BE
PRODUCED BY COMBINING THE VARIOUS KINDS OF OPSINS WITH
THE TWO KINDS OF RETINALS (ADAPTED FROM WALD, 1959)

	Retinal$_1$	Retinal$_2$
Rod Opsin	Rhodopsin λ_{max} = 500	Porphyropsin λ_{max} = 522
Cone Opsin R	Iodopsin$_1$ = erythrolabe λ_{max} = 555 or 570	Cyanopsin ?
Cone Opsin G	Iodopsin$_2$ = chlorolabe λ_{max} = 525 or 535	
Cone Opsin B	Iodopsin$_3$ = cyanolabe λ_{max} = 445 or 450	

chlorolabe, erythrolabe, and cyanolabe. This entire system has been summarized in Table 4.1, which is a modification of a taable originally presented by Wald (1959).

The general model we have of the primary sensory action in vision can be summarized as follows. It is simply a photoisomerization of a very particular part of the photosensitive molecule. A kink at the 11th carbon atom in the carotenoid is straightened by light changing retinal from a stereoisomer that bonds stably to opsin to an isomeric form that spontaneously disassociates itself from the protein. Although the carotenoid may be either one of two kinds, and the protein may be any of several different kinds found either in different receptor cells or different species of animals, the story seems to be essentially the same in all instances. Differences in absorption spectra are explicable on the basis of these chemical differences in the two moieties. Once stereoisomerization occurs, the rest of the sequence of breakdown stages is a dark reaction; that is, it occurs spontaneously without further photic stimulation. Now that we have considered this remarkable story, we can move on to the next stage —how is it that this chemical reaction can produce a receptor potential?

C. The Production of the Visual Receptor Potential
So far in this discussion, we have been mainly concerned with the characteristics of the retinal part of the large photosensitive molecule. The structure of this relatively small portion of a molecule of rhodopsin, or any of the other photopigments, determines the characteristics of the primary sensory action—the decomposition of the pigment due to the

photoisomerization of the retinal to its all-trans form. To explain the next step in the chain, however, the production of the receptor potential, we shift our attention to the opsin moiety. It is this much larger part of the photosensitive molecule that is now thought to be critical in the actual production of the receptor potential. The source of much of the material to be discussed here is once again George Wald's work.

The bonding between the retinal and opsin moieties can be described by the following chemical equation:

$$C_{19}H_{27}HC=O + H_2N-opsin \rightleftarrows C_{19}H_{27}HC=N-opsin + H_2O \qquad (4.1)$$
$$\text{11-}cis\text{-retinal } + \text{ rod opsin} \rightleftarrows \text{rhodopsin} \qquad\qquad + \text{water}$$

The key portion of this reaction is the substitution of all of the retinal molecule (with the exception of the oxygen atom) for the two hydrogen atoms that had been attached to the nitrogen atom on the opsin. While the oxygen and hydrogen form a free molecule of water, the opsin and the retinal are attached by a carbon to nitrogen double bond—a condition that can remain stable only if the retinal remains in the 11-cis stage. However, in addition to the availability of the double bonded oxygen on the retinal molecule and the H_2N group on the opsin as indicated in this equation, another atomic sidechain known as a sulfhydryl group—SH—is also required for the combination to occur and is likewise exposed when decomposition occurs. Under the action of the stimulating light, the rhodopsin molecule fractures and "exposes" two of these highly reactive sulfhydryl groups. At a later stage, in the sequence of the intermediate breakdown products, a hydrogen bond is also exposed, but apparently this occurs too long after the time the actual excitatory process occurs to play a very significant role in the actions yet to follow. Specifically, the opsin fragment with its exposed sulfhydryl groups is supposed to directly affect membrane permeability, even though it must penetrate the disk membrane to get to the cell membrane.

"Exposure" of the sulfhydryl groups is a somewhat ambiguous notion, for they apparently are not part of the actual bonding reactions holding retinal to the opsin. Wald suggests, in one of his figures (see our Figure 4.5), that the exposure is almost a function of the stereo-geometry of the opsin moiety. Where previously the sulfhydryl groups had been buried deep within the molecular structure of the rhodopsin molecule, the structural changes occurring in the structure of the opsins during the photodecomposition actually bring them to the surface, where they are available for chemical interaction. Whether this sort of geometrical change is a metaphor for a much more complicated catalytic or direct chemical reaction is hard to say. The important fact is that shortly after the initiation of the bleaching process, the opsin is no longer an inert and unreactive part of the rhodopsin complex, but is altered to a reactive structure capable of participation in other processes by mechanisms other than the rupture of C=N bond.

The process of immediate interest, of course, is the production of the graded electrical receptor potential. There are two possible mechanisms that might be invoked as explanations for the production of receptor

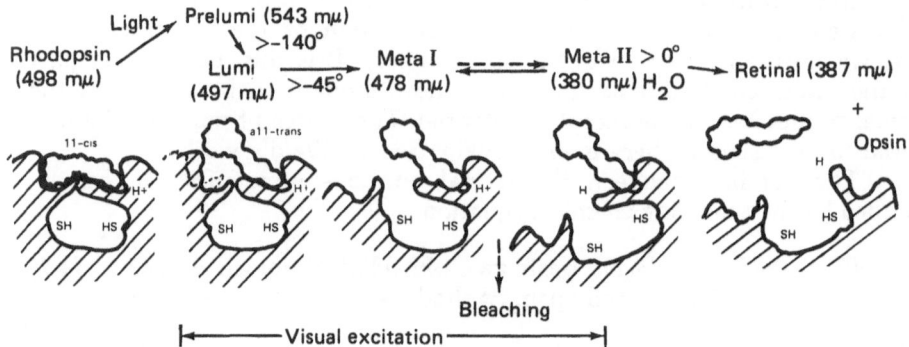

FIGURE 4.5 Wald's schematic model of the decomposition of a photochemical, showing the various stereochemical stages in the breakdown of the rhodopsin molecule. Note particularly the freeing of the —SH groups which, he believes, are associated with the production of the generator potential (from Wald, 1968).

potential. But it should be clearly noted that both of these are somewhat speculative, and there is still a great gap in our knowledge concerning which, if either, is the actual source of the receptor potential of the eye.

The first hypothesis is that the exposed sulfhydryl groups on the opsin immediately begin to chemically react with either the outer cell membrane of the receptor itself or with the more immediately available interior membranes of the lamella of the receptor outer segment we observed in the electron micrographs of Chapter 3. If the opsin, in some way, could change the permeability of either membrane, there would be a resulting depolarization or hyperpolarization as the passive forces redistributed, in at least this local region, the ions whose concentration differences produced the resting potential. A local current sink or source, which could lead to action at a distance—presumably at the synapse at the base of the receptor cell—would thus be produced. Such a hypothetical system would have another advantage. It would explain one adaptive reason for the presence of the platelike lamella in the outer segments of the photoreceptors. The lamella could be amplifiers of a sort. A local depolarization in one region might summate with those in others to produce a far greater receptor potential magnitude than that which possibly could be produced by the single cell membrane.

Hagins, Penn, and Yoshikami (1970) have recently suggested that the action of the photobreakdown products may be to suddenly reduce the permeability of the rod or cone membrane and thus to reduce a continuous ionic current that he observed when the receptors are in the dark. The decrease in permeability can lead to a hyperpolarization of the membrane potential, and it is indeed a hyperpolarization that is typically found in vertebrate photoreceptors when they are exposed to light. (In invertebrates the photoreceptor potentials are more usually found to be depolarizations.)

The second hypothetical possibility explaining the production of the visual receptor potential is based upon a recent discovery in electrophysiology. Brown and Murakami (1964) have shown that if one records the photically driven voltage (the electroretinogram) between the front and the back of the eye of a dark adapted vertebrate eye, and if one uses very high stimulus energies, there is a very rapid voltage shift, which seems to be associated with the initial stages of the breakdown photochemical. The reaction is very rapid, occurring with a latency of only a few microseconds, and is thus comparable to the latency at which the exposure of the sulfhydryl group is thought to occur. It also is compatible with the time at which it is thought the generator potential begins to appear. The fast visual response or the early receptor potential (ERP), as it is now known, is dependent upon parallel alignment of the rhodopsin molecules in the intact outer segments of the intact eye. It will not occur in solutions of the photochemical in a test tube (Cone and Brown, 1967). Almost no other change in the physics of the situation seems to affect the amplitude or latency of the response. Since the signal is measurable only at very high stimulus intensity, it is not clear what role it might play in normal vision or whether it is actually the generator potential. But nevertheless, it is of great interest, at least, in suggesting that there may be direct electrical action produced by various bleaching steps that is not mediated by an intermediate chemical membrane permeability change.

Cone (1967) feels that the ERP is a direct result of the redistribution of charges as the rhodopsin molecule goes through the various intermediary stages of decomposition following the initial photoisomerization. Cone and Cobb (1969) were able to evoke a different pattern of ERP at different times following a strong preliminary conditioning flash, and they believe that the shape of the ERP in these cases is characteristic of the presence of one or another of the breakdown products. Since, the threshold for the ERP is 10^6 greater than that of the receptor cell response, the ERP does not appear to be the generator potential *per se*, but it probably will continue to be an important measure of the photochemistry of retinal pigments.

In summary, it must be emphasized that this brief speculative interlude is only that. We still have no conclusive answers concerning the origins of the receptor potential in the visual process. It looks as if we will just have to wait for some scientist more particularly interested in those neural processes to devise a system of tho e critical experiments, which are so necessary for the advance of our knowledge.

III. TRANSDUCER ACTION IN THE EAR

A. Nonneural Stimulus Modifications

Airborne acoustic energy is modified in a number of important ways by the nonneural apparatus of the ear. The external ear, or pinna, and the auditory meatus, or ear canal, act very much like an old-fashioned hearing horn to collect and concentrate the energy emitted by a sound source. The energy so concentrated impinges upon a delicate tissue—the tympanic membrane—which separates the outer ear from an air-filled middle ear

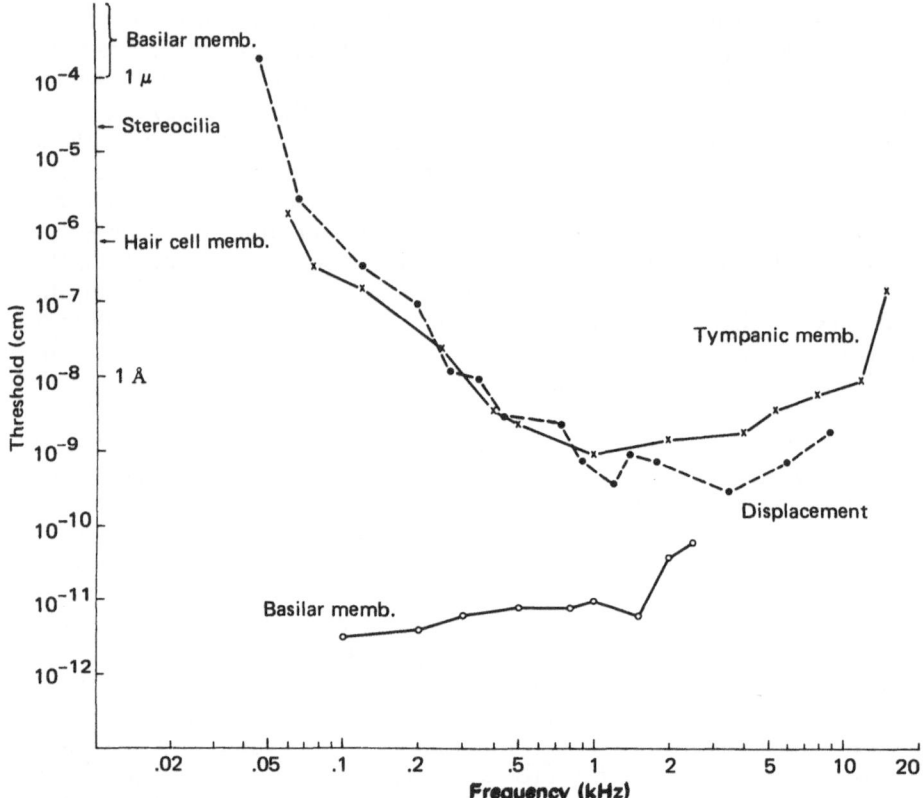

FIGURE 4.6 A graph comparing the dimensions of the apparatus of the basilar membrane and the threshold movement for acoustic sensation at the tympanic membrane and the basilar membrane. Two curves are given for the tympanic membrane. One curve, drawn as a solid line, is theoretical and based upon calculations, while the curve drawn with a dotted line is based upon empirical measurements. The curve for the basilar membrane is a calculated value only. Note that the calculated threshold movement for hearing at the basilar membrane is more than 10 million times smaller than the thickness of the basilar membrane itself and has a value approaching one-tenth of the diameter of a hydrogen atom! (from Lawrence, 1965).

chamber. In the middle ear a system of tiny bony levers performs one of the most important nonneural modifications of the incident acoustic energy. The mallus, incus, and stapes (the three ossicles) form a lever system, which reduces the magnitude of movement and increases the force of the applied acoustic signal. The inner end of this string of ossicles is connected to another membranous tissue—the oval window—which separates the air-filled middle ear from the fluid-filled inner ear, the detailed anatomy of which has already been described in an earlier chapter.

The very small displacement to which the hydromechanical system of the ear may respond is truly amazing. Figure 4.6 (from Lawrence,

1965) shows the displacements at the tympanic membrane and at the basilar membrane for threshold signals plotted as a function of the frequency of the stimulating sound. Some of the data points plotted are calculated and may be subject to some criticism, but the data of Wilska (1935) are direct measurements and confirm that these ultrasmall movements are at least of the correct order of magnitude. It is most interesting to note, as Lawrence points out, that the mean free distance traveled at 20°C by a typical atom of one of the gases of air is as large as 10^{-5} cm. Comparing this value with the values given in this figure, we see that the threshold movement of the basilar membrane is a million times smaller than even this small value—10^{-11} cm! In fact, threshold acoustic signals are 1/10 the diameter of a hydrogen atom! These values specify a signal to noise situation, which is very severe, and yet almost all of us can easily detect information patterns under these extreme conditions. Indeed, the dimensions of these threshold movements are such that we are no longer conceptually dealing with gross mechanical systems, but really must think at a molecular level at which the vibrations might even be considered to have almost direct chemical effects.

The nonneural processing of the incoming auditory signal continues even after the transmission of the signal beyond the oval window. In fact, nonneural processing plays what may be the key role in acoustic frequency discrimination. The historical development of the theory of auditory quality has typically been one that asked whether the analysis of the component frequencies of a signal occurred peripherally or centrally. In large part, current theories of hearing are place theories attributing the analysis function to the mechanical action of the fluid-filled cochlea. Maximal displacements of the acoustic wave are localized at various places on the cochlea in patterns that differ for the different frequencies.

Early theories of place encoding had assumed a set of tuned resonators, which vibrated separately in tune with a particular input frequency. For reasons we shall discuss in greater detail in Chapter 10, which is devoted specifically to the problem of auditory quality coding, resonance place theories have had to be, in general, discarded. In their place has arisen a set of hydraulic theories, which are based on the mechanical analysis of wave patterns set up in fluid-filled tubes by the acoustic stimulus fluctuations. The process is nonneural in the sense that the manner in which the place localization of different frequencies occurs is dependent only on the physics of the cochlear tubes and the acoustic wave, and no change is involved in the kinds of energies involved.

We should also note that the structural mechanics of the middle and inner ear play important roles in specifying the bandpass characteristics of the acoustic receptor. The three auditory ossicles—the malleus, incus, and stapes, for example—are important in the maintenance of the high-frequency bandpass characteristics of the mammalian ear. In animals like lizards, in which a single cartilaginous strut replaces the chain of ossicles, the high-frequency response characteristics are markedly attenuated.

Another form of nonneural modification of the incoming signal is, in fact, mediated by some highly interesting neural feedback links. Two tiny muscles in the middle ear, the tensor tympani and the stapedius, are connected to the ossicles and the surrounding wall of the bony cavity in such a way that they can reduce the amplitude of acoustic movement when the ear is overloaded with very large sounds by providing a counteracting force to the ossicles. Thus, their action is analogous to that of the pupil, which also acts as modulators of the stimulus intensity.

We shall defer our discussion of the most remarkable and important of these mechanical functions—the conversion of temporal frequency information to spatially localized patterns on the basilar membrane—to the later chapter on sensory quality coding. There we shall see how such a mechanism plays a major role in the differential encoding of stimuli of varying frequency. We shall now consider the next steps in the transductive process—the primary sensory action and the actual conversion of the mechanical movement induced by a sound wave into neuroelectric energy.

B. The Primary Sensory Action in Audition

The primary sensory action in the cochlea is thought to be the shearing action on the receptor hairs created by the movement of the tectorial membrane along the hair cells. This simple statement, however, is ambiguous and inadequate, for there are many ways in which such a mechanical shear could be detected. The response could be a direct function of the amplitude, velocity, or even acceleration produced by the force. A detailed explanation of the mechanics of primary sensory action has come from the work of Georg von Békésy. Von Békésy received the Nobel Prize in 1961 for his work on the mechanics of the ear, and much of our discussion of modern auditory theory as presented in this book will be based on his contributions.

For the moment we have to consider a specific question. Given that the ear is sensitive to mechanical forces, is it a deformation, velocity, or an acceleration transducer? Von Békésy (1951) approached this problem in a novel way. He recorded the cochlear microphonic potentials, produced by a trapezoidal acoustic waveform such as that shown in Figure 4.7 (a). If the cochlear microphonic, which, as we shall see in the next section, is thought by at least some investigators to be the actual receptor potential, is dependent on the deformation, then the response should follow the trapezoidal shape of the stimulus itself as shown in Figure 4.7 (b). If, as one other alternative, it is a velocity detector, then it would be expected to produce a differentiated waveform, producing signals only when the basilar membrane is moving, like that in Figure 4.7 (c). If, on the other hand, it is an acceleration detector, then the waveform observed should follow the double differentiated shape of the stimulus as shown in Figure 4.7 (d). Von Békésy's (1951) observations with "carefully prepared cochlea(s)" led him to conclude that the cochlear microphonic in this case is, in fact, trapezoidal like the position of the basilar membrane. Therefore, the transducer action is one that is dependent upon the displacement, rather than the velocity or acceleration created by the acoustic stimulus.

Where do these displacement detectors reside? The answer to this question seems to be clear. All investigators agree that some part of the

FIGURE 4.7 A schematic drawing of the possible observations that might have been obtained in von Békésy's experiment to determine the specific nature of the primary sensory action. (a) Shows the nature of a trapezoidally applied stimulus. (b) Shows the cochlear microphonic response that would be expected if the primary sensory action was dependent only on the displacement. (c) Shows the response that would be expected if the primary sensory action was based on a velocity sensitive detection process. (d) Shows the response that would be expected if it was an acceleration sensitive response. Direct observations indicated that the waveform was most like (b), and thus the hair cells act as displacement detectors (adapted from von Békésy, 1951).

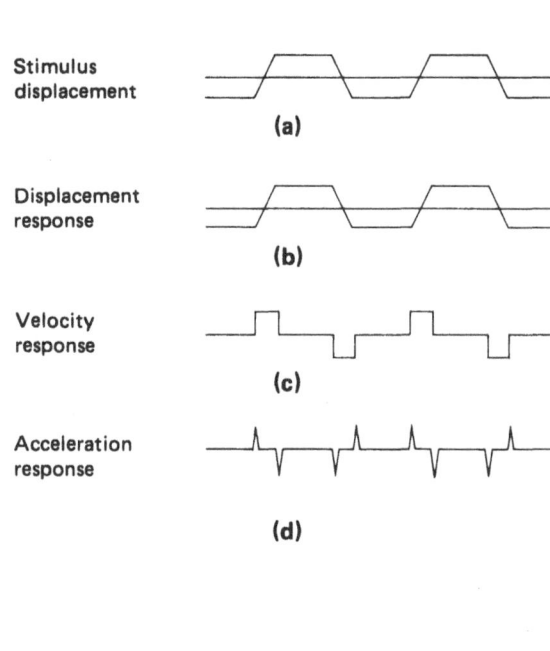

cochlear hair cell is the acoustic transducer. Apparently, although this is not so certain, the hairs or cilia transmit the mechanical forces of the stimulus to the cuticular base plate at their basal end. This base plate, it is often presumed, is the actual mechanosensitive tissue and is specialized for the conversion of the mechanical energy to the electroneural membrane fluctuations. How this energy conversion may be accomplished is the tale told in the next section.

C. The Production of the Auditory Receptor Potential

Although there is a very complete and detailed story concerning the production of the auditory receptor potential told by one distinguished scientist, Hallowell Davis, there is still some controversy surrounding this particular theory. In addition to the fact that there are the usual difficulties in understanding what are the exact processes going on at the ultramicroscopic level of molecules and membranes, there is also another problem which has complicated this issue. This problem arises out of the fact that it is not yet agreed by all concerned that the receptor potential has been unequivocally identified. The lack of agreement is not due to a shortage of possible candidate voltages, but rather to an abundance of electrical signals of one kind or another that can be detected in the inner ear.

When the cochlear microphonic was first detected by Wever and Bray (1930), it was immediately assumed to be the neurally transmitted acoustic signal. During subsequent experiments, however, these same workers showed that the cochlear microphonic was a most unusual nervous response. It had enormous high-frequency following capabilities (up to many thousands of hertz) and was so independent of the metabolism of the body that it could be detected long after the death of the animal (Wever, Bray, and Lawrence, 1941). Since nerve impulse rates were known to be limited to about 1000 Hz, and mammalian nerves were known to be so sensitive to anoxia, the microphonic clearly could not be the result of a propagated nerve impulse pattern. For many years following their discovery, the cochlear microphonic was, therefore, considered to be merely an artifact, perhaps of the orderly crystalline structure of the array of hair cells. In recent years, as our knowledge of sensory mechanisms has grown, and the general necessity for the identification of a receptor or generator potential has become more apparent, there is renewed interest in assigning this role to the cochlear microphonic. Perhaps the most modern theoretical statement of the origin of the cochlear microphonic is that presented by Davis (1965). His theory is, therefore, also an important one in defining the nature of the auditory transduction process, if, as seems possible, the cochlear microphonic is indeed the acoustic receptor potential.

Davis' theory should be separated into two parts. In the first part, a most compelling theory of the production of the cochlear microphonic is presented. In the second part, there is a somewhat longer logical leap. There, his assumption is that this cochlear microphonic is indeed the receptor potential and that it is directly responsible for the release of some transmitter substance at the synaptic junction between the hair cell and the dendrites of the fibers of the cochlear nerve. To fully understand the difference between the two parts of the theory, we have to look at Davis' statements in detail and consider where observation becomes speculation.

Davis' theory, in brief, states that the cochlear microphonic, or the ac potential, as it is otherwise known, is generated by a gating action of the acoustic signal. A substantial standing or direct current voltage difference between the interior of a hair cell and the fluid of the scala media is known to exist, and it is this dc voltage that Davis looks upon as the pool of energy tapped to produce the microphonic. Figure 4.8 (taken from Davis' paper) shows the general scheme of the endocochlear voltages within the inner ear. The two connecting scalae, the scalae vestibuli and the scalae tympani, are filled with a single fluid—the perilymph. The perilymph is continuous throughout the two scalae via a tiny opening—the helicotrema—which is located near the apex of the cochlea. Though both have nearly the same potential with respect to the lymphatic fluid or blood, there is, surprisingly, a slight discrepancy between the two. The scala vestibuli usually exhibits a potential 2 or 3 mV more positive than the +5 mV typically recorded in the scala tympani. This slight potential difference is probably due to local differences in the ionic composition of the perilymph in each case, but the source of this difference is obscure. In any event, the potential difference between the two scalae is so small that it is not considered to play a significant role in the auditory process.

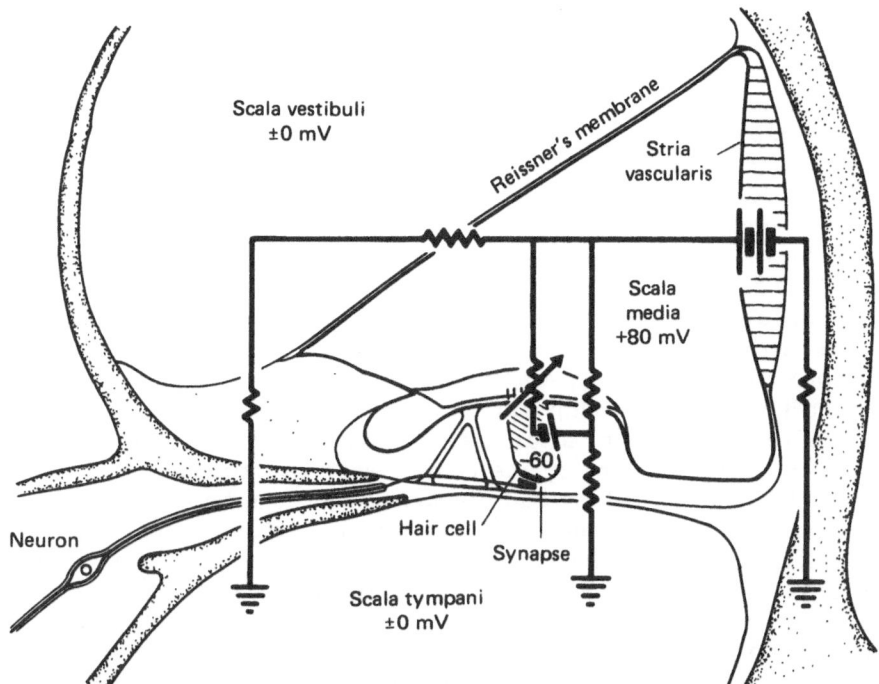

FIGURE 4.8 Davis' "resistance microphone" theory of the generation of the cochlear microphonic is diagrammed in a way that emphasizes the voltage values found in the inner ear. According to Davis, the hair cell acts as a valve to gate the very large bioelectric potential difference between the inside of the hair cell and the scala media to produce a current that is observed as the microphonic. See text for complete details (from Davis, 1970).

On the other hand, a different situation obtains in the scala media. There, a positive potential of +80 mV with respect to blood is recorded with dc measuring systems. Another important potential difference is also present in this situation. That, of course, is the very large negative voltage, which is typically found inside any nerve cell, and in this case we are specifically referring to the receptor hair cell itself and its −80 mV intracellular potential.

It is not certain what the mechanism is for the establishment and maintenance of so large a positive potential in the scala media. But it apparently has something to do with a very great surplus of K+ in comparison with the ionic composition of the perilymph in the scala vestibuli or tympani, or the typical ionic composition inside a cell.

Whatever the origin of the endocochlear potentials and the receptor intracellular potential, there is no disagreement that they exist and can summate to give a very large total potential across the hair-cell membrane. The total voltage across the cell membrane of the hair cell in particular, therefore, is about 160 mV—an extraordinarily large potential for a single cell membrane and, in fact, probably the largest transmembrane potential found in the human body.

Davis suggests, quite correctly, that this potential difference would have to be associated with a substantial dc resting current because of the finite impedance of the cell membrane. It is his further suggestion, and this is the key assumption in his theory—that the cuticular plate underneath the hairs is capable in some undefined way of varying its impedance under the influence of mechanical deformation. As the impedance varies, the resting current would be altered. In this manner the current flow driven by the large transmembrane potential can be modulated or gated in such a way that the total effect can be quite a bit more energetic than the energy that initiated the action. This process would be analogous to the processes involved in electron tube or transistor amplification of electronic flow, though certainly not homologous.[1]

There are a number of advantages to Davis' theory of cochlear microphonic generation. The theory meets the necessary criterion for energy amplification that von Békésy had previously shown to be necessary, and the microphonic clearly, therefore, reflects the behavior of an active metabolic system. While the problems in this first part of Davis' theory are relatively minor, we might draw attention to the fact that it is not exactly clear what "resistance" or "impedance" means when one is talking about ions flow through semipermeable membranes, but this is a reductionistic detail, which is not terribly germane to the essence of his argument.

Criticisms of the Davis theory, however, may be directed at the second much more highly speculative portion. The explicit assumption in this latter part is that the cochlear microphonic, produced as described in the first part of his theory, is, in fact, the receptor potential. That is, he assumes that the cochlear microphonic is specifically responsible for the triggering of the synaptic action, which leads to the spike action potentials in the second-order neurons. Davis does state that the same processes, which account for the modulation of the resting dc current, may also, in some separate way, increase the release of neurochemical transmitter substance. What, then, is the role of the gated current? Is it merely a concomitant of and, in fact, irrelevant to the critical processes involved in neural activation, or does it play some direct role in transmitter substance release? Furthermore, does this thus account for the fact that already high levels of resting current do lead to a moderately high level of sustained activity on top of which threshold signals must be detected? Similarly, it is well known that microphonics of this same sort are produced by a large number of other tissues in the body. Many of them are sufficiently separate from any sensory transduction process that it is sure that they are not involved in neural transmission. The real question concerning the identification of the cochlear microphonic with the receptor potential is: is there

---

[1] It is interesting to note that a similar gating process has been suggested by Hagins, Penn, and Yoshikami (1970) for the vertebrate photoreceptor and that a gating theory of nerve membrane potentials has wide currency in contemporary neurophysiology.

any experimental evidence that it alone is sufficient to initiate synaptic activity? The answer to this question is that Davis, at least in 1965, felt there was none, and he himself looked upon this as the most speculative link in his argument.

We might speculate further and point out other possibilities. The release of transmitter substance by the acoustic hair cell may be the result of some other voltage mechanism hidden in the cochlear microphonic. It might even be a direct effect of the mechanical deformation on some locus of the cell membrane and not require any electrical intermediary. This other locus, for example, could be the presynaptic portion of the membrane itself, and the presynaptic potential itself could be the equivalent of the receptor potential if this were so. For all practical purposes, however, it is unlikely that a separate membrane potential could ever be measured in the presence of the larger cochlear microphonic. At least, no one yet has found a way to disassociate the separate receptor potential if, indeed, it does exist.

Davis is very much aware of such criticism. Nevertheless, it is also probably true that even within these limits, his theory is better structured and more plausible than any competing one. It is for this reason that we give it prominence in our discussion.

IV. TRANSDUCER ACTION IN SOMESTHESIS

A. Nonneural Stimulus Modifications

Unfortunately, detailed investigations of the transductive mechanism in the wide variety of cutaneous and proprioceptive receptors have not been abundant. There simply are too many sensitive microstructures and too few neurophysiologists to provide the kind of data that are necessary to develop a complete description of each kind of receptor. For this reason, we shall turn to one typical somatosensory receptor, which seems to display many of the characteristics that are probably common to all somatosensory mechanoreceptors. The work we shall describe is that of W. R. Loewenstein and his colleagues.

Loewenstein has taken advantage of the existence of a very large Pacinian corpuscle in the mesentery of the cat. He has used this receptor as a "model system" to investigate some of the important questions that arise when one studies transduction from mechanical forces to neuroelectric energy. As we saw in Chapter 3, there are a very large number of different morphological types of somatosensory receptors. It was also noted in that section that the differences in the structure of the end organ were thought by some to be important in defining the specific sensitivity of the receptor to a particular kind of stimulation. Others, however, reject end-organ morphology as an important factor. The question thus arises: what is the role of nonneural structures encapsulating the receptive neuron terminal in defining the properties of the transducer? Does it affect the threshold, the specific tuning to a certain adequate stimulus, adaptation characteristics or any other important stimulus-response function?

Loewenstein and Rathkamp (1958) have searched for an answer to

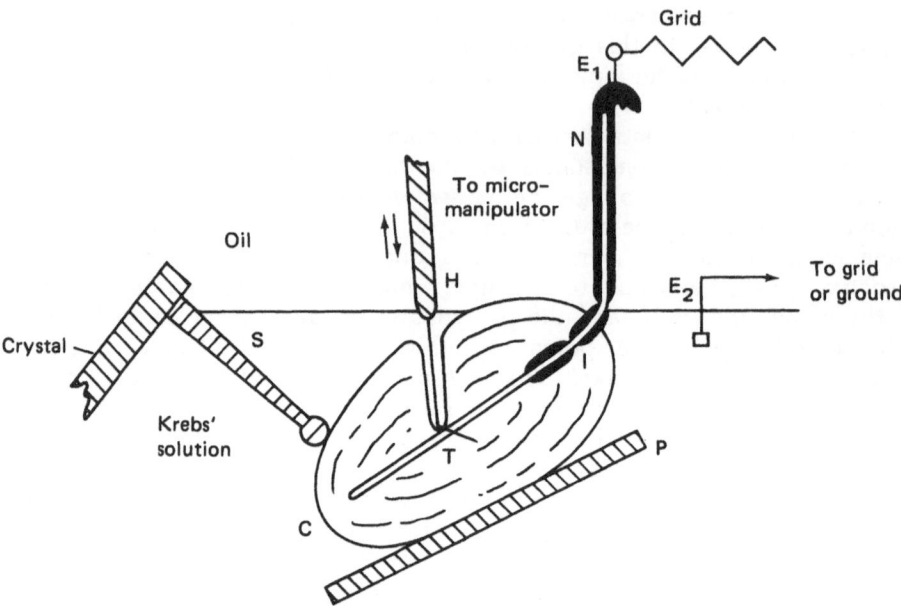

FIGURE 4.9 Schematic drawing of the preparation of a Pacinian corpuscle and the recording techniques used for the analysis of the transductive process. Where S is the Stimulator, C is the Pacinian corpuscle, P is a glass plate, H and T are wires used to block the receptor and E_1 and E_2 are electrodes. (From Loewenstein and Rathkamp, 1958).

this question in a most remarkable way. They have concluded that the encapsulation of the Pacinian corpuscle, at least, plays only a nonneural role in the transductive process. Thus, its role is more analogous to the preneural absorption of the ocular media or to the amplification of force by the auditory ossicles than to that of a participant in a primary sensory action. We shall now consider their evidence for this conclusion.

The Pacinian corpuscle of the cat's mesentery is an extraordinarily large receptor structure. Nevertheless, it is still a single cellular structure, and even the largest are microscopic at best. The reader should restudy Figure 3.36 to remind himself of the nature of the layers of the capsule around the terminal portion of the sensory nerve fiber. Loewenstein and Rathkamp's technique was to isolate a single Pacinian corpuscle along with a length of its nerve fiber. These were immersed in an appropriate physiological solution and loosely attached to a glass plate as shown in Figure 4.9. Ultrafine dissection techniques using tiny hooks and slivers of glass controlled by micromanipulators were used to strip away successive layers of the corpuscle. Careful recording of the generator potential showed that the corpuscle itself seemed to play no role in the determination of the peak magnitude of the Pacinian corpuscle's generator potential response to an impulsive stimulus. For the moment let us anticipate this finding and consider what other role, if any, the corpuscle might play in effecting preliminary nonneural modifications of the stimulus.

Mendelson and Loewenstein (1964), and more comprehensively in Loewenstein and Mendelson (1965), report a most interesting experiment, in which the results exhibit such a nonneural role for the capsule. Figure 4.9 also shows the position of the recording electrode used in that experiment. With only a single electrode, both spike action potentials and the graded generator potentials could be recorded by imposing appropriate bandpass restrictions on their amplifying system. The design of their experiment involved the recording of both of these neuroelectric signals simultaneously under two different conditions. In the first condition, the corpuscle was intact, but in the second, it had been totally dissected away. Figure 4.10 (a), (b), (c), (d) shows the electropotentials recorded in the various parts of this experiment. Figure 4.10 (a) shows the generator potential when the corpuscle was intact, and Figure 4.10 (b) the double spike produced at the onset and offset of the elongated stimulus. Figure 4.10 (c) shows the generator potential pattern when the cell was stimulated in the same way but after the corpuscle had been removed, while Figure 4.10 (d) shows the single spike produced in this case.

A number of important points are immediately obvious. First, the total system acts as a differentiator with a very short time constant. That is, the long stimulus duration is ineffective in producing more than a single spike. Subsequent studies showed that the Pacinian corpuscle will produce a single spike action potential for each pulse stimulus in a train up to a frequency of nearly 1 kHz, but there is almost no way of producing more than one spike for each pulse with any reasonable stimulus intensity unless the duration was as abnormally long as described above. The conclusion that must be drawn from Figure 4.10 is that while there is no change in the characteristics of the spike response whether or not the corpuscle is intact, there is a very substantial change in the generator potential waveform. Where that potential had been relatively sharply differentiated with the corpuscle intact, responding only at the onset and offset of the long duration stimulus, with the corpuscle removed, it displays only a slight amount of adaptation during the course of the stimulus.

The main finding of Mendelson and Loewenstein's study is thus that there is a dual differentiation mechanism in action in the Pacinian corpuscle that keeps the neuron from firing more than once at the onset or at the offset of each impressed stimulus no matter how long the stimulus. One of the two differentiators is some sort of a neural process, which prevents the continuous generator potential from eliciting more than a single spike. Little is known of this mechanism. The other differentiation is a nonneural one and acts by peaking the generator potential waveform at the onset and offset of the stimulus. It is not immediately obvious why the two back-to-back differentiation mechanisms are necessary, although it is clear that such mechanisms contribute to the establishment of a coding mechanism in the Pacinian corpuscular transducer, which is essentially a high-pass filter sensitive only to stimulus variations.

How can a mechanical system such as the external corpuscle "dif-

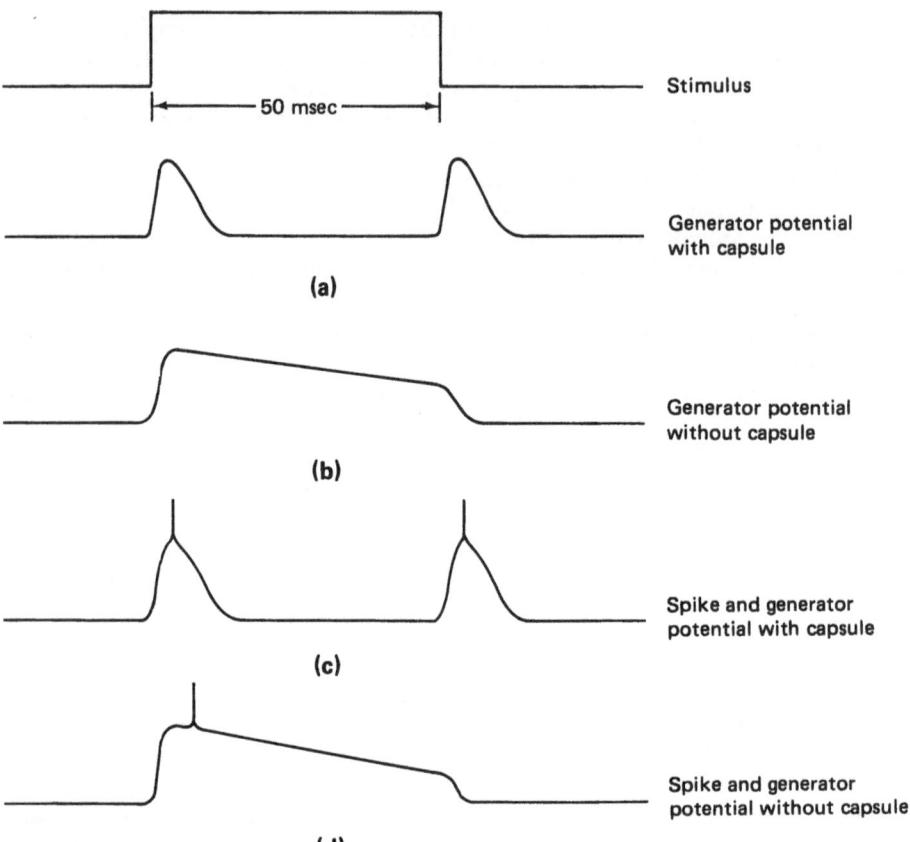

(a)

(b)

(c)

(d)

FIGURE 4.10 Schematic drawing of the effect of the removal of the corpuscle on the generation of the generator and spike action potential patterns for long lasting stimuli. See text for details (adapted from Loewenstein and Mendelson, 1965).

ferentiate" an input stimulus? The answer to this question seems to lie in its elastic properties. Mechanical deformations are transmitted to the neural membrane by the physical mass of the corpuscle. However, after the initial compression, the corpuscle is able to adjust its shape and, by redistributing its mass, release at least some of the deformation on the membrane, thus inactivating the mechanism that produces the generator potential. A formal theory to this effect in terms of the viscous and elastic flow of the corpuscular structure has been presented by Loewenstein and Skalak (1966).

B. The Primary Sensory Action in Somatosensation
The wide variety of cutaneous and proprioceptive receptors is probably stimulated through the medium of a number of different primary sensory

actions. Hensel, Ström, and Zotterman (1951) have shown that neurons in the lingual nerve leading from the cat's tongue exhibit properties that suggest that there is a direct sensitivity to temperature. Some fibers, which responded only when the static temperature was maintained within a certain narrow region, were observed, while others seemed to respond only to transient changes in the temperature of the cat's tongue. Some fibers seemed to respond best to cooling and others to warming, while those that responded to ambient or steady levels also seemed to be separated into cold and warm systems. Quite complicated patterns of response were often observed among these steady discharge fibers, which these workers thought differentially encoded warmth and cold on the one hand, and warming and cooling on the other. In general, however, it is fair to say that we have little knowledge of the primary sensory action of those somesthetic receptors, which lead to such thermal sensations or to such complex experiences as pain, itch, or tickle. Most of the answers that we have to this question for somesthesis are based upon research on mechanoreceptors like the Pacinian corpuscle.

Based upon the discussion of the preceding section, we can see that the question of the primary sensory action for the Pacinian corpuscle is one that has to be answered in a carefully qualified way. If we consider the normal situation, with the corpuscle intact, one might initially be led to believe that the primary sensory action is the transient change of a deforming stimulus. We might initially conclude, therefore, that the Pacinian corpuscle is a velocity detector, since responses were elicited only at the onset and offset of the stimulus. If, on the other hand, we decided that we shall not include nonneural modification and shall concern ourselves only with the neural aspects of the transducer, then we would want to look at the pattern of the generator potential after the removal of the corpuscle. Under these conditions, the Pacinian corpuscle exhibits exactly the same properties as does the cochlear hair cell. It responds relatively continuously to a continuous deformation.

In this context we would have to conclude that the Pacinian corpuscle is also a static deformation detector rather than a velocity detector. A deformation detector would also be consistent with the fact that a differential or gradient of force is necessary for the elicitation of cutaneous sensations. (Remember the finger in the pool of mercury: the sensation occurs only at the line of demarcation between mercury and air.) Pressure applied equally to all parts of the skin or the underlying receptors does not produce a response. It is only when there is a differential force that the membrane is deformed and sheared, and nervous activity is generated. This is, of course, also the reason deep-sea fishes are able to use delicate mechanoreceptors at great depths without a constant flow of background neural impulses. There simply is no stimulus gradient, no matter how great the uniform pressure, until an object is touched.

C. The Production of the Somesthetic Generator Potential

Loewenstein's laboratory has also provided the most up-to-date explanation of the production of the generator potential in a somesthetic receptor preparation. Unfortunately, as with the acoustic receptor, there is a great gap in our knowledge of the details of this process. It seems clear, as we have seen, that the primary sensory action is a mechanical deformation of the nerve membrane itself. Furthermore, measurements can be made of the generator potential produced by a given deformation and the functional relationships between it and a stimulus elucidated. But, unfortunately, we have no idea yet how the graded generator potential is actually produced. No physiochemical theory, which can explain for either the acoustic hair cell or the somesthetic receptors how a mechanical deformation can alter the permeability of the membrane to ion flow, has yet been forthcoming. Once membrane permeability has been altered, it is a direct calculation to compute the variation in the resting potential, but the initial step is still shrouded in the mystery of molecular permeability. So we can only say that ion redistributions occur as the membrane permeability changes, producing the depolarization we call the generator potential.

But how indeed does a mechanical deformation alter membrane permeability? Are these specialized tissues stimulated to release substances that act on membrane permeability in some chemical manner? Are "pores" enlarged or altered in shape in a way that allows some ions previously incapable of crossing the membrane barrier to do so now? Are charge distributions altered so that electrostatic forces repelling and attracting certain ions are now of a different pattern? Are active transport mechanisms, which actively move ions from one side of the membrane to the other, now brought into play? These and other possibilities are typical of the explanations that might be invoked to account for the actual transduction, but no one, to this time, has yet been able to come forth with a theory that is convincing and compelling. One of the reasons why it has been difficult is that the level of analysis is an ultramicroscopic one. It is not at all certain, for example, exactly what might be meant by such concepts as "pores" or even "membranes" in a situation such as this, in which the role of participants of atomic dimensions must be considered.

Thus, while the work we are about to discuss cannot clarify the exact nature of the conversion process at the subcellular level, Loewenstein and Rathkamp (1958) have at least clearly shown where in the membrane several of these very important processes occur. Their technique and results were generally as described above; total microdissection of the corpuscle led to little observable diminution or alteration of the generator potential other than the increase in duration as the differentiating properties of the corpuscle were removed. Impulsive stimuli continued to lead to generator potentials and spikes, which were indistinguishable whether or not the corpuscle was present. (See Figure 4.11.)

At this point in their studies, Loewenstein and Rathkamp introduced a new technique—the pressure block—in order to determine the role of specific portions of the receptive tip of the axon. When a fine wire was used to compress the neuron at the first node of Ranvier (as shown in Figure 4.9), the spike action potential disappeared, even though the generator potential was still present and normal. The effect of the block on the spike action potential can be seen in Figure 4.12, showing the spike before, during, and following the compression block. Compression blocks

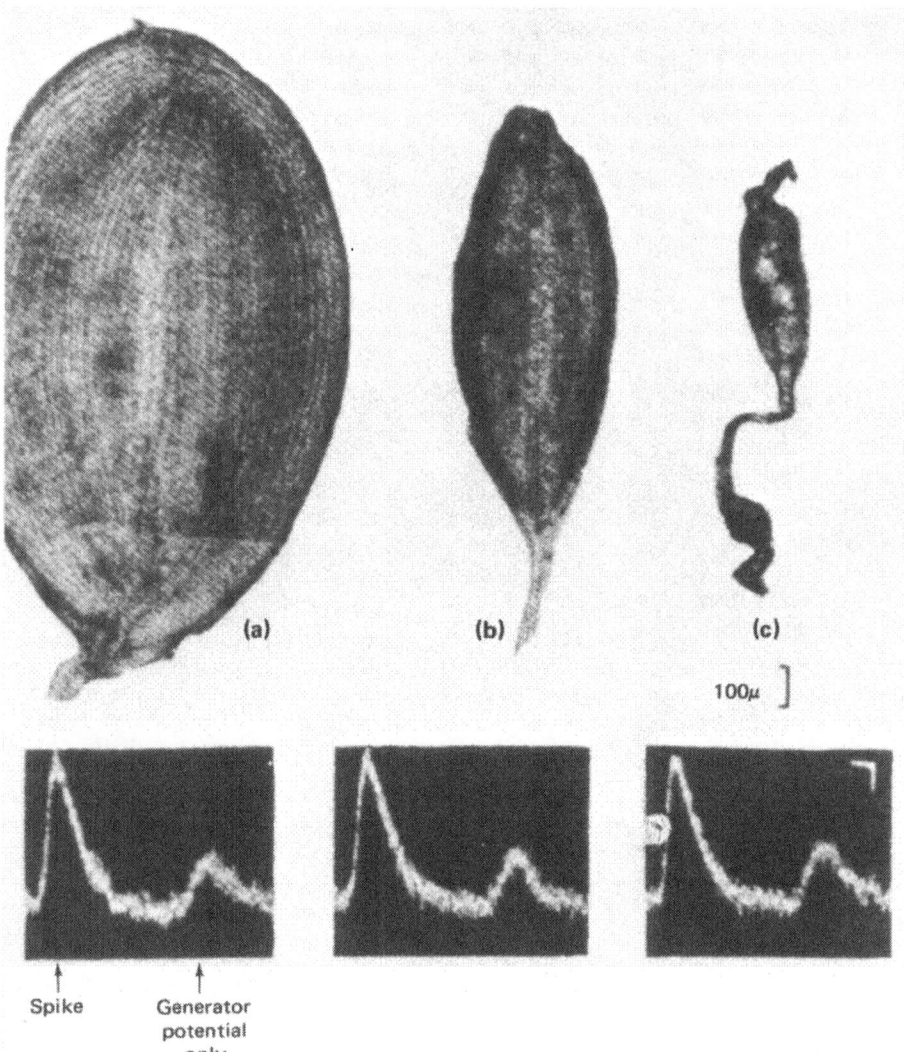

FIGURE 4.11 *Photographs showing the relation between the state of encapsulation of the Pacinian corpuscle and the resulting electropotentials. Two stimuli, one suprathreshold for spikes and the other subthreshold, but each very brief, have been presented, and despite substantial removal of the many-layered capsule, neither the spike response nor the brief generator potential changes in any observable way (from Loewenstein and Rathkamp, 1958).*

applied at other more central nodes of Ranvier do not show a corresponding drop out of the spike action potential. The conclusion that was drawn by Loewenstein and Rathkamp is that it is the first, and only the first, node of Ranvier that is specialized for the conversion of generator potentials into spike action potentials.

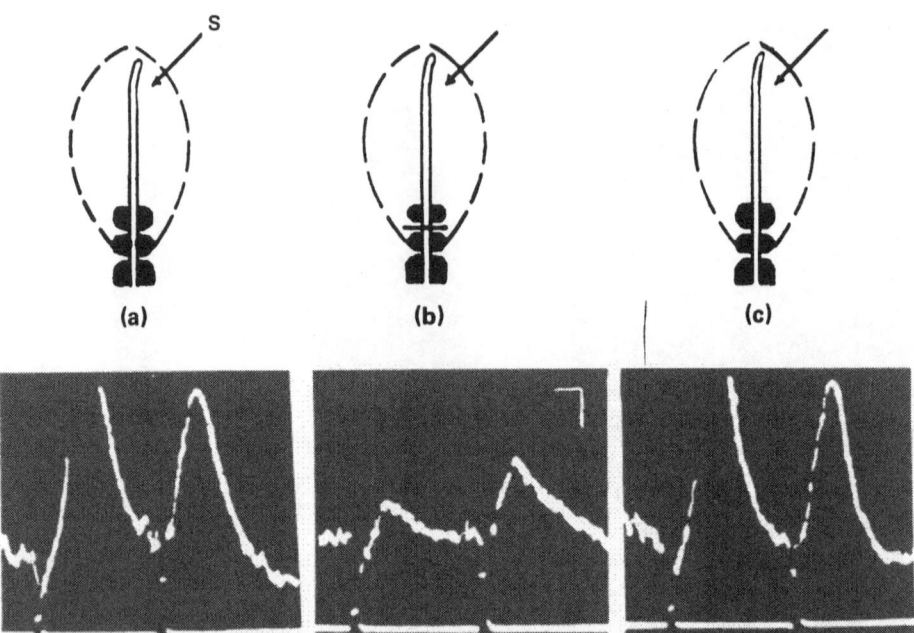

FIGURE 4.12 *Loewenstein and Rathkamp's pressure block experiment, which demonstrated that the first node of Ranvier is the critical point for the conversion of the generator potential into the spike action potential. The arrows in this figure show the point of presentation of two brief mechanical stimuli. In (b) a pressure block is applied at the point indicated with the horizontal line. Only the generator potential is seen in this case, but both before and after the block [(a) and (c)], the stimuli produce a pair of spikes (from Loewenstein and Rathkamp, 1958).*

The next question, then, and the one of most direct relevance to the topic of this section is: what is the site of origin of the generator potential itself? The pressure block technique was also used to answer this question, but in this case the pressure block was applied to the unmyelinated portion of the nerve ending at the tip of the axon. The result obtained by Loewenstein and Rathkamp, in this experiment, was that the closer to the tip of the neuron the block was placed, the larger was the generator potential and the more normal looking. Figure 4.13 presents these experimental results. The major conclusions that have to be drawn from this important experiment are: (a) it is the unmyelinated terminal end of the nerve fiber that is uniquely capable of converting mechanical energy into generator potentials, and (b) this capability is not localized. Rather, it is distributed over the entire receptive portion of the terminal, and the magnitude of the potential generator depends upon how much of the terminal portion of the neuron is stimulated.

An important general point that emerges from the Loewenstein and Rathkamp experiment is the high degree of specialization different por-

FIGURE 4.13 Loewenstein and Rathkamp's pressure block experiment, showing that the amplitude of the generator potential is a function of the amount of the terminal end of the nerve that is available. The arrows indicate the point of application of a single stimulus. The horizontal lines indicate the point of the mechanical block. In (a), (b), and (c) progressively smaller portions of the terminal are involved, and the generator potential gets progressively smaller (from Loewenstein and Rathkamp, 1958).

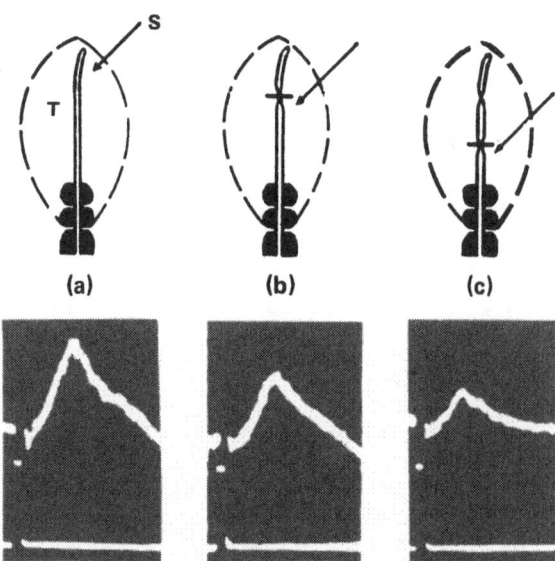

tions of the nerve membrane exhibit, even though these portions might be located within a few micra of one another. The most terminal portion of the axon can produce generator potentials, but cannot be stimulated in any way to produce regenerative spike action potentials. The narrow collar of membrane at the first node of Ranvier, on the other hand, cannot be stimulated directly to produce generator potentials. Yet this collar is the only portion of the nerve that seems to be capable of converting the generator potential to the regenerative spike for long-distance communication. More central portions of the axon, while perfectly capable of propagating spikes, cannot convert the graded generator potentials, unless abnormally large, into spikes.

This, then, is a description, as we know it today of one of the somesthetic sites involved in the transduction of mechanical energy to electrochemical neural energy. There is, of course, an immediate urge to compare this process to those occurring in the cochlea. And, indeed, there are fundamental similarities in the processes, but there are also dissimilarities which would strain any such analogy. The very high positive endocochlear potential in the scala media has no counterpart in this somesthetic receptor system. Thus, the notion of an impedance reducing mechanism capable of gating exceptionally large biopotentials, as suggested by Davis for the cochlea, has no exact equivalent beyond the usual intracellular-extracellular fluid potential difference. Furthermore, the specialized subcellular microstructure of the cochlear hair cell, the hair, and the cuticular base plate (or equally well, the equivalent structure of the cells of the vestibular epithelium) have no corresponding components in the neuronal terminal within the Pacinian corpuscle. The special role thought to be played by the cuticular base plate, therefore, would have to be played by some other membrane mechanism, and no specialized substructure is yet known in the end organ of these cutaneous receptors.

Another consideration is that it is not at all certain that the story that has emerged from the work of Loewenstein and Rathkamp for the Pacinian corpuscle is generalizable to all other mechanoreceptors. Nevertheless, there is a strong presumption that it is and that the corpuscular sheaths, as varied in shape as they are, do not play a direct role in the differential encoding of any other cutaneous or proprioceptive signals. Thus, the notion that the transducer function is actually an evolved sensitivity of the terminal portion of the anatomically undifferentiated neural membrane itself seems to be the best explanation for most somesthetic receptors.

V. TRANSDUCER ACTION IN OLFACTION

A. Nonneural Stimulus Modifications

Nonneural stimulus modification in the nose seems to be relatively simple and straightforward. Wafts of vapors of volatile chemical substances are introduced by inspiration into the nasal cavity and, by convection and diffusion, are carried to the olfactory receptor epithelium.

Yet some attempts have been made to explain olfactory quality coding on the basis of the differences in the locus at which different stimuli exert their effects. Adrian (1954) noticed that there were spatial patterns apparent in gross potential recordings from the olfactory mucosa. He speculated that these spatial patterns were true codes for olfactory discrimination and were produced by differential distribution of various odorants across the olfactory epithelium as a result of differences in their physical properties. Mozell (1967) has recorded responses from different branches of the olfactory nerve of the cat and has found evidence that the magnitude of a summated nerve discharge recorded from the most medial and most lateral nerve branches were "in a ratio (lateral nerve branch discharge/ medial nerve branch discharge) which was dependent upon the chemical presented." Recently Mozell (1970) has expanded his ideas to include a new theory of chromatographic separation, which places different olfactory stimuli at different locations on the olfactory epithelium. We shall discuss this place notion of olfactory quality coding in detail in Chapter 11.

While it is possible that such a differential spatial distribution might play some secondary role in olfaction, most workers now believe that the primary sensory action is, in fact, determined by the nature of the chemistry of the odorant molecule rather than some sort of locus effect due to the physical properties of the stimulus.

B. The Primary Sensory Action in Olfaction

Although it seems certain that the olfactory primary sensory action is a chemical interaction between the chemicals of the stimulating odorant and constituents of the olfactory epithelium, we lack a convincing statement of the nature of this chemical process. Chemicals differ in several different ways, and we are not yet certain which one is key. The problem is complicated by the fact that some apparently antithetical hypotheses put forth by different investigators may be, in fact, not quite as far from each other as they might initially seem. Very often superficially competing theories really represent alternative ways of looking at chemical reactions. Thus, for example, Amoore's (1952, 1964) theory of stereoisomeric shape coding, while at first glance quite different from some of the binding type theories, may actually be based upon ideas of shape, which are in fact derivable from the fundamental nature of the chemistry of molecular binding. The confusion is compounded by the fact that conventional chemical interactions (specific reactions occur between specific ions) are not capable of explaining why many different chemicals with similar shapes, but dissimilar structures, can produce similar olfactory experiences.

Modern theorizing about the primary sensory action of olfaction, as summed up by Adey (1959), has considered that it may not be the specific chemical composition but, rather, some more general feature of a molecule's makeup that accounts for its differential action. Adey notes that Hill and Carothers (1933) suggested that the matter was as simple as the number of atoms in an organic ring molecule directly determining olfactory quality, but there were many exceptions, which led to the rejection of this simple idea. Legge (1953) suggested a modified shape theory, which was based upon the rupture of specific bonds as odorous materials interacted chemically with the olfactory epithelium. Both Alexander (1937) and Kistiakowsky (1950) supported the view, on the other hand, that the action was based on catalytic modification of organic reactions by odorous substances. Kistiakowsky actually developed a theory based specifically upon inhibitory action in this case, but it, like other catalytic theories, was unconvincing. Smell thresholds are typically so low that inhibitory catalytic reactions seem unlikely candidates because of their large energy requirements. Sumner (1953) hypothesized a model theory of olfaction based upon Pauling's notion of bonding, which suggested that the bonding angles of some chemicals resident in the olfactory epithelium were altered in the same way as the bonding angles of 11-cis retinal molecules in the retina were altered by light. Presumably spontaneous processes would follow analogous to the dark decomposition of the series of intermediary breakdown products of rhodopsin.

Dravnieks (1967) has emphasized an important fact regarding the bonding of odorants to the olfactory receptor tissue. He noted that electron donor-acceptor characteristics of the olfactory material and the receptor tissue may have very important roles to play in setting the absolute thresholds for odors. While his work was specifically concerned with the threshold of olfaction, Dravnieks feels that it also is possible to extend the notions of electron donor-acceptor action to qualitative distinctions at higher intensity levels. Dravnieks also has discussed the possibility that differential rates of absorption of different liquid-sol-gel phases scattered across the olfactory epithelium may account for some facets of olfactory quality discrimination.

Davies (1965, 1970) has suggested a model of olfactory transduction, which he refers to as the "Puncture and Penetration" theory. The main idea in this formularization is that molecules of odorous substances are absorbed by some relatively poorly defined mechanism into the lipid surface of the olfactory receptor cell membrane—but only temporarily. After a brief period, these molecules may either escape outward from the membrane, a process which is most properly referred to as *desorption,* or diffuse through it. Because of the molecular properties of the membranes, however, the hole that is left after the odorant leaves cannot be immediately filled, and there is, therefore, a temporary gap through which Na^+ and K^+ ions can diffuse under the influence of the usual passive forces. This redistribution of ions across the cell membrane leads to the direct generation, according to Davies, of the generator potentials and ultimately to propagated nervous activity.

According to Davies' puncture and penetration theory, the differentiation of odorous qualities is a result of the specific diffusion properties of olfactory stimuli. He postulates that the quality of a sensation will depend upon the relation between the diffusion rate of the stimulus molecules away from the hole and the hole's healing rate.

Over the years a number of other investigators have attempted to link the infrared or ultraviolet optical absorption or emission properties of chemicals to the primary sensory action. Early theories suggested that it was direct absorption of infrared energy by the receptor tissue from the odorants (or vice versa), but this notion was disqualified as a possible mechanism by Ottoson (1956), who showed that no smell could be induced through a membrane transponent to the hypothesized critical wavelengths. Direct chemical contact was required for olfactory perception.

The most important of the modern optical theories is Wright's (1964) postulate of vibrational coupling. He believes that the molecular basis of olfactory discrimination lies in the fact that specific chemical structures have specific vibrational patterns, which are incidentally reflected in their infrared spectra. Wright believes that the primary sensory action in olfaction is a coupling of the nearly resonant frequencies of vibration of substances in the olfactory pigment with those of the odorant stimulus molecules. Thus, substances with identical vibration patterns should smell alike. Unfortunately for his point of view, some recent experiments (Russell and Hills, 1971; Friedman and Miller, 1971) have shown that enantiomeric forms of some chemicals (that is, molecules that have identical structure with the exception of being mirror images of each other, and thus which would be expected to have identical rotational and vibrational energies) do not always smell alike. The enantiomeric forms R- and S-carvone, for example, smell like oil of spearmint and caraway, respectively. These recent experiments were carried out with particular attention to the control of impurities. By interconverting between the two substances, the smell could be systematically changed. These two controls overcame earlier criticisms of impurities as a source of error in experiments with enantiomeres. As the journal *Nature* put it, these data are "death" to any theory that attributes olfactory specificity to the optical or vibrational properties of the macromolecule.

The safest conclusion, however, to be drawn at the present time is that there is no theory of olfactory primary sensory action that is universally accepted. If any one theory can be singled out as at least having received more attention recently, it is certainly the development by

Amoore (1952, 1964) of a suggestion made by Moncrieff (1949) referred to as the stereochemical configuration theory of olfaction.

Before we discuss Amoore's work, it might be well to review a bit of basic organic chemistry nomenclature. As we saw in our discussion of visual transduction, chemical compounds can vary in their shape as well as in the proportion of the constituent elements. Thus, we saw that retinal, for example, could assume a large number of different shapes, depending upon where bends occurred in the string of carbon-to-carbon bonds. On the other hand, many different chemicals can assume almost the same stereoisomeric shape, even though they have very different chemical formulas. The similarity, however, may also reflect some similarity in underlying structure, which may be more profound than simple shape similarities and which may produce common chemical reactivities. It is for this reason, as we noted above, that several different measures of the nature of odorants may all correlate with olfactory quality, even though none is a unique key to the primary sensory action.

In this light Amoore's theory probably should be considered to be something of a metaphor. While it is not yet convincing in terms of the specific mechanisms that bind a particular molecule to a particular receptor site, it does illustrate one systematic factor, which may be used as an indicator of common odorous quality. The statistics associating shape and sensory quality, which he presents, are fairly vigorous and suggest that if shape is not the critical factor, it is at least a pretty good sign of the true mechanism.

Amoore's theory was originally based upon a number of indirect pieces of evidence. His original approach was based upon an assumption which, *a priori*, might have seemed to be somewhat of an oversimplification. He simply assumed that if there were specific receptor sites, there would have to be a finite, and perhaps even a very small number of different basic smells. Such a notion has been supported by the fact that very specific anosmias (smell "blindnesses") are known to exist. Such specific insensitivities suggest the presence of a set of specific receptors, one type of which may be missing to produce the deficit. Amoore turned to a literature search to determine what basic smell names were used by chemists more often than any others. These, he presumed, would be characteristic of the set of basic smells. The literature search did turn up a surprising fact! A very large proportion of the smells reported by chemists could be accounted for by only seven smell names. These were:

Camphoraceous
Musky
Floral
Minty
Etheral
Pungent
Putrid

Amoore continued his literature search and examined the structural shape of a large number of chemicals that were routinely described as having

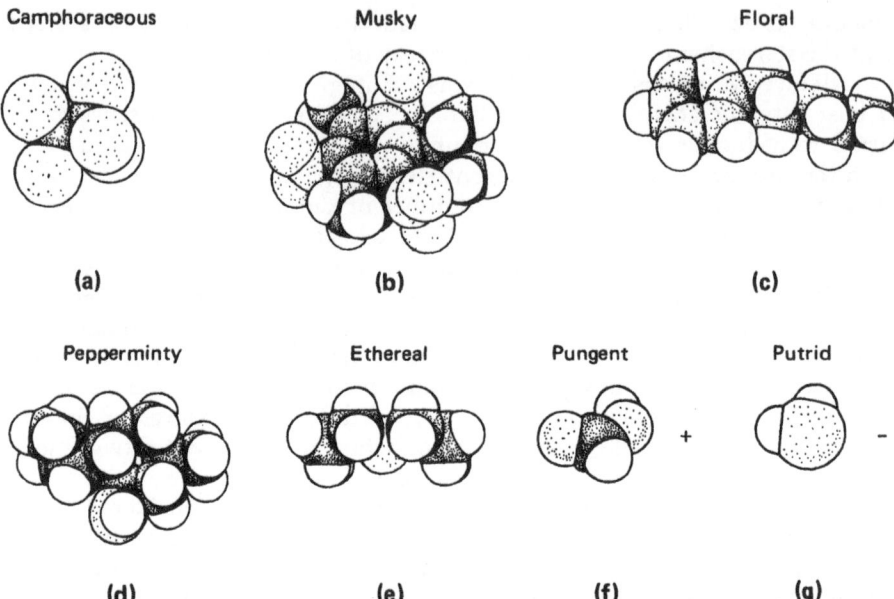

FIGURE 4.14 Amoore's suggestions of the stereogeometric forms of the seven basic smell substances and the names commonly associated with these stimuli. Five of the basic smell chemicals are individually shaped. Two are based upon the electrical charge of a relatively small molecule (from Amoore et al., 1964).

one or the other of these smells. He found that, indeed, there was a rough correlation of shape and odor! Each of the seven basic smells (except for pungent and putrid) was associated with one of the archetypical shapes shown in Figure 4.14. Camphoraceous smells seemed to be associated with chemicals whose stereoisomeric shape was ovoid. Musky smells were characterized by oval disks; floral smells by mace-shaped molecules; minty smells by oval wedges, and etheral smells by rod-shaped molecules. The two exceptional smells, pungent and putrid, were not consistently of one shape or another, but, rather, Amoore observed that pungent smells typically tended to be positively charged objects (indicative of an electron deficiency someplace in their structure), and putrid smelling objects typically tended to be negatively charged objects (a surplus of electrons).

The next step in the development of Amoore's theory required him to make a speculative leap, which is both ingenious and, as it turned out, treacherous. He assumed that if the molecules of the odorants were of such specific shapes (or charges), then the way in which they would be captured by the olfactory receptor site might also depend upon similar specificity in the shape of the receptor sites. Figure 4.15 displays the set of the five shaped and two charged receptor sites, which Amoore thought conceivably could be sufficiently specific so that one basic type of odorant fits in better than any of the others.

Before we proceed to a further discussion of this idea, which as the reader can see emerges as a sort of "key-and-lock" theory, it would

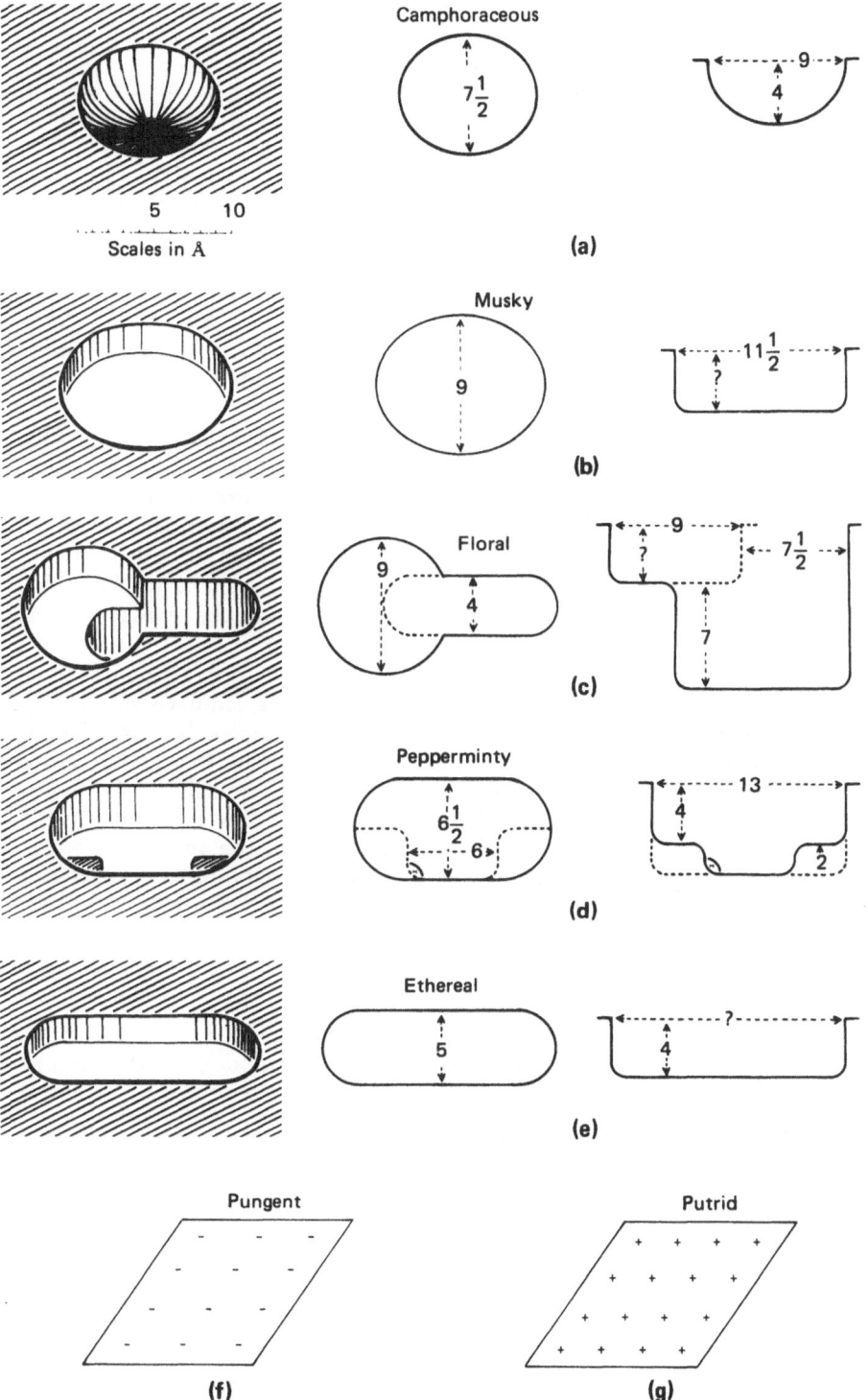

FIGURE 4.15 Amoore's suggested shapes and dimensions for the five shape sensitive receptors and the two charge sensitive sites on the olfactory receptor (adapted from Amoore, 1962).

be well to consider that this notion of shaped receptor sites might also be a sort of a metaphor. Receptor site shape might be a description of a region that has a very specific sort of chemistry, just as molecular shape of the odorant may be a metaphor for a specific form of chemistry. The main features of Amoore's theory, then, are not so much the exact nature of the site as they are the general notion that there are small localized spots, which have a heightened receptivity to one of the several types of odorous molecules. There is no reason why these localized spots need be exclusively of a single type on the microvilli of a single receptor cell. Thus, while a spot may be very specific, it would still be possible to have receptor cells that were more or less broadly tuned to a wide variety of different odorous substances.

Amoore was then faced with the problem of how to go about testing the theory. He has, over the years (Amoore, 1965; Amoore and Venstrom, 1967), carried out a number of very interesting experiments, which have elaborated and modified the original notion. Laboratory-synthesized molecules of the appropriate shape were sensed by expert observers in an attempt to find out whether the smell associated with the shape of the molecule held true for newly developed molecules. Generally the answer was in the affirmative.

In one of his most recent papers, Amoore (1965) reports the development of two highly precise ways of measuring shape similarities—a step considerably beyond simple statements of whether molecules were ovoid or rod shaped. The first of these techniques involved the manufacture of solid models of the molecules and plexiglas "tank" models of the hypothetical receptor sites. The model of the molecule was then immersed in the water-filled receptor site model and measures taken of the amount of water displaced by the model molecule. The complementarity (C) or degree of fit was then defined as:

$$C = \frac{V_d{}^2}{V_s \times V_m} \tag{4.2}$$

where V_d was the volume of water displaced by the model, V_m the volume of the model, and V_s the volume of the site. The better the fit, the closer the complementarity would approach 1. However, because all models could not be immersed completely and because of the "knobby" shape of these molecular models, the actual ratios varied from a high of 0.44 to a low of 0.03.

Unfortunately for his theory, these complementary scores did not correspond very well with an associated set of psychophysical tests of odor similarity. Many different molecular shapes with complementarity scores that were quite alike smelled quite differently, and many with very dissimilar scores smelled quite alike. "In fact," as Amoore says, "for the etheral and camphoraceous sites, the results were downright disappointing."

It should be remembered though that in this particular case, the comparison is being made between molecular shapes that are well known

TABLE 4.2   A STANDARD SET OF ODOROUS CHEMICALS THAT
WILL PRODUCE THE SEVEN "BASIC" (ACCORDING TO AMOORE) SMELLS*

Standard Odor	Representative Compound
Etheral	1,2-dichloroethane
Camphoraceous	1,8-cineole
Musky	15-hydroxypentadecanoic acid lactone
Floral	d,1-β-phenylethylmethylethyl carbinol
Minty	d,1-menthone
Pungent	formic acid
Putrid	dimethyl disulfide

and hypothetical receptor sites of which virtually nothing is known. For
this reason Amoore tried an alternative method to compare shapes. Silhouette diagrams were made of the top, front, and side view of each
of the test molecules. This time these silhouettes were compared not
against a hypothetical receptor site, but against similar silhouettes of a
standard set of odorous chemicals. Table 4.2 lists these standard odorants
as chosen by Amoore.

Metrics of the similarity of a test and a standard molecule were then
computed in the following way. Amoore first physically determined the
center of gravity of the cutout silhouette. The radial distance from this
center to the periphery was then measured each 10 deg of arc. Comparisons
were then made by subtracting each distance on a sample from an equivalent measure on the standard and computing the mean deviation $\bar{\Delta}$ of all of
the 108 angular radii (108 radii are present because each of the three silhouette views of a single molecule had 36 different measured radii). The
similarity index was then computed as the ratio:

$$\text{similarity} = \frac{1}{\bar{\Delta} + 1} \tag{4.3}$$

Correlations were then computed between psychophysical tests of
odor similarity and these measures of shape similarity. Relatively high
degrees of correlation between odor and shape similarity were found for
107 different substances.

The main thrust of these geometrical analyses is that a major modification was required of the original stereoisomeric theory. Amoore still

believes, on the basis of the silhouette similarity measures, that the basic discriminating characteristic of olfactory chemicals is molecular shape. But he has had to soft-pedal the notion that equivalently shaped receptor sites account for the differential receptivity. The simple three-dimensional geometry of the receptor sites seems clearly not to be able to explain the selective action of molecules of a given shape.

If a key-and-lock notion cannot be used to explain different sensory effects of molecules of varying shapes, then we once again must face the possibility that shape alone is merely an epiphenomenon. It is a measure indicative of some more fundamental characteristic of the interactive forces that hold molecules together, and it is that more fundamental property, rather than shape, that must explain receptor specificity.

In summary, we can say that it now seems most likely that the primary sensory action in olfaction is a chemical interaction of the molecules of the odorant with more or less specific receptor sites on the surface of the olfactory epithelium. The nature of this chemical reaction is, for all practical purposes, unknown. With the rejection of the lock-and-key aspects of Amoore's theories,[2] the single strong fact remaining is that the shapes of the molecules, whatever they may mean, are highly correlated with psychophysical discriminations. Future research will have to unravel how this shape difference is discriminated by olfactory receptors.

C. The Production of the Olfactory Generator Potential

Since we do not know the nature of the olfactory primary sensory action, the mechanism of the production of the olfactory generator potential must be equally obscure. We can only speculate that in some way, the chemical action leads to a change in the permeability of the membrane of the receptor cells of the oldfactory epithelium. This permeability change allows the ionic equilibrium to shift in such a way that a graded potential, which is capable of initiating spike action potentials further down the filia olfactoria, is produced.

This simple and speculative statement, however, is complicated by another problem. There is a great deal of controversy concerning whether or not the olfactory generator potential has actually been detected and recorded. A family of slow potentials is known to be generated at the olfactory epithelium by odorous stimulants. Nevertheless, like the auditory situation, it is not clear whether any of these are, in fact, the true generator potential. Ottoson (1956) has made extensive studies of a graded negative potential, which occurs with moderate latency and a very slow time course after the application of a stimulus. Figure 4.16 (a) shows a typical negative electroolfactogram recorded with the apparatus shown in the inset. This signal is now commonly referred to as the "Ottoson" potential in honor of its discoverer.

However, there is also a positive-going potential of similar temporal characteristics observable under some conditions. Takagi, Shibuya, Higashino, and Arai (1960) observed that with certain stimulants, the

[2] For the most recent statement of his ideas, see Amoore's (1970) book entitled *The Molecular Basis of Odor.*

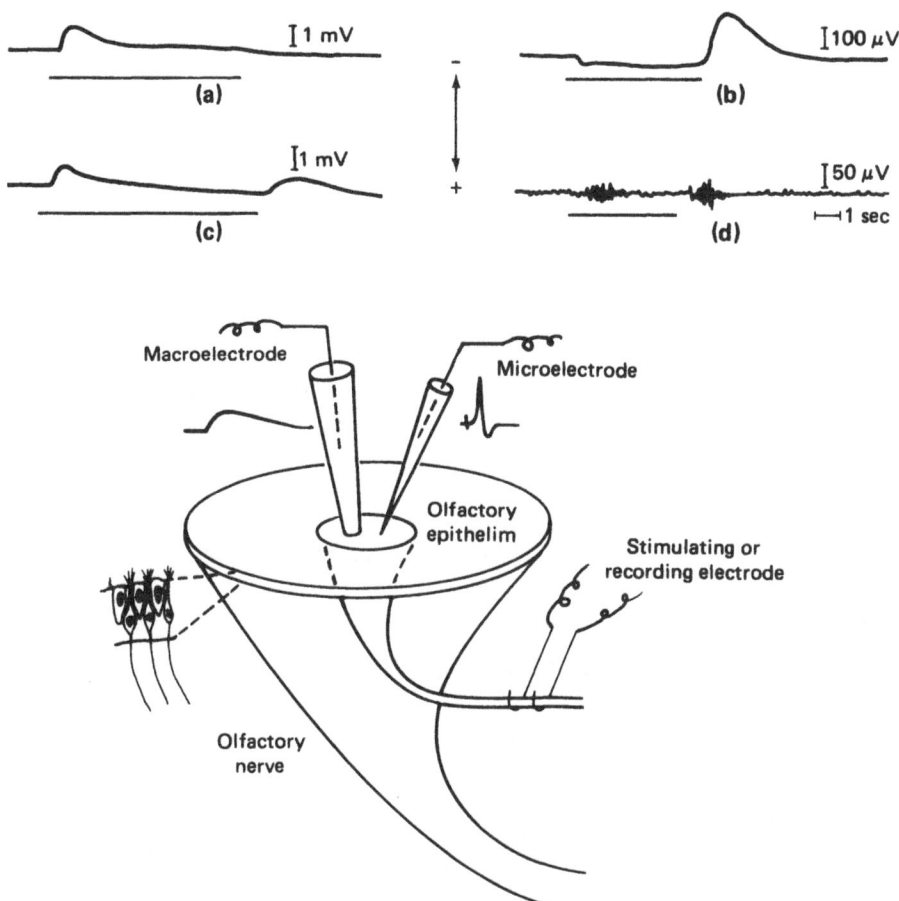

FIGURE 4.16 Records of the variety of electroolfactograms (presumably an integrated form of the olfactory generator potential) recorded when different stimuli are used. (a) Shows a typical negative-going (upward) "on" response reported by Ottoson. (b) Shows a positive-going "on" response and a negative-going "off" response. (c) Shows a negative-going "on" and a negative-going "off" response. (d) Shows that spike activity that is induced by (b) and indicates that either polarity is effective as the generator potential, or alternatively that neither is the generator potential. There is, however, nothing special about the negative-going Ottoson potential. The underlines indicate the stimulus duration producing the various potentials. The insert shows the recording apparatus (adapted from Takagi, 1967).

polarity of the graded Ottoson potential was reversed [see Figure 4.16(b)]. In addition, Takagi and Shibuya (1959) showed that there was often also a negative-going off-potential associated with the typical negative-going Ottoson or the anomalous positive-going on-potential, as shown in Figure 4.16(b) and (c). Figure 4.16(d) shows the associated spike activity in the olfactory bulb and its relation to some of these graded potentials.

Unfortunately, there are a number of discrepancies, which prevent confirmation of either one or some of the system of graded potentials as generator potentials. Takagi (1967) spells out some of the discrepancies in an interesting review of the problem. Among others, one of the most damaging is the report by Shibuya (1964), which showed that the Ottoson potential could be eliminated (by wiping off the mucous usually spread on the olfactory epithelium) without any diminution of olfactory bulb spike action potentials. Takagi goes on to suggest that at least some of the system of graded potentials may be no more than secretory potentials produced by the sustentacular cells of the olfactory epithelium. If so, it would be a somewhat disappointing state of affairs, because no known candidate for the generator potential role would then be left. Clearly, there certainly is much more to be learned about the transductive process of olfaction both with regard to the generator potential and its origin and also with regard to the mechanism for the conversion of generator potentials to spike action potentials. Unfortunately, this latter conversion is probably a function of a region at the base of the olfactory receptor cell, where its axon emerges, and the olfactory axons are so small that technical difficulties probably will prohibit any substantial progress in unraveling this mystery in the foreseeable future.

VI. TRANSDUCER ACTION IN GUSTATION

A. Nonneural Stimulus Modification

Taste is probably simpler in regard to its nonneural components than any of the other senses. Substances are placed in the mouth, munched and crunched and presumably must go into aqueous solution in saliva in order to be effective taste stimuli. No one has suggested that there is any other nonneural modification that serves any useful function in quality coding other than a sort of spatial localization of receptors found across the surface of the tongue. Receptors most sensitive to salty solutions are found mainly on the tip. Bitter receptors, on the other hand, seem to be located mostly at the back part of the tongue, while sweet receptors are found in greatest density along the sides. Whether there is any adaptive utility of such a spatial pattern is moot, but it seems unlikely that there is any differential way of distributing varying substances to specific places on the tongue on the basis of their chemical structure or physical properties.

B. The Primary Sensory Action in Gustation

Gustation is a sense that seems to be mediated by direct chemical interactions between the molecules of the stimulus and the constituent molecules of the receptor cells. Yet the very directness of this chemical action makes our knowledge of the primary sensory action less complete than for some other less directly activated modalities. The primary processes involved in taste are so microscopic that it is not yet even clear exactly where the site of the primary action resides. Presumably, and this is a point which is quite speculative, the significant chemical action occurs on specialized portions of the microvilli of the migrating gustatory receptor cells we described in Chapter 3.

Because of this sort of uncertainty and difficulties with stimulus control, research in the area of gustatory transduction has concentrated on problems that are amenable to chemical analysis. For example, attempts have been made for many years to find chemical correlates of the four classic fundamental tastes mentioned above. Before we discuss some of the associations that have been made, it would also be well to consider the fact that even this notion of a "fundamental taste" is an idea that has been drawn from only the loosest analogy between visual color mixing ideas and gustation. While it may have some useful and convenient pedagogic value, the lack of a single dimension of variation comparable to photic wavelength makes the analogy a weak one. This is particularly so in light of the fact that the correlations between chemical structure and taste have been incomplete, at best. Furthermore, up to now, taste scientists have generally found it most difficult to create complex tastes from mixtures of the four fundamentals: sweet, sour, salty, and bitter. There is, apparently, much more going on than simple additive mixture of this set of fundamentals.

Pfaffmann (1959), in a comprehensive review of the taste literature through the 1950s describes the tentative and inconsistent nature of the associations that have been made between tastes and chemical structures. The sourness of substances seems to be a function of the pH or acidity of the solution. The greater the amount of the hydrogen ion that is present, the greater the sourness of a substance. But, to confuse the issue, not all acids are sour. Amino acids are sweet, and picric acid is bitter.

A sensation of sweetness results from stimulation with a wide variety of very dissimilar substances. Typically, however, organic molecules are the ones that taste sweet, but heavy metal salts of lead and beryllium also taste sweet. This probably accounts for the high incidence of lead poisoning in children in poverty situations. Lead salts from painted walls are used as a dangerous substitute for the sucrose or lactose of candy or milk.

Dzendolet (1968) has suggested that a common feature of the sweet tasting substances is that they have some molecular bonding arrangement, which makes them proton (hydrogen ions) acceptors. This is a mechanism that would be approximated anytime a hydroxyl (OH^-) or even a hydroxyl-like ionic structure is created by some chemical action. For example, Dzendolet believes that the metal ions of inorganic salts created upon dissolution become surrounded with water molecules, that is, become hydrolyzed. However, since the metal ions are positively charged, they tend to repel some of the hydrogen atoms of the hydrolyzing water that become lost or trapped by other proton sinks such as saliva. In some instances the loss of these protons leads to an OH^- group becoming sufficiently free from one of the repelled hydrogen atoms to act as an acceptor of some other hydrogen ion. If this new hydrogen ion comes from the gustatory receptor sites, the sensation of sweetness is presumed to be evoked. Heavy metals such as beryllium and lead, which are also

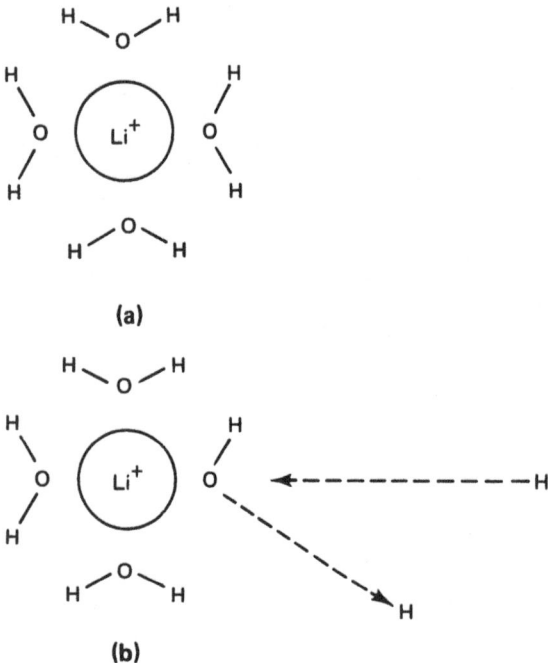

(a)

(b)

FIGURE 4.17 Dzendolet's scheme of H^+ ion replacement, which may lead to specific sensitivities for sweet tasting substances. He proposed that when ions like Li^+ become surrounded by water molecules, the positive charge of the Li^+ tends to force a H^+ ion away from one of the water molecules. At some subsequent time, the resulting OH^- molecule may be released and become a H^+ acceptor. It is that attraction for H^+ ions that Dzendolet believes is common to all sweet tasting substances (from Dzendolet, 1968).

known to be sweet, are presumed to operate in this same manner. Figure 4.17(a) and (b) displays in two plates the initial hydrolyzing reaction of a typical metallic ion and the resulting repulsion of a positively charged hydrogen ion from one of the water molecules.

Dzendolet goes on to explain how proton acceptor sites are also potential explanations of the sweetness of such diverse materials as organic molecules such as sucrose, saccharin, and urea. In all of these cases, the primary sensory action is the removal of hydrogen ions from the receptive tissue by one of these materials that have a strong affinity for this ion. The affinity, though common to all of these substances, may be due to any one of several different bonding mechanisms.

Many chemical classes contain substances that are reported to have a bitter taste, and typically as the weight of inorganic molecules increases, they taste increasingly bitter. Very often, bitter substances contain nitrogen.

Salty tasting substances are usually the ones that ionize in solution. Saltiness seems to depend on the ionization of soluble salts, which are usually made up of a metallic cation and, also usually, a halogen anion. The metals usually involved are sodium (Na^+), potassium (K^+), Lithium

(Li$^+$), magnesium (Mg^{++}), and calcium (Ca^{++}). But the ammonia radical (NH$_4$$^+$) is also often found as the cation in salty tasting substances. Typical anions include chlorine (Cl$^-$), bromine (Br$^-$), iodine (I$^-$), the sulfate radical (SO$_4$$^{--}$), the hydrocarbonate radical (HCO$_3$$^-$), and the nitrate radical (NO$_3$$^-$). Salty tasting substances are of particular interest, because they often include, among their constituents, some of the ions involved in the maintenance of the transmembrane resting potential. The addition of these species of ions could conceivably be expected to influence ionic equilibria very directly, but as we shall see, this appears not to be the case.

Beidler (1967) has presented one of the most comprehensive contemporary views of gustatory transduction. He summarizes one modern view of the cell membrane as a sandwich of lipid molecules between two layers of protein. (It should be understood that this is but one of several models of the membrane. For example, see also Singer and Nicolson (1972) for an alternative model.) The lipid molecules, according to Beidler, are perpendicular to the surface of the membrane, while the protein molecules lie transversely along the parallel surface. Because of differences in the reactivity of the inside and the outside protein layers, the two layers are not considered to be identical, and the membrane is of assymetrical permeability. Figure 4.18 is a drawing (modified from Beidler), which shows the general arrangement of one of the outer layers and the lipid central core only.

The main idea is that the transverse protein chains, which make up the surface of the membrane, are linked together by several different kinds of bonds. Furthermore, because of imperfect bonding, there are a wide variety of available bonding sites that can be linked to appropriately reactive substances that might be in the neighborhood. The membrane may also have locally charged sites and even a cumulative charge over all of its surface.

It is not possible to go into the electrochemistry of bonding in detail. For our purposes, it will be sufficient to merely point out that Lifson (1957) [as cited by Beidler] lists four different ways that sites can bind ions:

1. *Attractive interactions between small ions and the electrostatic field of the individual membrane polyelectrolytes.*
2. *Attractive interactions between small ions and the cumulative negative membrane potential, which results from the overall excess of anions in the protein network.*
3. *Joint bonding of one ion with a number of reactive groups.*
4. *Bonding of a single small ion with a single reactive side chain of the protein.*

Figure 4.18 also depicts these several kinds of binding action.

The net impact of the presence of this variety of binding types and sites is that many different solutions can be bound in many different ways to many different places on the receptor surface. Beidler goes on to point out that it is not only the charged ions that are capable of this sort of interaction, but also many other nonelectrolytes such as sugars,

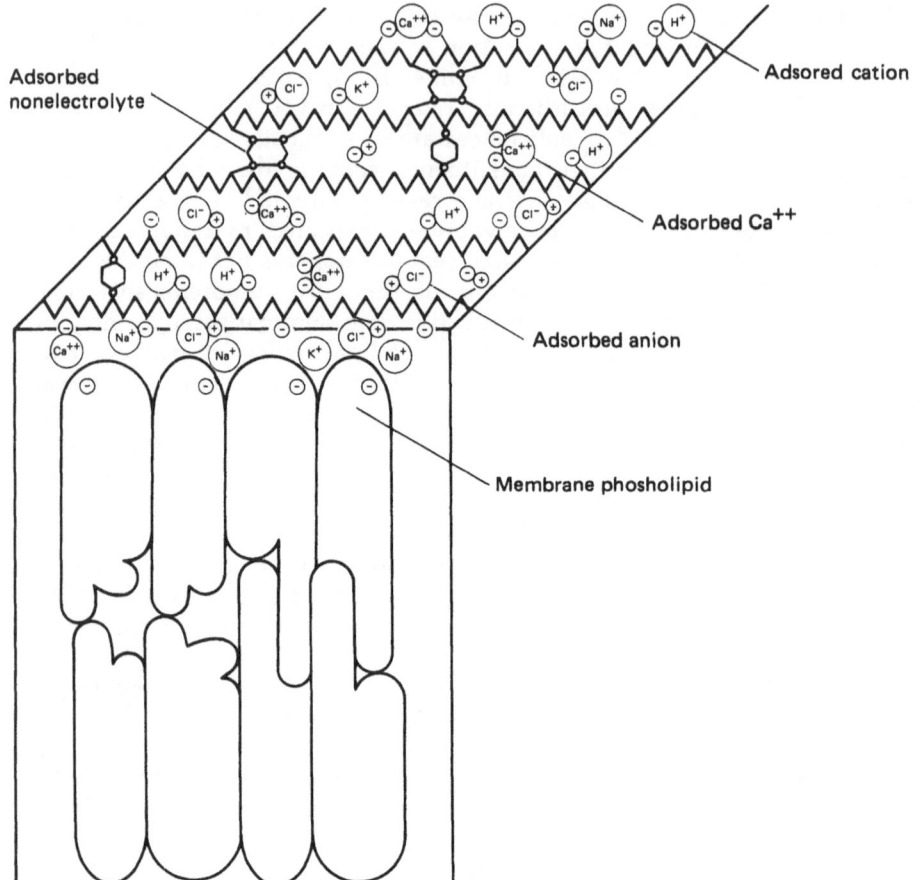

FIGURE 4.18 Beidler's schematic drawing of the variety of receptor sites on the gustatory receptor (from Beidler, 1967).

steroids, and urea are capable of being bound to the proteinaceous outer coat of the cell membrane. He also suggests that other organic molecules may be capable of being bound directly to the lipid phase beneath.

Beidler's notions are extremely interesting and most certainly will be important in the development of future understanding of the primary sensory action in gustation. But at this stage of the game, they are distressingly incomplete. No specific statement can be made of the particular types of bonds that are necessary to produce a given sensation. Simple correlations between chemicals and tastes seem to remain elusive. Different acids, different cations, and different large organic molecules all bind in ways that are specific to the particular ion, and little of a truly general nature seems to appear at the present time.

The story is further complicated by the fact that not all of the bound ions serve to excite. Some seem to inhibit sensory activity, and some seem to play no direct role, but merely alter the charge distribution

on the membrane, an alternation which could, presumably, have substantial indirect effects on the binding of other more directly effective
agents. In general, but again not exclusively, anions tend to bind to the
charged regions on the membrane in a manner which generally inhibits. Cations, on the other hand, generally tend to excite. Perhaps the
essence of Beidler's current ideas can be best summed up by quoting
him directly.

> The relative number of anionic and cationic membrane sites, as well as
> the concentration and effectiveness of each kind of cation and anion
> in the taste solution, determine not only the magnitude of the taste
> response but also its direction, whether inhibitory or excitatory.
>
> (BEIDLER, 1967, p. 532.)

But the exact nature of the specific primary response for the various
taste senses is yet to be worked out.

A step in this direction has been taken by Dastoli and his co-workers.
Dastoli and Price (1966) and Dastoli, Lopiekes, and Price (1968) have
reported that it is possible to extract a substance from the tongue of cattle
that exhibits a weak binding action to various sugars in much the way
predicted by Beidler and in a manner that is highly correlated with sweetness psychophysics. The sweet sensitive substance appears to be a protein with a molecular weight of about 150,000. More recently, Dastoli
(1969) has reported that he was also able to extract a protein, which
seemed to be relatively specific to bitter tasting substances. The type of
interaction between these proteins and the sapid substances seemed to be
best described in terms of the weak electrostatic binding actions we have
already discussed.

The reader should also refer to the discussion of Ozeki's (1970)
work in Chapter 11, in which the specific membrane permeability changes
resulting from gustatory stimulation are considered.

C. The Production of the Gustatory Receptor Potential

It is clear that the story of both the site and the mechanism of the generator potential production process is far from fully understood. The
various binding actions, which we have described, certainly lead to
changes in the characteristics of the receptor membrane. It must be assumed that there is an alteration in the permeability of the membrane
to the specific ions involved in the maintenance of the resting potential
as the binding interactions occur. As the Na^+, K^+, and Cl^- ions change
their steady-state conditions across the membrane, a depolarization (the
receptor potential) probably occurs. The effects of this depolarization presumably might be to release transmitter substance at the base of the
olfactory cell or to directly depolarize the postsynaptic regions, thus leading to activation of the initial fibers in the various gustatory nerves.
Beidler suggests that the transmission of the information contained in the
receptor potential could possibly be a result of a quasi-physical effect like
the reorientation of the molecules to the membrane. But this is speculation,
and the effect might also equally well be a simple electric sensitivity of

the regions supplying the transmitter substance. Again we must simply admit that in this present discussion, we are at the frontier of contemporary knowledge, and no more definite information other than these vague speculations has as yet been forthcoming.

Empirically, some graded potentials, which may actually be the gustatory receptor potentials, have been observed with dc amplifiers and microelectrodes inserted into individual receptor cells of the taste bud. Kimura and Beidler (1961) have found that the amplitude of these signals varied as a function of the nature of the chemical used as a stimulus as well as with its concentration (see Chapter 6). Whether this particular graded potential is actually the receptor potential or is merely another example of a chemical reaction, concomitant but irrelevant to the transductive process, cannot yet be definitively established.

This, then, brings our discussion of the prerequisite materials to a close. We have considered the philosophical implications, the physics of stimuli, the relevant anatomy of receptors, and their transductive properties. These are the classical materials, that are absolutely essential for an understanding of the remaining topics in this book. Clearly though, at this point in this book, we have reached a line of demarcation beyond which our attention is going to shift to a new orientation. That orientation is characterized by correlative studies between psychophysical and neurophysiological data. To understand the implications of this new set of material, we now turn to a discussion of what it is that we mean by coding and coding dimensions.

SECTION TWO: SENSORY CODING

CHAPTER 5: AN INTRODUCTION TO THE BASIC CONCEPTS OF SENSORY CODING

I. INTRODUCTION

So far in this book we have dealt with materials that were organized in a more or less conventional fashion. With this chapter we begin to deal with the problems of the neural coding of sensory experience—a set of topics that have only begun to emerge as a coherent scientific subtopic in the last decade or so. Prior to the 1960s, only a few workers had dealt with the specific subproblems of what we now appreciate as a much more complex and general inquiry into the relationship between experience and nervous action.

The word *coding*, itself, is clearly a borrowed one, and we have to make clear to what it is that we refer in this second half of this book. This is the main purpose of this chapter. The term has been used in communication theory and cryptographics, as well as in contemporary studies of the representation of genetic traits by large molecules. Nevertheless, the word coding, as various as its use is in all of these sciences, has a relatively constant meaning. It is the subject matter of inquiries into the nature of *representation*. In all of the sciences the following question is asked: how do signals or symbols from one universe of discourse represent patterns of information from another? The major theoretical notion that underlies coding theory is that there are invariants of organization, pattern, or meaning, which can be conveyed from sources to destinations even though represented by different symbols and in different kinds of physical energies in the communication process.

Perhaps this point can be clarified by a few simple analogies. Imagine a line of people each of whom is capable of translating the information presented to him in one language into a different language, and then passing it on to the next person in the chain. The idea communicated, barring linguistic anomalies, can usually be regenerated in the original language at the end of a chain by an appropriate translator. At the end of the chain, however, it is probably the case that the exact sentence structure will not have been maintained, and furthermore there is always the possibility that mistranslations or misinterpretations, either intentional or accidental, may have occurred. (This sort of "noise" is a constant by-product of all but the most perfect of communication systems.) But, with a bit of good luck, the meaning of the communicated idea will be more or less reproduced, in spite of the fact that it has been represented by several different languages at several different stages of the communication process.

Languages are the analogues of codes in the lexicon of the sensory-coding theorist. Words are the analogues of the variety of different neurophysiological signals. Grammatical rules are the analogues of the rules of transformation and encoding. On the other hand, it is often not so easy to discern what the analogue of the message is in the case of sensory coding. We may either assume that the physical geometry and timing pattern of the stimulus initially define a message or perhaps, more properly, we may assume that the dimensions of sensory experience are the real components of the message. As is well known, it is not always the case that the two are direct correspondents. Illusions produced by conflicting cues and outright hallucinations are both common categories of experience in which there is a lack of correspondence between the percept and the stimulus.

What, then, is a formal definition of a code? We may define a code as a set of symbols that can be used to represent message concepts and meanings (patterns of organization) *and* the set of rules that governs the selection and use of these symbols. For example, the representation of the amplitude of a stimulus or of a sensory magnitude (the message) by a train of nerve impulses (the symbols), whose frequency is related to the stimulus magnitude by a logarithmic compression law (the transformation rule), is a fairly complete statement of at least one coding situation. In previous chapters we have been discussing mainly the characteristics of the symbols of neural coding. Now we turn our attention more to the transformation rules.

Sensory-coding mechanisms have several peculiar properties, which distinguish them from the communication links in, say, telegraph wire. Perhaps the most subtle and important difference is that there really is no requirement for any decoding of the message at its destination. We certainly do not yet know what aspects of neural action are identifiable (see Chapter 1) with experience, but it seems almost certain that all that is required is that there *exist* some representation of the pattern at some appropriately high level of the nervous system. It is not necessary to assume the existence of a central decoder or in Bullock's (1961) words, to find out "who reads ensemble codes." All that is necessary is that the coded information pattern arrive at its destination. We may then assume that the pattern of neural activity so constituted is identifiable, in at least some manner, with the experience. No homunculus, no separate nonneural mechanism of any kind, need be invoked, merely the establishment at some center of a given state or pattern of neural action.

While it is clear that there are profound philosophical implications to such a perspective, no matter how technically or esoterically the statement may be phrased, these are matters for others to discuss and ponder. The notion that the mental life is equivalent to the state of neural activity at some appropriate center is presented as an axiom of the discussion that follows.

Another important notion that emerges from that analogy of the line of translators is an equally significant axiom of sensory coding theory. In the line of translators, there was no single language that was more fundamental than any other. In the nervous system, there are also chains of encoders and neural translators, and there is also no best or more fundamental single code for a message any more than there was a single best language for the representation of the whispered message.

We often refer to the steps in the sequence of neural representation as the levels of encoding because of the general "ascending" directionality to sensory communication. Two coded representations of the same stimulus pattern at two levels of the nervous system, although transformed into different sets of symbols, must represent at least the critical features of the original external stimulus pattern. Indeed, these two coded representations can also be considered to be transformations of each other. The main limitation of this generalization is that not all features of the original pattern may be retained throughout the sequence of transformations—later stages may contain less information, or more, or simply differ more from the original pattern than earlier stages. Nevertheless, the important point is that at each stage in the chain of nervous transmission, the same information may be represented by almost unrecognizably different patterns of physical and electrochemical energies. Thus, when we talk about "the" nervous code, it is absolutely critical to define the transmission link or level about which we are speaking.

In general, the second law of thermodynamics requires that there be degradation of the information content at each stage of neural transmission and at each sequential recoding stage. A main function of the nervous system, as is clearly evident from many kinds of investigation, is to accomplish a degradation of the information content of the stimulus in a selective fashion, gleaning from among the environmentally or evolutionarily irrelevant only those patterns that are biologically useful. Degradation of the information pattern in this case does not mean only the loss of components of the signal. It also refers to additions to or alterations of the pattern on the basis of stored information that might have previously entered into the memory of the organism, or on the basis of the injection of other spurious signals. Degradation is more properly considered as a measure of the fidelity of the system, with either information loss or spurious information addition contributing equally to message quality deterioration.

In the context of our present discussion, two further examples of signal degradation may be useful to elucidate this point. A flash of light, which is a trigger for some more elaborate behavior pattern, clearly carries much less information than the observer subsequently attributes to it. A flash is simply that—a brief impulse of light. However, the observer may have learned through previous experience that a flash is associated with some more complicated percept, and the flash thus may recall a complex system of memories. Clearly, the original message in this case has been degraded in the sense that far more "meaning" is attributed to it than it really contains. This additional meaning is noise, in the view of the coding theorist.

On the other hand, a complex visual stimulus field may be processed by the nervous system in such a way that only its contours or gradients are communicated to higher centers. In this case, the information is also degraded, not by adding additional information, but rather by deleting certain of the informational components, which were part of the original stimulus. This, too, is a degradation of the stimulus, but in this case by subtraction rather than addition.

The multiplication of levels and coded representations and the problems introduced by message degradation suggest that it may be difficult to find coding principles of great generality. There is, however, a great simplifying notion present, which suggests that general principles may emerge. That idea is that there are probably common functions at comparable levels of the various sense modalities. The organization of this book, in particular, is based upon an attempt to elucidate those features that appear to be common to all modalities. An alternate emphasis, which might have been used but which, it is believed, would exaggerate the unique attributes of the different sensors, would be to organize the book along the classic pattern of the sense modalities themselves.

Another important point that must be made now is that the general problem of sensory coding is a much more complex and multifaceted one than the simple problem of determining the functional relationship between stimulus intensity and nerve impulse frequency, which is so often presented as "the" sensory-coding problem. While such an oversimplification is not as frequently the case as it has been in the past, there still is some tendency to emphasize this single aspect of sensory coding in the current literature.

The reasons for this emphasis are not hard to find. The dramatic size and explosiveness of the propagated spike action potential made it a far more visible and interesting signal than the much more delicate graded synaptic and receptor potentials. In addition, the usual technology in a single cell electrophysiological experiment involves the use of a micropipette and an oscilloscope. For all their virtues, these instruments are limited in scope. The micropipette responds to events at but a single place, and the oscilloscope (at least until some of the recent developments of some highly ingenious spatial display techniques) had usually been used as a simple plotter of time functions. Experiments based on this particular methodology, therefore, tended to overemphasize the importance of time functions at a particular point in space. It has not been until recently that it was realized that there are many other possible neural codes of equal importance. This is certainly an example of the tremendous constraining influence on one's perspective that can be produced by one's technology.

In the following sections we shall try to spell out a view of the coding problem, that is based upon the correlation of two groups of dimensions. The first group of dimensions describes messages. As we have noted, there are two ways in which the characteristics of the message may be discussed. One way is to assume that the key reference is, in fact, the physical stimulus and that it is sufficient to merely talk about physical stimulus dimensions.

On the other hand, our earlier discussion of the transductive processes should have forewarned us that physical dimensions may be very quickly re-encoded into entirely different stimulus dimensions even within the receptor itself. A temporal dimension might be converted into one of magnitude, and a spatial one might become a temporal one under the appropriate conditions. An alternative scheme in which such conversions could be accounted for is desired.

An eminently feasible alternative is to base our discussion on the dimensions of the sensory experience rather than the stimulus. In this case, we would deal with a dimension of the experience rather than the dimensions of the stimulus, that might have produced that sensory fluctuation. This alternative scheme might well be called the set of discriminable dimensions of the physical stimulus or, alternatively, the set of common sensory dimensions. This latter nomenclature emphasizes the fact that this schema is modality independent. The same set of common sensory dimensions can be used to describe patterns as well in one sense as in any other.

This point can be made somewhat more concrete by a specific example. Consider the auditory sense. A stimulus with a certain physical intensity produces, at a given level of the ascending pathway, a neural fluctuation along some dimension. This neural fluctuation is interpreted by the nervous system in such a way that in a psychophyscial experiment, subjects may report that the stimulus was associated with a certain loudness or perceived magnitude. It is the prime premise of the remainder of this book that the relationship between the subjective experience and the neural fluctuation is the key problem that must be unraveled in psychobiological coding theory. It is not the relationship between either the stimulus and the neural fluctuation or the stimulus and perceived magnitude.

This discussion of a schema of sensory dimensions also reminds us of another fact. If a stimulus dimension can be varied without producing any behavioral change in either the short run or the long run, it is, for all practical purposes, not a dimension of interest to students of the psychobiology of sensory coding, but only to the neurophysiologist. An example of such an indistinguishable dimension change would be a shift in wavelength of the emitted radiation from an infrared or ultraviolet source. Though there is a great change in the characteristics of the physical energy, this change simply would be undetected by the sensory mechanism.

Fluctuations within the differential threshold or beyond the absolute thresholds would also presumably fall outside of our category of discriminable physical stimuli. From this sensory or biological point of view, two stimulus patterns that are not discriminated by the organism as being different are identical. It is possible that a variation in a neural coding dimension itself may be incapable of conveying behaviorally useful information. From the point of view of coding theory, such a non-functional dimension must also be considered to be of less significance than one that can be shown to affect behavior. As we shall see, one of the most important issues in the study of sensory coding will be to determine what dimensions of the neural response can pass tests of psychophysical discriminability. This is the only way to distinguish between the relevant and the irrelevant.

It is appropriate to mention again that this notion of the dimensionality of both discriminable stimuli and a set of possible neural codes has had a long and distinguished history. The attributes of psychological experience long used by psychologists encompass one similar notion. In recent years, Piéron's (1952) most interesting book on the dimensionality of sensory experience has been especially important to the development of the thinking of the author of this present book. Furthermore an insightful analysis by Rosenblith and Vidale (1962), which concentrated mostly on the visual and auditory senses was especially impressive. Piéron's book is rather infrequently cited in the American literature, but its discussion of what we have called common sensory dimensions has apparently had an important indirect influence on the development of the concept of sensory codes.

Once having defined the common sensory dimensions, the second part of this task is to identify the relevant neural parameters. In an earlier publication of this conceptual model (Uttal and Krissoff, 1967), the words "possible dimensions of the neural code" were used to catch the intended flavor of this plan. A better phrase has come into use in recent years; Perkel and Bullock (1968) refer to the possible neural dimensions as "candidate neural codes." A candidate neural code may be defined as any neural signal that varies as a function of some stimulus variable. To be a candidate does not require that it be demonstrably associated with any behavioral dimension. A candidate neural code is entered on this list purely on the basis of having been observed to vary concomitantly with some variation in a physical stimulus dimension. As we shall also see, a candidate code can be accepted as a true code only after it has passed certain tests of necessity and sufficiency not usually carried out in neurophysiological experiments. Nevertheless, additions to the list of candidate codes lie purely in the domain of the neurophysiologist. The list presented here is based upon the earlier list (Uttal and Krissoff 1967), but has been expanded and modified under the influence of Perkel and Bullock's (1968) recent tabulation.

It is important to remember that there is a dual air of uncertainty concerning the dimensions that are entered on the list of candidate codes. First of all, there is no assurance that the list is complete. New dimensions of variation are constantly being discovered and are being added to the

FIGURE 5.1 The relationships among the stimulus world, the neurophysiological responses, and the psychophysical responses. Neurophysiologists and psychologists have traditionally considered separate sets of problems from those now scrutinized by psychobiologists. But much of the older data are of relevance and provide suggestive, if not direct, evidence toward the solution of psychobiological problems.

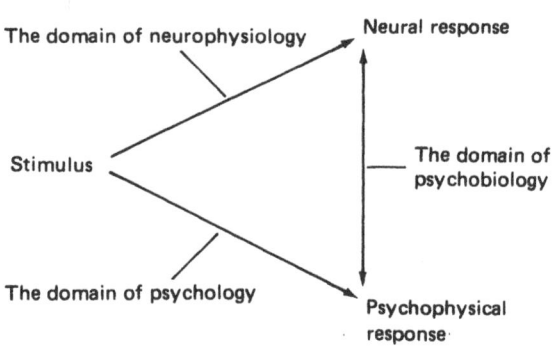

list of candidate codes. For example, it is only in the last decade that we have begun to be aware that not only the conventional mean frequency dimension of nerve impulse trains is a candidate code, but that the independent higher-order statistics of interimpulse interval might also be candidate codes. Other possible additions to the list might also be lurking just offstage, awaiting only the development of some new measuring instrument or an insightful investigation by some ingenious experimenter.

Another element of uncertainty concerning dimensions entered on the list of candidate codes is that certain dimensions, which have single metrics in some external measuring system, may have alternative and independent ways in which they might be decoded. For example, frequency is an ambiguous dimension—it may be decoded by either measuring the average interval between two impulses or by counting the number of intervals in some integrating period. In this case, also, we must wait for some further experimenter to resolve how the influence of a particular dimensional variation is exerted.

Now to conclude our introduction, we can sum up much of what we have said by noting that it is clear that the problem of the relationship among the stimulus, the neural response, and the percept has many aspects. As we have noted before, neurophysiologists mainly are concerned with the relationship between the stimulus and the neural response. They, therefore, bear the main responsibility for the establishment of the list of candidate codes. Psychologists, on the other hand, are mainly concerned with the relationship between the stimulus and the total systems behavior of the organism. Psychobiology, as we define it in the context of this book, is mainly concerned with the classic mind-body problem itself—the relationship between the neural response dimensions and the dimensions of experience. Figure 5.1 summarizes these three domains.

It is clear that the psychophysical problem and the neurophysiological problem are quite a bit more simple conceptually than is the psychobiological one. A host of new philosophical and logical problems is introduced when one attempts to make a psychobiological comparison than in the other two domains. This book, it should be repeated, is primarily a consideration of the psychobiological domain; however, it is clearly not possible to ignore the other two sets of contributions. In fact, the plain fact of the matter is that we are more likely to find neurophysiological data reported in the literature rather than psychobiological data, and in many instances our comparisons will be, in this sense, indirect. The true aim of this book should, however, be kept in mind as one proceeds through the subsequent material.

II. DISCRIMINABLE DIMENSIONS OF THE PHYSICAL STIMULUS[1] (THE COMMON SENSORY DIMENSIONS)

A. Perceived Quantity

The sensed intensity or magnitude of a physical stimulus has long been an area of concern to the psychophysical cryptographer. We might have initially considered referring subjective magnitude solely to stimulus intensity, but our discussion so far makes it clear that this is not the thing to do. While most subjective magnitudes vary with stimulus intensity to a degree, there are also any number of other ways in which the receptor or neurological mechanisms can introduce variations in subjective magnitude even with constant stimulus intensities. For example, consider that the brightness of a photic stimulus varies not only with the number of photons, but also with the wavelength of the spectral component that is utilized. Similarly, it is equally well known that the loudness of a sound is dependent on the acoustic frequency as well as the sound pressure level. Pairs of electrical pulse stimuli applied to the peripheral nerves (Uttal, 1960) produce sensations of varying amplitudes as the interpulse interval varies. Thus, in general, stimulus intensity is not the only correlate of sensory magnitude.

Conversely, stimulus intensity variations are not always sensed purely as sensory magnitude shifts. Increasing stimulus intensity beyond certain limits can produce substantial quality changes—in hue, in saturation, in pitch, or even in the production of pain.

Sensory magnitude, therefore, seems to be a more comparative dimension for the coding problem than stimulus intensity. The solution of the coding problem is a process which, as we have said, requires comparisons of psychophysical functions and candidate codes rather than of stimulus characteristics and candidate codes.

B. Perceived Quality

The kind or quality of a sensory experience is, of course, the other classic area of sensory research. Yet again, there is an ambiguity in the interpretation of this term or of its closely related biological equivalent, sen-

---

[1] Some of the following material has been adapted from a paper entitled "The response of the somesthetic system to patterned trans of electrical stimuli: An approach to the problem of sensory coding." W. R. Uttal & Madelon Krissoff; in D. R. Kenshalo, ed., *The Skin Senses.* Springfield, Ill.; Charles C. Thomas, 1968.

sory modality. At its most gross level, the problem of modality is trivial. It is clear that the receptor organs make an initial analysis of incident physical energies by virtue of a lowered threshold to one kind of physical stimulus. There is no question that the human eye is best able to detect radiant energy between 400 and 800 nm, or that, among the sense organs, the ear responds maximally to pneumatic pressure fluctuations within the range of 30 to 15,000 Hz. This is the "adequate stimulus" basis of gross "place" coding of the senses.

The second part of this dual interpretation is not trivial and has been the major point of attack of sensory theoreticians for the past century. The problem in this case concerns those different kinds of stimuli discriminable within a given modality. The nature of color vision and pitch perception, each representing families of micromodalities within vision and hearing, respectively, is a problem of this level.

In the case of vision and hearing, the specifications of the physical stimulus are very highly developed. We have a single physical dimension in each case, which can be systematically varied to alter the microquality of the visual or auditory sensation. However, when one deals with senses such as somesthesis, olfaction, and gustation, another complication arises. The separation of the various modalities into their families of micromodalities is based upon popular, historic, and nonscientific traditions. The complexities of subjective quality, in the cutaneous senses, are probably not adequately described by a statement mentioning only the classic categories of touch, pain, pressure, warmth, and cold, and an open-ended group of "derived" sensations. The electrical stimulation of the skin, for example, gives rise to sensations, some of which mimic some of these qualities, but also some for which these older classification schemes have no descriptive term.

It is surprising how difficult it is to give a good definition of quality. It might well be defined as the discriminable changes, which are left over after one has accounted for the magnitude, temporal, and spatial differences between stimuli. The best we can do here is a statement that, at least, hopefully will leave the reader with the notion of discriminable differences between kinds of stimuli.

C. Temporal Discriminations

We now leave the classic problems of quality and quantity and move into an area of discussion that is far less familiar to most students of sensory processes. There appear to be many different kinds of temporal discrimination, and these may be interpreted in manners common to several modalities. For very long durations and intervals, the temporal judgments made by an observer may be considered to be modality independent, since the stimulus events merely serve to delimit some other internal timing process. On the other hand, for very short times, within a modality, specific timing considerations are critical. For example, the ability of the nervous system to use a frequency code for intensity is bounded at the upper end by the threshold for temporal acuity. At the lower end, theoretically there is no bound, but practically, as interpulse intervals increase, there arrives an interval beyond which the neuronal circuitry can no longer wait to do its counting. Fraisse (1966) has recently published an important volume dealing with the perception of time. Beyond the scholarly presentation of a wealth of studies of temporal discrimination, his main contribution is an elucidation of the complexity of the family of time senses. Our categorization includes the following temporal discriminative abilities.

1. *Relative Temporal Order.* The ability to determine which of two different stimuli arrived first is of a high level of biological significance. This parameter of the stimulus may be dealt with in purely temporal terms by the observer, but, surprisingly, it is more often interpreted spatially. One of the most familiar of this latter class of discriminative abilities is the auditory system's use of differential time of arrival (and for higher-frequency tones—relative intensity) to localize a sound source in space. The timing precision of binaural localization is astonishingly high, corresponding to only a few microseconds of asynchrony in the arrival times.

Relative temporal order of two spatially disparate stimuli can also be a major determinant of the spatial localization of the resultant combined thermal, tactile, and gustatory sensation. Von Békésy (1963b) has demonstrated many instances of these effects and has shown that very slight differences in the relative temporal order of the two stimuli can substantially change the apparent position of the fused sensation.

2. *Temporal Acuity.* Temporal acuity is defined as the ability to distinguish two identical stimulus events, sequential in time, as being separate, rather than a single event. Temporal acuity is, of course, directly related to the relative temporal order sense, for to specify one stimulus as having preceded another, they must have been distinguished as separate events temporally. Yet we believe that these two capabilities are distinguishable from each other, since the former capability requires an ordinal judgment in addition to the more primitive resolution capability of temporal acuity. Hirsh and Sherrick (1961) demonstrated just such a distinction between simultaneity and order in their study of temporal order by showing situations in which it was possible to precisely state that two events had occurred even though the subject was confused about relative temporal order.

3. *Duration or Interval.* Another temporal sense involves the ability to replicate the sustained duration of an event or the interval between two events. This sense requires the organism to be capable of clocking time. How this is accomplished is a problem of much current speculation, since so many biological rhythms, which could serve as bases for the clocking operations, have been discovered. It is clear that there is probably no reason to distinguish between a marked interval and a continuous event, since the true stimulus information is only that included in the initiation and termination of the interval or event.

All three of these temporal discriminative abilities probably play an important role in what might be called complex temporal pattern recognition. Whether there are other temporal abilities that must be added to fully describe all aspects of temporal discrimination is yet to be determined.

D. Spatial Discriminations

The recent visual research of Hubel and Wiesel (1959), Lettvin, Maturana, McCulloch, and Pitts (1959), and of Barlow and Hill (1963), among others, have emphasized the importance of special codes for dynamic spatial parameters. In each case, stimuli were shown to produce different nerve messages when the stimulus pattern differed geometrically, even though all other stimulus dimensions were held constant. On a simpler level, it is clear that spatial localization of stimuli applied to different points of the receptor fields must be accounted for, and although we have a good deal of evidence to suggest that this is carried out by a corresponding place code within the nervous tissue, there still remain two other major problems. First, how does one explain the pseudolocations made of interacting patterns, such as those summarized in von Békésy's (1958) paper on funneling on the skin? Second, how does the mapping of spatial localization by a place code overlap with those theories of quality coding or of other stimulus dimensions that also require spatially distributed codes?

In the study of interactions between different spatial areas, a great deal of progress has been made. Ratliff (1965) reviews the work of the last century, not only describing the spatial codes for contours, but also giving a detailed electrophysiological analysis of the transformation processes, which lead from the original spatial stimulus pattern to the evoked pattern of neural signals. We shall discuss all of these problems later in Chapters 7 and 8 in great detail.

However, we do want to emphasize briefly, at this point, that there are specific types of spatial perceptual experiences that must ultimately be explained by some sort of neurological coding model. We must determine how it is, for example, that different stimulus locations are discriminated from each other. We must determine what the neural codes are that allow us to discriminate size differences and enhance contours or even see textures. It is clear that we do not have all of the answers to these questions yet. The purpose of this section is only to list and categorize the dimensions of the sensory experience, which must be so explained.

These, then, are among the most prominent of the sensory dimensions that we know to be discriminable, and that must be accounted for in any attempt to define the complete neural code. We shall now consider the possible dimensions of the nervous activity—the candidate codes—which might provide symbols for the representation of these sensory variables.

III. POSSIBLE DIMENSIONS OF THE NEURAL CODE (THE CANDIDATE CODES)

To associate common sensory dimensions accurately with neural response dimensions, one must be cognizant of as many of the likely neural dimensions as possible. The purpose of this section is to list and describe the more important of these dimensions without either resorting to a meaning-less class inclusive of all classes, such as "the spatio-temporal pattern," or to biologically unlikely possibilities.

There are, however, two important cautions, which should be noted before we consider the items in this list. First of all, the list has its origins primarily in the observed dimensions of neuroelectrical signals. It is quite clear, however, that many of these electrical signals may not be themselves the active agents, but, rather, may only be indicators of say, chemical processes, which are more directly involved in the information flow.

For example, at the synapse, the information flow is signaled by the amplitude of both the graded presynaptic and postsynaptic potentials. The actual synaptic transmission, on the other hand, is mediated by the number of packets of transmitter substance that migrate across the synaptic cleft. Both of these types of representation, the amount of the transmitter substance and the amplitude of the synaptic potentials, are presumably related, and each is a continuous function of input signal magnitude. Nevertheless, the code actually read by the postsynaptic tissue is not usually an electrical one, but a chemical one. Whether electrical signals generally represent similar indicators of more basic chemical processes elsewhere is still moot.

The second important caveat is that this list is necessarily incomplete, and new items are being added to it almost every year as new candidate codes are uncovered by neurophysiologists. New instruments, new experiments, and, perhaps most important, new insights all suggest new candidate codes which must be fitted into this scheme. By accentuating the dimensionality of the signals rather than their specific physics, however, a considerable amount of generality and flexibility is achieved, and the list remains open-ended.

It should be repeated here that the compilation of the list of candidate codes at this stage has nothing whatsoever to do with the psychophysical dimensions. It is, rather, a task that must be carried out by the neurophysiologist and, as such, is independent of any perceptual significance that the candidate code might later be shown to possess. Once a code has been identified as a candidate, then its relationship to perceptual dimensions must be separately assayed by persons who are best operating in the domain we have referred to as psychobiology.

A. Place

The particular location or place activated by an incoming signal is one very important means of representing some attribute of the input signal. There are several different kinds of spatial codes so far suggested. One of the most common is referred to as the notion of *labeled lines*. In neuronal communication systems, the mere fact that a given nerve is activated is often said to be associated with sensory quality by virtue of the specific characteristics of the transducer. There are many conceivable ways in which one particular neuron or group of neurons might be selected for the transmission of information by an incident stimulus. Lowered thresholds to particular types of physical energy or specific temporal pattern sensitivities are among the most interesting possibilities.

Müller's (1840) theory of the specific energy of nerves is a formal statement of place coding, which seems to hold true in a gross way for the representation of sensory quality. Activation of the optic nerve, for example, by any stimulus, no matter of what form, always does produce a visual sensation. In a more microscopic sense, however, the coding of microquality (hue, pitch, and so on) by place codes seems to break down and depend more on some sort of a relative temporal code—a phenomenon to which we shall pay considerable attention later in those chapters dealing with quality coding.

Another form of spatial coding, which is firmly entrenched in the sensory literature, is the notion that particular loci in the central nervous system are uniquely associated with one or another of the great sense modalities. The localization of acoustic function on the temporal lobe, visual function on the occipital lobe, and somatosensory functioning on the postcentral gyrus of the cerebral cortex all presumably represent place codes for these particular sensory macroqualities.

In recent years we have seen that these spatial codes are not absolute. Activation of a given locus is interpreted in different ways if the pattern of activation is highly localized or if it is broadly distributed. The topography of the spatial distribution of the activity, therefore, can be expected to play an important role, perhaps even in the representation of nonspatial stimulus dimensions such as sensory magnitudes.

B. Number of Activated Units

Another possible dimension of neural coding is, simply, the number of activated fibers or cells in a given nerve tract or ganglion. Magnitude is the sensory dimension, which is most often considered to be mapped, at least in part, by the number of responding neural elements. Since an increase in the number of responding units also means that more places must have been activated, it is expected that there would be strong interactions between stimulus dimensions that are coded by place and those that are coded by number.

In addition to the number of fibers that fire, we may also consider that the number of times that a given fiber fires or the duration of a burst may be a code in some instances. Thus, the number of activated units may be really a subclass of a more general candidate code—the number of impulsive responses occurring in a given volume in a given period of time.

Thompson, Mayers, Robertson, and Patterson (1970), for example, have shown that some neurons in the association cortex of the cat are capable of emitting a response if, and only if, a certain characteristic number of stimulus inputs has occurred. This ability to count did not depend upon anything other than the characteristic number for each cell. Individual cells would produce a response to the appropriate number (in various cases 2, 5, 6, and 7) of auditory or visual stimuli of any intensity, even when each individual stimulus was separated by relatively long

(1 to 5 sec) periods of time. This is an instance in which a number code at one level may be converted into a place code at another level.

C. Neural Event Amplitude

The discovery of the all-or-none law effectively removed the amplitude of the response of a single axonal spike potential from among the list of candidate coding dimensions. It appears certain now that the all-or-none law is generally valid for axonal spikes, and that the amplitude of the individual nerve impulse is related only to the metabolic state of the axon and not to any characteristic of the stimulus once the spike threshold is exceeded. However, it should be remembered that in other parts of the neuron, it has been equally clearly established that slow potentials of graded amplitude and prolonged duration are the significant information symbols.

The amplitude of the neural signal appears as an important information carrying code in many different contexts. We have already become acquainted with two of the most important: the receptor-generator potential and the potentials that are recorded from postsynaptic tissues.

In another context, we must also consider some of the amplitude measures recorded from peripheral nerve compound action potentials to be closely associated with one or another discriminable stimulus dimension. Very often, however, differences in such compound neuroelectric amplitudes merely reflect more fundamental processes. For example, the compound action potential recorded from peripheral nerves is most probably a cumulative index of the number of constituent axons that are responding in an all-or-nothing fashion (Uttal, 1967).

Another possible example of a situation in which compound action potentials encode amplitude is found in the set of measures associated with the cortical evoked potential. Here, also, there is considerable evidence that the evoked potential amplitude is a sum of the individual responses of a large number of other neural action potentials. However, there is some controversy over the origin of these signals. Some believe them to be the sum of many millions of dendritic graded potentials. Others feel that they are the summation of equally large numbers of spike action potentials. In either case, it is clear that the amplitude of the signal must be a highly indirect measure reflecting an integration of the cumulative activity of several other subpopulations of neural responses. The interesting question, of course, is: are the statistics of summation used in the production of the evoked brain potential the same as those used by the nervous system to define the perceived experience?

D. Temporal Pattern

Naming "temporal pattern" as one of the dimensions of neural coding is almost as weak a statement as naming a class of "spatio-temporal patterns"; each notion is so vague as to be almost meaningless. In the following paragraphs, we strive for more precision by specifying exactly what the dimensions are under consideration.

1. Graded Potential Time Functions—The shape of the response. Graded potentials of all kinds, receptor-generator potentials, compound action potentials from peripheral nerves, evoked brain potentials, and even free-running electroencephalographic recordings can all be described as having certain shapes. Shape is a vague term, of course, and what is usually meant by shape is a function or set of measures that describes the amplitude fluctuation of the graded potential as a function of time. Some of these parameters are relatively straightforward. For example, the simple latency pattern of the various amplitude deviations following the presentation of a stimulus can be used as a first approximation to shape. But superimposed on these simple latency measures can also be descriptions of the characteristics of the rise of the waveform. Does it abruptly appear or does it rise gradually in either a linear or exponential fashion? These are the sorts of questions that we have to answer precisely in attempts to use shape as a descriptor of the initial portion of a graded response.

Another class of time function dimensions, which has often been of importance in the representation of sensory phenomena, deals with the steady-state or quasi-steady-state portion of the response. For example, one might want to know: does the stimulus maintain a constant amount of activity or is there a significant amount of adaptation or neural accommodation over the time course of a constant stimulus? For those signals, such as the free-running electroencephalogram, which are varying spontaneously (the word "spontaneously" must, of course, be read in this case as "under the influence of unknown stimuli"), such shape parameters as the rate of change, the frequency spectrum, and the rise and fall pattern of specific waveforms must all be considered as candidate codes. In general, though, "shape" is a relatively loose term and, like macrotemporal pattern (see below), must be further qualified before being of any real use.

The following temporal candidate codes all are descriptors of the pattern of regenerative spike action potentials. Here, in accord with the all-or-none law, there is no suggestion that the amplitude of an individual spike can carry any useful information. Spike amplitude merely reflects local metabolic conditions. The temporal parameters of importance are, rather, those that describe the pulse frequency modulation characteristics of groups of spike potentials.

2. Frequency of Firing. While place and the number of activated neural elements are relatively unambiguous measures, which can be evaluated without confusion (even though the technical details may be cumbersome), frequency is an ambiguous dimension of neural activity. Frequency, or the number of responses per unit time, may be evaluated in one of two different ways by a subsequent decoding mechanism. The first way is one in which time measurements are made of the intervals between each pair of sequential responses. The alternative form of decoding possible for frequency is one in which a count is made of the number of neural events occurring within some basic integrating unit of time. As Anatol Rapoport

(1962) pointed out, the interval-sensitive procedure would be essentially an analogue process, since the range over which the interval varied could be continuous. On the other hand, the counting procedure is essentially a digital process dealing only with integral values of the number of events.

3. Macrofluctuations in Frequency Pattern. Wall and Cronly-Dillon (1960) suggested that a specific code for somatosensory quality, at certain levels, might be the macropattern of the frequency of neural discharge in afferent pathways. Thus, a frequency pattern, in which the nerve impulse rate goes from a minimum frequency to a higher frequency very rapidly and then slowly diminishes, would be perceived differently than a signal in the same pathway and with the same average frequency, but whose frequency pattern slowly increases and then rapidly diminishes. These macrofluctuations are regularly observed in many types of neurophysiological recordings from single cells and might be of significance in the encoding of stimulus dimensions other than quality.

4. Microfluctuations in Frequency Pattern. An important related question is whether or not the nervous system is able to detect microfluctuations in frequency, and whether such an arhythmia is significant as a neural coding. A microfluctuation would be defined as a transient change in the frequency pattern. A missed pulse or an extra one, or a momentary gap in the train of spikes, all might be codes for one or another common sensory dimension.

5. Temporal Comparisons Between Two or More Places. Another important class of candidate codes includes those situations in which comparisons are made in some neural center between temporal patterns which arrive on spatially separate channels. The auditory system, for example, certainly operates in some fashion that takes into account the phase and amplitude differences of neural responses to the synchronized stimuli applied to the two cochlea. Mountcastle, Poggio, and Werner (1963) have reported a similar temporal comparison process in position indicators in the cat thalamus. Furthermore, Pfaffmann (1959) has suggested that a similar kind of relative activity detection process might underly gustatory quality coding. A related idea is the volley principle (Wever, 1949), which has been invoked to explain high frequency following by the auditory system. According to this principle, spatially separate neural structures are capable of cooperatively conveying a frequency that exceeds the capacity of any individual neural structure. Such a process would require a high degree of synchronization detection ability on the part of the neurons involved and a precise comparison of their firing rates—an ability that somewhat surprisingly does seem to occur. In any of these cases, the important fact is that the critical information is not absolutely contained in a single channel of information, but rather depends upon comparison of relative amounts of activity in parallel channels. This is the basic idea of what are generally called pattern, cross-neuron pattern, or ratio theories of sensory quality.

6. Derived Statistical Measures. When we spoke of macrofluctuations, we were referring to relatively continuous changes in the frequency pattern. When we spoke of microfluctuations, we were referring to transient changes in the frequency pattern. There is, however, another possibility. There may be long-term fluctuations in the statistics of the pulse pattern that depend upon an evaluation of the microtemporal fluctuations, but in a summarized fashion over long periods of time. Thus, the standard deviation and the range of the interval histogram of individual units in the cochlear nucleus of the cat have been shown to exhibit a specific signature by Rodieck, Kiang, and Gerstein (1962). Mountcastle, Poggio, and Werner (1963) have also shown similar effects in thalamic cells representing joint position and have given an interesting analysis of how this information could be used as a code.

Furthermore, other derived statistical measures are common descriptors in statistics. In addition to the mean frequency and the variance (or standard deviation) of the interval pattern, higher-order moments can also be calculated, which can be used to compute such characteristics as the skewness or kurtosis of an interval histogram. These derived statistical measures may also conceivably play a role in neural coding. Unfortunately, there have been no attempts to determine if these derivatives of the higher moments actually vary systematically with stimuli. Thus, no progress has been made in testing their role as candidate codes, much less in determining how they might be associated with common sensory dimensions.

IV. CAUTIONS IN THE ASSOCIATION OF SENSORY DIMENSIONS AND CANDIDATE CODES

From the vantage point which has been provided by the preceding discussion, it should be apparent that the general solution of the sensory-coding problem contains a number of substeps. First, the dimensions of sensory experiences must be elucidated by psychophysical experiments on man and animals. Second, the neurophysiologist must identify dimensions of neural activity for inclusion in the list of candidate codes by determining which dimensions are functions of stimulus variations. Third, preliminary associations can be made between common sensory dimensions and candidate codes at various levels of the ascending pathway.

These associations, however, are at best only tentative. There are a number of conceptual constraints, which make final confirmation of the association—the fourth step—very elusive indeed. These constraints place limits on the assurance with which we can accept any sensory-coding association. In the following paragraphs we shall try to point out some of these potential conceptual and technical pitfalls, which impede final confirmation of tentative associations between candidate codes and common sensory dimensions.

A. A Distinction Between Signs and Codes—The Merely Concomitant Versus the Truly Relevant

The experimental paradigm in most neurophysiological experiments is such that correlations and functional relationships between stimuli and candidate neural codes can be directly established. Psychological experiments, on the other hand, typically correlate stimuli and experiences or sensations as reported behaviorally. The association of a given sensation and a specific candidate code, therefore, is generally indirect, both being functions of the third aspect of the situation—the stimulus pattern. While it seems obvious in retrospect, it is surprising to see how often physiological models of sensation ignore the fact that there is no *a priori* reason why a neural dimension, no matter how well correlated with stimulus parameters and thus indirectly with the sensory experience, should necessarily play the role of an identity function in the coding process. Philosophical considerations of parsimony (why should a neural fluctuation occur if it does not do anything?) aside, it is logically incorrect to assume that the existence of a correlated candidate code is proof that it is a true code.

To make this distinction clearer, we shall introduce a set of distinguishing definitions, expanding on the general definition of a sensory code mentioned earlier. We have defined a neural code as a set of symbols and transformation rules that allows an economical representation of a corpus of information, in a way amenable to decoding by some interpretive mechanism. To be a true code, we must add the key idea that it is also necessary that the code actually be interpreted by some subsequent mechanism. In other words, to remove some neural signal from the list of candidate codes and place it on the list of true codes, we must demonstrate that it is both necessary and sufficient for the concomitant variation of some behavioral (psychophysical) experience. A representation, which is not so interpreted, but is lost at some more central level of information processing, is, in this context, a *sign*. A sign may be useful to a neurophysiologist who may decode it or measure its properties as an indication of the current state of the stimulus environment or of the neural communication system. However, within the behavioral framework of sensory coding, such undecoded fluctuations represent little more than concomitant variations of reduced interest.

For example, in some central nervous tissues, there are cells in which a high degree of correlation exists between the variance of the intervals between successive action potentials and stimulus amplitude. Under conditions of minimal external stimulation, the intervals are both widely spaced and vary considerably. On the other hand, when high stimulus levels are imposed, the intervals both shorten and decrease in variability about their new mean value (see, for example, Hagiwara, 1949, 1950; Poggio and Viernstein, 1964). This change in interval variability has been shown to exist, but it is its effect on subsequent stages of the nervous system that must ultimately help us to distinguish this variability as either a code or a sign. If fluctuations of interval variability affect subsequent levels in such a way that they differentially influence some behavioral function, then this candidate code may be considered to be confirmed as a *code* for that function. If, on the other hand, the influence of the interval variance is lost at some subsequent synapse and cannot be shown to affect any behavior, such a candidate is defined to be only a *sign* of the external environment.

In addition, it is useful to distinguish between two kinds of signs. The first category includes those signs that are completely stimulus determined, but that lose their influence because of the insensitivity of some subsequent portion of the nervous system to their particular kind of fluctuation. We may refer to these as *stimulus signs*. On the other hand, *systemic signs* include those fluctuations that are introduced into neural signals by factors other than external stimuli, but that still do not affect all subsequent levels of the nervous system. An example of such a systemic sign is a change in the amplitude of an evoked potential caused by a metabolic deficit or a posture which, though altering the signal, does not affect the behavior. It should be noted that there can also be *systemic codes*. Systemic codes include stimulus-unrelated fluctuations in the neural state that affect behavior. Such a variable as memory would be a typical example of a systemic code.

This dichotomy between the terms *systemic* and *stimulus* is similar to the distinction suggested by Sutton, Braren, Zubin, and John (1965). They referred to *exogenous* or stimulus-related influences and *endogenous* or internal influences on the evoked potential. The distinction made here between *signs* and *codes*, however, speaks to an entirely different matter than that with which they were concerned. In a discussion of evoked brain potentials, a careful distinction between the two kinds of signs is as important as the distinction between a sign and a code.

In peripheral nerves the distinction between a sign and a code can be more easily conceptualized. Assume that we set up two known patterns of nerve impulses with electrical stimuli. In the context of this discussion, an adequate demonstration of the psychophysical *discrimination* of these two neural signals is operationally sufficient to define it as some sort of a code, since discrimination indicates a sensitivity equivalent to interpretation. But, while the family of potential signals in peripheral nerves can be easily categorized, the complex interactions of the net of neurons that constitutes the central nervous system are far less well understood. In each case, however, the sufficiency test for a code is the same. It requires that we use the entire efferent action—a complex and multi-influenced process which has been generally called *behavior*—as the measuring instrument. It is important to emphasize the point that no neurophysiological measurement, no matter how sophisticated and no matter at what high level of the nervous system it is carried out, can substitute for the behavioral test to distinguish a sign from a code. Therefore, the sensory scientist must consider the behavioral response as the ultimate test of whether or not some complex neural process actually is the basis of some awareness or experience.

How does one go about actually performing the necessary tests to distinguish between a sign and a code? It is not at all clear that it can actually be done in all cases, but there is a general paradigm, which might prove to be useful. The critical element in such a test is that it is necessary to drive the nervous system to respond in a precisely defined manner, and then compare the dimensions of this known neural response with the dimensions of some appropriate psychophysical response.

It is not always possible to do this, of course, but there are situations in which such tests can be performed. One example will be discussed in greater detail in Chapter 6, but a brief description of another procedure here may help to clarify this notion of the necessary paradigm for distinguishing between signs and codes.

Dawson and Scott (1949) have developed a technique for recording compound peripheral nerve action potentials from human beings without any surgical intervention. Electrical pulse stimuli were used to elicit, on a one-for-one basis, a compound action potential in a human nerve. Using this electrical pulse stimulation technique, specific inquiries can be made into the effect of given patterns of interpulse interval on the psychophysical experience. The great advantage is that the experimenter is able to bypass the transducer and deal with known, rather than unknown, nerve action potential patterns—he is in full control of the dimensions of the nerve action potentials and can make direct comparisons between the nerve action (not the stimulus) and the experience. Similar techniques can be used in animal studies to study the efficacy of the variations in a given dimension of neural experience [see our discussion of the work of Segundo, Moore, Stensaas, and Bullock (1963) later in Chapter 6] on subsequent encodings such as those occurring at a synaptic junction. Of course, simply the fact that a candidate code does differentially effect a synaptic transmission is not alone a conclusive test of its acceptability as a true code, but in conjunction with the psychophysical test, the evidence does become compelling.

B. Dimension Alterations

It must be expected, from what we already know of the coding of sensory information, that there will be very drastic changes in the coded form of a stimulus pattern at various levels of the afferent nervous system. For example, as noted, the most current theory of auditory encoding assumes that there is a transduction from temporal (frequency) stimulus patterns to a spatial code by a hydraulically mediated cochlear place localization of different frequencies. It is not too surprising, therefore, to learn of other specific neural structures that respond spatially to a specific temporal pattern of stimulus input. The existence of temporal "keys"—particular temporal patterns capable of activating specific loci, thus converting time to space—has been suggested by recent results. On the psychophysical side of the ledger, McKay (1961) has also reported several instances of spatial patterns that give rise to flickering changes in the visual field, suggesting the conversion of spatial to temporal patterns. Presumably, these affects are related to eye movements. Thus, we should expect spatial-to-temporal, as well as temporal-to-spatial, transformations. The caution inherent in these results is that we should not demand dimensional constancy throughout the afferent pathways, and that codes, at one level, need not be identical nor even of the same dimensional category as codes at another level. All that is required is that the information pattern be represented in one way or another at all levels. Thus, a stimulus pattern might be represented at one level by a temporal code, at another by a spatial code, and at another by an amplitude code. No topographic or isomorphic consistency is really necessary, nor is there any need for linear (or nonlinear) representation of functions that appear to the perceiver to be linear (or nonlinear). All that is required is some representational scheme, which transmits the critical information of the input pattern in some available language. (Remember the metaphorical line of speech translators.)

For these reasons, it is important to avoid the narrowing of perspective, which would arise from the false requirement that temporal stimulus pattern be represented by temporal candidate codes, and other similar but equally incorrect isomorphisms. A most important corollary is that there is no one coding scheme which can be identified for each dimension of each sense, but only local definitions of codes at specifically defined levels.

C. Boundary Condition Results
Another caution relates to the fact that many results are significant only in the sense that they represent limiting cases or boundary conditions. The determination of a threshold in a psychophysical or a neurophysiological experiment is a case in point. The threshold may impose a limit on the availability of a certain dimension to serve in some particular coding operation, but it does not necessarily completely define the functional variability of such a dimension as the corresponding stimulus dimension is varied. Different coding mechanisms may come into play at different stimulus amplitudes, for example.

D. Multiple and Overlapping Coding in Two or More Dimensions
The old phrase "spatio-temporal pattern," naive and virtually meaningless as it was, did reflect a certain problem. Many complex stimulus patterns are not unidimensional, and it is sometimes misleading to expect a given stimulus dimension to be associated with only one candidate code. In fact, such a separation may not be possible without considering interdimensional interaction, since some dimensions may act to modify some other dimensions. It is probably misleading to presume a one-to-one relationship between all stimulus dimensions and a single candidate code. As we shall see, there appear to be relatively large numbers of redundancies in the coding schema.

There are two different ways in which multiple coding may be exhibited. The first way might be best called *redundant coding*. In this situation, the variation of a single stimulus dimension may lead to the simultaneous variation of two or more candidate codes. An example of such a phenomenon is the now well-known simultaneous variation of mean frequency and variance of a spike action potential pattern as stimulus amplitude is varied.

The second way in which multiple coding may be exhibited might best be called *overlapping coding*. In this situation, two or more stimulus dimensions may be capable of altering a single dimension of neural coding. For example, both the intensity and wavelength of a photic stimulus are known to affect the rate of firing of a ganglion cell axon in the optic nerve. Of course, in this case of a single neuron, such overlapping coding would lead to an ambiguous situation, since the change in wavelength could always be compensated for by a change in intensity. This ambiguity can be resolved only on the basis of other parallel neural communication lines that convey similarly coded information, but with slightly different coding characteristics. In fact, this is probably the basis of color coding and perhaps of quality coding in general. We shall discuss such overlapping codes in great detail in Chapters 9, 10 and 11, where we shall consider the special importance of the concept of temporal comparisons between different places to quality coding.

A related matter of concern is produced by the very high degree of convergence within the nervous system. Signals at higher levels may not reflect the influence of a single input alone. Rather, such a higher-level signal may be the result of the integration and processing of patterns of inputs from several sources. The matter is further complicated by the fact that feedback signals from more central portions of the nervous system can also alter the pattern of activity at peripheral levels. This and related kinds of centrifugal effects often lead to responses of great complexity, since input-output relations now become subject to both regenerative and degenerative effects of positive and negative feedback. The difficulties and surprises of signal tracing encountered in systems with elaborate feedback loops are well known to electrical engineers.

E. Species and Intraindividual Variability

While ideally we would like to be able to generalize as much as possible to keep sensory theories as simple as possible, it is probably also important to keep in mind the fact that not all organisms, either within or among species, operate in exactly the same fashion. Furthermore, there is also the possibility of what Perkel and Bullock (1968) refer to as "labile coding." At different times, it is conceivable, the different coding mechanisms serve a single function at some place in the nervous system. Varied maturation processes in a wide variety of species, including man, may result in different coding mechanisms being utilized at different stages of individual development. Analogous differences in coding mechanisms may be expected to exist at different stages of the evolutionary scale.

F. Attentional Limits on Our Perspective

We have, several times in the course of this book, referred to the fact that the attention of the scientific community is directed to small portions of the total problem by accidents of technology and of style. The overemphasis on the frequency factors of spike action potentials as codes for intensity has been the classic example. The development of the more general notion of the coding problem was inhibited until new instruments and new experimental paradigms widened our perspective. A very complete study of the general problem of paradigms of consensus and the ways in which revolutions in scientific perspectives occur has been made by Kuhn (1970) and may be of interest to the more philosophically oriented reader.

G. False Analogies

Another conceptual pitfall, which has become particularly evident in the last few years, is the oversimplified physiological modeling by some scientists interested particularly in perception. This is not the place to discuss this issue in detail, but the interested reader may want to look at a recent paper (Uttal, 1971b) or skip ahead to Chapter 8. Both discussions spell out the pertinent considerations of what often happens when physiological data become psychological models. The crux of the matter is that some physiologically oriented perceptual psychologists have developed explanatory models of some visual phenomena, which are based almost exclusively on the mistaken notion that similarity in the form of the process is tantamount to identity in structure.

Mathematical model making is also subject to this same sort of pitfall. Descriptive mathematical models do not directly imply specific structural mechanisms. The general nature of the methods of solution of most complex mathematical methods makes it possible for many different mechanisms to produce essentially the same sort of behavior or, at least, analogous behavior. But analogies of response form are not the same as homologies of structure, and similar patterns of behavior in a neurophysiological net and a behavioral trait need not necessarily lead us to the conclusion that the two are identical in their underlying neural mechanism.

For example, lateral inhibitory interaction has been used as a model to explain several different kinds of visual metacontrast. While there certainly is some sort of mutual inhibition in metacontrast—mathematical models may be made which describe pretty well the sort of data obtained (Weisstein, 1968)—some now feel that the metacontrast situation is vastly more complicated, and mutual inhibition among semantic symbols, which are more alike in meaning than geometry, may be a more appropriate model than mutual inhibition in spatially distributed nerve nets. Recent results indicate that these perceptual events are modified by such factors as shape similarity and even word meaning. The implications of these cognitive processes, almost certainly mediated at a very high level in the metacontrast situation, rule out simple nerve net interactive explanations based upon the geometry of the stimulus material. We shall speak in greater detail of this material later when we discuss the spatial coding problems.

V. A SUMMARY

It should now be clear what we mean by a theory of sensory coding. Though there are a number of cautions that have to be observed, the general task involved in the unraveling of the codes of the nervous system is the precise definition of the associations between common sensory dimensions and what are known to be the candidate neural dimensions. To simplify this matter, we might consider this task to be one in which we are required to fill in the entries on a correlation matrix such as that shown in Table 5.1.

A table such as this, as we have said, will have to be developed for each level of neural coding. As we have also pointed out previously, this means that there may be several different levels of coding even within a single cell and many within the entire course of the ascending pathway. This need for a multiplication of coding matrices would be somewhat discouraging if it were not for the fact that we may also expect to find some common features at equivalent levels as comparisons

TABLE 5.1 A SAMPLE OF THE SORT OF CORRELATION MATRIX
THAT MUST BE FILLED OUT FOR EACH LEVEL OF NEURAL ENCODING*

		Neural Response Dimensions (The Candidate Codes)			
		Place	Topographic Pattern	Number of Activated Units	Neural Event Amplitude
Common Sensory Dimensions		Quality				
		Quantity				
	Temporal Parameters	Relative Temporal Order				
		Temporal Acuity				
		Duration				
	Spatial Parameters	Spatial Localization				
		Spatial Interaction and Patterns				

* By judicious choice of what constitute equivalent levels, such a table may be usable for equivalent levels in all of the senses, thus establishing the foundation of a general theory of sensory coding.

are made across the senses. This places the severe requirement on the sensory-coding theory to be sure that all of the comparisons being made are between truly comparable levels of encoding.

It is not too difficult to be led astray and to make false comparisons in this search for a general theory. A classic example has been the oft-repeated statement that the frequency discrimination of the skin is far poorer than that of the ear. In fact, however, the frequency discrimination capability of the ear, from a neural coding point of view, is more comparable to spatial discrimination capability on the skin than to its frequency sensitivity. The analysis of acoustic frequencies into spatial patterns on the cochlea confuses the issue and illustrates some of the problems that can develop when one depends too much on the potential physical stimulus as a referent. On the other hand, when the acoustic nerve is driven electrically (Simmons et al., 1965), comparisons of the frequency discrimination capabilities of the ear and the skin turn out to be very similar.

Table 5.1 (*cont.*)

Neural Response Dimensions (The Candidate Codes)				
Temporal Parameters				Temporal Comparison Between Two Places
Frequency	Frequency Macrofluctuations	Frequency Microfluctuations	Derived Statistical Measures	

This, then, concludes our introduction to what it is that is meant by a "theory" of sensory coding. In this chapter, we have attempted to stake out the issues and the specific nature of the problem. In the following chapters, we shall look in detail at some of the progress that has been made in the association of candidate neural codes with common sensory dimensions.

It would be most satisfying if we were able to say that all of the material to be presented in the following chapters was the result of exhaustive tests of candidate codes, but of course this is not the case. We have had to depend, to a great extent, on the conventional physiological and psychological data—the classic paradigms of experimentation. There is simply not yet an adequate corpus of psychobiological knowledge to rigorously observe all of the cautions mentioned above. Some of the experiments that we shall discuss are clearly ones that do no more than define a candidate code; others associate a given neural dimension and a common sensory dimension only putatively. From all of this, however, it is hoped that a clearer picture and an intelligent appreciation of the state of the science of sensory coding will emerge.

CHAPTER 6: THE CODING OF SENSORY MAGNITUDE

I. INTRODUCTION

The general subject of this chapter is the relation between the quantitative aspects of stimuli, neural events, and experiential dimensions. However, we are immediately faced with the need to define the term "quantity" with respect to each of these three universes of discourse to fully understand the material we shall discuss.

What do we mean by stimulus intensity, psychophysical or neurophysiological magnitude, or the more general rubric "quantity"? The least precise of these three terms is the most general one—quantity. It refers simply, and not too definitively, to "how much" in the physical, physiological, and psychological universes of discourse with which we have been dealing so far. In Chapter 2 we presented and discussed the metrics of stimulus intensity. The definition of the quantity of these physical units is relatively direct and easily understood, because there is a pool of common agreement in the community about the operations that are necessary to precisely define them.

The definition of the dimensions of variability of neurophysiological signals is also associated with rather clear-cut operations. However, it must be remembered that the main intent of sensory-coding theory is to determine which of these relatively well-defined dimensions is actually associated with or representative of the intensive perceptions. It need not be the magnitude of the neurophysiological response which is so associated, for as we shall see, temporal codes and even spatial loci can represent psychophysical magnitude. The important point to remember is that there is no *a priori* reason why a quantitative neural dimension is necessarily more likely than any of these other candidate codes to represent psychophysical magnitudes.

When we cross over, however, to the sensory or perceptual universe and begin to consider "subjective" common sensory magnitudes, agreement is not quite so quickly forthcoming. A new set of terms such as brightness, loudness or, in general, the "perceived magnitude" of any of the other senses begins to appear in our discussion with less than crystal clarity of definition. The definition of these terms is far less direct and far less easy to get across to the reader, primarily because the operations necessary for their definition are less well agreed upon. Furthermore, the intrapersonal privacy of sensation precludes a definition that is free of average values and references, in some way, to the unobservable internal standards of the observer. In practice, sensory magnitudes are always defined in terms that stress the idea that if the temporal and spatial characteristics of the sensation and the kind of sensation remain constant, then the dimensions along which changes still can be sensed are those of subjective magnitude—a definition by exclusion rather than inclusion. Modern operationalism would thus have us identify sensory magnitudes with certain experimental manipulations.

If this sort of approach to the definition of subjective magnitudes seems to be unsatisfying, at least the reader can be assured that he is in good company. Some of the difficulties, which the most distinguished of workers can get into in attempts to define subjective intensity, are exemplified in the following quotation.

> *I intend to distinguish between intensive and extensive sensations, depending on whether they concern the sensory perception of something whose magnitude can be judged intensively or extensively. For example, I shall include as an intensive sensation the sensation of brightness, as an extensive sensation the perception of a spatial extent by sight or touch; and accordingly I shall distinguish between the intensive and extensive magnitude of a sensation. When one object appears to us brighter than another, we call the sensation it arouses intensively greater; when it appears larger than another, we call it extensively greater. This is merely a matter of definition and implies, as generally understood, no specific measure of sensation.*
>
> *With every sensation whatsoever, intensive as well as extensive, magnitude and form may be distinguished, although in the case of intensive sensations magnitude is often called strength and form quality. With sounds, the pitch, even though it is a quality of the sound, has also a quantitative aspect insofar as we can distinguish a higher from a lower pitch.*
>
> (FECHNER, 1860, p. 14.)

or more recently:

> (1) *The Character of Intensity*
> *For any process of sensory excitation, there is a quantitative charac-*
> *ter in the stimulus, which governs the variation of the intensity*
> *of excitation, and to which modalities of reaction can be linked.*
> *Thus the sound of a tuning-fork vibrating a fixed distance from the*
> *ear will be judged to be more intense, or to be less intense, accord-*
> *ing to whether the vibration amplitude of the branches of the fork*
> *has increased or decreased.*
>
> (*PIÉRON, 1952, p. 36.*)

A search through some more recent textbooks of sensory psychology leads to the conclusion that the question of the definition of intensity is avoided entirely, and the authors simply assume that there is some form of community understanding of what is meant by sensory intensity, based on certain common agreements rather than precise definition. Thus, these definitions leave the reader with a paucity of operational links to the meaning of subjective magnitude.

Another difficulty with this point of view is that it forces sensory scientists into a situation in which they tend to make the stimulus intensity the sole referent for studies of sensory magnitude coding, and this association is well known to break down in many different situations. Nevertheless, it appears that we are not going to be able to resolve this matter any better than some of our predecessors, and thus we shall simply assume in the words of one colleague, "that magnitude differences exist whenever reliable judgments can be made of the brightness of visual stimuli, loudness of acoustic stimuli or of the appropriate intensive sensory dimensions in any other modality." Our attention will, therefore, be directed at specific experimental paradigms that have attracted the attention of psychologists and neurophysiologists over the years. Specifically, this chapter will concern itself with two important issues: the nature of the physiological mechanisms that might help us to understand the detection of low-level stimuli—the "threshold" problem—and the relationship between physiological correlates of stimulus intensity, on the one hand, and the magnitude of suprathreshold sensations on the other. In addition to these topics, we shall also consider some of the descriptive mathematical models that are most relevant to these problems of intensity coding.

II. THRESHOLDS AND SIGNAL DETECTION

Thresholds have always been of basic concern to sensory scientists, because they represent the origin of any perceptual or neurophysiological intensive dimension. The classic view of sensory thresholds held that there was a lower energy limit below which signals were not capable, under any conditions, of producing a response. It was assumed that these thresholds might vary under certain conditions (such as the state of adaptation or the metabolic state of the organism), but that given a certain state, the line between a subthreshold and a suprathreshold stimulus was sharp and was constrained only by the physical statistics of the external stimulus. A stimulus below the threshold could never elicit a response—if it did, this simply meant that there had been an incorrect definition of what constituted the threshold.

Over the years as new psychophysical techniques were developed and further exploration made of what actually constitutes a stimulus, it became increasingly clear that this deterministic definition of the threshold was inadequate. Thresholds varied with technique, and more important threshold measurements often seemed to be characterized by probabilistic response functions rather than by sharply defined stimulus energy considerations. Stimuli, well below what was thought to be the threshold, in some instances did give rise to a response. Thus, there was introduced, into the concept of a threshold, a family of such notions as "false positives." The impact of all of these findings has been to force statistical considerations into the thinking of both neurophysiologists and psychophysicists who were concerned with thresholds and to even raise the question of the existence of a hard-and-fast "threshold" of any kind.

In the following sections, we shall introduce thresholds from a newer perspective—one that is based primarily on a statistical rather than a deterministic notion of what constitutes the lower bound of the intensive dimension. We shall then show how these ideas can be used in both neurophysiological and psychophysical theory, and by emphasizing the dual use and the similarities in findings once again remind the reader that the main purpose of this book is to relate neurophysiological candidate codes specifically with certain dimensions of the experience.

A. The Theory of Signal Detection

The problem of the measurement of absolute or minimum thresholds in psychophysics is directly analogous to the problem of signal detection in noisy electronic systems. It, therefore, was a natural development that some of the mathematical notions developed by engineers to describe the sensitivity of communication systems (see particularly Peterson, Birdsall, and Fox, 1954) would be applied to psychological detection problems. A number of important changes in the basic philosophy of the two approaches, however, make it important for the novice to understand the unique approach of modern psychological signal detection theory in the form first presented by Tanner and Swets (1954) and more fully developed by Green and Swets (1966). The situation has been complicated further by the fact that some of the older engineering ideas have reevolved from the psychophysical notions when signal detection theory was applied to similar problems in neural systems.

To illustrate the impact of this set of conceptual complications, we must note that signal detection theory, as it was originally developed, was a procedure for the analysis of the efficiency of transmitters, communication links, and receivers with *known* noise characteristics. Thus, signal and noise amplitudes were directly observable and could be used to quantitatively define the detection characteristics of radar and radio sets. The theory of signal detection as it has been applied by psychologists, however, is an attempt to do something quite different with the same mathematical machinery. Psychologists using signal detection theories are, in general, attempting to infer what the invisible signal-to-noise characteristics are and what the detection characteristics of an invisible communication system are on the basis of measures of its external behavior. Their use of the theory of signal detectability, therefore, is based upon a number of assumptions that are not part of the original theory. It is, in a sense, a form of mathematical backtracking from a solution to a problem! Many of these supplementary assumptions, incidentally, are no longer necessary when one starts discussing signal-to-noise ratios in neural systems in which the original notions of detectability measurement from known values of noise and signal strength can be applied.

The idea of "noise" takes on quite a different meaning in the psychological context than it does in the electrical engineer's world. To the psychologist, "noise" includes such factors as variability in the decision criteria that are being used from trial to trial, spontaneous noise in the neural communication links, as well as subjective estimates of the likelihood and payoffs involved in any given decision. Clearly, this is quite a bit more complex than the communication noise in a radiotelegraph. Nevertheless, the processes can be considered to be analogous.

It should be noted that the only data that are needed for most psychophysical signal detection experiments are the proportion of the total responses to which a subject said "yes" when there was, in fact, a signal present (the hit rate), and the proportion of times in which he said "yes" when there was, in fact, no signal present (the false alarm rate). From these two simple sets of data can be derived useful and significant characteristic measures of the subject's performance. Furthermore, if certain assumptions are made, the characteristics of the signal-to-noise ratios with which he seems to be operating can also be estimated.

An important advantage of the signal detection model is that it allows the psychologist to distinguish between *sensitivity* measures and *decision* measures. To understand fully how these factors may be derived, we shall have to consider in detail the meaning of some of the basic concepts used in the system. First, let us consider the form in which data are generated and analyzed in a signal detection experiment.

An important general notion, which has been introduced by the signal detection theorists, is that there are probability values that characterize the number of times a target will be correctly detected, as well as equivalent functions for the number of times false alarms will be reported. These probabilities are reflections of the invisible noise distributions in the system. As stated above, there are two possible responses, which can be given with varying probabilities in a simple yes-no type of psychophysical experiment (Yes, I saw it—No, I did not see it) and also two possible stimulus conditions that must be considered (There was a signal present —There was no signal present).

Four probabilities are thus defined:

1. The probability of reporting a signal when one was present
$P(S/s)$ A Hit

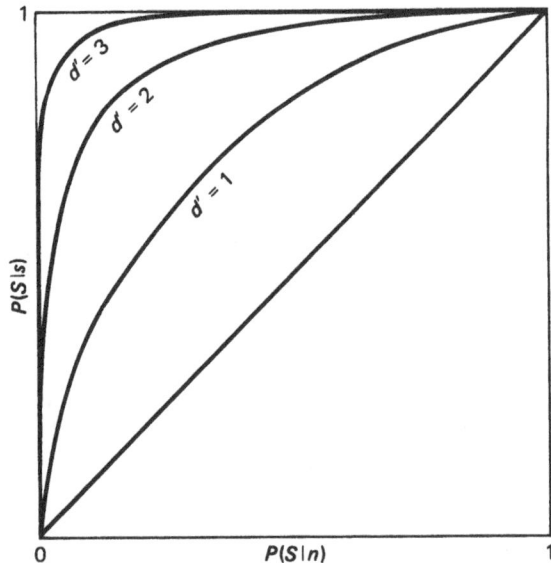

*FIGURE 6.1 Receiver oper-
ating characteristic (ROC)
curves plotted for three different levels of* d', *assuming
equal variances of the two
distributions of Figure 6.2.
Unequal variances would
tend to make ROC curve
asymmetrical (from Green
and Swets, 1966).*

2. The probability of reporting a signal when none was present
   $P(S/n)$ A False Alarm
3. The probability of not reporting a signal when one was present
   $P(N/s)$ A Miss
4. The probability of not reporting a signal when none was present
   $P(N/n)$ A Correct Rejection

This information could be represented in a two-dimensional table, but
there is a much more graphic and explicit means of more fully representing the relationships of the response probability functions as various parameters of the situation change. This is the now well-known ROC
(receiver operating characteristic) curve, a sample family of which is
shown in Figure 6.1. The ROC curve simply plots the hit rate against
the false alarm rate. Thus, points at the lower left-hand corner of the
graph represent the performance of a subject who is essentially responding so conservatively that he is, in fact, saying no to almost everything.
Thus, while he is rarely making the error of the false alarm, he is also
rarely correctly reporting the presence of any true signals. As the subject's
criteria change, perhaps as a result of the instructions given to him, he
may become more and more liberal. Points would then be plotted which
tend more toward the other end of the graph where his hit rate is very
high, but where his false alarm rate may also approach 100 percent.
Thus, where the subject is performing on a given ROC curve at any
given time is a measure of his decision criterion rather than his sensitivity.
   The formal measure that is used to describe this criterion level or response threshold in the theory of signal detection is β (beta), which is a
measure of the level of the tendency to report a signal at which the sub-

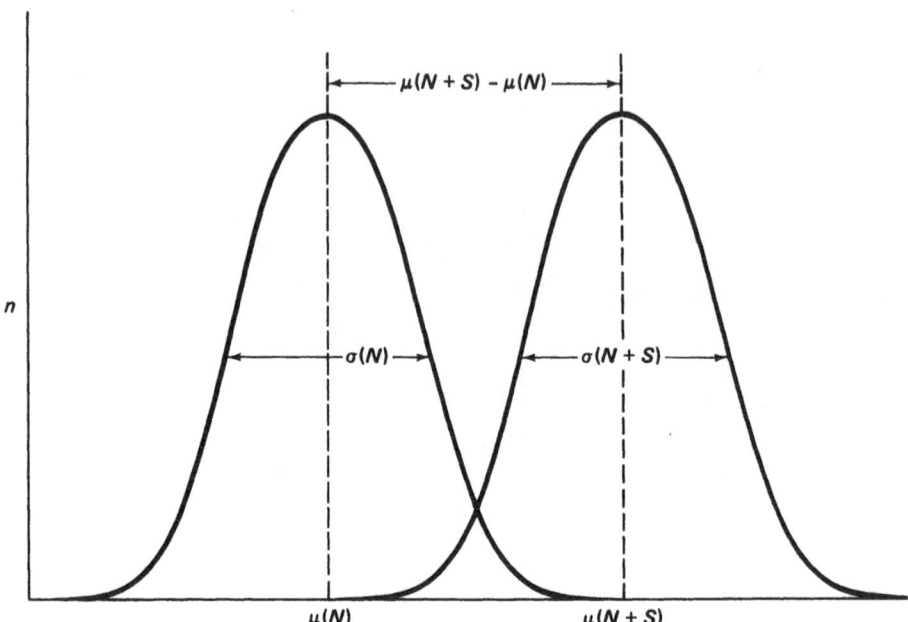

FIGURE 6.2 *A plot of the distribution of a hypothetical variable with and without noise. This is the basic model from which most signal detection descriptions of experimental data are derived.* $\mu(N)$ *is the mean of the distribution containing noise alone;* $\mu(N + S)$ *is the mean of the distribution that contains both signal and noise;* $\sigma(N)$ *is the standard deviation of the distribution containing noise alone; and* $\sigma(N + S)$ *is the standard deviation of the distribution that contains both signal and noise. Note the region of overlap of the two curves, in which it is uncertain from which distribution a particular event was obtained. The horizontal axis represents the range of possible scores while the vertical axis represents the number of times* (n) *a score occurred.*

ject expects he can maximize the value of his decision. It is, in other words, a variable threshold beyond which the subject will say that a signal was present. The measure β, then, is determined by the subject's conception of the odds and of the values he associates with the possible outcomes, and is presumably selected by the subject to maximize his return. β may be varied experimentally by varying the instructions and the payoffs given to the subject.

The other major descriptor required is a measure of the sensitivity of the system. Remember that in the old electrical engineering world, the conditions of signal and noise were observable directly. The experimenter could then plot a pair of curves such as those shown in Figure 6.2. The first curve represents the distribution of the noise alone, while the second curve represents the distribution when signal and noise are both present. For example, the first curve might represent a histogram of the intervals between random noise pulses in a pulse modulated system. When a signal is added to this noise, the interval distribution would shift as spikes occurred more frequently due to the presence of the signal pulses. The band-pass of the system might or might not change, and thus the standard deviation of the curve representing signal plus noise might also change or not. For the purposes of most of our discussion, it will be a useful simplification to assume that the standard deviation remains constant as well as that the two curves are both normal. In this situation an objective measure of the discriminability of the signal can be given in terms of the relative degree of overlap of the two curves. Formally, a useful discriminability measure for this situation in which all of the parameters are known could be expressed as:

$$d = \frac{M_1 - M_2}{\sigma} \qquad (6.1)$$

The ability of a given instrument to distinguish signal from noise could be calculated with this equation, in which M_1 is the mean of the pure noise distribution, M_2 is the mean of the signal-plus-noise distribution and σ is the common standard deviation.

It should be intuitively obvious that d is a measure of the overlap of the two curves. When the two means are close together, and there is only a small difference between them, then there will be a substantial amount of overlap of the two curves, and it will be most difficult to determine if a particular instance belonged to the noise or the noise-plus-signal distribution. Sensitivity is, therefore, said to be low. When the difference is great, then there is a lessened probability that instances drawn from each distribution will lie in the common overlapping region, and sensitivity will be high. Similarly, the narrower the distribution (the smaller its standard deviation), the less likelihood of overlap for a given M_1 and M_2. The important thing to remember is that d is an estimate, which can be made purely and uniquely on the basis of message characteristics if they are known.

In the psychological situation, however, we usually do not know all of the characteristics of the noise; it is invisible and is only indirectly reflected in our observations of the responses made by the subject, but it is assumed that there is an equivalent sort of probabilistic distribution and an equivalent sort of noise and, furthermore, that a measure of discrimination sensitivity that will operate in exactly the same way can be defined. This analogous measure of discriminability (d' pronounced "dee prime"), which includes the effects of all of the "invisible internal noise" as well as any external stimulus noise, can be defined as:

$$d' = \frac{M_1 - M_2}{\sigma} \qquad (6.2)$$

where M_1 and M_2 are the means of the two psychological distributions, one containing the signal and one not, and σ is their common standard deviation.

The crucial point to remember is that in the application of the theory of signal detection in a psychological experiment, the two hypothetical distributions, which we are discussing, are really implicit in the behavior of the subject and usually cannot be made truly explicit. Thus, M_1, M_2 and σ are values which, for all practical purposes, can never be really precisely defined or measured. What we can do is extricate from our data an estimate of d', which tells us something about discriminability and information about the shape of the ROC curve, which is suggestive, but not definitive, of the form these hypothetical distributions might take.

Nevertheless, the analysis can be pushed somewhat further if we are willing to make certain simplifying assumptions. Specifically, we may assume that the two distributions have some standard shape. We may make assumptions about their normality and the equality of variance, for example. When we have done so, we are assuming a shape for these distributions and, therefore, may apply normal probability tables or other statistical tools to make further estimates of the nature of the invisible noise. It is most important to remember, however, that these simplifying assumptions are only that and are not rigorous solutions to the problem.

Differences in effective d' will show up as shifts in the position of the entire ROC curve as shown in Figure 6.1. Increased discriminability reflected by a larger d' puts more and more of the area of the ROC graph underneath the curve.

What "discriminability" or d' actually means in a given experiment depends upon what the experimental design was. In a detection experiment, it might be a measure of the ease with which a given stimulus can be correctly detected with any one of a number of different psychophysical techniques. But it can also have a slightly different connotation in experiments on recognition, intelligibility, and even memory. Although the particular shape of the ROC curve and the area included under it empirically specifies a particular d', that d' cannot be used to characterize the mean and standard deviation of the invisible noise distribution without making the simplifying assumptions mentioned above. Rather, d' is used as an empirical dependent variable in experiments in which the effects of varying some stimulus parameter on a subject's performances are desired to be measured. It can, furthermore, be used to compare the sensitivity of a set of subejcts when the experimental conditions are held constant.

Since it is possible to compute from known stimulus characteristics the best that any internally noise-free observer who is operating as an ideal statistician could do, signal detection theorists have also developed the notion of an *ideal observer*. This theoretically ideal observer can be used as a standard to estimate the additional effects introduced by the invisible noise within the subject. The ideal observer would typically have a d'_{ideal} equal to the square root of twice the signal-to-noise ratio in the external stimulus.

An index of efficiency η' can be formulated for any situation in which we know the specific characteristics of the stimulus and thus d'_{ideal} and in which an experiment can provide an estimate of the subject's sensitivity d'_{subj}. This index of efficiency is usually defined as:

$$n' = \left(\frac{d'_{\text{subj}}}{d'_{\text{ideal}}}\right)^2 \tag{6.3}$$

One of the very important notions introduced by the theory of signal detection is the idea that the threshold, once almost the *sine qua non* of psychological theories of sensory performance, may, perhaps, no longer be a valid psychological construct. As we review the details of the preceding discussion and, in particular, the probabilistic notions of discrimination between signal and noise, the idea that there is a critical lower limit on the sensitivity of an observer may seem somewhat hard to justify. As an alternative, the signal detection theorists have suggested that we may want to consider the possibility that what, in fact, "threshold" determinations measure is not so much a lower limit of sensitivity as it is something about the decision criteria, which are being momentarily used by a subject. Thus, where the classical psychophysicist would place the blame for the lower bound of sensitivity on the characteristics of d', the signal detection theorist would consider "thresholds" to be a characteristic of β, in other words, response rather than sensory thresholds.

Green and Swets (1966) discuss this point and note that there are several reasons to consider that the notion of the absolute sensory threshold is either an artifact of some of the older experimental paradigms, or of shifting decision criteria. First, they note that the threshold is a construct, which is highly variable in several different ways. There is the matter of variability in values obtained even when precision of measurement is rigorous. For example, even in neurophysiological experiments, the "threshold" for spike elicitation seems to vary from moment to moment. Second, there is also a matter of criterion or psychological variability in many different detection experiments, which add substantial amounts of variance. Third, differences in psychophysical technique give substantial differences in threshold estimates. Fourth, there is a set of situational factors that influence detectability: the contrast between the target and the background, the time since the last stimulus, and the general status of the subject. In many situations the detection of signals is one that is not so much a matter of the absolute energy of the stimulus as it is a matter of the relative amount of energy in the stimulus and the background and the history of both.

A further complication we may also note is that under certain conditions, the "threshold" may turn out to be so very low indeed as to make the notion of a lower limit almost meaningless. Hensel and Boman (1960), for example, have shown that a single spike action potential elicited in the peripheral somatosensory nerve of a human subject can be psychophysically detected. Hecht, Schlaer, and Pirenne (1942) have shown that under appropriate conditions, as few as 5 to 8 quanta of light can give rise to a visual experience in a measurable proportion of the presentations, and only 1 quantum be absorbed by a given receptor for this threshold experience.

Simply considered from an empirical point of view, we must also note that new values of the estimates of thresholds are always falling as new psychophysical procedures are applied. The notions of coding may be relevant here. We so often find that the differential effects of some stimulus pattern previously thought to be "below threshold" can be detected in some new situation in which a judgment is demanded along some other sensory dimension. Though this is not a compelling argument for the absence of thresholds, it does suggest that, at least historically, we have been almost always wrong in our estimates of the lower limits of sensitivity to one or another stimulus dimension, except in those instances in which the threshold is assumed to be as low as it can theoretically be. Unfortunately, it is not possible to resolve the issue completely at the present time. It is a complicated controversy, which depends also upon exactly what kind of a theory of the threshold one is discussing. Perhaps the best statement of the implications and importance of the problem has been given by Green and Swets (1966) in a few paragraphs, whose special lucidity makes quotation in full worthwhile.

> *Do sensory thresholds exist? If they do exist, can they be measured precisely enough to serve as a cornerstone for psychophysical science? It will be clear that the care given here to the concept of the sensory threshold is necessary for several reasons. One reason is the great durability of the concept. As indicated, it was among the first quantitative concepts established in experimental psychology and, despite considerable criticism almost from its inception, it is widely used today. The notion of some limit on sensitivity is, of course, highly likely on a priori grounds, but whether or not there exists a limit in the sense of the threshold is a very intricate question. That a crucial experiment has not been devised is indicated by the fact that when the classical view appeared again recently to be in jeopardy, several modified versions, consistent with the new data, were soon developed. Clearly, a blanket denial of sensory thresholds of any sort is not to be accepted in advance of a protracted period of study. However, if the classical view of the threshold is incorrect, then it is important to spell out the ramifications of this result, since they are many and not all are obvious. Perhaps the most important implications are for measurement. Suffice it to say now that the classical threshold is not merely a statistical construct; the conceptual neurophysiology on which it is based is directly reflected in some popular forms of psychophysical methods and measures; if the concept is not valid, then these methods and measures are inappropriate. The classical threshold concept has also had an extensive influence on theory in several areas. Estes (1962) has recently reviewed its place in learning theory. To take an example from sensory theory, one pursued further in Chapter 9, the concept has supported for years a prediction which has been applied to multiple observations, multiple observers, and multicomponent signals, although a large share of the data relevant to the prediction are contradictory to it. It may also be noted that the classical view of the threshold has fostered the large literature on subliminal, or subthreshold, perception.*
>
> (GREEN and SWETS, 1966, p. 120)

Signal detection theory helps to alleviate many of these problems by focusing attention on d' and β rather than on the threshold. More complete descriptions of the procedures and implications of modern psychophysical version of the theory of signal detection can be found in Coombs, Dawes, and Tversky (1970), Corso (1967), or for what is perhaps the most rigorous discussion, Green and Swets (1966) itself.

Signal detection theory, or rather a reverted form of it very similar to the old engineering techniques from whence the psychological model evolved, can also be used to study neurophysiological problems. The terms noise, signal, and discriminability all have relevance in that context too, but the meaning of the terms may be slightly different than in a psychophysical experiment.

Perhaps most important is the fact that it is no longer necessary to deal with "invisible" noise situations. In a neurophysiological experiment, the observer can make measurements of the variability and spontaneous activity in a way that is much more closely analogous to the electrical engineer's analysis of communication systems than to the situation in which the psychophysicist finds himself. The noise and signal-to-noise ratios and other characteristics are no longer invisible, and it is only necessary to assume some sort of criterion for distinguishing between noise, on the one hand, and signal plus noise, on the other hand, for the neuro-physiologist to have a complete and unique story. The psychophysicist can deal only with the molar behavior of the system, and only by making certain assumptions, not all of which are always perfectly plausible, is he able to draw nonunique conclusions about the underlying signal and noise properties.

But in a neurophysiological experiment, it is also clear that some measure of the system's detection of a signal other than a psychophysi-cal response must, of course, be found. Such a measure might be a shift in the mean rate of spontaneous firing, the latency of a response, or the elicitation of a criterion amplitude of some integrated signal like the electroretinogram. Any of these measures might be adequate descriptors of the local responsiveness of the system. Since all of these measures will be subject to noisy variability, the general neurophysiological prob-lem of threshold detection also depends upon the detection of a signal of some sort hidden in the spontaneous neural noise. The nature of neural spontaneous noise is a topic of considerable importance in this regard as well as being of intrinsic interest, and it is this topic to which we now turn.

B. Spontaneous Neural Activity

As we have seen, psychophysical thresholds have now come to be looked upon as probabilistic rather than deterministic functions. We have also suggested that this new approach emphasizes the notion of the detection of a signal against a background of noisy or quasi-random activity. This model can quite easily be transferred to neurophysiologi-cal paradigms, for in most neural systems there are also backgrounds of neural activity. While some of the differences we have just noted between psychophysics and neurophysiology must be kept in mind, the appli-cability of signal detection theory should be becoming clear. To clarify it even further, we shall now discuss the nature of neural "noise" and then discuss an outstanding example of an application of signal detection theory to visual thresholds.

The nervous system is never entirely quiet until the organism has died. The brain continues to give off some sort of electroencephalographic signals during all stages of sleep, anesthesia, or stimulus deprivation. Cells are active at all levels from the receptors onward. This activity has typically been called spontaneous, but perhaps a fairer definition would be couched in terms of stimuli, which are not under the control of the experimenter. These uncontrolled stimuli may either by extrinsic or intrinsic to the neuron. In even the best designed experiment, there is always the possibility that sensory systems can be activated by stimuli not directly produced by the experimenter. The body itself, for example, is capable of producing mechanical stimuli, which are capable of activating the acoustic or somatosensory receptors. The pulse, muscular twitches, and, given the exquisite sensitivity of the acoustic receptor, even the Brownian motion of the air must be considered to be sufficiently energetic to produce or modulate neural activity.

Finely tuned electrochemical systems also probably do activate themselves in ways that are closer to the common notion of the term spontaneous. The probability of activation is probably never really zero, even if the experimenter were able to control all possible stimuli. Perhaps the best example of this true "spontaneity" is given by Eccles (1964), who summarizes the work done on the miniature end-plate potential and other postsynaptic potentials by a number of investigators. Miniature postsynaptic potentials are relatively small depolarizations of the postsynaptic tissue that show some surprising characteristics. First, they are very regular in their size, with either uniform fundamental amplitude or multiples of that basic quantal value. This should be a surprising statement in light of the oft-repeated statement, in this text and elsewhere, that postsynaptic potentials are continuously graded. However, the continuous gradation is a characteristic of higher amplitudes of synaptic activity and is, perhaps, something of an artifact of the scale of observation. Miniature postsynaptic potentials, at the next lower level of discussion, seem to exhibit quantal characteristics. Eccles points out that this quantal characteristic is probably due to the fact that each miniature postsynaptic potential is produced by a packet of a relatively constant number of molecules of some synaptic transmitter substance. Thus, while the freqency of the miniature postsynaptic potentials can be altered very significantly by alterations of the ionic composition of the extracellular fluid, or by forcing appropriate transmembrane potential shifts, the amplitude of the miniature potential itself appears to assume only certain discrete values, varying only as a function of the state of the postsynaptic membrane.

In the context of the present discussion, the most interesting part of this tale is that the rate of occurrence of the miniature postsynaptic potentials appears to be a highly random process unrelated to any known antecedent condition. At this level, and if there are similar miniature potentials in the analogous portions of receptors, it may be that we are dealing with responses that are indeed either truly spontaneous, or at least de-

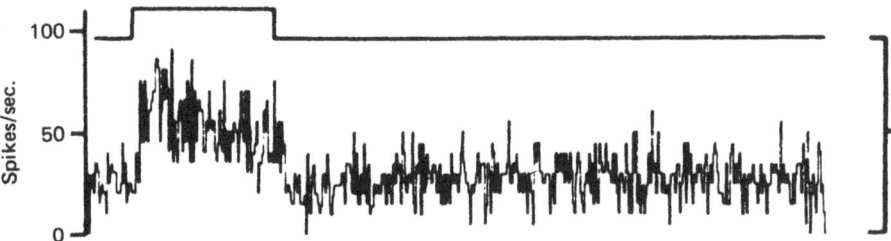

FIGURE 6.3 A record from a cat's retinal ganglion cell, showing the rate of spike firing as a function of the presence or absence of a stimulus. Note that there is a spontaneous nonzero level of activity even without the stimulus. When the stimulus is turned on, an increase in the level of activity occurs, but a statistical test must be used to determine what is noise and what is signal plus noise when the response level is low (from Barlow and Levick, 1969).

pendent upon molecular phenomena at a statistical level of which we know very little.

Spontaneous spike action potentials in axons are also known to be ubiquitous at almost all levels of the nervous system. Barlow and Levick (1969) have studied visual detection processes in the presence of spontaneous noise by looking at the responses of the retinal ganglion cell. Their figures show dark firing rates varying from 20 to as high as 50 spikes/sec. Figure 6.3 shows a sample poststimulus histogram plot of this spontaneous activity. This figure also clearly shows the transient change in frequency when a pulse of light was applied to the cat's eye.

Kiang (1965) has studied the problem of spontaneous activity at a similar level in the auditory system and has demonstrated equivalent levels of activity in the acoustic nerve. Figure 6.4 is a plot of the spontaneous activity of three different acoustic nerve fibers, and it can be seen that this activity varies over even wider ranges than those indicated by Barlow and Levick for the visual system. In a later figure in his book, Kiang presents data showing spontaneous rates as high as 100 spikes/sec. Once again the activity seems to be relatively random, although it is important to remember that quasi-random activity can be generated by the pooling of responses, which are themselves highly periodic (Cox and Smith, 1954).

At a higher level of the nervous system, Mountcastle, Poggio, and Werner (1963) have studied the response of the somatosensitive cells of the ventrobasal nuclear complex of the thalamus to variations in joint position. They were also concerned with the spontaneous activity of these cells, and their report contains references to spontaneous levels varying from 12 to 25 spikes/sec.

The cerebral cortex has been studied extensively by Burns (1958), who attempted to determine if, in fact, cortical cells exhibited spontaneous activity. He concludes that it is not possible to answer this question in this complicated net because of the difficulty of cutting off nervous input without simultaneously damaging the circulation. But in addition,

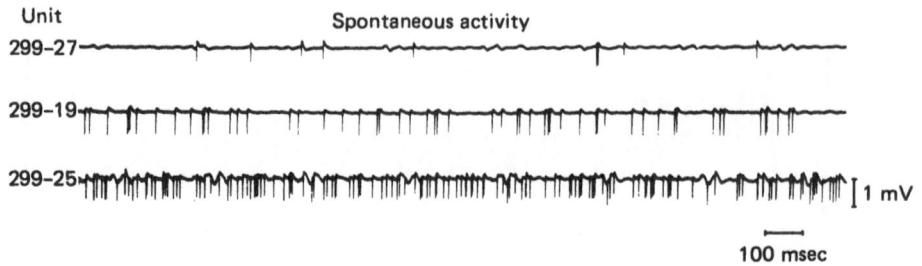

FIGURE 6.4 Sample records of spontaneous activity in auditory nerve fibers (from Kiang, 1965).

it is difficult to avoid confusion between spontaneous activity and circulating discharges if, indeed, there is any difference between the two in this context.

Nevertheless, in the light of the ubiquity of "spontaneous" activity at so many levels of all sensory pathways, it is clear that the detection process in neural systems is probably not so much a matter of the criterion activation of some critical unit someplace in the nervous system as it is a criterion change in the rate of ongoing activity there. This criterion change may either be an increase or a decrease—each is as good a candidate code as the other. We shall now consider the features of some plausible mechanisms, which could possibly explain how it is that nervous decoders might be able to perform the sort of signal detection task required in this situation.

C. The Detection of Threshold Visual Stimuli

Barlow and Levick (1969) have presented a notable analysis of the detection problem of low-level signals in the visual pathways. Recording from ganglion cells in the cat's retina, they obtained histograms of the number of spike action potentials in each time epoch following a stimulus, as well as corresponding records from nonstimulus conditions. The task was a classic example of a signal-to-noise detection problem. The observer (the neurophysiologist in this case) had to decide, on the basis of some criterion, whether or not a transient shift in the histogram was really a "response" or merely a statistical fluctuation of the spontaneous activity.

Barlow and Levick are scrupulous throughout their paper in pointing out the limitations and unusual features of their approach, and certainly many psychobiologists should heed their warnings. But perhaps the part of their work that we should emphasize is their overall concept and perspective. They did not look at any behavioral performance measure to determine whether a pattern of neural impulses was "detectable" or not. Rather, they substituted their own analytical and observational tools for the sensory-decoding mechanisms of the cat. Thus, their experiment models notions of signal detectability that are more analogous to an "ideal observer" looking at the train of nerve impulses than to the psychophysical theory of signal detectability. Their measurements are of information-processing capabilities that would more or less constrain the optimal behavior of the cat if he had been connected to and attending to the information coming along the optic nerve. They, thus, can specify an ideal discrimination measure d for this sensory system, but do not actually estimate the cat's d'. Most properly we should say that the detection capabilities of Barlow and Levick's instrumentation and analysis procedure and a sort of ideal detectability d of the nerve impulse pattern are being estimated in this situation. What they did accomplish, therefore, is a clarification of the sort of signal and noise conditions that are naturally present in the cat's visual pathway and that must be handled by the cat's central nervous system when incoming messages occur.

The experimental procedure utilized by Barlow and Levick involved the insertion of extracellular glass coated metal microelectrodes into the retina through the sclera and stimulation with lights of various durations and luminances. Recording techniques of this sort, as we have seen, concentrate on the time pattern of recorded single cell responses. Automatic data-processing techniques, which plotted interval histograms to summarize the data, were used.

The unconventional and novel portion of Barlow and Levick's experiment was the analysis and determination of what constituted a detectable threshold neural response. Two of the several techniques they used are of special interest. In the first case, Barlow and Levick simply observed the record with their naked eyes and judged subjectively whether or not a sufficient deviation in the histogram had occurred to be considered a response. The other technique, which we shall examine in more detail, depends upon the application of the formal axioms of signal detection theory. An important result of their study was that the formal signal detection procedure did not work any better, that is, give either lower or higher thresholds than the subjective one.

The mathematical assumptions that underly this work are numerous and, as we have seen, often subtle, but so, indeed, are some of the procedural strategies used by Barlow and Levick. For example, one of the most important details of their analysis was the selection of the duration of the period following the stimulus within which they would search for a response. The strategy they used to determine the appropriate length of this period for a stimulus of a given duration was to average the responses elicited in a large number of trials. Implicit in this technique, of course, is a very specific assumption, namely, that this sort of averaging (or some analogue of it) is also part of the nervous system's repertoire of strategies. Such a supposition is plausible, for the visual system most certainly pools the responses of a very large number of cells to determine a psychophysical response rather than depending solely upon the activity pattern of a single cell.

The mathematical advantage achieved when one averages signals is due to the fact that random noise (the nonstimulus variability of the interval histogram in this case) averages toward zero, while the time locked activity (in this case the deviation of intervals due to the stimulus) tends to average toward some nonzero value. In this fashion, Barlow and Levick were able to determine the total duration over which the effects of the stimulus could be detected, and then, armed with this information, return to the single stimulus situation with a known period in which they must look for the effects of the stimulus.

The formal signal detection procedure for the determination that a response has occurred in a single trial was based, once again, on the difference of the means of two distributions. The first distribution was that of the number of impulses that occurred in a period of time, prior to which there had been no stimulus. Many samples of stimulated trials had to be measured to give an estimate of the overall statistics. One typical distribution of this sort is shown in Figure 6.5 as modified from Barlow and Levick's Figure 5. We have labeled this Distribution I. Overlapping with this distribution to a greater or lesser extent will be another distribution labeled II, displaying the number of impulses in an equally large set of periods of equal duration τ, but following a stimulus. This second distribution would look something like the one drawn with the smooth curve, which we have added to Barlow and Levick's original graph. This second curve is a hypothetical distribution of the number of impulses that occur when both a response (the signal) and noise are present.

Each of these two distributions has a mean, and each has a standard deviation, but the criterion for a response is not directly the mean or the standard deviation. It is, rather, the particular point on that second curve, above which Barlow and Levick were willing to accept a given sample count as indicative of a suprathreshold response. This point was defined to be the sum of the mean of Distribution I, $\mu(N_0)$, and some critical number N_c. A response was considered to have occurred when the number of impulses # was as large or larger than:

$$\# = \mu(N_0) + N_c \tag{6.4}$$

In other words, single instances would be considered as part of Distribution II and will be considered to reflect a suprathreshold response to the stimulus only if the count of the number of nerve impulses is greater than this criterion sum. In this case, N_c is defined as:

$$N_c = k\sigma(N_0) \tag{6.5}$$

where $\sigma(N_0)$ is the standard deviation of Distribution I, respectively, and k is a standard score of the normal curve. Thus, Barlow and Levick were able to select a confidence limit of a certain magnitude by the judicious selection of an appropriate k such that the false alarm rate could be adjusted to be as high or as low as desired. A false alarm rate in this case would be the percentage of the total number of times the small tail of Distribution I extends beyond the criterion value $\mu(N_0) + N_c$, the criterion chosen for the acceptance of a response.

Barlow and Levick have made an arbitrary choice of a value of k (which they call the signal-to-noise ratio) to allow only about 0.2 percent

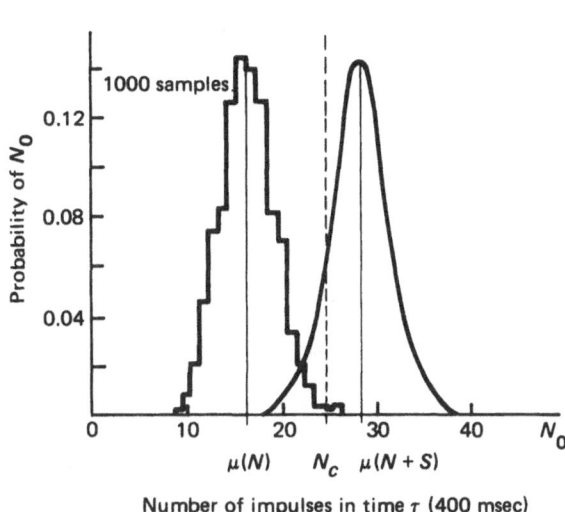

FIGURE 6.5 A diagram similar in concept to Figure 6.2, but adapted to the specific case of neurophysiological response detection in the cat retinal ganglion cell. The stepped curve is actual data recorded from measurements of spontaneous activity and plotted as an amplitude histogram. The smooth curve is an approximation to the distribution of signal plus noise in the event of a visual stimulus. N_c is a criterion (indicated by the dotted line) value above which a particular measure will be assumed to belong to the $N + S$ distribution (adapted and modified from Barlow and Levick, 1969).

false responses. This value of k ($k = 2.88$) can be substituted into Equation (6.5) to give a value for N_c, which can then be used as an objective cutoff point for those counts that will fall above or below the threshold and thus for the specification of whether or not a "response" had occurred.

There are a number of interesting points with regard to this analysis that are directly relevant to the neurophysiology of the situation. First of all, the higher the variance of the spontaneous activity, the greater the change in activity required for a given histogram to be accepted as a true response. Similarly, the duration of the period τ is also a critical factor in the determination of the size of N_c—the criterion increase in the number of spike action potentials.

Barlow and Levick also attended to other problems in their paper, such as the quantum/spike ratio—a measure of the number of quanta that are required to produce a single additional spike. This measure, of course, varies enormously, depending upon a large number of variables. Nevertheless, the important point, which they make in this most important study, is that the threshold, the lower boundary condition of the intensive continuum, depends upon the statistics of the spontaneous activity as well as on the absolute level of the signal. This is a much more precise expression of the older notion of thresholds.

We can now briefly sum up the material of the previous sections. Classical threshold theory has been, in large part, replaced by a newer perspective, which is characterized by probabilistic notions of signal detection in noisy environments. This approach can be used to describe and analyze the data obtained in both neurophysiological experiments and psychophysical experiments. Signal detection theory has the enormous advantage of being able to provide a mechanism for handling the occasional occurrence of the detection of signals very much below any possible deterministic threshold—data that previously had simply been thrown out. Barlow and Levick's work was introduced as a particularly important example of the application of this approach to a very likely neural correlate of the visual detection of low-level signals. Whether the concept of a threshold has any value at all from this new perspective depends primarily upon how well we are able to modify it to take into account these new probability notions. We shall continue to use the word threshold, but its connotation is now always intended to include the notions of overlapping signal and signal-plus-noise distributions, and "shifts in threshold" are intended to imply shifts in either the criterion or the nature of the noise.

In the following section, we consider another important aspect of low-level signal detection—that of the change in sensitivity as a function of previous stimulation. We shall try to describe the representation of adaptive processes by emphasizing the vigorous contemporary issue of the neural or biochemical locus in which their properties reside. An additional important aspect of this material is that it illustrates a situation in which a neural coding mechanism and a biochemical one jointly contribute to the final psychophysical phenomenon.

D. Adaptation of Visual Thresholds

The neural response to a very long lasting stimulus is not constant over the course of the stimulus. Furthermore, previous conditions of stimulation can alter the responsiveness at a later time. This general property of all nervous tissue to respond to an altered extent following prior stimulation is called *adaptation*. Adaptation is one of the ways in which the nervous system accentuates the properties of changing rather than constant stimuli. As a typical example of neural adaptation, consider Figure 6.6 from Kiang (1965), which shows the progressive decrease in the response of an acoustic nerve axon over a period of about 13 min, even though the stimulus during this period remains quite constant. In addition to this diminution in response to constant suprathreshold stimuli, the absolute threshold for a response also typically shows adaptive features in all sense organs. As a consequence of previous activity, all receptor systems are typically found to have elevated thresholds.

Perhaps in no other sensory modality is adaptation more dramatically illustrated than in the visual system, where the absolute threshold can increase by as much as a million times when the eye is light adapted compared to the lowest level achieved under conditions of prolonged dark adaptation. There is a most interesting story that must be told about dark adaptation, which is closely related to some of the notions of thresholds and signal detection that we have been considering so far in this chapter. The problem concerns how much of the visual threshold dark adaptation cycle can be attributed to the decline in the amount of photochemical during exposure to light, and how much can be attributed to neural events occurring in the retina.

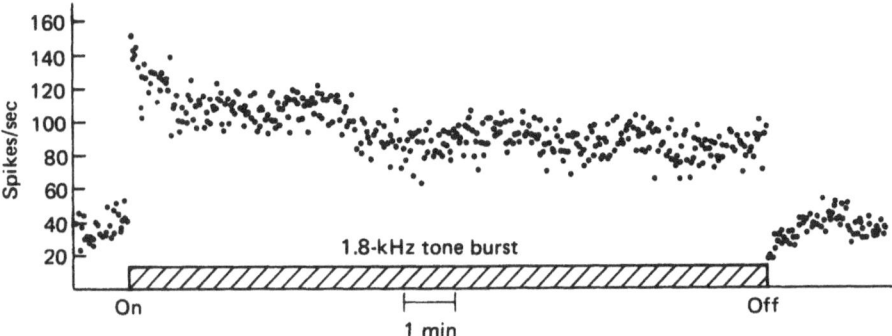

FIGURE 6.6 *Adaptation in a auditory nerve fibers when it is continuously stimulated with a tone at its center or best frequency (from Kiang, 1965).*

Dark adaptation, in the present context, is defined as the increase in sensitivity that occurs when the visual receptor is unstimulated for a period of time. This period may be very brief, or it may be very long, but it is generally true that the degree of dark adaptation will depend upon the length of the period of darkness. *Light adaptation*—a decrease in sensitivity—on the other hand, is the result of a set of converse processes that occur when the visual system is stimulated by light. One can measure an increase in the threshold, which is dependent upon the intensity of the stimulating light. Light adaptation, however, occurs so rapidly that it is almost independent of the duration of the stimulus.

Dowling (1967) has presented what is probably the most comprehensive explanation of the interaction of the photochemical and the neural factors, which affect threshold shifts during adaptation in the vertebrate retina. His work was based upon the use of the electroretinogram as an indicator of retinal sensitivity. The electroretinogram is a rather large graded neuroelectric potential elicited by photic stimulation, which can be recorded by placing electrodes in any one of a number of positions near, on, or in the eye. This sort of retinal electrical activity can most easily be detected with electrodes placed on opposite sides of the retina, that is, one outside the eye and the other inside, if the experimental animal is suitable for this sort of surgical intervention.

Figure 6.7 is a typical vertebrate electroretinogram recorded in this manner. Four portions of this waveform have been tagged with identifying names in order of increasing latency of appearance. The *"a wave"* is negative going and a very small voltage deviation of brief latency. It is immediately followed by the most striking portion of the response, the positive *"b wave,"* and then by the very long lasting positive *"c wave,"* and finally the little negative-going notch known as the *"d wave."* Each of these waveforms behaves quite differently with respect to certain experimental manipulations. The *a* and *d* waves, for example, are not affected by temperature, but are diminished by the presence of alcohol. The *b* wave, on the other hand, is actually enhanced by alcohol, but abolished by the infusion of KCl. These and other differences in the behavior of the dif-

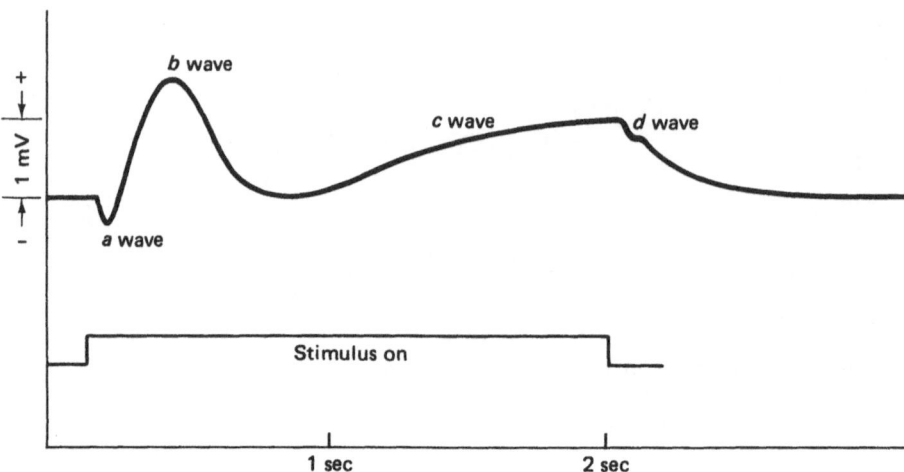

FIGURE 6.7 *A drawing of a sample electroretinogram, showing the various components and their relation to the stimulus period.*

ferent waves have made it clear that the different waves actually reflect the effects of fundamentally different biological processes in the operation in the visual mechanism and that each probably originates at a different place in the retinal network.

The *b* wave of the electroretinogram was of special interest to Dowling, because it alone, of the four components, appears to exhibit electrophysiological behavior corresponding to findings obtained from psychophysical tests on human subjects. For example, the *b* wave seems to have roughly the same dynamic range as human dark adaptation measurements. It appears at about the same threshold stimulus values and disappears when a stimulus is no longer reported. Furthermore, it alone is diminished in amplitude in a monotonic manner as the brightness of a stimulating field is reduced. Using the electroretinogram as an indicator of retinal function had a number of other important advantages for Dowling's analysis. First, it is a measure that could be used on animals, a fact which thus opened up the application of such other important comparative techniques as the direct measurement of the amount of photochemical present at any given time or at any stage of dark adaptation. The animal of choice in Dowling's experiments was the common laboratory rat, an animal whose retina is somewhat simpler to understand than that of man, since all of its photoreceptors are rods.[1]

Given this introduction, let us summarize the intricate system of interlocking experiments that Dowling carried out. His main goal was to determine the underlying biological basis of visual adaptation. It had

[1] These days, things change very fast. Green (Science, 1971 V.174, pp. 598–600) now reports the presence of something other than a conventional rod in the rat retina. Whether it is a cone or not is not certain but it does have "threshold, spectral and speed" characteristics quite distinct from the usual rod.

long been assumed that the amount of rhodopsin was the single important variable in this process. If much had been bleached away, then little visual sensitivity remained. If much had been regenerated, then visual sensitivity was again high. Dowling and others had proposed over the years that, in fact, these photochemical concentration factors were not sufficient to explain all facets of the problem—there probably were also other neural network effects on adaptation. The experiments, which we shall now discuss, were designed to separately assay the effects of the photochemical and neural effects to see which features of the visual adaptation process could be explained by each. Furthermore, while photochemical effects can be simply assigned to a single locus—the outer segments of the rods—the neural effects are not as easy to localize, and, therefore, this also became an important secondary goal.

Dowling used two dependent variables in studies we shall discuss. The first was a direct measure of the amount of light required to produce a criterion (50 μV) b wave amplitude in the electroretinogram. The intensity of this criterion visual stimulus was determined as a function of the various levels of the adapting stimulus. The second dependent variable was a direct extraction and measurement of the amount of rhodopsin—the rod photopigment—present at corresponding levels of the adapting stimulus. Using these two measures, Dowling performed a set of three different experiments, the results of which have all been combined into one now-famous graph, which helps us to understand the respective contributions of the neural and photochemical factor to light and dark adaptation. Unfortunately, because it is so rich in information content, this graph is complex, and the way in which this graph is constructed is usually difficult to comprehend. Therefore, we shall build the graph up by separately describing the results of the three experiments contained in it, and then consider the significance of the comparisons which then can be made.

First, let us consider the effect of light adaptation on the electroretinogram. Dowling's experimental procedure in this experiment was to provide a controlled background illuminance for a preconditioning period, and then determine what the luminance of an additional incremental light source had to be to produce a criterion b wave amplitude. The results of this experiment were found to be almost totally a function of the luminance of the background and not of duration because of the brevity of the light adaptation process (probably less than 100 msec).

Figure 6.8(a) shows the results of this first experiment. It is clear that the relationship between the necessary stimulus increment for a criterion electroretinographic b wave and the background luminance is a linear one with a slope of $+1$.

Dowling's second experiment was the determination of the shape of the more prolonged dark adaptation curves. Because dark adaptation, unlike light adaptation, occurs at modest speeds (that is, has a prolonged time course), the function that is to be plotted is a matter of the background illuminance in only one special detail. That detail, of course, is the initial point at which the dark adaptation process starts. The first point of any dark adaptation curve will be the same as the single measure

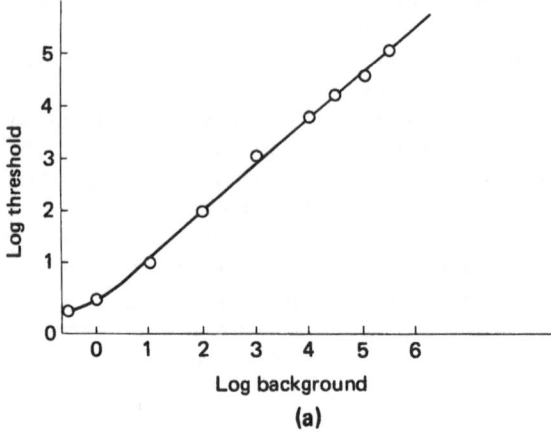

(a)

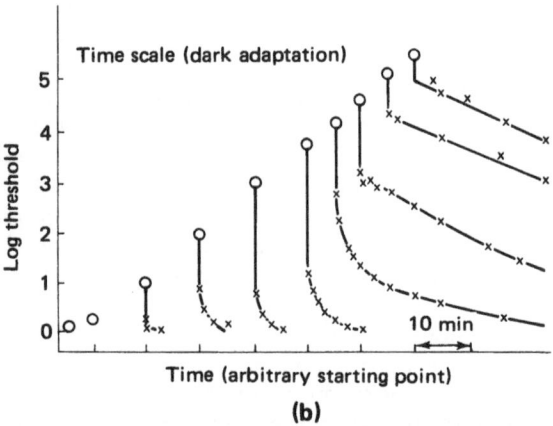

(b)

FIGURE 6.8 Dowling has compared the dark adaptation, light adaptation, and photochemical absorption curves to show that there are both neural and photochemical components to the dark adaptation curve. In this series of figures, we have broken up his complicated final graph to show how it was constructed (a) The light adaptation curve. Since light adaptation occurs in 1 or 2 msec, this can be plotted purely as a function of background light intensity. (b) A set of dark adaptation curves, each of which starts from a point on the light adaptation curve corresponding to the same background illuminance. Since this curve is very much a function of time, it must be plotted along a time axis. (c) Measures of the absorbance of light by photopigment extracted from the eye at various background illuminances. (d) The final curve is composed by scaling the light and dark adaptation curves and the photochemical absorbance curve to comparable scales. The overlap of the photochemical absorbance curve and the dark adaptation curve points of inflection are the key to the conclusion that both neural (fast) and photochemical (slow) factors are involved in dark adaptation. See text for full details (adapted and modified from Dowling, 1967).

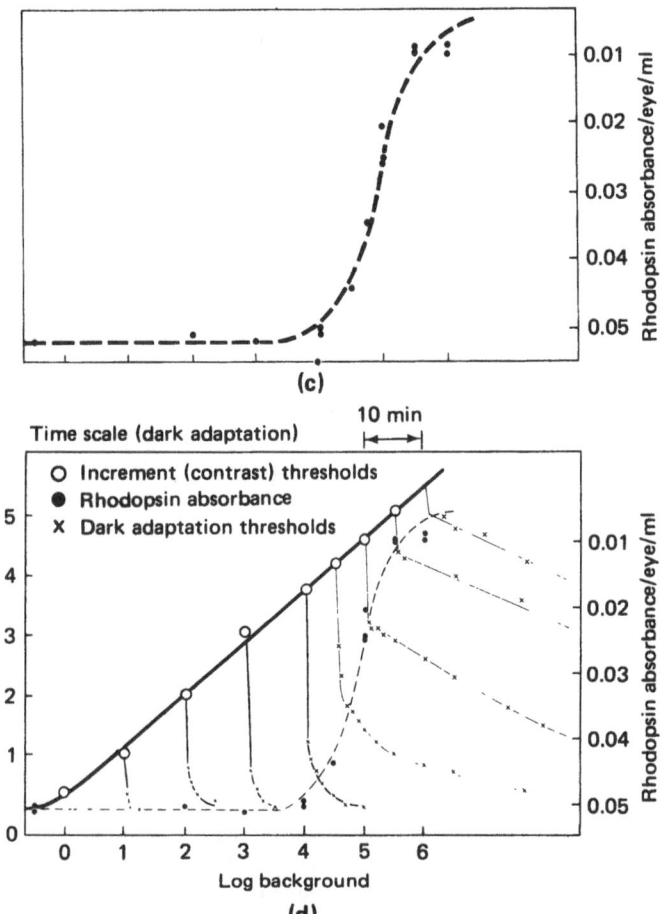

(c)

(d)

of the luminance determined level of light adaptation in the first experiment, thus providing a linking mechanism tying the two sets of data together. The important variable in dark adaptation is time, and it is against that dimension that it must be plotted by testing the level of dark adaptation at various intervals following the begining of the dark period. Once again using the criterion of a 50 μV b wave, the set of curves shown in Figure 6.8(b) is obtained, showing the dark adaptation for varying initial levels of stimulus luminance.

The third experiment was of quite a different sort. In this case, direct measurements were made of the amount of photochemical that remained in the rat's eye after illumination with a given background illuminance. Dowling's dependent variable in this third experiment was the amount of light absorbed by the extracted residual rhodopsin. The greater the absorbance, the more rhodopsin remained. Low values of absorbance indicated that more rhodopsin had been bleached into various breakdown products. To make this chart directly comparable with the previous two, the vertical coordinate (absorbance/ml) has to be plotted upside down as shown in Figure 6.8(c). The key point being made here, of course, is that the amount of light absorbed is a good measure of the amount of rhodopsin present.

The superimposition of the three graphs on top of one another is relatively straightforward. The light and dark adaptation curves are linked by the log background illuminance. The initial points of the family of dark adaptation curves fall without further scaling directly on the points of the single light adaptation curve. The rhodopsin absorbance curve, however, has to be adjusted in its vertical scale to fit into the picture properly. This was simply done by extending the vertical scale until it covered the same range as the other two curves.

The composite of the three curves is displayed in Figure 6.8(d). A number of additional points of special interest are immediately apparent. All of the dark adaptation curves can be seen to exhibit two important properties. First, there is a point of inflection on each curve, representing high background illuminances, and each of these curves, therefore, is composed of two segments. The first segment falls very rapidly, while the second segment displays a much more gradual fall, which may take as long as an hour to return to the original level of dark adaptation. Second, each of the dark adaptation curves associated with a lower level of background luminance is composed of but a single segment, displaying a very rapid recovery to the original levels of sensitivity.

The key feature of the superimposed graphs of Figure 6.8(d), which explains the shapes of the dark adaptation curves, is the superimposed rhodopsin concentration curve. The points of inflections on the two-segment dark adaptation curves are seen to occur at locations that are comparable to those on the rhodopsin concentration curve. The major implication of the similarity of the points of inflection and the rhodopsin concentration curve is that the dark adaptation process is a joint effect of the amount of rhodopsin present—a relatively slow mechanism—and some other mechanism, which adapts far more rapidly. This latter rapid mechanism is, according to Dowling, a neural one, which depends upon the recovery of some synaptic sensitivity somewhere more central in the retina than in the receptor layer. Much of the remaining discussion in Dowling's paper is aimed at identifying the locus of this fast neural adaptation process. We shall now consider the evidence he gathered to identify the locus of the fast adaptation process in the bipolar layer of the retina.

The first step taken by Dowling in the localization of the fast adaptation process was to determine whether it is a central or peripheral effect. Dowling and some of his colleagues had discovered that the electroretinogram was almost entirely normal even after the optic nerve had been severed. Such drastic surgery not only cuts off the possibility of centrifugal communication, which might have been capable of signaling gain control information from the central nervous system to the retina, but also leads to degeneration of the ganglion cell bodies of the retina. Even after substantial numbers of the ganglion cells have degenerated, the b wave of the electroretinogram still remained relatively normal. Thus, the locus of the fast neural process must be more peripheral than the ganglion cell layer.

Approaching from the other end, another possible locus of the neural adaptation process could be the receptor cells themselves. But Dowling cites Lipetz (1961), who showed that illumination of cells anywhere in a given receptive field leads to a decrease in the sensitivity (as reflected by the fast dark adaptation process) throughout that entire receptive field. Thus, the process seems not to be dependent upon the condition of individual photoreceptors, but rather upon an interconnecting neural net, which is more central than the receptor layer.

These two findings, the lack of effect of a transection of the optic nerve and the independence of the stimulus position in a receptive field, direct attention toward the middle layer of the retina—the bipolar cell layer. Another very important fact supporting the notion that the bipolar layer is, in fact, the locus of the fast process is based upon the close association between the b wave of the electroretinogram and the psychophysical functions. Dowling notes that previous studies clearly identified the b wave as having its origin in the bipolar layer, and thus the dark adaptation process is also most likely located there. Finally, Dowling has suggested that the mechanism underlying these fast adaptation processes may be mediated by reciprocal feedback among bipolar and amacrine and ganglion cells, whose synaptic contacts all occur in very close proximity to one another.

In the preceding discussion, we have dealt with the possible ways in which fluctuations in threshold measurements can be mediated. Two processes, a fast one dependent upon neural activity and a slow one dependent upon the available number of molecules of the photochemical, were implicated as contributors to the overall dark-light adaptation process. There are many unanswered questions concerning the details of the neural processes that underly the fast adaptation process in particular, but Dowling's analysis gives us what is probably a satisfactory picture of where things are happening.

However, more recently, some of the premises of Dowling's analysis have been subject to some question. Miller and Dowling himself (1970), have recently reexamined the problem of the origin of the b wave of the electroretinogram, using the large celled retina of the amphibian known as the mud puppy. They believe now that the b wave, rather than coming from the bipolar cell layer, actually is generated by Müller cells—large glial or supporting cells that run across virtually the full thickness of the retina. Thus, while Dowling was correct in stating that the b wave was not produced by the receptors or by the ganglion cells, he may have been incorrect in directly attributing their origin to the bipolar and horizontal cells. The question of how these electrical responses originate in the nonneural Müller cell, however, is still open. No known photochemical process within the Müller cells could directly explain the electrochemical responsiveness of their cellular membrane. Miller and Dowling have, therefore, suggested that the Müller cell potential is, in fact, produced by the indirect action of the neurons (the bipolars and horizontals) in the distal portion of the inner nuclear layer of the retina. Thus, while the b wave may not be a true code but only a sign, that is, not signal carrying but only concomitant, it is still a pretty good indicator of the action of those neurons through which the true coded information passes. No major change in the analysis of Dowling's 1967 paper would be required other than the assignment of "sign" status to the b wave.

Furthermore, Boynton and Whitten (1970) have also made an important contribution to this problem by showing that there may be some sort of neural adaptation in the receptor itself, in addition to the slow component of adaptation attributable to photopigment bleaching. In sum, this is an exciting and interesting area, in which considerable progress is being made, but which also has a number of remaining problems.

We can sum up the material in this section by reemphasizing Dowling's conclusions, which still seem to hold in spite of the doubts of the origin of the components of the electroretinogram. There are, he concludes, two different processes affecting the dark adaptation of a photoreceptor. One is a very slow process, which seems to be closely associated with the regeneration of rhodopsin following the cessation of a visual stimulus. The other is a very fast process, which is apparently encoded by the action of neural factors, which are capable of being reversed in the dark much more rapidly than rhodopsin can regenerate. This leads to a two-segment dark adaptation curve (even in the rat's retina, which contains mainly rods) whenever the stimulus intensity gets high enough to bleach a substantial amount of the rhodopsin.

In the present section, we have emphasized the neural and photochemical processes underlying visual thresholds. Presumably, the neural processes we have discussed are not specific to vision alone, but comparable mechanisms exist in the other sense modalities. The special characteristics of the visual mechanism make it clear exactly what the issue is in this case, and interest in vision has led to a great deal of specific data. But there is little comparable knowledge about the other senses. We now turn to another topic concerning the intensive dimension, however, in which there is a great deal of information available for many of the sensory modalities. We shall consider problems, not of thresholds, but of the continuum of sensory magnitudes ranging from the threshold as a lower limit up to regions of stimulus intensity, at which qualitative changes (such as the introduction of pain) begin to appear.

II. THE RANGE OF THE INTENSITY DIMENSION AND THE RESPONSE DYNAMIC

A. Introduction

So far we have only considered one point on the intensive dimension— the threshold—its lower limit. We shall now consider the rest of the range. It is well known that all of the sense organs can operate over enormous ranges of stimulus intensities. In many cases this range is much wider than even the best of man-made instrumentation. For example, the dynamic range of the human ear for a 1-kHz tone extends from threshold stimulus values of about 0.0002 dynes/cm^2 to a pain threshold about 140 db (decibels) higher. This is a range from minimum to maximum of

100 trillion to 1 (100,000,000,000,000 to 1)! The visual system is similarly able to operate over a range in which the largest stimulus that can be handled is as great as 10 billion times the minimum detectable stimulus. The olfactory system is sensitive in certain instances to incredibly small concentrations [although as Geldard (1953) points out, this may represent a very large total number] of certain molecules like mercaptan. Thus, even though it is obscure what the upper limit of the olfactory range is, it is clear that it is extremely large.

In contrast to these enormous ranges of sensitivity to variations in stimulus intensities, there is a curious narrowness of the response range of most candidate neural codes. The frequency of spike action potentials, for example, can vary only from perhaps 800 or 1000 Hz down to a point at which the intervals between spikes are so large as to be virtually meaningless. Certainly 1 spike/sec would be considered noise in most systems, while as we have seen, perhaps even as many as 40 or 50 spikes/sec, must also be considered in many instances to be spontaneous activity. Thus, spike action potential frequency, one of our most important candidate codes, is limited at most to a range of 100 to 1.

Graded potentials, on the other hand, can vary over wider ranges. The lower limit of the cochlear microphonic, for example, which can be reliably detected as a response to a low-level stimulus with good equipment, is 0.020 to 0.030 μV as measured at the round window (McGill, 1959). At the upper end of the scale, potentials as large as a few millivolts have been recorded. Thus, the dynamic range of this particular graded candidate code can be as large as 100,000 to 1, a reasonably wide range, but one still considerably less than the enormous range of the whole auditory system.

The issue to which we now turn concerns the characteristics of the intensity functions of the various modalities within these response ranges. We shall be concerned with the relations that obtain between intensive stimulus dimensions and either psychophysical and neurophysiological intensive responses. Such a function we shall refer to as the intensity stimulus-response dynamic or more simply as the response dynamic. Because the stimulus ranges are, in general, wider than either of the two response ranges, there will often appear to be a compression of the former by the latter, and the logarithmic coordinates so often used reflect this biological fact. However, as we shall also see, this is not always the case, and some stimulus ranges are often expanded by psychophysical measures and occasionally even by neurophysiological response transformations. The very general exponential notation introduced by Stevens in his discussion of the psychophysical power law can be seen, therefore, to play an important role in the generalization of this notion of the response dynamic.

In the following sections of this chapter, we shall discuss the two most important mathematical models relating stimulus intensity and either psychophysical or neurophysiological response. We do so, however, from the point of view of a disinterested observer—disinterested, that is, in championing the cause of either specific formulation. Neither model is from a purely empirical point of view, able to fully handle all of the data. Clearly, the Fechnerian expansion of the Weber idea is not able to cope with the abundance of psychophysical data, which are not only non-logarithmic, but not even compressed. The Stevens power law model, while providing a convenient descriptive approximation to much of the data, has, as we shall see, also been criticized on empirical grounds with regard to its ability to adequately describe data.

In subsequent sections, we shall deal with the neurophysiological data relating stimulus intensity and neural response in detail. An important aim of this review will be to identify the anatomical levels within each sensory system at which the total system response dynamic originates.

B. Mathematical Descriptions of Response Dynamics

1. The Weber-Fechner Relation—a logarithmic law. It was not too many years ago that the Weber-Fechner description of the relationships between stimulus amplitudes, incremental thresholds, and subjective magnitudes was considered *"The* Psychophysical Law." In the context of the more general notions we now have of the multidimensional aspects of sensory-coding theory, it is clear that the formulas relating these dimensions represent only one aspect of a much more extensive universe of discourse. It is essential to remember that the Weber-Fechner law is but one of a family of coding rules, which collectively describe the relation between dimensions of the stimulus and the family of common sensory dimensions. Sensory coding is not limited to quantity, but also includes quality, space and time discrimination and representation.

With regard to subjective magnitudes, however, the Weber-Fechner formulization is of particular interest for two reasons. First, historically it represented one of the fundamental notions in the development of both the psychophysical and neurophysiological aspects of the sensory sciences, and second, it is so very often today the specific critical target of some of the newer approaches. Although it is quite clear that the Weber-Fechner law is no longer able to adequately model the abundance of data obtained in the last century, it is important to understand the assumptions that underly its formulation. In the following sections, we review the history of Fechner's mathematical development of some empirical observations made by Weber and the impact these ideas had on many decades of sensory research.

In the middle of the nineteenth century, E. H. Weber reported the results of some experiments on differential thresholds, which asked the general question: what is the size of the increment that has to be added to a given stimulus intensity to produce a just noticeable difference? Weber's experiments were initially carried out using weight estimations as a model experiment, even though there was no applied interest in this particular type of judgment. His experiments involved the measurements of the differential weight that had to be removed from or added to a standard weight for the change to be detected with either active (with hand movements) or passive (without hand movements) examination.

Weber's general conclusion was that the amount of weight that had to be removed was a constant proportion of the total weight originally in hand. In other words, Weber's law may be formulated as:

$$\frac{\Delta I}{I} = C \tag{6.6}$$

although Weber himself never used this equation. It was Fechner who quantified the qualitative notion expressed in Weber's verbal statements. Indeed, Weber was probably not even the first to mention the ratio relationship in sensory studies. Fechner (1860) mentions that the mathematician Euler, 100 years earlier, had noted the relationship for the musical scale. Fechner also noted that Steinheil and Pogson had appreciated the relationship for the scales of stellar magnitudes. Nevertheless, Weber was the first to proclaim its general applicability to sensory magnitudes in many different modalities. Fechner himself, however, was among the first to notice that the relation was not of general applicability and that there were limitations and instances in which it was not valid, a portent of some criticisms to be made 100 years later.

Approximation though it might be, Weber's Law, nevertheless, does emphasize the nonlinearity of the response dynamic, and it is for this reason, rather than its precision as a predictor, that it probably has maintained attractiveness as a psychological construct over the years.

Fechner carried out a number of experiments verifying the generality of Weber's law for brightness and loudness. He also studied temperature sensitivity, but discovered that the constant ratio law held only as a rough approximation in the middle temperature ranges and did a woefully poor job of prediction for very high and very low temperatures. Moreover, unlike Weber, who was only concerned with specific and well-defined instances of sensory magnitude, Fechner extended some of the implications of that work to apply the psychophysical law in the realm of the barely quantitative by a number of imaginative leaps. For example he used it, at one point, to account in a pseudoquantitative form for the magnitude of "mental wealth."

> *A dollar has, in this connection, much less value to a rich man than to a poor man. It can make a beggar happy for a whole day, but it is not even noticed when added to the fortune of a millionaire.*
> (FECHNER, 1860)

Fechner's extension of the Weber relation took other bizarre turns beyond this surprisingly broad application. Fechner, a mathematical physicist by training, also chose to derive another distinctly different notion by manipulating his algebraic expression of the Weber statement mathematically. To do so, however, required several very important assumptions that have made his derivation controversial for many years. Fechner, first of all, assumed that since the just noticeable *stimulus* difference ratio was constant, then changes in the *subjective magnitude* should be also directly proportional to the Weber ratio. He expressed this idea in the following relation:

$$\Delta\Psi = K \frac{\Delta I}{I} \tag{6.7}$$

where $\Delta\Psi$ is the actual change in sensory magnitude for a just noticeable difference; K is a scaling constant; ΔI is the change in stimulus intensity for a just noticeable difference; and I is the absolute magnitude of the stimulus. This equation is not, and this is most important, directly derivable from the Weber relation of Equation (6.6). It is a separate notion and one of the two key assumptions in Fechner's development. Most important, it implies that all just noticeable differences $\Delta\Psi$ are equal in size.

The other key assumption in Fechner's development is that this statement [Equation (6.7) above] formulated at the level of macroscopic finite differences, can be taken to the limit and reduced to the infinitesimal differential form:

$$d\Psi = K \frac{dI}{I} \tag{6.8}$$

From this point on, all of the mathematics is straightforward enough, even if the final equation is empirically invalid. Equation (6.8) may be integrated on both sides to give:

$$\int d\Psi = K \int \frac{dI}{I} \tag{6.9}$$

or

$$\Psi = K \ln I + Q \tag{6.10}$$

where Q is a constant of integration. Q may be removed by formulating the equation in terms of the absolute threshold. At threshold $\Psi = 0$ and $I = I_0$, therefore:

$$0 = K \ln I_0 + Q \tag{6.11}$$

or:

$$-Q = K \ln I_0 \tag{6.12}$$

which may be substituted into Equation (6.10) to give:

$$\Psi = K \ln I - K \ln I_0 \tag{6.13}$$

or:

$$\Psi = K \ln \frac{I}{I_0} \tag{6.14}$$

which is a final form of what has now become well known as the Weber-Fechner relation. This expression states that the subjective magnitude of a sensation is a function of the logarithm of the ratio of the stimulus intensity and the absolute threshold stimulus intensity.

Admittedly, the derivation is a peculiarly indirect one with a pair of equivocal assumptions critical to its development. Many current mathematical psychologists claim that both of the assumptions are, in fact, invalid. Nevertheless, as we have said before, the compression function implicit in the logarithmic relation between stimulus intensity and perceptual magnitudes has given it wide currency for many years.

2. The Stevens Power Law. In recent years, some of the discrepancies of the Weber law as an experimental predictor have begun to emerge. Not all psychophysical intensity functions turned out to be logarithmically compressed, and therefore new formulations have been suggested. Perhaps the most vigorous champion of a systematic new point of view has been S. S. Stevens (1961),[2] who has proposed that intensive functions are better modeled by a power law. Stevens' formularization of his "psychophysical law" is considerably different than the Weber-Fechner relation in that it allows both expansive and compressive response dynamics and, further and most important, it involves few of the lengthy logical leaps of Fechner's derivation. In fact, there is only one real assumption of any consequence in Steven's model, and even that is almost an *ex post facto* explanation of the data rather than a necessary condition for the development of the empirical power law. That assumption is that equal sensory ratios require equal stimulus ratios. The major argument for Stevens' "psychophysical law" has, clearly, always been an empirical one, and it is on the basis of the data alone that it will ultimately be accepted or rejected.

Stevens' theory, if one can call his descriptive model a theory, is that all sensory magnitudes can be described by the following form of a generalized power function:

$$\Psi = K(I - I_0)^n \tag{6.15}$$

where all of the terms have the same meaning as in Equation (6.14) above. The only new term n is simply the exponent or power to which the stimulus term is raised. A key notion is that the power for each sensory modality (and for that matter many different tasks in the same modality) may differ from one case to another.

Before we consider the implications of this idea in detail, let us consider for a moment the effect of variations of the exponent. If the exponent is equal to 1, sensory magnitude is simply a linear function of the stimulus intensity scaled by the coefficient K. If the exponent is less than 1, however, the function is compressed or decelerated so that the same absolute incre-

---

[2] S. S. Stevens passed away early in 1973. He was one of the most important sensory scientists of the 20th century as this chapter clearly exemplifies. We all shared a sense of loss at the news of his untimely death.

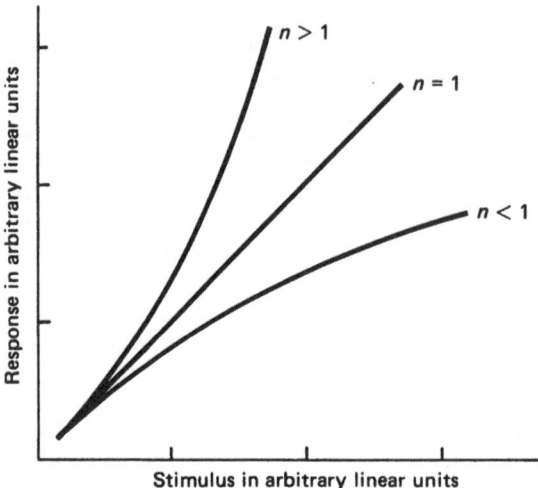

FIGURE 6.9 A drawing of a linear (n = 1), compressed (n < 1), and an expanded (n > 1) power function plotted on linear-linear co-ordinates.

ment at low levels of stimulation produces a greater differential response than when the intensity is high. If, however, the exponent is greater than 1, we have a situation in which expansion of the response occurs. That is, a given increment ΔI in stimulus intensity at high stimulus levels causes a larger change in sensory magnitude than when the stimulus intensity is low. Figure 6.9 illustrates on a linear-linear[3] scale the effect of varying the exponent. Much of the recent data reported by Stevens and his colleagues are well fit by power functions with exponents ranging from as low as 0.3 for relatively large visual stimuli to an unexpectedly large 7.0 for electrical stimuli applied to the teeth—electrical stimuli and pain being a combination that produces a highly expanded response dynamic. Table 6.1 is a recent compilation of exponents, which have been observed in a surprisingly varied spectrum of experiments exploring intensive-response dynamics.

There is a convenient graphical test to distinguish among the three types of response curves that we have so far discussed: the linear, the logarithmic, and the power function. A linear curve will appear as a straight line on graphs in which both coordinates are plotted on linear scales—a linear-linear plot. A logarithmic function will appear as a straight line on a graph in which the vertical coordinate is plotted linearly and the horizontal axis is plotted on a logarithmic scale—a log-linear scale. A power function, on the other hand, will appear as a straight line on a graph in which both axes have been plotted along logarithmic scales—a log-log plot. The slope of the straight line representing a power function on a log-

[3] In much of the following discussion, we shall be dealing with graphs that are plotted on axes that may be scaled linearly or logarithmically. The nomenclature we shall use to differentiate them involves a hyphenated expression. The first term in the expression will refer to the nature of the scale of the horizontal axis. The second term in the expression will refer to the scale of the vertical axis. Thus, a log-linear scale, for example, will be one with a logarithmic horizontal scale and a linear vertical scale.

TABLE 6.1 PSYCHOPHYSICAL MAGNITUDE
EXPONENTS OF POWER FUNCTIONS DESCRIBING THE
RESPONSE DYNAMICS OF THE VARIOUS SENSES*

Exponent	Paradigm
0.33	Brightness of 5° target in dark (continuous)
0.5	Brightness of brief flash
0.6	Smell of heptane
0.6	Vibration of 250 Hz on finger
0.67	Loudness of 3000–Hz tone
0.7	Visual area
0.8	Tactual hardness
0.95	Vibrations of 60 Hz on finger
1.0	Temperature
1.0	Visual length
1.1	Duration of white noise stimulus
1.1	Pressure on palm
1.1	Vocal sound pressure
1.3	Thickness of blocks
1.3	Taste of sucrose
1.4	Taste of salt
1.45	Lifted weights
1.5	Temperature (warmth on arm)
1.5	Tactual roughness
1.7	Handgrip
2.0	Electric stimulus in hearing
3.5	Electric stimulus to skin
7.0	Electric stimulus applied to teeth

* This table has been adapted from Stevens (1971) by placing the exponents in order, adding one value, and indicating the demarcation between compressed and linear or expanded functions with the dotted line.

log plot is equal to the exponent of that power function. Thus, when the slope of a linear function is 1 on a log-log scale (and its exponent is also 1), a straight line will, in fact, represent a true linear function. The relationship among the expanded, linear, and compressed functions on the linear-linear and log-log plots can be seen if one compares Figures 6.9 and 6.10. Expanded curves are accelerating, while compressed curves are decelerating on a linear-linear plot. All are straight lines on a log-log plot, but with slopes that vary according to the degree of curvature. Accelerating (expanded) curves have slopes greater than 1; decelerating (compressed) functions have slopes less than 1.

Logarithmic functions also come very close to overlapping some of the power functions with exponents much less than 1, and in certain instances some investigators have had to make careful statistical tests of the closeness of fit to determine which function is, in fact, able to account for more of the variance.

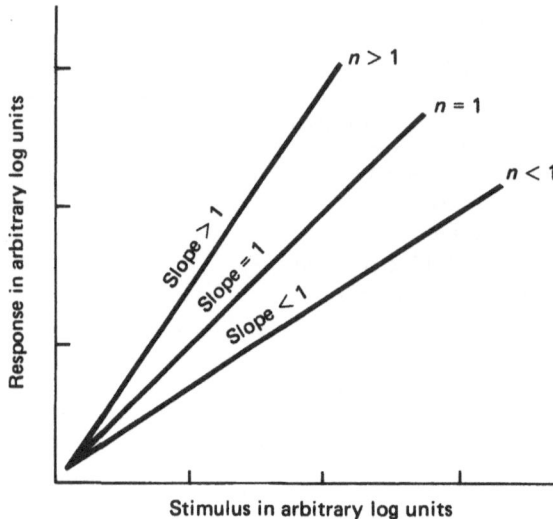

FIGURE 6.10 A drawing of a linear (n = 1), a compressed (n < 1), and an expanded (n > 1) power function plotted on log-log coordinates.

Stevens' notions have been extremely influential in stimulating research in the last few years, to say the least. In fact, as Zinnes (1969) puts it, "The number of papers purporting to show that the correct psychophysical law is a power law or a logarithmic law is probably increasing exponentially."

In spite of this enormous amount of activity, it cannot be said that there has been general agreement forthcoming about the validity of the power law, and Stevens' formulation has been challenged on many grounds. Even though his theory is a descriptive one and is not based on any specific mathematical assumptions comparable to those of the Fechner formulation, power function fits often seem to be dependent upon a rather specific experimental procedure. Stevens had developed the classical psychophysical method of fractionation into a newer procedure which he called the method of direct magnitude estimates. (See Chapter 7 of Corso, 1967, for a complete discussion of this method.) This newer procedure had the advantage of being capable of collecting enormous amounts of data in a very short time, but the specificity of the method required to produce power functions has led some workers to challenge the generality of the data so obtained. Many observed exponents vary considerably when other psychophysical procedures are utilized. This variation with procedure is something that Stevens himself has been aware of, and he has repeatedly made much of the fact that "valid" measurements can only be obtained when certain standardized procedures are used.

Stevens has suggested that all stimuli should be spaced in equal ratios along their intensive dimensions. While originally the method of magnitude estimates was supposed to require the use of a standard presented at the beginning of the experiment, Stevens now feels that it is better not to use a standard, but simply let the subjects use whatever magnitude estimating numbers they please. He further suggests that only a few presentations of each stimulus intensity should be allowed and that geometric means should be used to estimate central tendencies. If all of these conditions are met, it is his belief that all intensive dimensions will be well fit by some power function. But these special conditions have led many workers to wonder if the power law reflects the methodology of the experimenter rather than the biology of intensive coding.

The Stevens version of the "psychophysical law" has been subject to a number of other criticisms over the past decade. Since it is primarily an empirical law, the criticisms have had to be directed pimarily at the "goodness of fit" of the straight line on a log-log scale to sensory magnitude data. Zinnes (1969) has reviewed much of this data and feels that the power law often does not describe the data very well. A very germane criticism has been made by Ross and DiLollo (1970). They show that the magnitude estimate curves for lifted weights exhibit double inflections—a feature which is very uncharacteristic of power curves, and which must necessarily either be monotonically accelerating or decelerating if they exhibit any nonlinearity at all. Ross (personal communication) has also pointed out that the effect of plotting data on a log-log scale is to obscure many of the points of inflection and deviations of complex curves and that almost any function, if plotted with sufficiently large symbols on a log-log scale, gives a straight line. Figure 6.11 is an illustration of just how far this sort of information loss can go. What Ross is saying is that while all power functions do plot up as straight lines on log-log scales, all curves that are relatively good fits to straight lines on such scales do not necessarily represent power functions.

Furthermore, the situation may be very much more complicated than either the proponents of the log or power law hypothesis seem willing to admit. Barlow (1965), for example, has considered the nature of the function, relating the incremental threshold reported by human subjects as a function of background intensity as measured by the number of quanta in a visual stimulus. The data for his experiments are plotted in Figure 6.12. The Weber type of function (which would imply, as we have seen, a log law of subjective magnitudes) can be seen to hold over a middle portion of the range of stimulus intensities. At lower background intensities, Barlow feels that a square root law holds, which is directly the result of the increased role that "retinal noise" plays as the average background intensity decreases. That is, the square root rule derives from signal-to-noise discrimination considerations, which are emphasized at low levels of illumination where the quantum noise is still significant. At higher levels, the point of inflection suggests that a third "law" may better describe the data. The main implication of this sort of data for our discussion is that if one looks closely enough, there may, in fact, not be a single simple expression that can describe all behavior over the entire dynamic range of the visual system.

Thus, there is some question whether or not the power law is even an empirical fact. There is, further, a question of whether or not logarithmic and power functions are quite as different as one might initially suspect. Both Fagot (1966) and Stevens (1971) himself have also pointed out that, with small exponents, power functions come very close to ex-

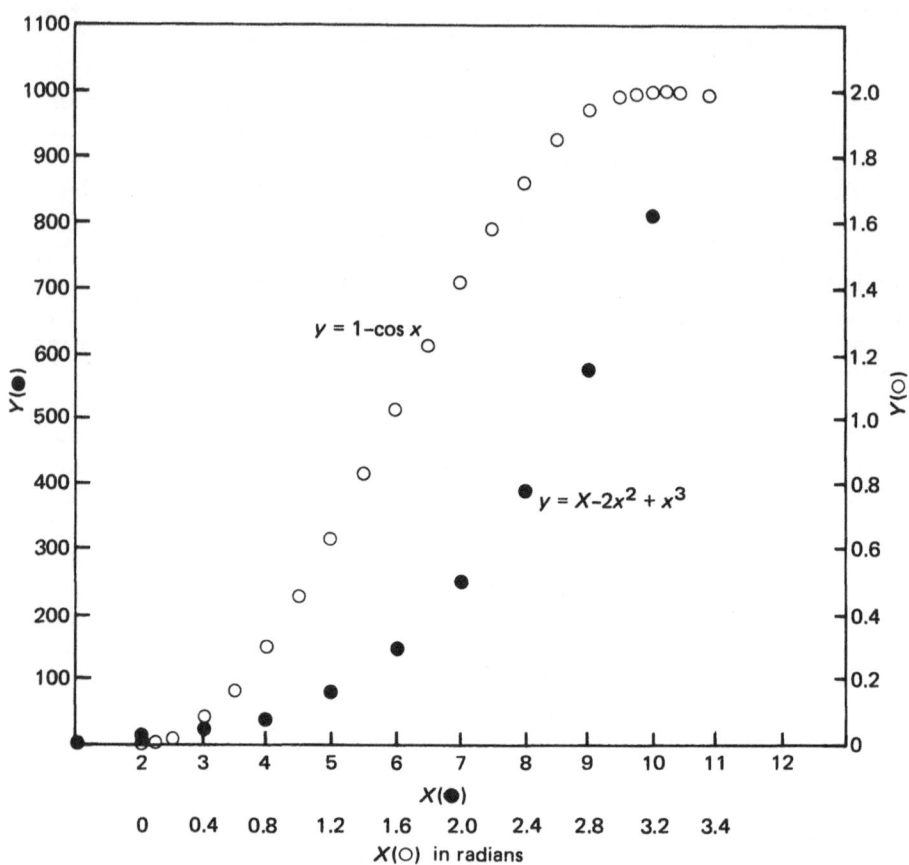

(a)

FIGURE 6.11 Two examples $(y = x - 2x^2 + x^3$, a polynominal, and $y = 1 - \cos x$, a trigonometric function), which are not power functions but which do appear to be well fit by straight lines when converted to log coordinates over much of their range. The curves are plotted on (a) linear-linear and (b) log-log coordinates. Note that not all points are plotted on both (a) and (b) because of the great difference in scaling (courtesy of Dr. John Ross, University of Western Australia).

hibiting the same functional shape as the log functions when plotted on linear-linear coordinates. Therefore, strongly compressed power functions (exponents considerably less than 1) may be indistinguishably different than log functions, and each of the psychophysical laws may simply represent an equally valid, but alternative, mathematical model for the representation of the data.

Another type of criticism has been directed at the procedure of pooling data from the large numbers of subjects usually used in magnitude estimation experiments by Luce and Mo (1965). The doubt they raise is: if the power law fit only holds for groups of subjects and not indi-

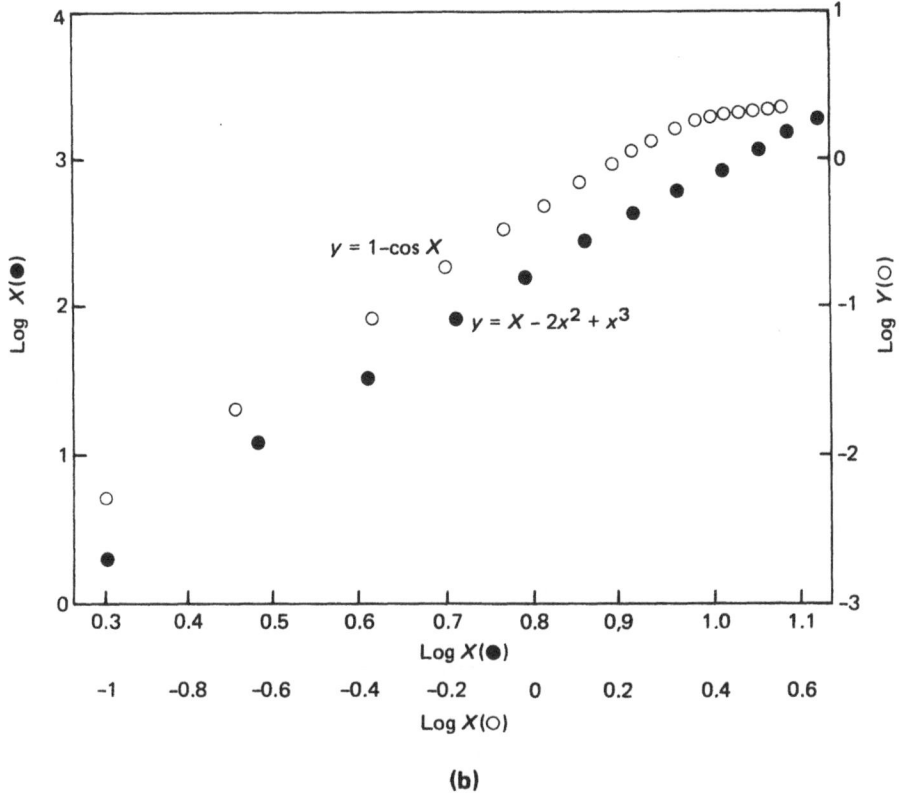

(b)

vidual subjects, then is it possible that what the power law represents is a manifestation only of the statistical pooling and not of the biological processes that underly the magnitude estimates of individual subjects.

Luce and Mo collected magnitude estimate data for subjects on two sensory continua—the magnitude of lifted weights and the magnitude of a 1000-Hz tone. Their data, rather than being pooled, were plotted individually for each subject on log-log scales. We reproduce their graphs in Figure 6.13(a) and (b). In their words,

> No subtle statistical analysis is needed to see that the plots shown in figure 1 and 2 are not well fitted by straight lines; moreover, even if we introduce the usual threshold correction on the independent variable, only Ss 1 and 8 appear to conform to power functions.
>
> (LUCE and MO, 1965, p. 7.)

The generality of the power law as a universally applicable function, therefore, seems to be also challenged by the fact that it does not appear in the performance of individual subjects.

Frankly, the author of this book finds the arguments for either power functions or logarithmic functions, or, for that matter, any single univer-

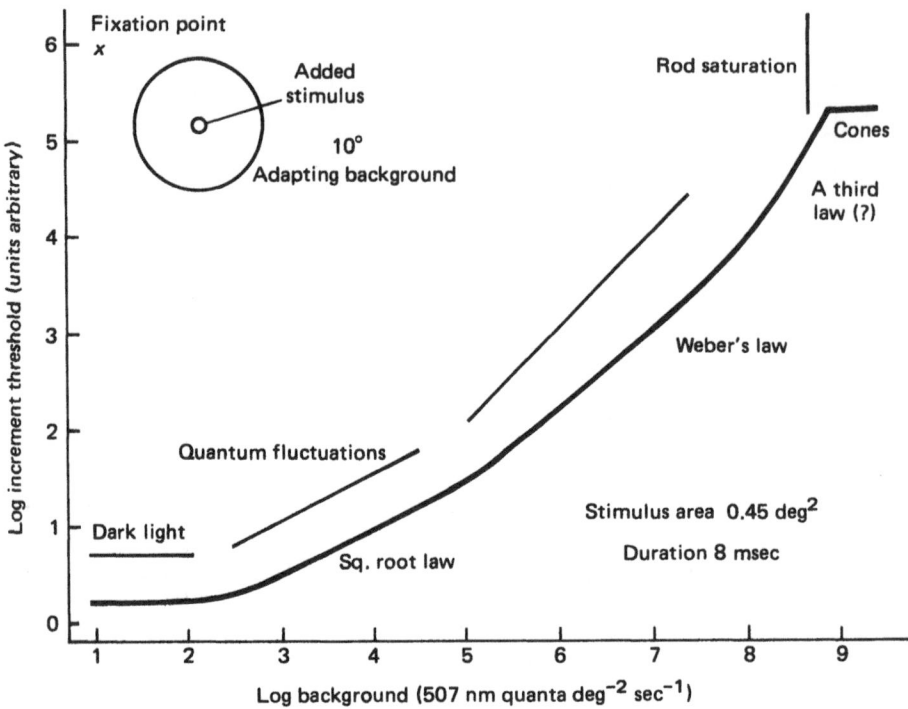

FIGURE 6.12 *A graph of the relationship between background intensity and the increment threshold in a human psychophysical experiment, showing the multisegmented nature of the curve even when plotted on log-log coordinates (from Barlow, 1965).*

sal function to be, at the present time, less than compelling. My hunch is that there is an enormous amount of complexity hidden, not only as one looks across the entire range of psychophysical experiments, but even as one looks at different intensity levels of a single stimulus dimension. The power function, however, is a very useful construct if one is interested in a simple metric of the general tendency of some intensive continuum. A single number, the exponent, gives an overall estimate of the rate at which it may be accelerating or decelerating. As such, it is a useful and convenient descriptor of both neural and psychophysical intensive dimensions, and it will be used in this sense later in this chapter. Its use in this context, however, should not be construed as an acceptance of the power law as a universal psychophysical or neurophysiological fact.

3. Other Models of the Response Dynamic. Though the Weber-Fechner logarithmic and the Stevens power functions are the best known of the mathematical models of the response dynamic, there have been, in recent years, other suggested formularizations of possible general laws. For example, a number of workers have suggested that the relationship between the stimulus intensity and both the neurophysiological and psychophysical magnitudes is described by the following formula:

$$R = \frac{R_{\max} I}{(I + I_{\frac{1}{2}})} \tag{6.16}$$

where R is the response for any stimulus level I $R_{\max}$ is the maximum response and $I_{\frac{1}{2}}$ is the stimulus intensity when the response is equal to one-half of $R_{\max}$. This relationship has been observed to hold for human

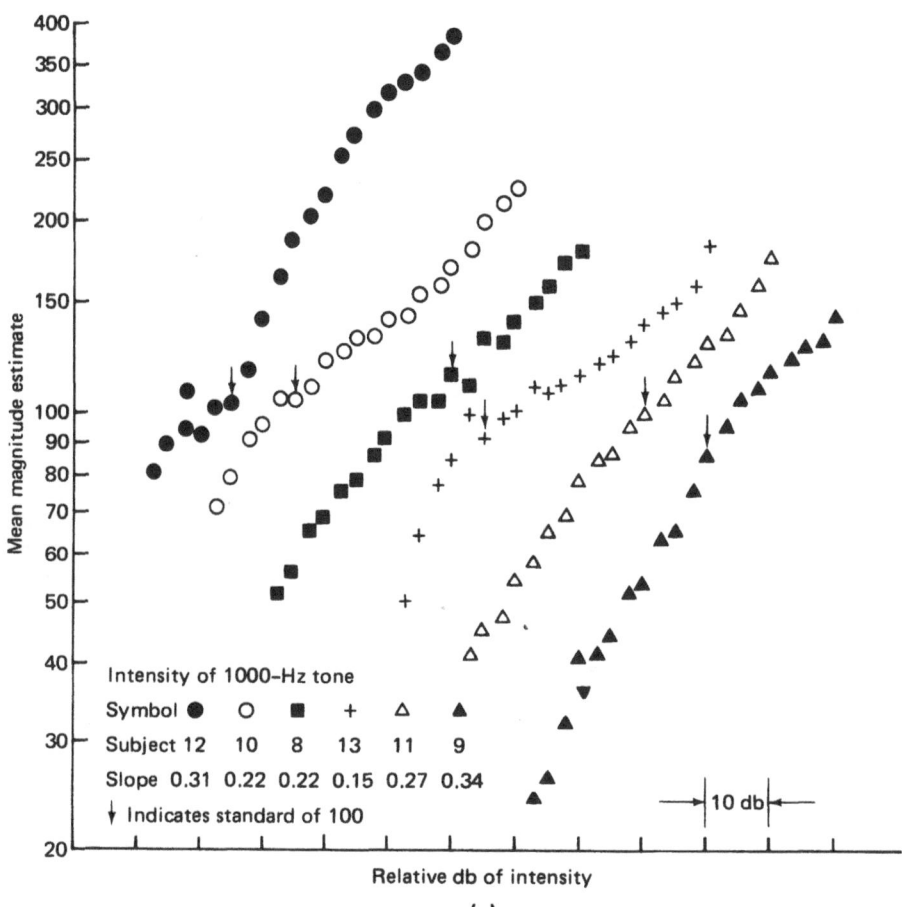

FIGURE 6.13 (a) Unpooled (individual subject) data for a loudness estimation experiment. (b) Unpooled (individual subject) data for a lifted weight experiment. Neither of these sets of data are well fit by power functions, even though the pooled data for many subjects are. This finding casts doubt on the general validity of the Stevens power law for individual subjects (from Luce and Mo, 1965).

FIGURE 6.13 (Cont.)

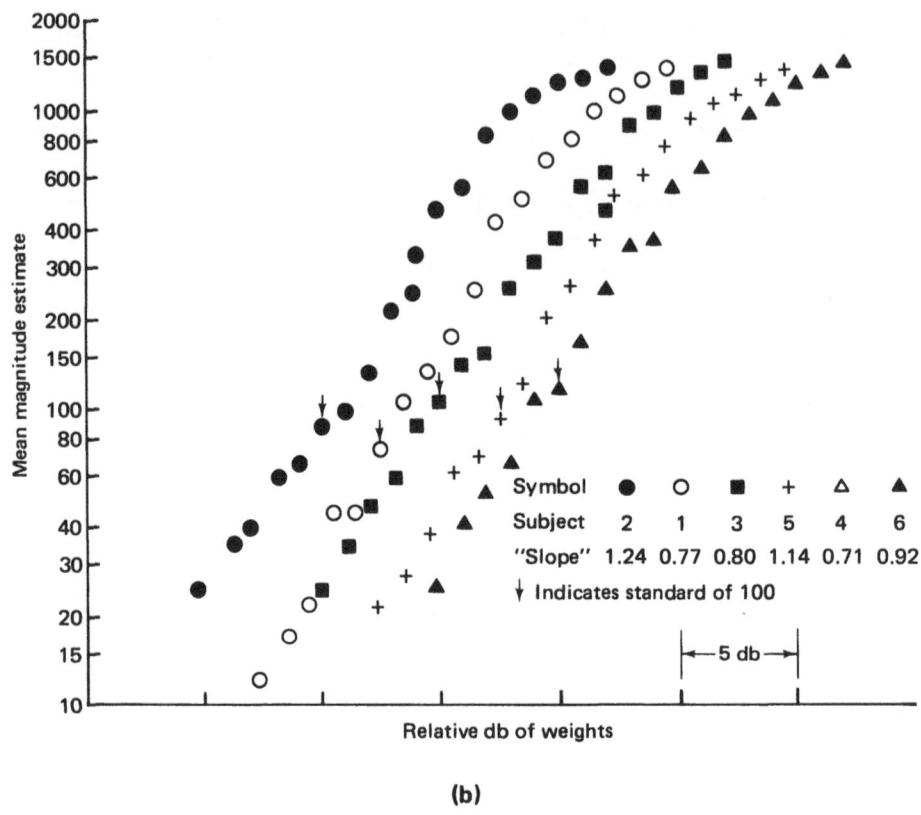

(b)

visual psychophysical experiments by Alpern, Rushton, and Torii (1970), for retinal bipolar responses by Naka and Rushton (1966) as well as by Werblin and Dowling (1969), and for cones by Baylor and Fuortes (1970). Interestingly, this equation and much visual data when plotted follow a sigmoidal curve, which has two points of inflection. They, thus, could not possibly be fit by any power function.

Lipetz (1971) has also suggested that the hyperbolic tangent function of the form

$$R = \frac{1}{2} + \frac{1}{2} \tanh w \tag{6.17}$$

(where R is the response produced by logarithmic units w of the stimulus intensity) may also describe a variety of response dynamics. This function has the property of closely approximating log and power functions over some portions of its range, but also fitting some data over larger ranges than can either of those functions. It is also a sigmoidal curve with two points of inflection [like that of Equation (6.16)], but this is not too surprising since it can be derived from that function.

Both of these functions have some advantages over the log and power laws, but it must be noted that it is also the case that they do not fit all data. As we shall see in the discussion that follows, there is probably more variability among the various response dynamics than any single function could possibly entail. A general law may simply not be in the cards in this domain.

C. The Neurophysiology of Response Dynamics

Whatever the nature of the mathematical function relating stimulus intensity and subjective magnitude, the empirical fact of nonlinearity (that is, compression and expansion) must be taken as a starting point. For the coding theorist, its existence raises two distinct problems. First, can we find candidate codes whose properties reflect the nonlinearity we find in the psychophysical data and which may be related to the stimulus by some function which approximates the psychophysical function? A second problem is the determination of the anatomical level at which these response dynamics are introduced into the coding process.

To answer these questions, it would be most satisfying if we could look at a body of comparable data from several levels within the same sensory system, as well as from a variety of systems. Unfortunately, however, no one has carried out such a systematic comparative neurophysiological examination of either the various levels or the various sensory systems using a single standard methodology. We shall have to put the story together piecemeal by gathering data, which have been collected under a wide variety of stimulus conditions and by many different investigators. To bring order to this compendium, it is best to deal separately with each of the sensory modalities for which we have data. We shall be interested in also comparing the shape of the response dynamic curve at different levels of a single sensory system. In the present section, we have chosen to separate our findings into only three categories. We shall look at the dynamic response of the generator or receptor potential, the peripheral nerve action potentials, and central nervous action potentials. In doing so, we shall be able to make only general comparisons of the response dynamics at different levels. For example, we shall be able to compare the degree of compression at the generator potential and at the level of peripheral nerves. While this has been done by individual investigators occasionally, more usually we shall have to draw the comparisons from unrelated experiments.

To facilitate this comparison, all data, insofar as it is possible, will be converted to power functions so that the exponents can be used as a simple metric of compression as described above. In doing so, it must be reiterated, no *a priori* assumption is being made that a power function is the best fit—that will have to be decided for each case individually—or that there is anything fundamental about the power law. The use of the power function in this context will be as a simple metric, which has the advantage of being able to succinctly characterize expansion, compression, or linearity of the response range with a single number even if the fit is less than perfect.

Indeed, many of the log-log graphs, which we have transformed especially for this discussion, do not appear to be well described by the straight lines, which represent power functions. Several of the curves display an early region at low stimulus intensities, over which an ex-

ponent somewhat greater than 1.0 seems to hold, and a later region for
high stimulus intensities, over which an exponent substantially less than
1.0 holds. Such bisegmented behavior appears to be relatively common.
It is of some special interest to look at the data that were collected prior
to the recent enthusiasm about the power law theory, for they do represent, from one point of view, the results of a "blind" experimental design.
More recent data collected and published in the light of the power law
"zeitgeist" may possibly represent something of a biased sample—those
that fit were published and those that did not were not.

In any event, the straight line approximations have been applied by
eye and hand rather than by some error minimization procedure, and the
reader may want to keep that in mind as he inspects each case.

The intended limitations of this approach cannot be overstated. There
will be a strong tendency on the part of the reader to assume that because
we are using the power law as a descriptor, that we attach to it some
special theoretical importance. *That is not the case!* Furthermore, there is
no reason to assume that even if the neurophysiological data are better fit
by one sort of law and the psychophysical by some other law that there
is any inherent contradiction. The basic notion of coding theory is that
information may be represented in any conceivable way as long as transformation rules or processes are available. The same question arises
with regard to linearity of relations between psychophysical laws and
neurophysiological laws. No congruence of function is required.

Despite such caveats, a preview of the data of the following sections
is very encouraging. There is, in fact, a great deal of uniformity and
agreement, not only within the senses, but across them. Generally, and in
sharp contrast to the psychophysical data, almost all neurophysiological
data do exhibit monotonically decelerating or compressed functional
behavior with regard to the stimulus.

1. Intensity-Response Relations in the Somatosensory System. a. Somatosensory generator potentials. We have already been introduced to the
work of Loewenstein and the techniques he used to explore the transduction properties of a type of Pacinian corpuscle found in the cat's mesentery. Once again, we must turn to his elegant experiments to provide us
with information about the intensity relations for this particular somatosensory receptor structure, which will serve as a model for this modality.
Loewenstein (1961a), using much the same techniques described in the
earlier paper (Loewenstein and Rathkamp, 1958), prepared a portion of
free nerve by peeling away the layered structure of the corpuscle. His
stimulator, in this case, was a glass rod attached to a piezoelectric crystal.
His recording electrode, equipped to record generator potentials, was
placed at a point just peripheral to the beginning of the myelin sheath.

The pertinent result of Loewenstein's 1961 study for our current discussion was the specification of the relationship between stimulus intensity
and generator potential amplitude. These data were obtained by varying
the intensity of the stimulus and observing the evoked amplitude of the
generator potential. Figure 6.14 displays the results of this experiment
on a graph, in which both stimulus and response are scaled linearly. For

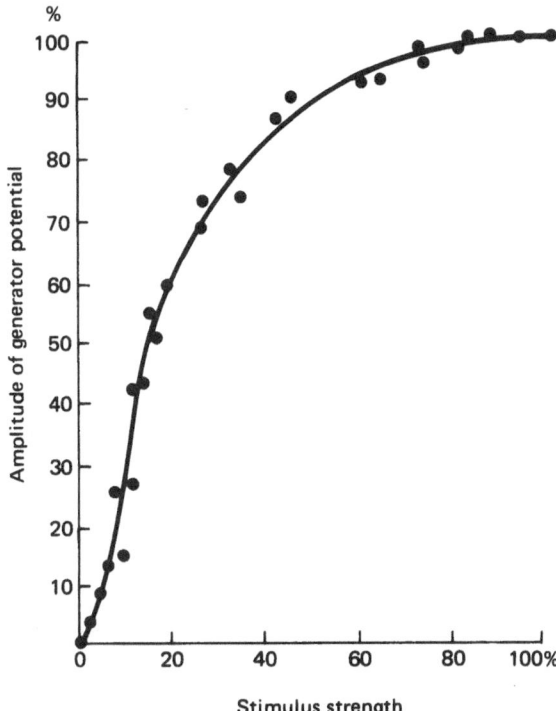

FIGURE 6.14 The somato-
sensory generator potential
as a function of stimulus intensity plotted on linear-
linear coordinates (from
Loewenstein, 1961a).

most of the course of this curve, it is obviously a compressed function, for
it does appear to be decelerating. However, there is also some suggestion
that there is a region in which this is not true. For low stimulus intensities,
the generator potential seems actually to be slightly accelerated, thus reflecting an expanded function.

But this brief statement is an oversimplification of the true complexity of the situation and of the richness of Loewenstein's results. Consider the fact that this receptor is a system in which the portions of the
neuronal membrane that produces the generator potential are mechanically coupled together. Loewenstein quite astutely pointed out that the
general increase in response could be produced either by a continuous
increase in permeability at the point of stimulation or by an increase in the
area of the tissue that is affected by the stimulus.

To determine which of these possibilities was the correct one, Loewenstein also carried out experiments to determine the relation between
area of the membrane activated and the generator potential amplitude. To
do this required using stimulators of differing sizes, but keeping the
displacement of the crystal at a constant amplitude. The curve shown in
Figure 6.15 depicts on a linear-linear plot the effect on the generator potential of varying the areal extent of this constant amplitude stimulus.
Clearly, the form of the response function for varying areas of activation is very close to that produced by variation in the stimulus amplitudes.
Loewenstein concludes from this comparison that the change in the

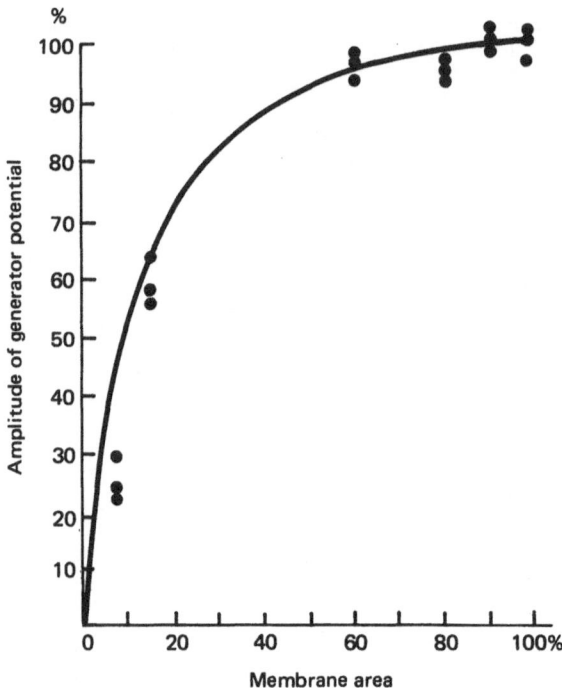

*FIGURE 6.15 The somato-
sensory generator potential
as a function of stimulated
membrane area plotted on linear-linear coordinates (from
Loewenstein, 1961a).*

generator potential produced by a stimulus of increasing amplitude is primarily a function of increasing area of activation, and that the flow of transmembrane ionic current at any given location is roughly constant over wide ranges of stimulus amplitude. Loewenstein's data, unlike that of almost all of the other studies we shall describe in this section, go far beyond a simple specification of the form of the relation. He has also analyzed the underlying membrane mechanisms, which account for the shape of the response, and has shown a rather surprising fact, namely, that in the Pacinian corpuscle the amount of generator potential produced at any specific microlocation on the receptive membrane is probably constant and almost independent of stimulus amplitude.

In Figure 6.16 Loewenstein's data relating stimulus intensity and generator potential amplitude have been replotted on a log-log scale to determine the exponent of an approximating power function. This plot suggests that a power function with an exponent of about 1.4 typifies the course of the response dynamic for the low intensity region, while an exponent of 0.38 typifies by far the larger portion of the dynamic range of this receptor.

This is a relatively frequent pattern, which we shall observe several times in the following discussion. It must be remembered, however, that because of the compression of the logarithmic scale, the one-log unit between 1 and 2 log units represents an actual stimulus range 10 times that of the less intense stimulus varying between 0 and 1 log unit. There-

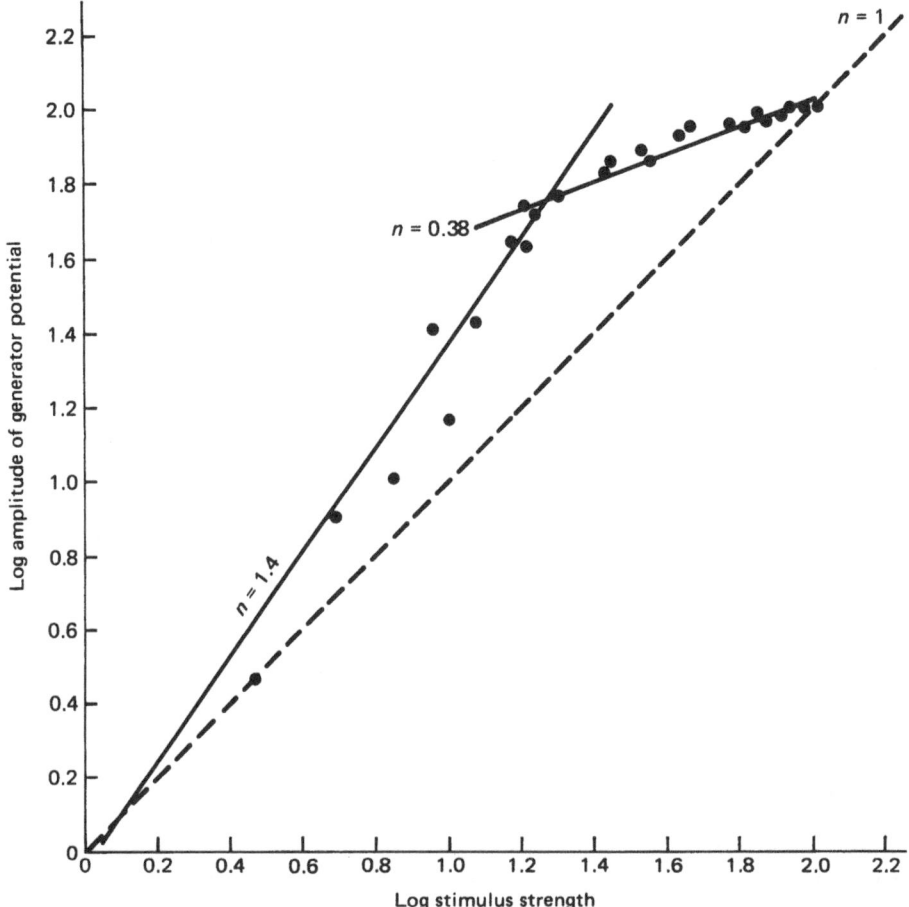

FIGURE 6.16 *The somatosensory generator potential as a function of stimulus intensity converted to log-log coordinates. This curve displays a two-limbed function with power function exponents of 1.4 and 0.38, respectively.*

fore, the upper portion of the curve is more characteristic of the total range of the function and is always the value we shall use in our summary analysis.

From a physiological point of view, this sort of finding suggests that for low intensity regions, the response dynamic may have evolved specifically as an expansive amplifier rather than a response range compressor, the latter being characteristic only of higher stimulus intensities. This dichotomy once again supports the notion expressed earlier in our discussion of the work of Barlow that rather than a simple power function relation over the entire stimulus range (as hypothesized by Stevens), more correctly, the dynamic response of the neural substrate may be said to vary from one portion of the range to another. Such a notion would probably be unacceptable to Stevens' theoretical formulation.

b. Peripheral somatosensory nerve action potentials. Werner and Mountcastle (1965) have carried out a study on the somatosensory peripheral nerve, which can be compared to Loewenstein's results. However, such a comparison is valid only if we note a major difference in the procedure of the two experiments. This difference is that Werner and Mountcastle were not studying the output of the deeply embedded cutaneous Pacinian corpuscle, but rather the response of fibers emanating from a cutaneous receptor known as the "Iggo corpuscle," a complicated bulblike cutaneous receptor structure originally identified and described by Iggo (1963).

Werner and Mountcastle used an ingenious stimulator, which electronically controlled the displacement of a lucite rod so that the displacement was entirely dependent upon the applied voltage and independent of the resistance encountered from the tissue being stimulated. In this manner, indentation of the skin, rather than applied force, was the independent variable, and the amount of displacement could be used as the measure of stimulus intensity.

The neurophysiological recording system measured the number of spike action potentials that occurred in a single axon dissected from the saphenous nerve of a cat. The number of impulses that occurred in some constant period of time following the stimulus was the measure of the response. Such a response metric does, acknowledgedly, obscure some of the fine detail of the response, since there is usually a vigorous response at the beginning of stimulation and a less active maintained response, but Werner and Mountcastle felt this was not important and simply counted spike action potentials over periods of time that ranged from 20 to 1000 msec.

In all, 21 fibers were studied in their experiments. Three of these axons, which were later found to be located over bone, responded peculiarly and were, therefore, not considered further. Of the other 18, 2 were unusual in that they did not exhibit response compression, but rather had a dynamic curve best represented as a power function with an exponent greater than 1 and thus were expansive. All of the other 16 did exhibit response compression to a greater or lesser extent. Figure 6.17 is a plot on both a linear-linear scale and a log-log scale of the pooled results of 10 of the fibers studied by Werner and Mountcastle. This subsample is believed by the authors to be representative of their total sample of fibers and will be the basis of the rest of our discussion.

Werner and Mountcastle, very much influenced by the work of Stevens in the preceding decade, have expended a significant amount of effort to establish whether or not the sort of curves they report is well fitted by power functions. They report statistical tests of the goodness of fit of both logarithmic and power functions for their data and quite conclusively show that the power functions account for a larger amount of the variance in this case. Correlation coefficients of the linear regression between stimulus and a power function representation of the response were 0.97 or higher. Needless to say, there was great variability in the power functions recorded from individual fibers. Exponents ranged from 0.26 up to 1.16, but a computation of the arithmetic average for the 43 runs

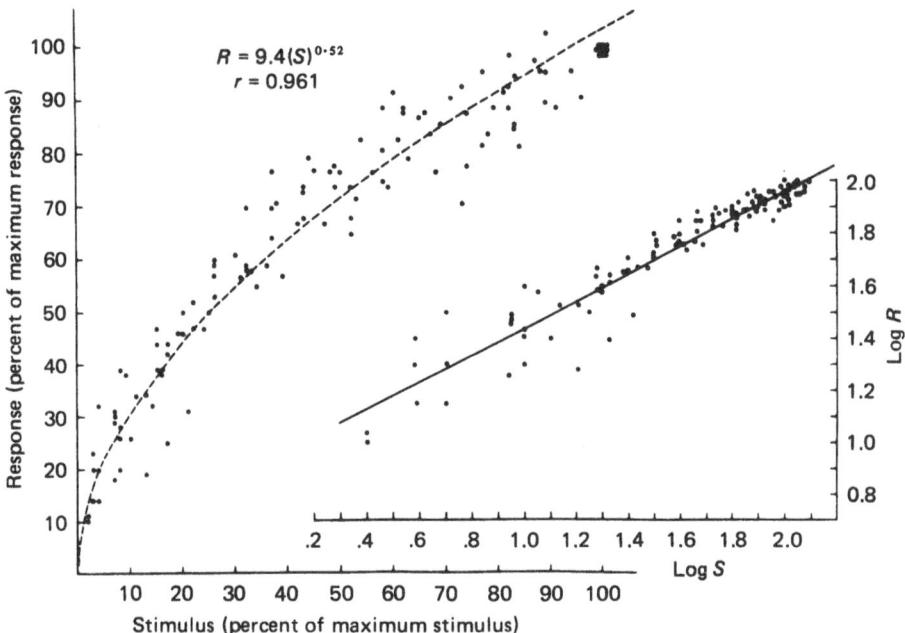

FIGURE 6.17 (a) The rate of spike action potential firing in peripheral somatosensory neurons as a function of the stimulus intensity. Both dimensions are in
terms of percent of maximum and plotted on linear coordinates. (b) The same
data converted to log-log coordinates, exhibiting an exponent of 0.52 (from
Werner and Mountcastle, 1965).

on the 18 acceptable fibers reported in one of their tables is 0.590. A
similar average of the particular 10 fibers that they felt were typical was
0.52. Thus, in the mean, the system of fibers is a compressed one. A comparison of this exponent with that obtained by transforming Loewenstein's data in the previous section shows that the peripheral nerve
response (at least as measured by Werner and Mountcastle's counting
methods) is somewhat less compressed (that is, the exponent is higher) than
the generator potential at the receptor level. Thus, even in light of all the
differences in method and preparation between the two experiments, it
does seem, at least, that there is no further compression beyond the receptor. To support this conclusion, we should also note (in preparation
for a discussion which will come later in this chapter) that some investigators have made direct comparisons, not between stimulus amplitudes and
the response dynamics of peripheral nerves, but between generator
potential amplitudes and the frequency of firing of the propagated spikes.
Katz (1950) has done this for a mechanosensitive muscle spindle in the
frog; Wolbarsht (1960) used this same experimental paradigm to compare
the generator potential and spike frequency in a mechanosensitive hair
of the blowfly; and Terzuolo and Washizu (1962) have also studied the
same relationship in the abdominal stretch receptor in the crayfish. All of
these experiments (as well as comparable studies in the visual system

which we shall discuss later) show a strong linear relationship between the generator or receptor potential on the one hand, and the spike action potential frequency, on the other. Studies of this sort are important in establishing at what neural level response compression is introduced into any sensory system, for they also indicate that there is little further compression at the mechanism that converts generator potentials to spike trains.

    c. Central somatosensory nervous activity. The author knows of no direct procedural analogue of either the Loewenstein or Werner and Mountcastle papers for the central somatosensory nervous system. Our search for neurophysiological data on the response dynamic of the central nervous system, therefore, has to turn to somewhat less direct comparisons.

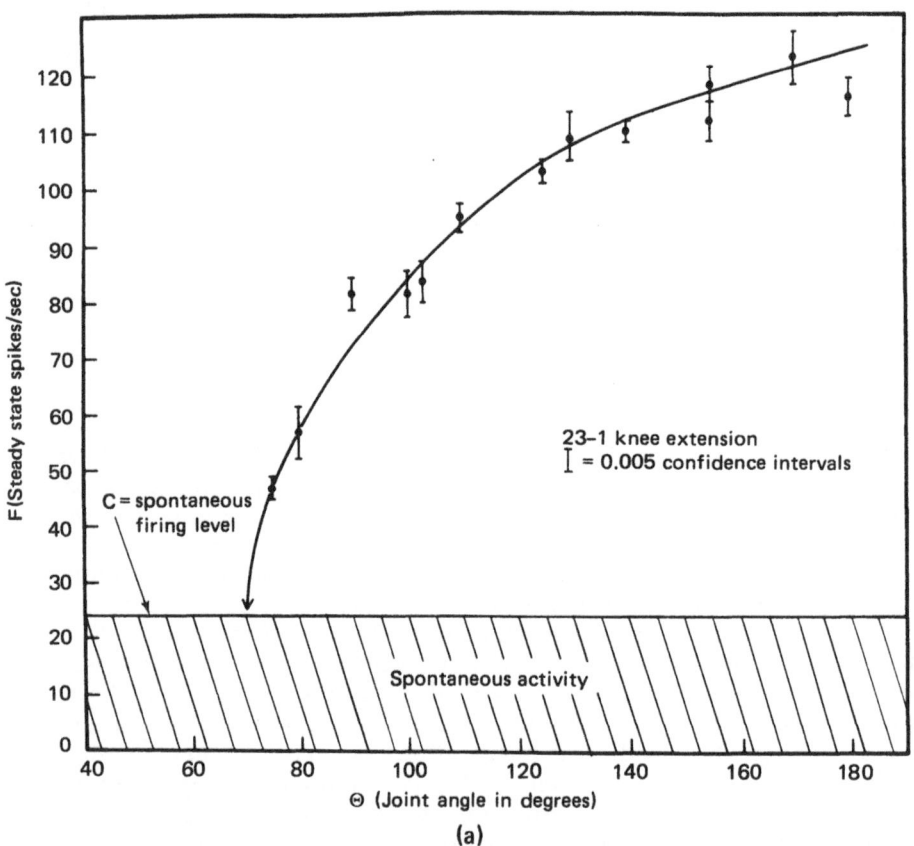

(a)

FIGURE 6.18 (a) The rate of spike action potential firing in thalamic neurons as a function of the angle of joint rotation plotted on linear-linear coordinates. (b) The rate of spike action potential firing in thalamic neurons as a function of the angle of joint rotation θ, less the threshold angle of rotation θ_t, and converted to log-log coordinates, exhibiting a power function exponent of 0.429. $F =$ driven rate; $C =$ spontaneous rate (from Mountcastle, Poggio, and Werner, 1963).

One of the most relevant studies is also from Mountcastle's laboratory. Mountcastle, Poggio, and Werner (1963) report a study in which extracellular microelectrodes were used to record the mean frequency of spiking in thalamic neurons of a Macaque monkey. However, the feature of this experiment, which moves it somewhat out of the context of the previous discussion, is that the stimulus was not a mechanical force producing a cutaneous or mesenteric displacement, but rather rotation of a limb joint. This experiment, therefore, somewhat contrary to what the authors themselves seem to assume, is an example of a situation in which the stimulus is spatial displacement and the candidate code is frequency of nerve impulse firing. Probably because it had been usual to associate spike action potential frequency with intensive stimuli, the authors, incorrectly from at least one point of view, state that their potential stimulus is varying along an intensive continuum. But, regardless of the semantics of the issue, their paper comes the closest to fitting the needs of this section.

Mountcastle, Poggio, and Werner report data that relate the joint angle of a limb of a cat to the mean frequency of firing of thalamic neurons. Figure 6.18(a) (reproduced from their paper) is a sample of the sort of data obtained as a function of joint angle for a situation in which the limb of the monkey was moved to different final angles very rapidly. In

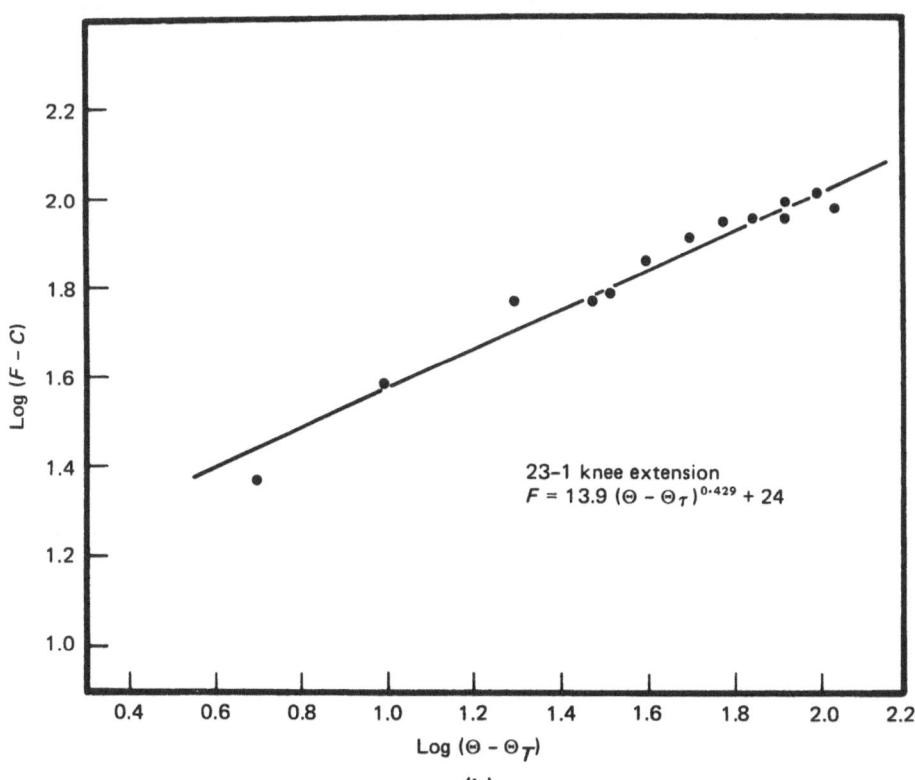

23-1 knee extension
$$F = 13.9 \, (\Theta - \Theta_T)^{0.429} + 24$$

(b)

Figure 6.18(b) (also reproduced from their paper), these data have been converted to a log-log plot and thus directly gives us the exponent of the best fitting power function ($n = 0.429$). In another table in their paper, these authors also report the exponents of the power functions obtained from a sample of 27 separate experimental runs on 12 different thalamic cells. The exponents in this large sample range from 0.30 to 1.60, although only 3 cells have exponents greater than 1.0. The average of these exponents is 0.730, a somewhat less compressed function (that is, a slightly larger exponent) than the one recorded for either the Pacinian corpuscle generator potential or the peripheral nerve function when activated with peripheral stimuli.

Another pair of studies, which are quite important in the establishment of the relative contributions of the various levels of the sensory pathway to the overall response dynamic, are two related inquiries into the dynamics of the evoked brain potential recorded from the human somatosensory system. The studies were nearly identical in design; both used, as a measure of the response, the amplitude of a particular component of the evoked brain potential. The studies differed in their choice of stimuli, however. In the first case (Uttal and Cook, 1964), an electrical stimulus was used. Electrical stimuli presumably act directly on the axons of a nerve, and thus bypass the receptors. In the second case (Ehrenberger, Finkenzeller, Keidel and Plattig, 1966), an actual physical vibration was applied by a mechanical stimulator quite similar to the one used by Werner and Mountcastle. In the latter case, therefore, the action of the normal transducers would be reflected in the evoked brain response since the receptors were not bypassed.

The main difference in the results of these two studies was that the dynamic range of the brain potential evoked by electrical stimuli (Uttal and Cook, 1964) was quite narrow. Responses saturated (that is, responded at maximum levels) at stimulus levels, which were only two or three times the level of a threshold stimulus after a nearly linear rise. (See Figure 6.19.) On the other hand, Ehrenberger and his colleagues found that with natural mechanical stimuli, the dynamic range was quite a bit wider—in fact, saturation occurred only after the stimulus was 70 db above threshold levels. When their data were plotted on a log-log scale, they found a straight line for each stimulus frequency provided a relatively good approximation, and that the slope of that family of straight lines averaged about 0.6, a number again quite close to that obtained for the generator potential, the average of the peripheral nerve power functions described above as well as the psychophysical power functions. Presumably then, most of the compression seems to be inserted into the system at the most peripheral levels. Figure 6.20 shows the three-dimensional graph Ehrenberger and his colleagues obtained, relating the evoked brain potential amplitude, stimulus intensity, and stimulus frequency. Franzén and Offenloch (1969) have recently replicated this study and found almost identical coefficients (0.57–0.58) for the power function that seemed to best fit the dynamic intensity function of the evoked brain potential. They also carried out a correlated psychophysical study, always an asset since identical techniques are used in the comparison studies

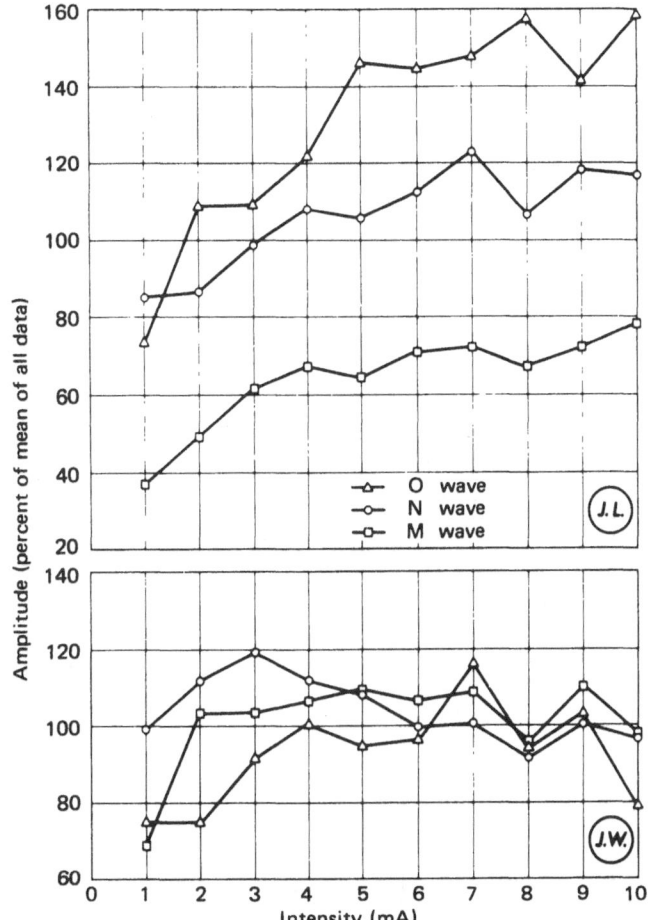

FIGURE 6.19 The response dynamic of somatosensory cortical potentials evoked with electrical stimuli displaying early saturation and narrow dynamic range. The M and N waves are early, contralateral, and modality specific. The O wave is a later response found over wide regions of the head (from Uttal and Cook, 1964).

of brain response and behavior, and found that a power function with exponents varying from 0.41 to 0.50 best described that data. There is, therefore, only a small discrepancy between the evoked brain potential and the psychophysical data in their findings.

All of these findings from research conducted in the somatosensory system are summarized in Table 6.2, along with results from the other modalities. We shall discuss these findings together later in this chapter, but some readers may prefer to look ahead to that table at this point.

2. *Intensity-Response Relations in the Visual System.* Considering the very large amount of work that has been done on visual neurophysiology,

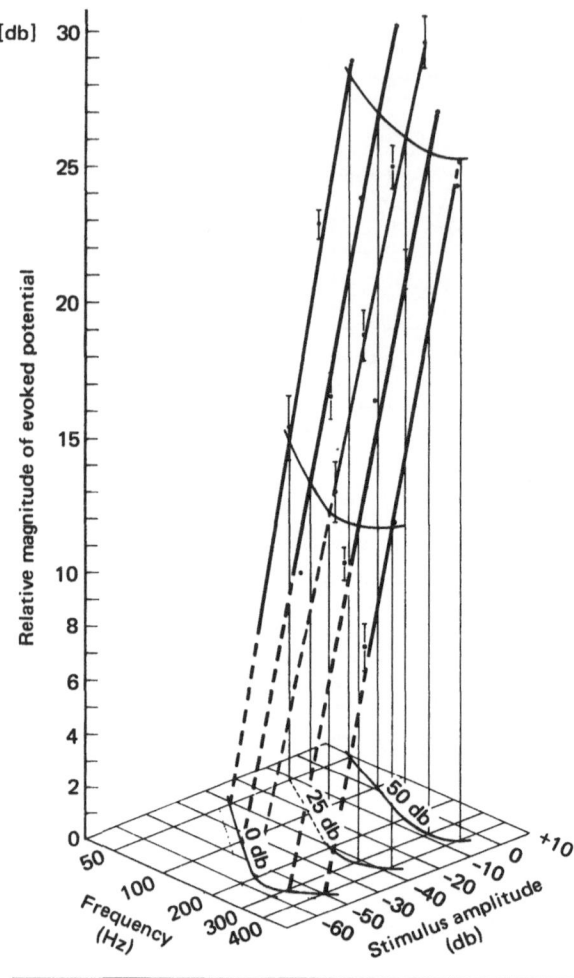

FIGURE 6.20 The response dynamic of somatosensory cortical potential evoked with natural stimuli of varying frequency (taps to the wrist), showing the very wide dynamic range typical of this sort of stimulation (from Ehrenberger, Finkenzeller, Keidel, and Plattig, 1966).

it is somewhat surprising to see how little relevant data, which specify the relationship between stimulus intensity and neural responses in the visual system, are available. In part, this is due to the fact that some of the responses in which we would be most interested are very difficult to measure indeed. Data on the receptor potentials in the human eye, for example, are simply not available, and it is only most recently that intracellular recordings from other vertebrate preparations have become available due to the small size of vertebrate visual neurons (see Witkovsky, 1971, for a comprehensive review of this newer material). Much of the work, which is of special interest and relevance with regard to intensities, therefore, has come from submammalian preparations. In particular, the eye of the horseshoe crab, of the turtle, and of the frog have been most productive model preparations in elucidating some of the intensity dynamics of visual systems, as well as some of the spatial features of neural interaction. The paucity of data in the higher reaches of the vertebrate visual system is, in large part, due to the fact that so many other stimulus dimensions seem to be producing strong effects, which override simple intensive effects at these levels.

In the following section, we shall also organize our discussion in ascending anatomical order. There are a few very new studies on vertebrate photoreceptor potentials, which are of particular importance and shall be presented first. We shall then consider in detail a very interesting and important study, which compares the generator potential and the spike train frequency in the eye of the horseshoe crab. This discussion will act as a bridge to studies of the peripheral nerve response of other animals. Finally, we shall briefly mention a study of evoked cortical visual potentials in man.

As a final word of caution, remember that we shall be jumping back and forth between vertebrate and invertebrate preparations with vastly different time constants, and there may be some controversy concerning whether this is justified. Whatever justification that can be mustered is based on the fact that many of the photochemicals in the visual systems of many different species seem to be based on a similar initial process—the retinal-protein photochemical and its spontaneous decomposition after photoisomerization.

a. Visual receptor potentials. Baylor and Fuortes (1970) have been able to record what is probably the receptor potential from single cones in the retina of the turtle by the use of an especially small micropipette. As usual, they found that a sustained negative resting potential, which hyperpolarized when stimulated with light, was recorded upon penetration. The hyperpolarizing receptor potential has been found to be characteristic of all vertebrate receptors, although most invertebrate receptor potentials seem to depolarize when stimulated as we have noted previously.

Figure 6.21 is a log-linear plot of the height of the potential, which was recorded for lights of various intensities relative to the maximum potential recorded with "very bright light." To compare this data with the other data discussed in this section of this chapter, we have, as usual, converted Baylor and Fuortes' data (as represented by the dotted curve) to log-log coordinates and replotted this converted data in Figure 6.22. Once again, the data are best fit by a two-segment power function with an exponent of 0.58 for lower intensities and one which is vanishingly small for higher ones.

Even more interesting from a phylogenetic and psychological point of view is the work of Boynton and Whitten (1970), to which we have alluded in earlier discussion. These workers studied the response dynamic of the receptor potential evoked from monkey cones and found that a power function with an exponent of 0.7 almost always describes the data obtained with an extracellular, but microscopic, electrode. With a pickup system such as this, they are, of course, not recording single cell responses, but rather the composite effects of many cones in the region of the electrode. Such signals are quite small, but can range up to about 2 mV. Clearly, the exponent they obtain is larger than that recorded at any other level—neurophysiological or psychophysical—in spite of the fact that it is obtained from a close relative of man.

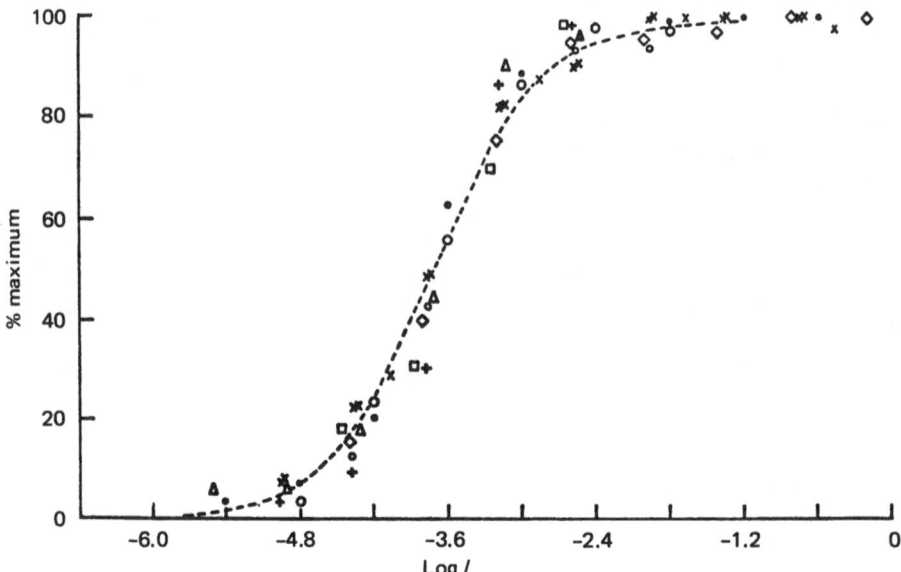

FIGURE 6.21 The visual receptor potential amplitude from turtle cones as a function of the logarithm of stimulus intensities (from Baylor and Fuortes, 1970).

Incidentally, a very good review of vertebrate photoreceptor electrophysiology has been writen by Tomita (1970) and may be of interest to the reader who would like to pursue this matter further.

b. A comparative study of the relations among stimulus intensities, receptor potentials, and peripheral nerve action. What is, perhaps, the classic study relating visual stimulus intensity, receptor potential amplitude, and spike action potential frequency was performed on the very large photoreceptors of the horseshoe crab eye by Fuortes (1958). The photoreceptor unit—the ommatidium—of this eye consists of a group of 10 to 20 retinula cells shaped and arranged like the slices of an orange and one peculiarly shaped eccentric cell (see Figure 7.27 in Chapter 7). The eccentric cell sends one projection up into the core of the group of retinula cells and one comparatively thick axon back along the optic nerve. It is now thought that the retinula cells are the actual photoreceptors and that any receptor potential is induced in them. These cells, however, are closely electrically coupled to the eccentric cell and activate it to produce the train of large spike action potentials, which are usually recorded when this preparation is stimulated with light. Smaller spikes, presumably from the small axons of the retinula cells which also make up part of the optic nerve, have also been reported.

Ommatidia and their constituent cells are sufficiently large so that Fuortes was able to insert fluid-filled micropipettes directly into the individual eccentric cell bodies. By selecting a sufficiently wide bandpass amplifier, it is possible to superimpose the spike activity being propagated along the axon upon the receptor potentials produced in the ommatidium.

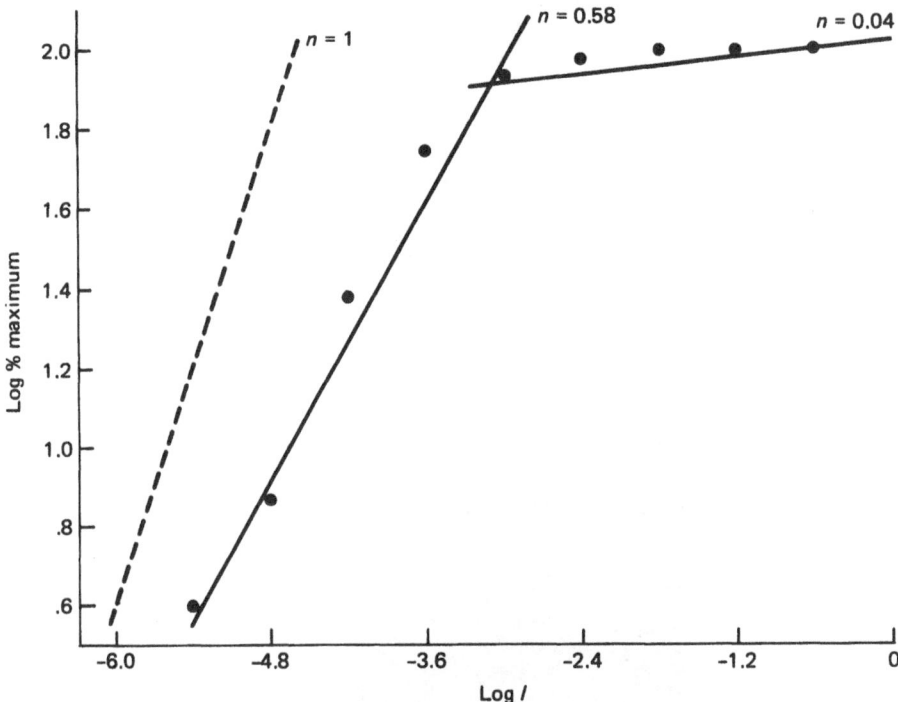

FIGURE 6.22 A sample of the data of Figure 6.21 converted to log-log coordinates displaying a two-segment range with power function exponents of 0.58 and 0.04, respectively.

Figure 6.23 is a sample set of this sort of combined response record, which allowed Fuortes to make a direct comparison of the two levels of coding. Following the initial transient burst, typical of turn-on effects we have already encountered in so many different sensory responses, the activity levels of both the generator potential and the firing rate of the spike activity in the axon settled down to a level, which was directly a function of the intensity of the stimulating light. As can be seen in this figure, there is very little adaptation over the course of a 2- or 3-sec stimulus. (This rather slow firing rate and minimum adaptation are characteristic of many of the invertebrate preparations that physiologists have used in their work. In some crayfish photoreceptor systems, as another example of these long time constants in invertebrates, the latency of the initial response to a flash of light may be as long as 5 or 6 sec.) Figure 6.24 reproduces Fuortes' data, summarizing the results of his experiments. This figure presents the functions relating the magnitudes of the generator potential and, separately, the frequency of firing of axonal spike action potentials to the intensity of the visual stimulus. The measurements, which are plotted in these figures, were always taken between 15 and 20 sec after the stimulus was turned on to allow the preparation to settle down following the turn-on transients. The data are plotted in the same form that Fuortes

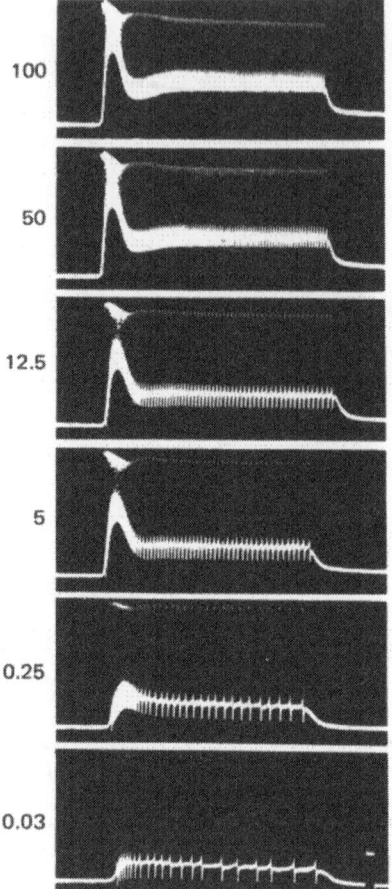

FIGURE 6.23 Sample, records showing the mixed generator potentials and spike action potentials recorded from the limulus ommatidium for visual stimuli of different intensities (from Fuortes, 1958).

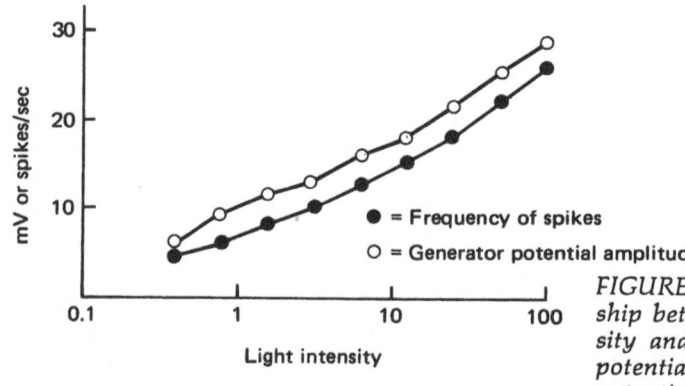

FIGURE 6.24 The relationship between the light intensity and both the generator potential and the spike action potential frequency in the limulus eye (Fuortes, 1958).

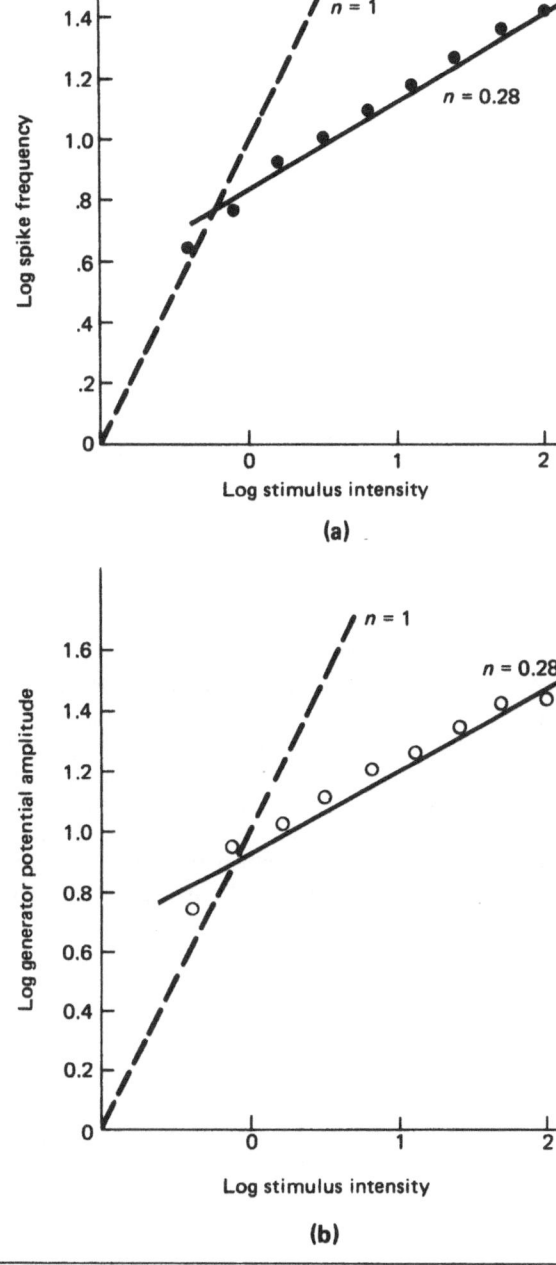

FIGURE 6.25 The data of Figure 6.24 converted to log-log coordinates. (a) Spike frequency. (b) Generator potential amplitude. Both functions display power function exponents of 0.28.

presented, namely, a log-linear plot. Fuortes noted that these scales were not perfectly straight lines on this scale and, therefore, were not strictly logarithmic functions. Fuortes' data have been replotted on log-log scales in Figure 6.25 (a) and (b). In this case, the data for both the receptor potential and the spike frequency are much more closely approximated by a

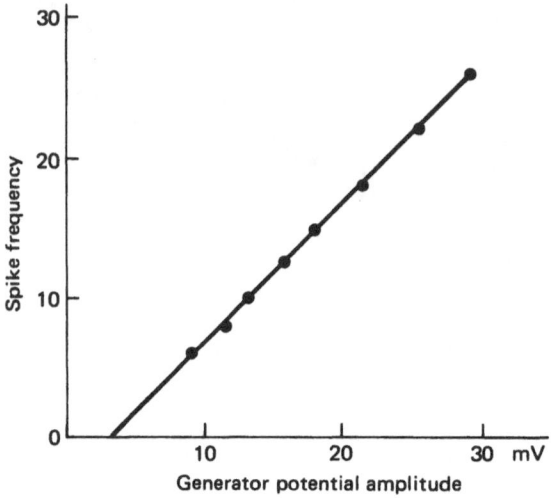

FIGURE 6.26 The linear relation between spike frequency and generator potential amplitude (from Fuortes, 1958).

straight line. Both functions are, therefore, better fit by a power function with an exponent of about 0.28 than by the logarithmic function originally suggested by Fuortes. (When two functions have the same exponent on a log-log plot, they must be linearly related, and therefore the frequency of spike firing is a linear function of receptor potential in this preparation.)

This improvement in fit, it should be noted, is not intended as a criticism of Fuortes' original analysis. It is simply a historic fact that much of the early work was influenced by the Fechnerian psychophysics, and it was not until the early 1960s that Stevens' demonstrations of the apparent ubiquity of the power function began to influence neurophysiology. Thus, many of the older reports, for example, Hartline and Graham (1932) or MacNichol (1956), report approximations to log functions, while more recent experiments (see below) seem most often to report power functions. It is hardly likely that the biology of the organisms has changed over the years. Rather, the perspective of the investigators and the mathematical models available to him changed in ways that have led to different descriptive models. This is, once again, evidence of the compelling force of a perspective or an idea in shaping even our view of raw data.

The most important result of Fuortes' experiment was that the receptor potential amplitude and the spike action potential frequency are linearly related. The extreme linearity of this relationship is evidenced in Figure 6.26, also a reproduction of one of Fuortes' graphs.

The implications of this important set of observations are clear. The response compression, which is observed in this system, is almost entirely accounted for within the initial transductive process.

c. Other peripheral visual nerve compression functions. As an additional example of the sort of response dynamics that can occur in peripheral nerves emanating from photosensitive receptors, let us consider a completely different invertebrate preparation. Uttal and Kasprzak (1962) studied the stimulus-response relationship in the axons conducting im-

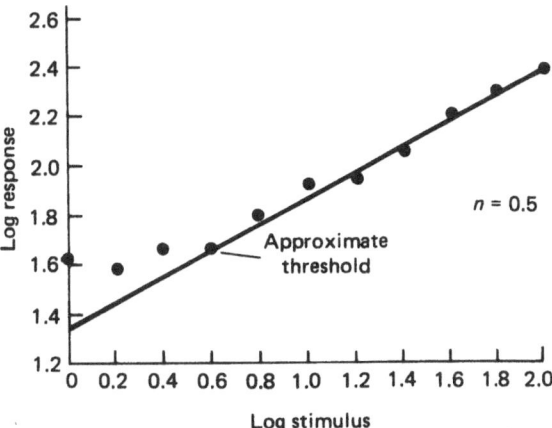

FIGURE 6.27 The relationship between the logarithm of the stimulating light intensity and the logarithm of the frequency of the spike response of the caudal photoreceptor of the crayfish, displaying a power function exponent of about 0.5 (from Uttal and Kasprzak, 1962).

pulses from a curious photoreceptor located in the most caudal ganglion of the ventral nerve cord of the freshwater crayfish. This unusual receptor organ has an absorption spectrum which is very much like that of the rhodopsin found in the human eye, but apparently the photopigment resides in only two cells, one on either side of the terminal ganglion in this bilaterally symmetrical ventral nervous system. A pair of scissors can be simply used to cut away the chitinous shell exposing the ventral nerve cord and the caudal ganglion. The entire nerve cord was then hung over a gross hooklike platinum recording electrode, which fed signals into an ac coupled preamplifier. Since there were only two cells present that were photosensitive, illumination of the crayfish's tail gives rise to spikes in only a pair of large axons in the ventral cord. The preparation could be made into a single rather than double cell one, even though no microdissection or microelectrodes were used, by simply splitting the easily separated nerve cord into two parts.

Illumination of the caudal ganglion gives rise to a stream of regularly spaced responses with, as we have mentioned before, very long latencies and relatively modest frequencies. Simple counting procedures were used to measure the number of responses that occurred in a period of 5 sec after the response had settled down from the initial turn-on transient. Figure 6.27 is a plot on a log-log scale of the number of responses that were obtained in that period as one varied the stimulus intensity. The form of the function is once again a straight line with the slope indicating an exponent of 0.53.

Similar compressed response dynamics are obtained in the visual system of vertebrates, as well as the invertebrate systems we have described. As convenient as invertebrate preparations are with their large cells and easy dissection procedures, it still would be more interesting to observe the same functions in an animal much closer in the phylogenetic tree to man than *limulus* or a crayfish. Hartline, who won a Nobel Prize for his extensive contributions to visual knowledge on the basis of his work on *limulus*, did not limit his career to that single animal. He has also done some very

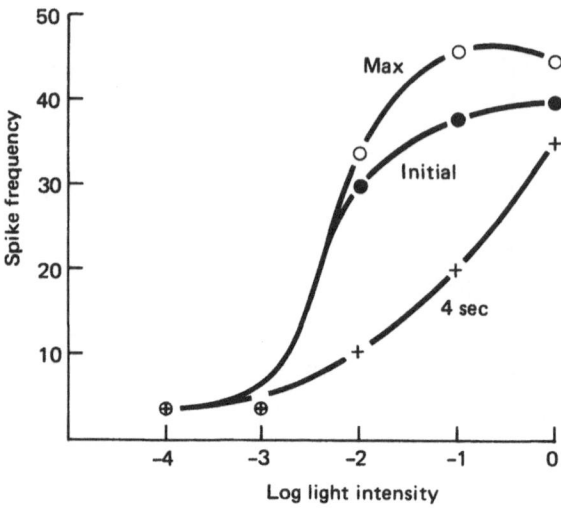

FIGURE 6.28 The relationship between the logarithm of light intensity and three different measures of the spike action potential frequency in the frog's optic nerve fibers. Data marked with circles are for the maximum frequency; data marked with solid dots are for the initial frequency spurt; and those marked with x are for a stable period 4 sec after the stimulus was turned on (from Hartline, 1938).

important work on the eye of the frog—another one of those extremely useful model systems in visual neurophysiology. Over three decades ago he published a paper (Hartline, 1938) reporting, among other characteristics, the relation between the spike action potential response of single axons in the optic nerve and stimulus intensity. This paper is still relevant and important in the context of our current discussions. Hartline dissected out small bunches of fibers from the frog's optic nerve and laid them across a wick electrode saturated with a conductive electrolyte. The wick electrode technique is not used very often these days, and the quality of the recordings, which were obtained with the galvonometric oscillograph used by Hartline, would not be considered to be of the same high level routinely achieved with metal or glass micropipettes and the modern oscilloscope. Nevertheless, his findings have retained their utility because of their clarity and insightfulness.

The general nature of the results of Hartline's experiments begins to give a hint of why some of the data that we would like to have, namely, simple functional relationships between stimulus intensity and response magnitude, are so difficult to obtain in the vertebrate visual system. The pattern of response is not as simple as the invertebrate data of the preceding discussion. Some cells were found to produce responses only when the light was turned on, others only when it was turned off. Others were found to produce bursts at both the onset and offset of the stimulating lights, while still others gave some combination of the two, with a more or less constant maintained response during the period of stimulation. Figure 6.28 is a reproduction of one of Hartline's graphs for a fiber that produces an on transient and then a maintained discharge during the course of the stimulus. The three curves drawn on this figure represent only three of the different measures that might be examined to determine the effect of stimulus intensity. The curve indicated by the open circles is based upon measures of the maximum frequency achieved during the brief

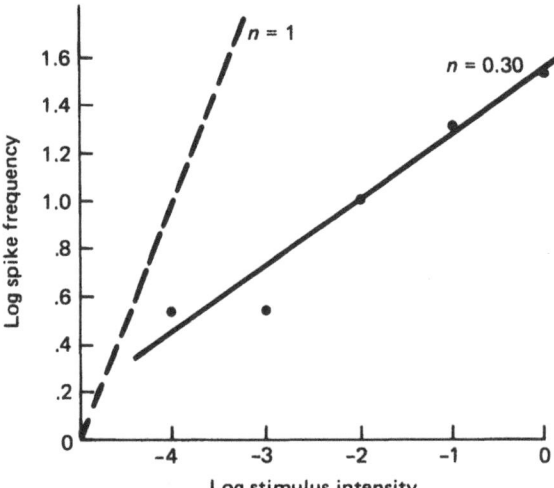

FIGURE 6.29 The data for the 4-msec stable period in Figure 6.28 converted to log-log coordinates, displaying a power function exponent of 0.30.

on burst. The curve indicated by the filled circles is for the initial frequency of the burst of spikes in the on transient, while the curve indicated with x is the function for the sustained activity after 4 sec of steady illumination. The curve for the sustained activity is the one that we have chosen to emphasize for the purposes of the present discussion.

But, is it fair to do so? Why this measure rather than any other, and why this type of cell rather than a simple on cell or a simple off cell? Is there anything special about the sustained activity? In general, we cannot answer these questions any better than to simply say that the choice of the maintained activity in this type of cell is more in conformity with both the subjective experience and the data from the simpler nervous systems of lower animals as well as the findings from the somewhat simpler structures of other vertebrate senses.

In Figure 6.29 we replot Hartline's data for this maintained activity on a log-log scale. It, too, appears to be well fitted by a straight line, suggesting a power function with an experiment of about 0.30, a low value typical of many visual systems.

According to Lipetz (1971), it is often the case in vertebrate preparations that the optic nerve ganglion cell axons do not respond in proportion to stimulus intensity. Rather, the responses of most of the cells seem to be dependent upon some specific feature of the spatio-temporal or quality pattern of the stimulus—a matter which we shall discuss in great detail in Chapters 7 and 8.

A few attempts to study the response dynamic of the ganglion cell have been made, however. Most notably Easter (1968) obtained this sort of data as an adjunct to a most interesting study of spatial summation among photoreceptors. He used isolated goldfish retinas in his experiments and limited his experimental samples to those ganglion cells that gave on responses to red light, thus simplifying what could have been a much more complicated set of findings. Flashes of light, which were no longer than 0.1 sec, were used as stimuli to minimize lateral inhibitory interactions between the two stimulus spots that were used in some other parts of the experiment. Easter's findings go far beyond the single point that we are interested in here, but for the purposes of our discussion, it is most significant to note that he found an average exponent of 0.55 for the 130 ganglion cells he sampled in this unusually rich experiment.

d. Central visual nervous activity. In spite of all the work that has been done on the central portions of the visual system, there is also little that can be specifically cited as pertinent to the problem of intensity coding. This is, perhaps, also due to the fact that so many variables other than simple intensity are important in the specification of the amplitude of the response, that in fact intensity actually plays only a minimum role. On the other hand, it may just be a matter of where the energies of neurophysiologists have been expended in recent years, and the pertinent data will appear sometime in the near future.

Perhaps the only study relevant to the specification of the response dynamic in the visual cortex is a report on the relationship between visual stimulus intensity and the response amplitude of the evoked cortical potential made by Loewenich and Finkenzeller (1967). They found that the response dynamic could be characterized by a power function with a very flat slope. The exponent of this function was only about 0.2. Low exponents of this sort also seem to be very characteristic of the few other studies of central visual intensity functions, according to Stevens (1971).

It should also be noted that the opponent mechanisms, which seem to operate in the central visual nervous system, make it difficult to specify the nature of the relationship between stimulus intensity and response amplitude. Some cells respond to increased light intensity by decreasing their rate of activity, while others respond by increasing their rates. The nonopponent cells observed by De Valois (1965), which are presumed to be associated with the representation of the overall brightness levels in the lateral geniculate body, seemed to be encoded with power function response dynamics, but the slopes could be either positive or negative in accord with the inhibitory or excitatory role played by a given cell. Again the reader's attention is directed to Table 6.2, where the key details of this discussion are summarized.

3. Intensity-response Relations in the Chemoreceptive Systems. In somewhat surprising contrast to the paucity of visual data, there is an extensive literature on olfactory and gustatory intensity functions. This is, at least in part, due to the fact that although we find considerable diversity of response as one samples from cell to cell in the chemical senses, there is little evidence of any of the very complex specific sensitivity to features of the spatio-temporal pattern of the stimulus as is found in the visual receptors. A related but contrary reason why the chemical senses have been particularly well-trodden avenues of research for studies along the intensity dimension is that it is very difficult to control the spatial and temporal aspects of their adequate stimuli. A puff of odorous vapor cannot be as easily limited to a duration of only a few milliseconds as can an acoustic, a visual, or even a somatosensory one.

Because of the very small size of some of the fibers conveying chemoreceptive information, many of the studies reported use summated or integrated measures of large numbers of spike action potentials recorded simultaneously from many different axons. This sort of measure is not the same as the conventional compound action potential, which is the result of a sort of physiological integration, but rather is a pseudocompounding produced by electronically integrating the observed neural activity. Thus, individual spikes, and perhaps also graded potentials, are synthetically accumulated into a single overall global estimate of the magnitude of the response.

a. Olfactory generator and gustatory receptor potentials. The classic studies of olfactory receptor potentials were originally carried out by Ottoson (1956). He first demonstrated the slow potentials now known as the electroolfactogram (EOG). We have already pointed out in our chapter on transducers that there have been some questions raised with regard to the validity of Ottoson's claim that the slow potentials recorded with his technique are, in fact, summations of the individual olfactory receptor-generator potentials; however, we shall still consider his results as the best possible candidate so far proposed for this role. In fact, as we shall see, the Ottoson potentials' response dynamics are sufficiently similar to those obtained with other better established generator potentials to add to the credibility of his hypothesis.

To briefly recall his technique, Ottoson simply placed silver-silver chloride electrodes on the exposed olfactory epithelium of a frog and led off the signals to a dc coupled amplifier system. Stimulation was usually accomplished in his experiments by simply blowing small quantities of air located with the odorous substances across the olfactory epithelium.

While Ottoson's monographs deal with a wide variety of different topics, we shall concentrate only on the relative magnitude of the response produced by varying concentrations of butanol—a substance chosen by him for extended investigation because of its high solubility in water. Figure 6.30 is a reproduction of Ottoson's data for concentrations ranging from those that were so low that only immeasurably small amounts of the stimuli were present in otherwise pure air to molar concentrations of the stimulus as high as 0.1. His original data are plotted on a log-linear scale in Figure 6.30 and can be seen to deviate considerably from a straight line, indicating that a logarithmic fit is not very satisfactory. In Figure 6.31 we have replotted these data on a log-log scale, and the fit to a straight line is much better. The slope of the data in this figure indicates an exponent of about 0.4 for the power function. This is comparable to 0.6 found by Stevens (1961) for olfactory subjective magnitude estimates for heptane and similar substances.

Kimura and Beidler (1961) have studied the intensity function of the receptor potential in the gustatory system. Using KCl-filled glass microelectrodes and dc coupled preamplifiers, they were able to evaluate the induced amplitude of the receptor potential as a function of the kind and concentration of the stimulating substance. They were able to show that

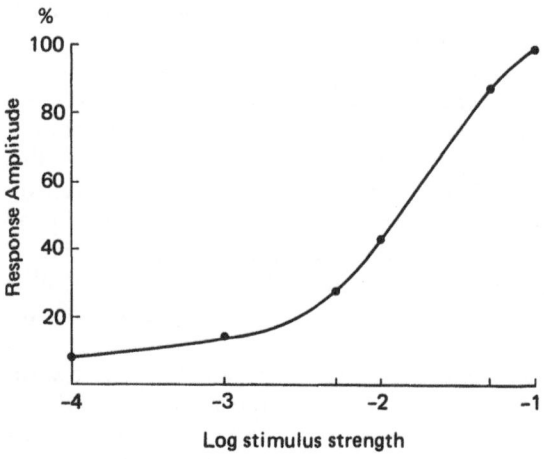

FIGURE 6.30 The relationship between the amplitude of the olfactory generator potential and the logarithm of odorant stimulus strength (from Ottoson, 1956).

even at the level of the receptor cell itself, there was sensitivity to a wide variety of substances in each and every cell, and the transductive mechanism can be said, therefore, to be broadly tuned (see Chapter 11). This is illustrated in Figure 6.32, which shows the responses to several basic taste stimuli by a single cell and also depicts the time course of the elicited receptor potentials. Since the stimulating substance was simply allowed to flow onto the tongue and was not immediately removed, the elongated duration of this response should not be misinterpreted as being equivalent to a prolonged response to a brief stimulus. The stimulus was simply present for that entire period.

All of the 10 cells studied by Kimura and Beidler were compressed in their response dynamics. Summary curves showing the average of both the receptor response amplitude and the integrated chorda tympani response to various concentrations of NaCl are plotted in Figure 6.33 on

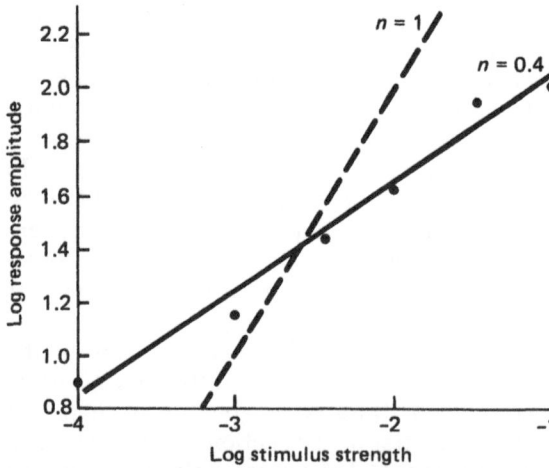

FIGURE 6.31 The data of Figure 6.30 converted to log-log coordinates, displaying a power function exponent of 0.4.

FIGURE 6.32 Receptor po-
tentials produced by NaCl,
quinine hydrochloride, sucrose, and HCl, respectively,
applied to the taste bud of
a hamster (from Kimura and
Beidler, 1961).

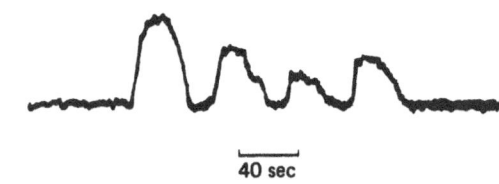

a linear-linear scale. These data are replotted on a log-log scale in Figure
6.34 (a) and (b) and are both seen to be rather poorly fit by a straight
line with a slope indicative of a power function with an exponent of approximately 0.31.

Thus, we see in both of these chemical modalities that the response
is already strongly compressed at the level of the receptor or generator
potential to accomplish response range compression.

b. Peripheral nerve action potentials. The relationship between olfactory stimulus amplitude and peripheral nerve spike activity has been
studied in two different ways by O'Connell and Mozell (1969). These investigators developed a highly precise means of presenting olfactory stimuli
of known concentration to the olfactory mucosa of frogs. Bursts of about
1 cm³ of odorized air were injected briefly into a more massive stream (about

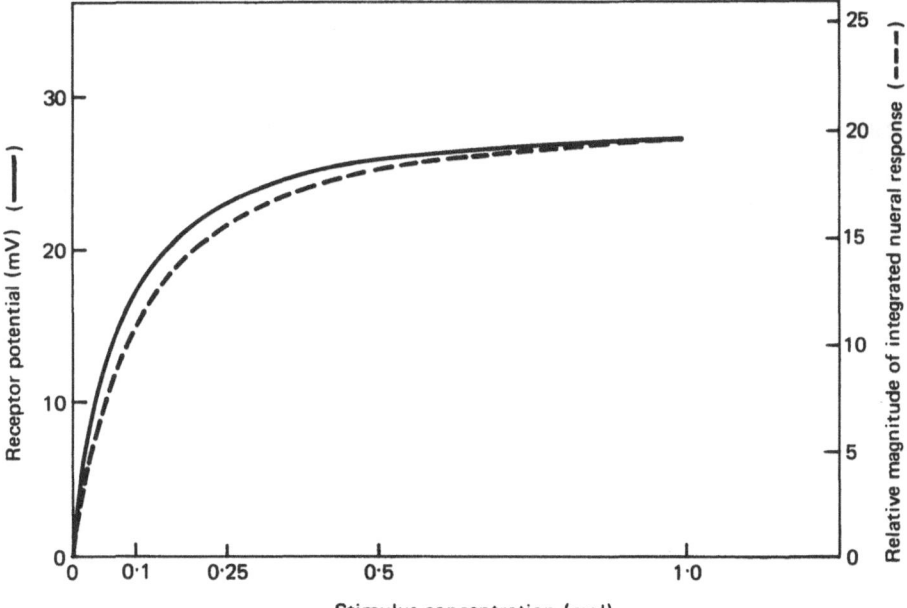

FIGURE 6.33 In this figure, both the receptor potential amplitude and the integrated neural response have been plotted as a function of NaCl concentration.
These data once again illustrate the near-linear relationship between receptor
potential and spike activity (from Kimura and Beidler, 1961).

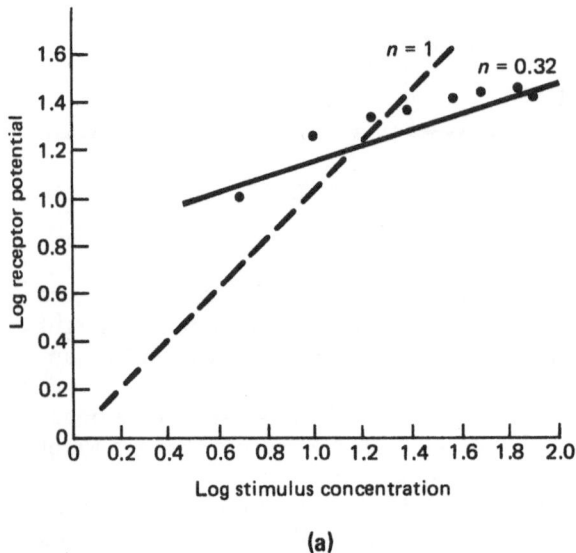

(a)

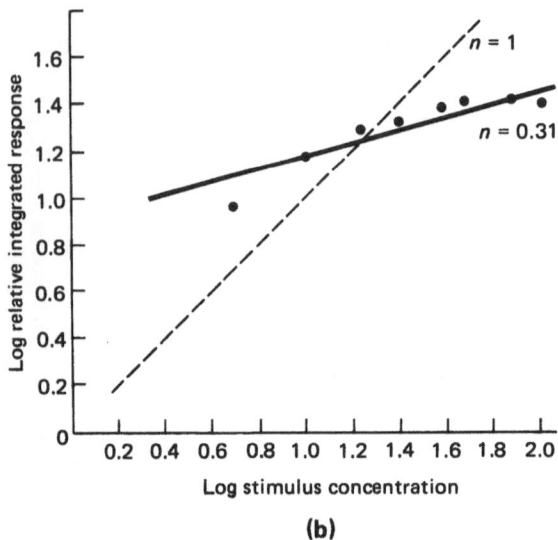

FIGURE 6.34 Data of Figure
6.33 converted to log-log coordinates. (a) The receptor
potential as a function of
NaCl concentration, indicating a power function ex-
ponent of 0.32. (b) The integrated response amplitude
as a function of NaCl concentration, indicating a power
function exponent of 0.31.

(b)

120 cm³/min delivered for ½ sec) of purified air. The combined airstream
was then passed over the frogs' olfactory epithelium. Concentration of the
odorant was controlled by varying the amount of pure air, which was mixed
with standard amounts of the odorized air before the final mixing.

In the context of our current discussion, we are interested in two
different aspects of O'Connell and Mozell's work. First, they describe the
characteristics of the spike activity recorded from about 20 different olfactory nerve cells to a single chemical (diethyl carbonate). Second, they have
used the electronic integrator described above to give a statistical estimate

of the overall pattern of activity in the whole olfactory nerve for several different chemicals.

Spike action potentials from single olfactory cells were recorded with metal filled glass microelectrodes and a plot made of the relationship between the stimulus intensity and the frequency of the evoked activity. Although the electrodes were inserted through the olfactory epithelium itself, the spike action potentials recorded were confirmed as having been generated in the axons of the olfactory nerve of the frog.

Figure 6.35 presents their results. The data are so variable that it is clear that the only real generality that can be drawn is that the responses of all of the cells are monotonic. Attempts to fit this family of curves with power functions would probably not be worth the trouble, but a quick glance at some of the responses on the linear-linear scale used in this

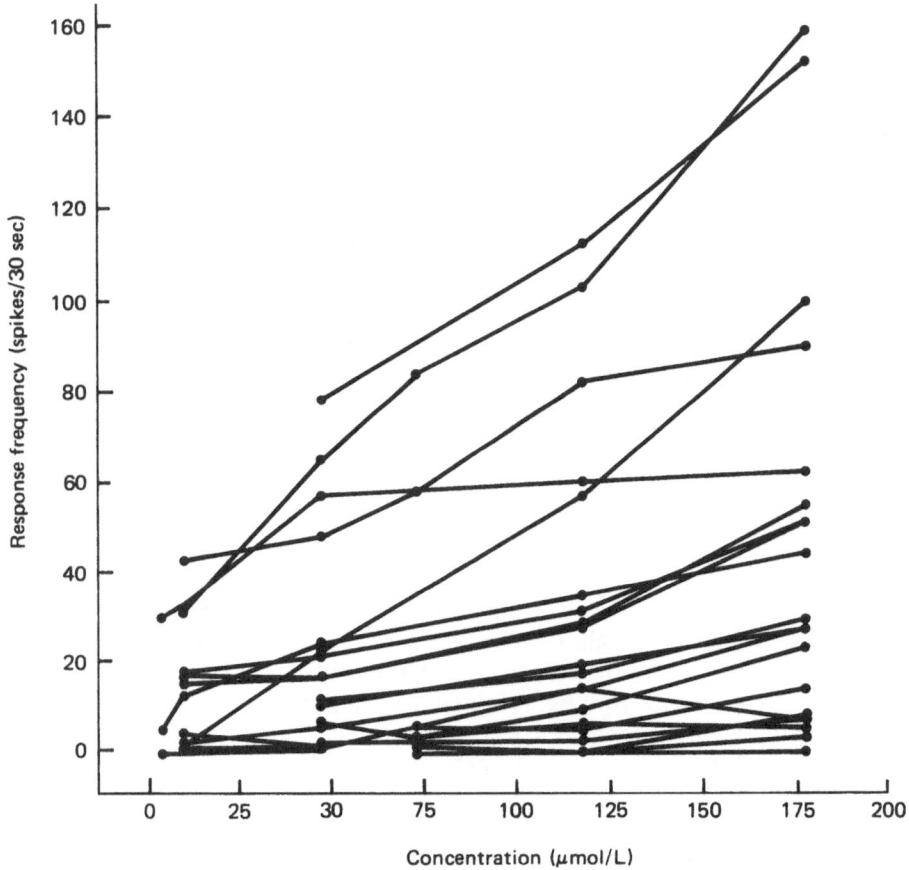

FIGURE 6.35 *A set of plots on linear-linear coordinates of the frequency of olfactory nerve spike activity as a function of the concentration of diethyl carbonate, showing the wide variety of response dynamics recorded for various olfactory cells (from O'Connell and Mozell, 1969).*

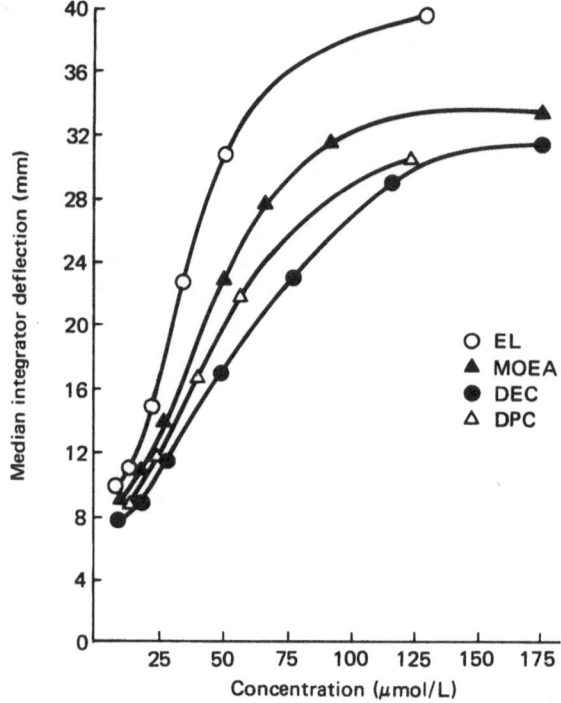

FIGURE 6.36 Olfactory fibers of the frog's nose respond differently to different chemical stimulants. In this case, the response dynamic has been depicted by plotting the integrated output as a function of the concentration of four different chemicals: EL = ethyl lactate, MOEA = 2-methoxyethyl acetate, DEC = diethyl carbonate, and DPC = dipropyl carbonate (from O'Connell and Mozell, 1969).

figure indicates that only a few cells have exponents slightly greater than 1, while many others have very low exponents indeed.

A better way to get a statistical picture of the activity of a large number of cells is to use a gross electrode and the electronic integration procedure. O'Connell and Mozell used a stainless steel wire of relatively gross dimensions (63.5 μ in diameter) to pick up the activity of a large number of cells, and then fed this pooled neural signal into an integrating circuit.

As we have indicated previously, the integral of the pooled spike activity is a good measure of the average or ensemble activity of the population of fibers. Even though a sample of large fibers may be contributing disproportionately to the output, it is probably still at least as unbiased as the average value that would be obtained by sampling a very large number of cells with microelectrodes—a procedure which can also introduce the same sampling errors due to the higher probability of probing larger cells.

The data obtained by O'Connell and Mozell with a gross electrode and with an integrated output are plotted in Figure 6.36 for four different odorants—ethyl lactate 2, methoxyethyl acetate, dipropyl carbonate, and diethyl carbonate. The data are plotted on a linear-linear scale, but we see, once again, that the function is strongly compressed with much larger differential stimulus intensities required at high levels than at low to produce an equivalent change in the response magnitude. By replotting the data on a log-log scale (as shown in Figure 6.37), once again the fit to a

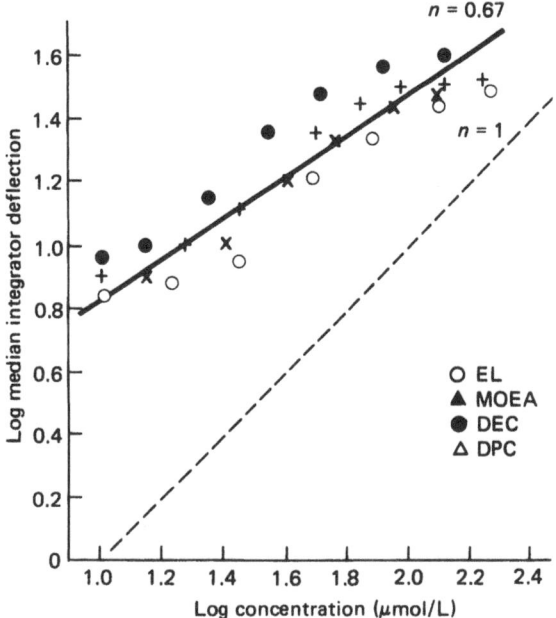

FIGURE 6.37 The data of Figure 6.36 has been converted en masse to log-log coordinates and replotted in this figure, indicating that it is well fit by a power function with an exponent of about 0.67.

power function is seen to be relatively good, and an exponent of about 0.67 seems to be a pretty good approximation for the four odorants.

Pfaffman, Fisher, and Frank (1967) have carried out analogous studies on various taste nerves in the rat. Stimuli (quinine hydrochloride, hydrochloric acid, sodium chloride, and sucrose) were applied through glass pipettes inserted directly into the cavities of taste buds. Recording techniques were similar to the second type used by O'Connell and Mozell; gross wire electrodes picked up the signals and fed them into an integrating circuit, the output of which displayed the integral of the total amount of activity. Figure 6.38 (a) and (b) are two of their raw data records, showing the integrated response (the upper traces) produced by stimuli timed as shown by the deflection of the lower traces. Figure 6.39 presents the summarized results obtained in the experiments for the four different sapid substances. These recordings were made from the chorda tympani. However, recordings from other nerve trunks often showed different response patterns, and our choice of the chorda tympani data is, admittedly, selective. These data, originally plotted on a log-linear scale by Pfaffman and his colleagues, are very similar to those reported by O'Connell and Mozell for the olfactory nerves, and when they are replotted on a log-log scale in Figure 6.40, they give relatively good fits to straight lines. The exponents of the power functions represented by these straight lines for the four stimuli are all very close to 0.53.

Another relevant study has been reported by Borg, Diamant, Oakley, Ström, and Zotterman (1967) and Borg, Diamant, Ström, and Zotterman (1967). This work is particularly rich in its implications for our analysis of the relationship between stimulus intensity, on the one hand, and neural

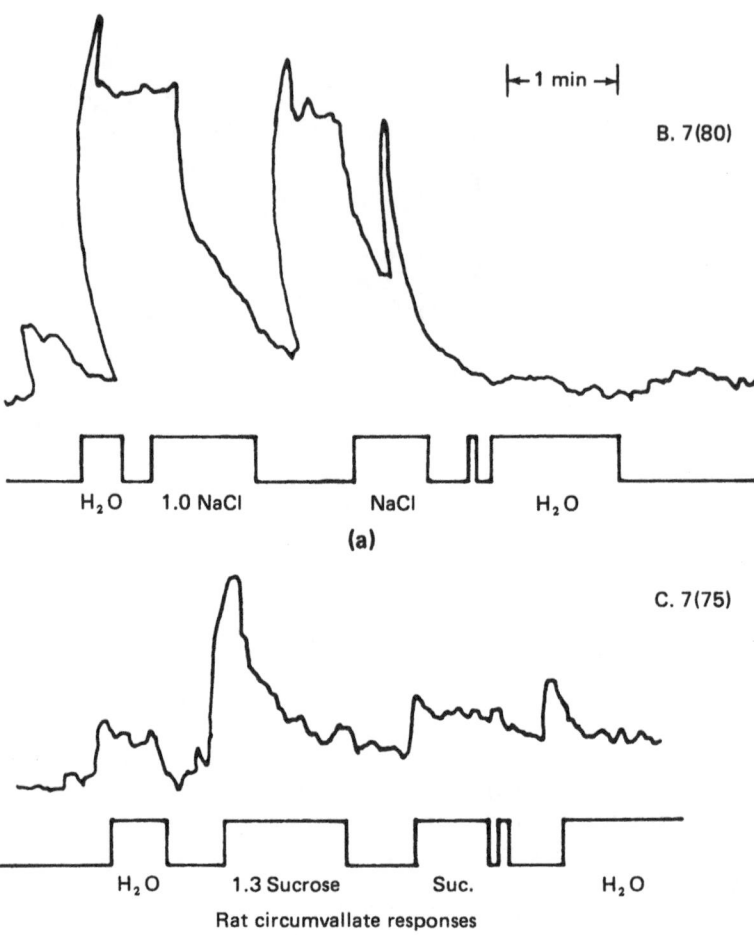

H_2O 1.0 NaCl   NaCl H_2O

(a)

C. 7(75)

H_2O 1.3 Sucrose   Suc. H_2O

Rat circumvallate responses

(b)

FIGURE 6.38 *Integrated glossopharyngeal nerve responses to NaCl and sucrose of various concentrations with water rinses at the indicated times. Note the difference in the time course of the response to the two different stimuli (from Pfaffmann, Fisher, and Frank, 1967).*

and psychophysical response magnitudes on the other, for an unusual experimental animal was used in this experiment—man himself! Certain middle ear operations require that the chorda tympani be cut, and it was only because of the therapeutic value of the operation that this extremely interesting data became available. This work is of special importance not only because Borg and his colleagues made general comparisons of neural and psychophysical responses under identical stimulus conditions, but also because both these types of data were collected on exactly the same subjects.

In the course of the corrective surgery, it was necessary to cut away

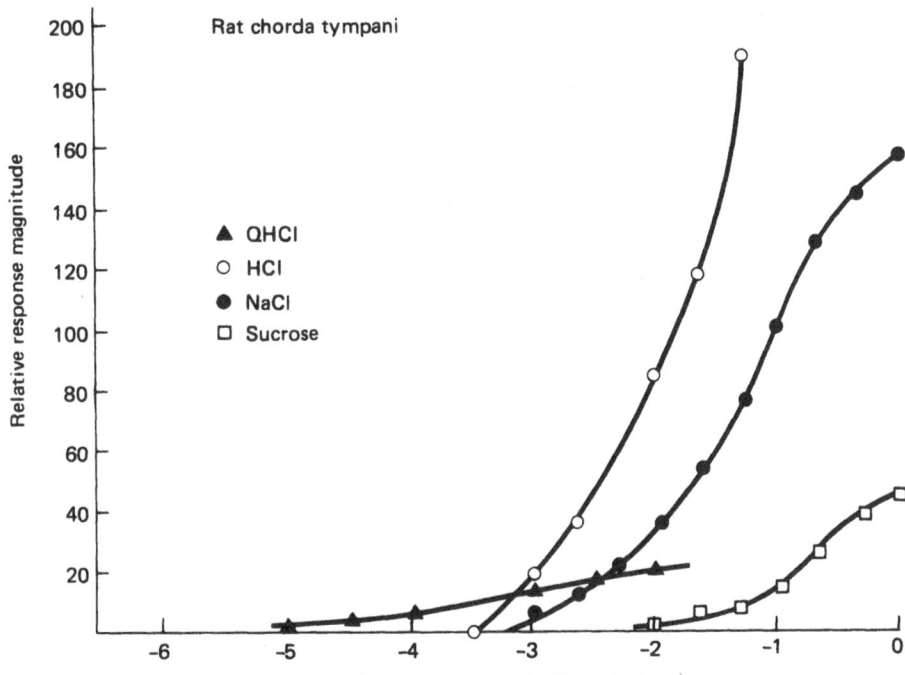

FIGURE 6.39 *Integrated response magnitude of the chorda tympani responses plotted as a function of the log of the gustatory stimulant intensity (from Pfaffmann, Fisher, and Frank, 1967).*

the tympanic membrane and then to sever the chorda tympani, a branch of which, fortunately for the purposes of the present discussion, runs through the middle ear. The nerve sheath was cut away, leaving the naked stump as it emerged on its way from the tongue to the central nervous system. Stimulating fluids were dispensed over the tongue by a mechanical system, which metered out a small amount of fluid. Recordings were made with relatively large electrodes inserted into the middle ear through the auditory meatus. Judgments of the magnitude of the sensation using Stevens' magnitude estimation technique were made to give the psychophysical data. Integrated recordings from the chorda tympani were used in much the same way as in the previous two experiments as the dependent variable. Figure 6.41 presents a sample of the psychophysical and electrophysiological results of an experiment, which used citric acid as a stimulus. Borg and his colleagues had been sufficiently alerted to the implications of Stevens' theory by the time this paper was published, and thus they plot their data directly on log-log scales. Their data also are generally well fit by straight lines and, thus, approximate power functions. Moreover, for a given subject, the exponents for the neural and psychophysical data agreed very well. Unfortunately, however, the variation of the exponents between the subjects was very large. For example, exponents given for the

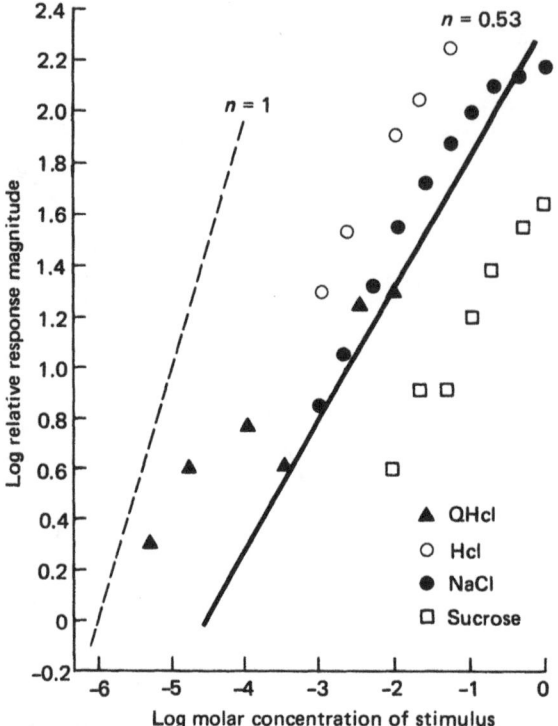

FIGURE 6.40 The data of Figure 6.39 have been converted en masse to log-log coordinates. All four functions are fairly well fit with a straight line with a slope of about 0.58—the exponent of the best fitting power function.

citric acid response dynamic range vary from 0.5 to 0.85. Borg and his colleagues also cite Ekman and Åkesson (1965), who found exponents varying from 1.11 to 1.97 for saltiness and 1.3 to 1.98 for sweetness (Borg et al. report somewhat lower values—1.0 and 1.1, respectively, for these stimuli). The small sample and wide variation in reported exponents in all

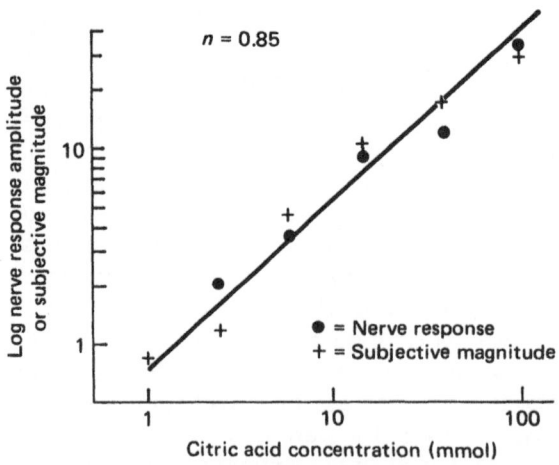

FIGURE 6.41 A comparison of neural and psychophysical power functions for the relationship between stimulus amplitude and human chorda tympani nerve responses (•) or psychophysical magnitude estimates (+) for citric acid. Both functions display power function exponents of 0.85 (from Borg, Diamant, Ström, and Zotterman, 1967).

of these experiments make it difficult to interpret their findings unambiguously.

    c. A possible central intensity function for the gustatory system. It is, in general, quite difficult to measure the response dynamics of the gustatory system at the level of the cerebral cortex. The gustatory area is not well defined, and the stimulus is quite difficult to manipulate in time and magnitude. Plattig (1969) believes that he has been able to do so, however, by using nonadequate electrical stimulation of the tongue as a surrogate stimulus. He thus avoided the problem of localization by using the compound evoked brain potential as his response measure. The dynamic function relating response amplitude to stimulus intensity was measured for several of the successive evoked brain potential waves. Only two of the waves so measured showed what Plattig refers to as "clear functions." The first negative wave displayed a dynamic response, which could be characterized by a power function with an exponent of 0.76, while the third positive wave was best represented by a power function with an exponent of 0.57. Neither one of these is very close to the 1.3 or 1.4 reported by Stevens for the sugar and salt subjective magnitudes, respectively, but both are fairly close to the higher-frequency vibratory dynamic exponent reported by Stevens (1970). It may have been that the evoked potential recorded by Plattig was in fact a tactual one, or it may have been that the psychophysical and central neural functions simply do not correspond, even though both are gustatory in origin.

4. Intensity-Response Relations in the Auditory System. a. **Auditory receptor potentials.** The acoustic modality has been left for last in our survey of the relationship of stimulus intensity and response parameters because it presents some special problems. We have already discussed the controversy that revolves around the identification of the receptor potential of the auditory mechanism. The most likely candidate, the cochlear microphonic (the cochlear ac potential), differs from other receptor potentials in a number of important ways. Most curious in the context of our present discussion is the fact that it is linear over a very large portion of its dynamic range. This is quite a different result than that obtained in all other receptors, even other mechanoreceptors like the Pacinian corpuscle. It is not possible at the present time to say whether this difference reflects the fact that the acoustic receptor potential producing mechanism is simply different, or whether the ac poential is, in fact, not the receptor potential, but an unrelated microphonic, which is so large that it will probably always obscure the true generator potential in the *in vivo* situation. Davis (1965), who has been the most vigorous champion of the ac potential's role as the receptor potential, was quite concerned about this discrepancy and has this to say:

> *Actually, I find one of the most puzzling aspects of the cochlear microphonic is its linearity over [a] wide dynamic range. . . . However, the cochlear microphonic is nonlinear with respect to sound pressure over even wider ranges of frequency and amplitude than those within which it is linear.*

> (*DAVIS, 1965, p. 188.*)

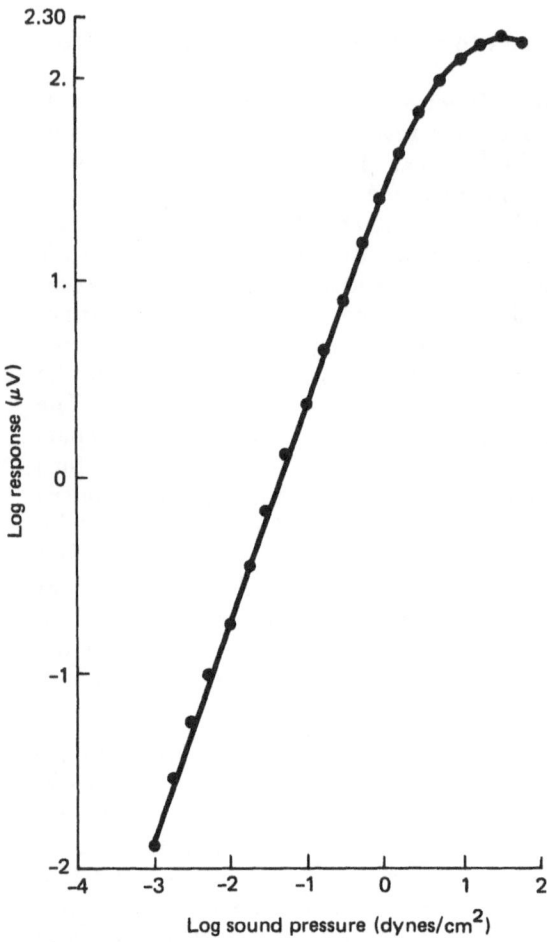

FIGURE 6.42 *The response dynamic relating acoustic stimulus intensity and the amplitude of the cochlear microphonic response in the cat. This curve happens to be a straight line for most of its course with a slope of 1, indicating a linear relationship between the stimulus and response. However, it should be noted that it is nonlinear over more of its range than over which it is linear, but that the logarithmic compression obscures this fact (from Wever, Rahm, and Strother, 1959).*

The definitive study of the stimulus intensity—response amplitude relationship of the cochlear microphonic was reported by Wever, Rahm, and Strother (1959). Using especially sensitive and noise-free amplifiers, these investigators recorded the ac potential picked up with a platinum foil electrode placed on the round window of a cat and obtained the data shown in Figure 6.42. The function was plotted by them on a log-log scale. The function has a slope of 1 even on this log-log plot from stimulus levels of about 0.001 to about 1 dyne/cm², but is nonuniformly compressed from about 1 to 100 dynes/cm². Along the other axis, the response displays linearity from about 0.1 to about 30 μV, but is compressed, again nonuniformly, from about 30 to 150 μV. Wever and his colleagues state:

> *Our conclusion is that the cochlear potentials bear a linear relation to sound pressure from the region of the behavioral threshold, perhaps below it, all the way to the level at which the ear begins to overload.*

(WEVER, RAHM, and STROTHER, 1959, p. 1449.)

Their data, however, as Davis points out, are not quite so unequivocal. From either point of view, either in terms of the stimulus range or in terms of the response range, Davis is correct in saying that it is nonlinear over larger portions of its range than over those over which it is linear. The overloading, of which Wever and his colleagues speak, may also be considered to be the region of compression—"overloading" merely being another term to describe the reduction in the efficacy of given changes in stimulus amplitude at higher stimulus levels.

Nevertheless, the function with its long region of linearity is certainly quite different from the continuous compression functions we have become acquainted with in this chapter so far and must be considered to be a deviant. It just does not fit into the scheme we have been developing throughout this section of this chapter. This is also one of the instances, furthermore, in which the integrated function of a large number of cells, as the signals recorded by Wever, Rahm, and Strother most certainly were, do not correspond well with the exponents of the psychophysical magnitudes. Stevens (1961) has shown power law compression with exponents of about 0.55 for auditory magnitude estimates. As we shall see in the next section, these generator response dynamics are not comparable with those of the individual fiber of the cochlear nerve either. However, as Lawrence (1965) has pointed out, the end points of this function do agree with the absolute threshold and upper acoustic limit obtained in psychophysical studies.

b. Peripheral auditory nerve action potentials. Kiang (1965) has studied the relationship between the single cell action potentials of the acoustic nerve and the intensity of an auditory stimulus. Glass pipettes filled with KCl solutions were driven into single axons of the exposed acoustic nerve of a cat. Here again, Kiang found that the picture is quite different in audition than that based upon data recorded in the peripheral nerves of other modalities. Figure 6.43 is a reproduction of Kiang's data for 12 acoustic nerve fibers. Responses were measured during stimulation with continuous tones of varying intensity. Clearly, no single cell has the dynamic range exhibited either by psychophysical results or by the ac potentials recorded at the oval window. For that matter, only a small proportion of the cells studied by Kiang were even monotonic as a function of stimulus intensities. Some fibers display an increase in their firing rate as the stimulus intensity increases, but only up to a point after which their frequency of response decreases. Some of the neurons have thresholds that are very high; the group of curves at the bottom does not begin to produce any noticeable change in their rate of firing until stimuli 40 to 60 db above threshold levels were attained. Because of these nonmonotonic functions, the application of the power function analysis would, of course, be inappropriate and meaningless.

Kiang's data on the narrow dynamic range of acoustic nerve fibers, while more complete and detailed, provide essential support for the similar data that were reported many years before on the intensity dynamic for single acoustic nerve cells by Galambos and Davis (1943). Their pioneering application of the newly developed microelectrode to acoustic neurophysiology was an important contribution and opened up rich new sources of

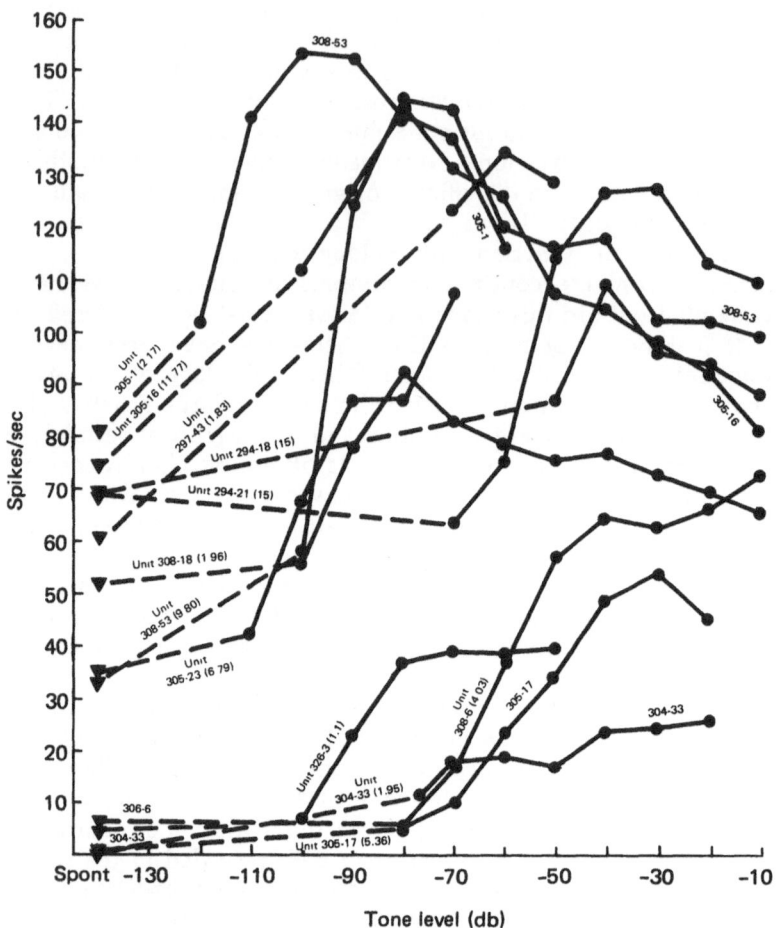

FIGURE 6.43 A sampling of the response dynamics of neurons of the auditory
nerve. Spikes per second have been plotted against a logarithmic (db) horizontal
coordinate. At best, this set of fibers is highly idiosyncratic, and most are not
even monotonic. Most cells also exhibit a rather narrow dynamic range. For these
reasons, conversion to log-log coordinates would be of no value. Dotted lines
connect spontaneous (▼) to driven levels. Numbers in parentheses are the best
frequencies of the neurons (in kH₂) (from Kiang, 1965).

information about neural coding. We shall have much to say about their
notion of tuning curves when we discuss pitch encoding in Chapter 8.

The major conclusion to be drawn from these data is that no single
peripheral fiber could possibly encode the enormous dynamic range over
which the acoustic system is known to be able to operate. Rather, relative
amounts of activity in families of cooperating neurons must collectively
signal intensity information.

One attempt to look at the response dynamic for the compound action
potential recorded from the auditory nerve has been made by Teas, El-

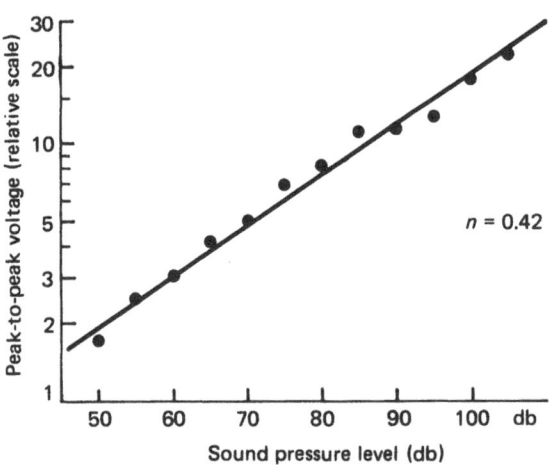

FIGURE 6.44 The relationship between the whole auditory nerve response and stimulus amplitude, displaying a good fit by a power function with an exponent of 0.42 (from Stevens, 1970, after Teas, Eldridge, and Davis, 1962).

dredge, and Davis (1962). They inserted macroelectrodes into the cochlea of a guinea pig, one on either side of the basilar membrane, and stimulated with brief tone bursts. This sort of recording electrode configuration responds to microphonics, summating potentials, and compound nerve action potentials. Stevens (1970) has replotted the data obtained by Teas and his colleagues on log-log coordinates to demonstrate the relationship between the amplitude of this compound spike action potential and stimulus intensity. These data, presented in Figure 6.44, show a reasonably close approximation to a power function with an exponent of 0.42, a value considerably less than the corresponding psychophysical power function, but at least one which is monotonic over a considerable range.

c. Central auditory nervous activity. The nonmonotonic and irregular nature of the acoustic nerve action potential as a function of stimulus intensity is also reflected as higher levels of the afferent pathway are examined. Rose, Greenwood, Goldberg, and Hind (1963) examined single cell responses in the inferior colliculus, one of the important midbrain relay stations for acoustic information. They found that over 50 percent of the cells in their sample had a nonmonotonic relation to stimulus intensity; these cells gradually increased, and then decreased their rate of firing as stimulus intensity continuously increased. Rose and his colleagues speculate that the decrease in firing rate at higher intensities is due to the simultaneous evocation of inhibitory and excitatory signals.

In contrast, working at the level of the medial geniculate body of the cat, Gross and Thurlow (1951) found that the responses they recorded with microelectrodes from a small sample of cells were monotonic, although, as in the periphery, individual cells exhibited the same narrow dynamic range at this level.

The acoustic response pattern, not unexpectedly, reaches its utmost level of complexity at the level of the cortex. Goldstein, Hall, and Butterfield (1968) have explored the patterns of responsiveness of single cells in the acoustic cortex to a wide variety of stimulus conditions and have con-

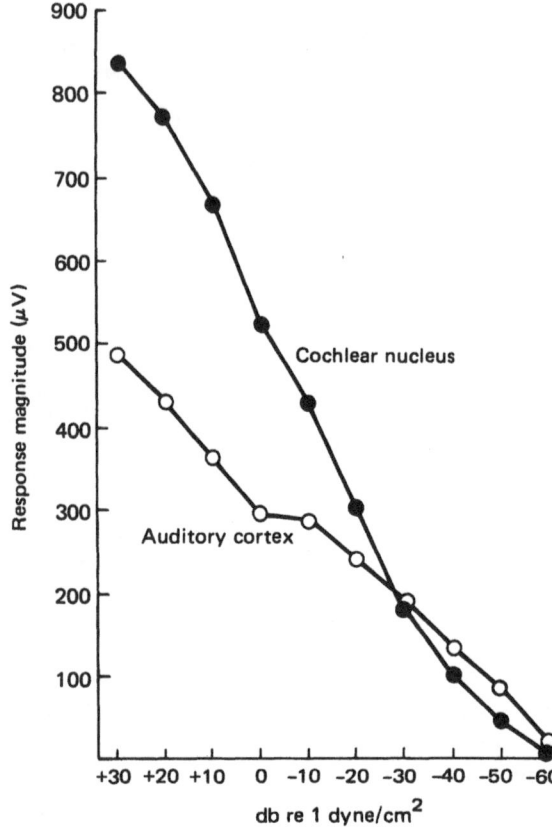

FIGURE 6.45 The relationship between compound potentials evoked at the level of the cochlear nucleus and at the auditory cortex and the log of stimulus intensity (from Saunders, 1970).

cluded that the behavior of these single cells is highly idiosyncratic. Some cells increased their activity; some decreased theirs; and others changed from increases to decreases as the frequency of the stimulating tone changed or as its intensity varied.

It seems apparent that simple stimulus intensity-response amplitude correlations may simply be inapplicable in the acoustic modality. The situation seems to be much more complex than found in the other modalities and depends upon interacting patterns of neural discharge at central levels as well as at the lower ones. The reader should rest assured that there is no need to throw out coding theory in general even if this is the case. We simply must acknowledge the fact that the intensity codes in the acoustic sense are unknown at the present time. The only other speculation that seems timely is that the difficulty encountered in an analysis of the temporal codes in the acoustic sense should not be too surprising if we remember that this sense, more than any other modality, must cope with the temporal dimensions of its adequate stimulus.

What about integrated response measures? In spite of the fact that the single cell data from the central auditory system are so idiosyncratic, is there any possibility that some collective measure like the evoked brain potential might reflect wide ranging monotonic intensity functions? Keidel

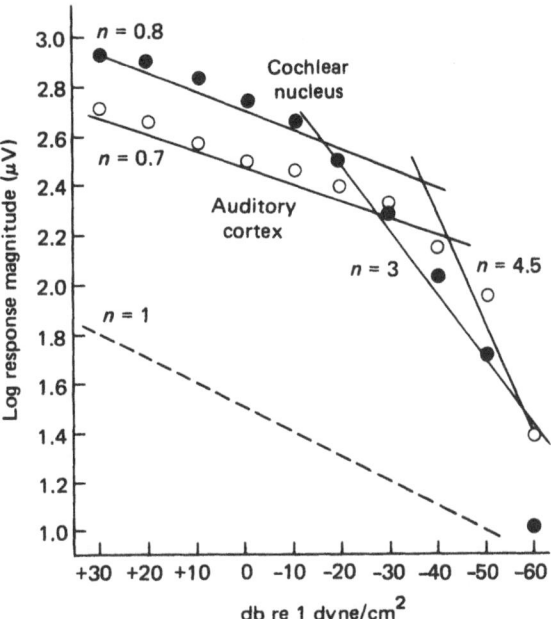

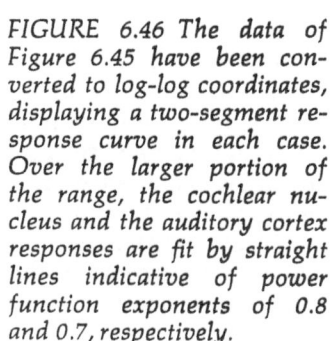

FIGURE 6.46 The data of Figure 6.45 have been converted to log-log coordinates, displaying a two-segment response curve in each case. Over the larger portion of the range, the cochlear nucleus and the auditory cortex responses are fit by straight lines indicative of power function exponents of 0.8 and 0.7, respectively.

and Spreng (1965) examined the rise of specific components of the acoustically evoked brain potential and found at least one of them—a late nonspecific component occurring at about 150 msec after the stimulus—had a fairly wide range of response (90 db) and also exhibited a response dynamic that could be well represented by a power function with an exponent of 0.36. However, other components with different latencies, or in different stages of adaptation, or even just different criteria of measurement, exhibited different exponents for their representative power functions. Whether Keidel and Spreng had actually discovered the key dimension or had simply found one that was fortuitously in agreement with the psychological data is moot.

Saunders (1970) has also used compound action potentials recorded with macroelectrodes as his measure of the activity level of both the cochlear nucleus and the auditory cortex in the cat. His findings, like Keidel and Spreng's, show that these potentials, evoked with auditory clicks of varying magnitude, covaried at least over a 90-db range and appeared to be fairly linear on a log-linear plot. Figure 6.45 shows his original data, and Figure 6.46 shows the data replotted on a log-log plot to give a general estimate of the trend of his data. These data, once again, exhibit a two-segment power function, but adhering to our previous criterion, we shall only consider the higher-intensity branches. These exponents were 0.7 and 0.8 for the auditory cortex and cochlear nucleus, respectively. It is quite clear that while individual cells seem to behave idiosyncratically and even nonmonotonically, as well as displaying narrow response ranges, there are cumulative bioelectric potentials associated with these levels of the nervous system that do seem to vary over a good portion of the auditory psychophysical range and to correlate with behavioral data to at least a first approximation.

5. *A Summary of the Neurophysiological and Psychophysical Data on Response Dynamics.* This, then, completes our survey of the relevant neurophysiological data relating stimulus intensities and response parameters. Admittedly, our selection of "relevant" studies has been restricted. In selecting the data used to exemplify the response of the various sensory modalities, there has been a bias on our choice, for we have almost certainly overemphasized those cells that do respond monotonically to changes in stimulus intensities, as well as steady-state conditions of response. The complexity of the findings in the acoustic system emphasizes that the picture may, in fact, be quite a bit more intricate than this sampling might suggest. For example, some cells in different nerves of the gustatory tract behave differently than the chorda tympani responses that we have selected for our discussion. Furthermore, in all sensory modalities there is clearly a very great degree of interaction between the quality of the stimulus and its intensity. There are, of course, also some further questions about the applicability of invertebrate data to theories of mammalian perception. But all in all, the depth of the coverage presented here does seem to support the conclusions we shall draw below.

Another reminder—our use of the power function nomenclature in these sections and our replotting of data into log-log plots are not to be considered to be equivalent to an acceptance of Stevens' power function theory. We have already noted that there are a number of problems in its general application. But, in a descriptive sense, it does provide a unique and simple way to characterize the general degree of compression (or of expansion), which any given function is exhibiting.

With these cautions in mind, it is still possible to draw certain general conclusions from our consideration of at least four of the five sensory modalities we have considered. Table 6.2 lists the sense modalities and the exponents of the power function used to describe their response dynamics for each of the several neural levels at which we have the appropriate data. The exponents have been noted for the level of the generator potential, and the single cell peripheral neuron action potential, compound or integrated peripheral nerve action potential, and central nervous single cell and compound action potentials whenever possible. Finally, we have also indicated those psychophysical power functions that are felt to be closely analogous to the electrophysiological experiment.

As we look over this summary table, a number of important points are immediately apparent. First, there appears to be no simple relationship between the neurophysiological exponents at any level of the nervous system and the psychophysical ones. There are virtually no neural exponents in this table or reported elsewhere in the neurophysiological literature that exceed 1.1 for any but a small portion of their total range. Second, the receptor potentials are typically as compressed or more compressed than any later stages in the neural processing. Therefore, most response compression apparently occurs in the peripheral transductive process. Third, even evoked brain potentials, presumably much closer to the behavior than the peripheral signals, do not correspond to the psychophysical exponents. The evoked potential exponents are typically lower and thus must be non-linearly related to the psychophysical functions. Fourth, there is a paucity of data of dynamic functions from the central nervous system. This is in part due to technical reasons, but also in part due to the biology of the respective situations in each of the modalities. Let us now consider the implications of these findings in more detail.

The fact that so much of the compression appears immediately at peripheral levels and the fact that there is relatively little further change as one ascends the sensory pathways compel us to conclude that the major portions of the response dynamic are accounted for by the very processes that produce the generator potential. It is probably the case that the specific mechanism of compression is quite different from one type of receptor to another, but whatever the underlying process, most of the compression appears at the transductive level.

We also see that even some cortical evoked potentials—the neural signal that some would say comes closest to being equitable to the psychophysical judgments—are usually compressed even though corresponding psychophysical judgments of the same stimulus dimensions often exhibit expanded power functions with exponents greater than 1.

A critical and germane issue is thus raised—is it necessary to assume isomorphism between the neural response functions and subjective magnitudes? The answer to this query is clearly no. The whole idea of coding is based upon the notion that symbols in one domain can represent information patterns in another if there are appropriate transformation rules. Thus, in the spatial domain, linear perceptions of the spatial relations on the body can be represented by wildly distorted but topologically constant spatial representations on the cortex. (See, for example, Woolsey, 1958). But even this topological constancy, as one goes from one point to another on the somatosensory cortex, is not necessary. There is no *a priori* reason why spatial relations need necessarily be maintained. As long as there is some sort of coded arrangement and the decoding mechanisms, whatever they are, were programmed with the rules describing the nature of the disorder, a spatially random system is as good as a linear and well-ordered one from the point of view of representation or coding theory.

From this same perspective, it can be seen that there is no *a priori* need to assume that compressed neurophysiological responses in the intensity domain could not represent or encode linear or expanded psychophysical functions. For example, the compressed response dynamic of the evoked potential may be an entirely valid representation of a linear or even an expanded psychophysical function or vice versa—isomorphism need not be maintained.

Another important consideration is that there may be a sort of bias on the psychophysical estimate that is not present in the electrophysiological data. The issue here is that the form of the function for psychophysical judgments may really be a mixture of several different phenomena. One influence on the psychophysical judgment would be the pure sensory magnitude as encoded by the incoming signals in the various manners we have already considered. In addition, and overlaid on top of this purely

TABLE 6.2 THE EXPONENTS OF THE POWER FUNCTIONS THAT
DESCRIBE THE RELATIONSHIP BETWEEN THE STIMULUS INTENSITY AND
BOTH NEUROPHYSIOLOGICAL AND PSYCHOPHYSICAL RESPONSES*

Modality	Generator or Receptor Potential	Peripheral	
		Single Cell	Cummulated
Vision	0.04, 0.28, 0.58 0.7	(4) 0.30 0.28 0.53 0.55	(1)
Audition	1.0 (then nonconstant)	(2)	0.8 0.42
Somatosensation	0.38	0.59 0.52	
Gustation	0.32	0.53	0.53 (All) 0.5 → 0.85 (Sour) 1.0 (Salt) 1.1 (Sweet) 0.31 (Salt)
Olfaction	0.4		0.67

* Data have been tabulated for each of the senses at several different levels of the ascending pathways. Numbers inserted in the tables are the power function exponents, which have been discussed earlier in the text, and entries have been made without regard to species differences. The conclusions that this table compels us to accept include: (a) Receptor or generator potentials usually have as low or lower exponents as any higher level. Most neurophysiological compression occurs, therefore, at that most peripheral level. (b) The exponents of evoked brain potentials are usually different from the corresponding psychophysical exponents, and thus the two sets of data are nonlinearly related. (c) In general, no simple isomorphic relationship exists between the psychophysical and neurophysiological data.
Note:
(1) In vertebrates, response magnitude is usually sensitive to temporal or spatial features rather than to absolute stimulus intensity.
(2) Often nonmonotonic, narrow range, and idiosyncratic.
(3) Depends on the specific component of the evoked potential measured.
(4) Barlow finds three different functions that describe different portions of the overall visual intensity range.

sensory influence, are fluctuations in the decision criteria, which are certainly operating in the production of magnitude estimates by the subject. Subjects may be thrust into quite a different operating condition when, as one drastic example, small increases in stimulus intensity at high levels suddenly begin to produce painful experiences or other qualitative changes. Simply put, subjects may simply use different decision criteria for strong

Table 6.2 (*cont.*)

Brain Stem		Cortex		Psychophysical
Single Cell	Cummulated	Single Cell	Cummulated	
			0.2 (3)	0.33 (5° target) 0.5 (Flash)
(2)	0.8	(2)	0.7 0.36 (3)	2.0 (elec.) 0.67 (mech.) 1.1 (vocal sound)
0.73 0.43			0.6 (mech.) 1.0 (elec.) (3)	0.6 → 0.95 (mech.) 2.0 →7.0 (elec.) 0.45 (mech.)
				0.5 →0.85 (Sour) 1.0 →1.9 (Salt) 1.3 →2.0 (Sweet)
				0.6 (heptane)

than for weak stimuli. In other words, the meaning or expected value of a stimulus may influence the magnitude estimate as much or more than its pure sensory value. Such a set of notions of the complete nature of psychophysical judgments is not meant to invalidate the subjective magnitude estimates techniques, but simply to point out that other factors than the most simple forms of sensory intensity representation may have to be considered in the analysis of the meaning of some of the data obtained with such psychophysical methods. There is no question that these techniques give rise to data that are reliable indicators of the way in which people behave (barring routine experimental confoundings), but the way in which people behave in estimating magnitudes may be only partially dependent upon sensory intensities.

In sum, psychophysical measures are believed to reflect the influences of several different processes. In addition to the contribution of the sensory magnitude, *per se,* there are also decisional and criterion influences that make the psychophysical data deviate from what one would obtain if there were some direct way to assess sensory magnitude in isolation.

It would be a grievous oversight if at this point we did not consider the viewpoint of S. S. Stevens himself with regard to this sort of data. Stevens has published two recent statements of his views (Stevens, 1970,

1971) concerning the neural correlates of the power functions, which he has found so frequently in the results of psychophysical experiments. In these papers Stevens discusses two points, which must be considered separately. First, he concerns himself with the question of whether or not the neurophysiological data are adequately represented by power functions. As we have seen, this is an empirical issue, which is clouded with some uncertainties, but which will ultimately be answered by critical tests of goodness of fit. Unfortunately, goodness of fit is only rarely tested in a formal fashion in most experiments, and future investigation will have to resolve this particular controversy.

The second issue, which is repeatedly alluded to by Stevens throughout his two papers, concerns an entirely separate point: the presence or absence of an isomorphic relationship between the psychophysical and the neurophysiological data. How congruent, he asks (as we have in the preceding portions of this chapter), are the findings from the psychophysical and neurophysiological laboratories when the stimuli are identical? Stevens' answer to this question is wisely equivocal. His analysis of the data from a number of senses suggests to him that in some instances there is isomorphism with regard to the exponents of the psychophysical power functions. In other instances, he acknowledges that there is no congruence and that the psychophysical data and the neurophysiological data do not agree. He says, for example, in various places in the two papers:

> . . . the cochlear microphonic with its exponent 1.0^4 is probably not the instigator of the loudness response with its exponent 2/3.
>
> (STEVENS, 1970, p. 1047.)

> Seen by electrodes in the cochlea, then the growth of the summated nerve impulses proceeds at a slower pace, with a lower exponent, than the growth of loudness in the human ear.
>
> (STEVENS, 1970, p. 1047.)

> It appears, then, that there are at least four sense modalities in which some particular aspect of the human cortical potential has been shown to follow a power function, and in which the four exponents exhibit the same relative values as those obtained in psychophysical experiments.
>
> (STEVENS, 1970, p. 1048.)

> The failure of the cortical V-potentials to exhibit growth functions having the same exponents that govern perceived sensory magnitude. . . .
>
> (STEVENS, 1970, p. 1048.)

And finally:

> That outcome has thus far proved to be the most general finding with averaged evoked potentials: in those rather numerous instances in

---

[4] As we have seen, this is not an entirely correct statement.

which the growth of a cortical response has seemed to follow a power function, the value of the exponent has fallen systematically below the corresponding value of the exponent obtained in psychophysical studies. When two power functions differ in exponent, they are non-linearly related.

(STEVENS, 1971, p. 237.)

Later after commenting on a study by Easter (1968), in which the goldfish retinal ganglion cell was shown to exhibit a power function with regard to stimulus intensity that had the same exponent as the human visual psychophysical data, Stevens says:

The temptation is great to conclude from the coincidence of exponents that a powerful method for the analysis of the operating characteristics of the visual transducer has at last been formulated by Easter's splendid experiments, and that the site of the psychophysical power law has been pushed into the retina. Caution must prevail, however, for the abundant richness of current physiological findings do no more, at the present stage of knowledge, than signal directions for future excursions.

(STEVENS, 1971, p. 239.)

Stevens' advice is well taken in part. Looking over the papers we have reviewed in this chapter and the additional papers cited by Stevens, it is quite clear that there is at best only a partial isomorphism between the psychophysical and neurophysiological data. Stevens makes no claims to the contrary and, in addition, implies in this last quotation that he, too, has doubts about the significance of what even perfect isomorphism among corresponding exponents from the two data domains would mean. We do, however, believe that the data do speak to the problem of the locus of neural response compression, the topic of our next section.

D. What Is the Site of Response Compression?

Finally, let us return to the question of the site of the compression. It seems safe to conclude that almost all of the compression measured in the neurophysiological studies is introduced by the receptor itself. Whenever specific comparisons are made of the generator potential amplitude with the rate of peripheral nerve spike activity, for example [in the visual system (Fuortes, 1958), in the gustatory system (Borg *et al.*, 1967, or Kimura and Beidler, 1961), or in mechanoreceptors (Katz, 1950, Terzuolo and Washizu, 1962, and Wolbarsht, 1960)], nearly linear relations obtain. The general fact that the values of the exponents in Table 6.2 for generator potentials are less than or equal to those measured for any of the later stages of neurophysiological processing also speaks strongly for the conclusion that the response dynamic of the generator potential can be credited with contributing most to the enormous dynamic range of all sensory systems.

As a final comment concerning the locus of the compression function, let us reconsider the specific comparison of somatosensory evoked potential data discussed above. When one compared the somatosensory cortical potentials evoked by electrical stimuli (Uttal and Cook, 1964) to those evoked by natural mechanical stimulation (Ehrenberger, Finkenzeller, Keidel, and Plattig, 1966), it was found that both the dynamic range and the exponent of the representative power function were quite different. Electrical stimulation produces a very narrow dynamic range with an exponent very close to 1, but stimulation with natural mechanical stimuli produces quite a wide dynamic range and an exponent of 0.6. The explanation of these differences was assumed to be based on the fact that the receptors had been bypassed by the electrical stimulus. Implicit in this assumption is the conclusion that the receptors are mainly responsible for the dynamic compression observed in the entire somatosensory system.

A similar sort of comparison had been made earlier by Stevens (1961) for the auditory system using a psychophysical indicator, the exponent of subjective magnitude scales, rather than the evoked brain potential. Stevens had noted that when one evaluated the power function relating variations in the intensity of natural acoustic stimulation to subjective magnitudes, the exponent was usually found to be 0.6. However, when electrical stimuli were used (Jones, Stevens, and Lurie, 1940) to directly stimulate the cochlear nerve in subjects without tympanic membranes, the auditory experience resulting was best described by a loudness power function, which had an exponent of over 2.0. Stevens' earlier conclusion was exactly the same as the point made here, namely, that the receptors are the major source of the compression function.

IV. IS INTERVAL IRREGULARITY A CODE FOR SENSORY INTENSITY? —A MODEL ANALYSIS

So far in our survey in this chapter on the coding of sensory magnitudes, we have concerned ourselves mainly with only two candidate codes—the frequency of the spike action potential train and amplitude of either some composite wave or some graded portion of the single cell's response. Both of these candidate codes have been seen to be associated with stimulus intensity in many different physiological experiments. A new question now must be considered. Are there any other of the candidate codes, which we discussed in Chapter 5, that might be conceivably associated with stimulus intensity and the related sensory magnitudes?

The answer to this question, in brief, is that the variance of the interspike interval of axonal spike action potentials does seem to correlate with the intensive dimension in a manner that appears to be independent of their mean frequency. Before we discuss the general point, though, we should note an important simple statistical fact. It is entirely possible for the standard deviation (one possible index of variability) to vary independently of the mean. To illustrate the implications of this statement, we have presented in Figure 6.47 two pulse trains. Each of these trains lasts for the same duration as the other, and each contains the same number of impulses. Thus, both have the same mean frequency. However, it is clear that the two trains are quite different along some other dimension.

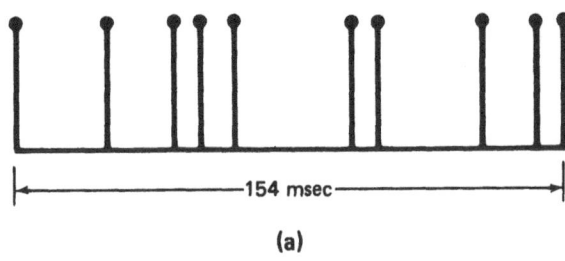

(a)

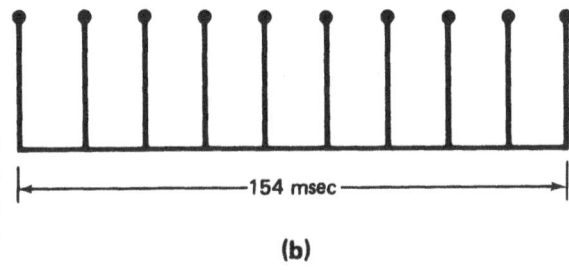

FIGURE 6.47 Two trains of spike action potentials (or stimuli) of equal mean interval but differing interval regularity.

(b)

That dimension is the interval irregularity or variability, or the "jitter" as it is often called, of the size of the interval between successive pulses. The fact that the mean frequency and the standard deviation of the spike train are statistically independent suggests the possibility that they may also be independent biologically, and each might act as a separate and distinct code.

However, before this hypothesis can be accepted, there are a number of questions that must be asked and answered in sequence. First, it is necessary to establish that the dimension of interpulse variability is indeed a candidate code; that is, it must be demonstrated that interval irregularity actually occurs in natural neurophysiological situations as a consequence of some stimulus manipulation. Second, we should also establish that this irregularity information has a differential effect on synaptic junctions as the degree of jitter varies. Otherwise the information, which is contained in the variability dimension, would be simply blocked at the first synapse encountered during its ascent along the sensory pathway. Third, as we have said so often, in order to fully establish this candidate code as a true code, useful to the system for the communication of sensory information, we must show that it has some sort of behavioral effect. In the following sections, each of these questions is discussed in turn and answered affirmatively. In doing so, it is hoped that this material will also serve as an illustration of the general procedure, which is necessary to confirm a candidate code as a true code.

A. Demonstrations of the Natural Occurrence of Interval Irregularity
The history and the theory of the general problem of spike action potential interval irregularity have been reviewed by Moore, Perkel, and Segundo

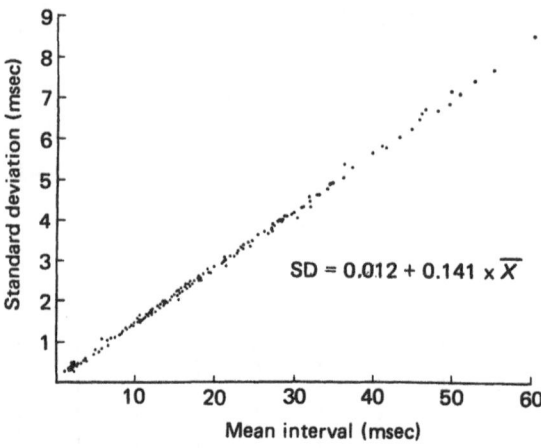

FIGURE 6.48. The linear relationship between the standard deviation of intervals between spikes and the mean interval for peripheral neurons driven by brief mechanical stimuli. The equation of the best fitting straight line is given in the slope intercept form (from Werner and Mountcastle, 1965).

(1966), who point out that Hagiwara (1949, 1950) was probably the first one to observe and recognize the possible importance of spike interval jitter. More recently, Werner and Mountcastle (1963), studying the somatosensory system's responses to joint rotation, observed variation of the regularity of interpulse intervals as a function of the magnitude of rotation. Microelectrodes were used to pick up the temporal pattern of spike activity from thalamic neurons in this experiment. Werner and Mountcastle observed that there was a monotonic variation in both mean frequency and the regularity of interpulse intervals as the joint position was changed, and these two measures were linearly related. In a later study (Werner and Mountcastle, 1965), these same authors found that the same sort of nearly linear relationship held between mean frequency and the standard deviation of the interval irregularity for impulses in the peripheral saphenous nerve of a cat, produced by brief cutaneous stimuli of varying intensity as shown in Figure 6.48. This finding should allay any concern whether joint rotation is properly to be considered an intensive dimension.

Monotonic increases in interspike interval regularity with increased stimulus intensity have also been observed by Goldberg, Adrian, and Smith (1964) for the auditory system and by Buller, Nicholls, and Ström (1953) for muscle spindle activity in the frog.

The main contribution of this sort of data is to provide an answer to our first question, namely, that interval irregularity of interspike intervals is functionally related to stimulus intensity in a variety of biological situations. However, another important aspect of the functional relationship shown by Werner and Mountcastle and others between the mean frequency and the standard deviation of interval is that the two are usually linearly related. This suggests the possibility that, perhaps, the variability is nothing more than an indirect product of the frequency of the elicited spikes and only indirectly a function of the stimulus. If this were so, clearly interval irregularity might not carry any separate and useful information, but might only follow the frequency code. An effective way of

determining the separate effectiveness of interval irregularity as a code
would be to drive the nerve with different frequency patterns and determine if interval variability was capable of producing different responses
even when the mean frequency was held constant. The next sections report neurophysiological and psychophysical experiments, which use just
this procedure and provide the answers to the subsequent questions in this
model analysis.

B. The Effect of Interval Irregularity on Synaptic Transmission

To demonstrate that interval variability can really carry useful information, separate from the covarying mean interval dimension, we must not
only demonstrate that it is functionally related to stimulus variation, but
also demonstrate that the information pattern so generated is, at least,
capable of being conveyed across a synapse. A study of the synaptic
effectiveness of variations in interval irregularity has been carried out by
Segundo, Moore, Stensaas, and Bullock (1963) on the synapses of the
visceral ganglion of another one of those wonderful model animals, the sea
hare (*Aplysia californica*).

The advantages of using a simple intevertebrate preparation to study,
in a reduced form, some response that would be quite difficult to isolate
in a vertebrate preparation, have already been discussed. The ganglia of
Aplysia, for example, are very much the same in structure from one specimen to another. In fact, many of the cells have been numbered and named
in such a way that any worker can agree which cell is being dealt with
in any given experiment. In addition to this standard nomenclature
for individual cells, this preparation has other advantages. The cells are
very large, and in many cases the individual details of their pre- and
postsynaptic connections are known. It is thus possible to provide an
input for a specific cell and observe the effects of its output on some
equally well-known third-order cell. Generally, this is impossible to do
with the smaller cells of the vertebrate nervous system, which are impaled "blindly" with microelectrodes and where little is known of their
specific inputs and outputs.

The particular cell that Segundo and his colleagues were working
with was the so-called giant nerve cell—an ultralarge cell which could
be easily penetrated with a glass microelectrode filled with KCl to record
the differential effects of driven presynaptic nerve impulses on both
postsynaptic graded and spike action potentials.

The general strategy in this important experiment was to apply electrical pulse stimuli to compound nerves containing axons, which fed into
synapses impinging on this giant nerve cell. Since the stimuli were precisely controlled in the time of their occurrence and one stimulus pulse produces one spike, the temporal pattern of the evoked afferent spikes was
precisely known. The postsynaptic potentials, both graded and regenerative, of the giant nerve cell were then analyzed to determine if there
was a differential pattern of response as a function of the timing of
the presynaptic neural spike potentials.

Two types of electrical pulse stimulus patterns were used by Segundo
and his colleagues. The first utilized trios or triplets of pulses, in which

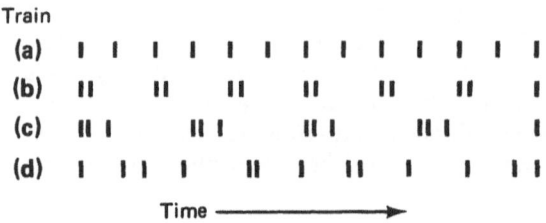

Train

(a)

(b)

(c)

(d)

Time ──────────────────▶

FIGURE 6.49 Sample stimulus patterns made up of trains of pulse electrical stimuli with varying interval irregularity and grouping as used in the Aplysia experiment (from Segundo, Moore, Stensaas, and Bullock, 1963).

the middle pulse was positioned at various delays following the first stimulus pulse and preceding the third pulse. The second type of stimulus pattern was a prolonged burst with a constant duration and a constant number of pulses. The mean frequency of all of these prolonged bursts was thus regulated to be the same, but as Figure 6.49 shows, the variance of the interval differs from one pattern to another. This same figure also indicates some of the measures used by these authors as dependent variables. For example, the amplitudes of the graded postsynaptic responses could be measured in two different ways. First, the incremental amplitude produced as a result of a particular stimulus pulse could be used. Second, total amplitude of the graded signal produced by all of the stimulus pulses presented up to a given time was an alternative measure. A third dependent variable could be defined in terms of whether or not a spike action potential was elicited by a given spike in the series, given the prior temporal history of the stimulus pattern.

A typical result for triplets of stimuli is shown in Figure 6.50. In this figure, the dependent variable measured on the vertical coordinate is the total graded postsynaptic depolarization recorded after the third of the three impulses in the triplet has been presented. On the horizontal coordinate, the interval between the first and second shock has been plotted. It is important to note that Segundo and his colleagues go out of their way to emphasize that these are data that are really only representative for an intermediate range of postsynaptic potential amplitudes.

Since the intensity of the electrical stimulus can affect the size of the volley (that is, the number of activated axons) along the stimulated nerve, and the size of this volley can affect the size of the postsynaptic potential (PSP), it is possible to vary the amplitude of the PSP by varying stimulus amplitude as well as by the temporal pattern of the stimuli. The effect of stimulus amplitude on PSP amplitude has also been shown parametrically in Figure 6.50.

The results obtained by Segundo and his associates indicate that the interval pattern of the three stimulus shocks is very important in determining the amplitude of the graded postsynaptic potential. The situation can be seen, however, to be rather complex, varying along at least two dimensions in an interacting fashion. If the amplitude of the individual pulses is too high, timing is irrelevant because each pulse will be strong enough to produce a spike. If the amplitude of the individual pulses is small or medium, however, then the timing becomes critical, but is dependent, to some degree, on such variables as the total duration of the

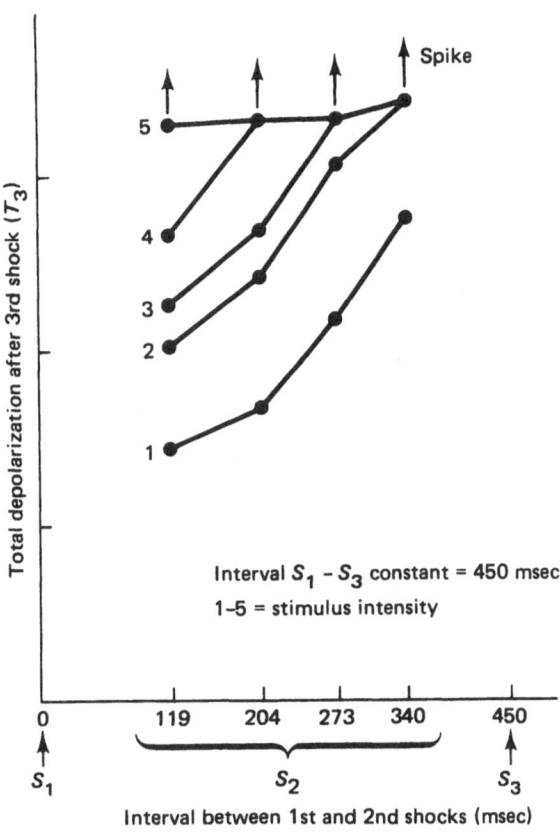

FIGURE 6.50 The effect of timing of stimulus triplets on the size of an excitatory postsynaptic potential (EPSP). For constant $S_1 - S_3$ interval, the position of the middle stimulus (S_2) is critical in determining the amplitude of the EPSP and whether or not a spike will be elicited (from Segundo, Moore, Stensaas, and Bullock, 1963).

burst. For example, whether a third presynaptic spike will be able to produce a postsynaptic spike will depend on what the interval was between the preceding pair of spikes as well as on its own amplitude. The fact that these parametric curves expressing postsynaptic potential amplitude are convex upward, however, suggests that the effect of the interval between the first two pulses becomes less important the more they are separated in time from the third.

A similar state of affairs obtains for long bursts of spikes with differing degrees of interpulse interval variability. Segundo and his co-workers assumed, in this case, that the efficiency of a specific burst pattern could be measured by determining how long it took to arrive at some criterion level of postsynaptic depolarization. The results of this type of experiment are illustrated in Figure 6.51 for two different stimulus patterns. When the intervals between the stimulus pulses (which can be seen as downward going artifacts) were regular, it took a longer period of the time before the criterion level was reached than if the intervals were irregular (for example, presented in pairs). This difference occurred, it must be repeated by way of emphasis, even if the mean frequencies of the two bursts were identical.

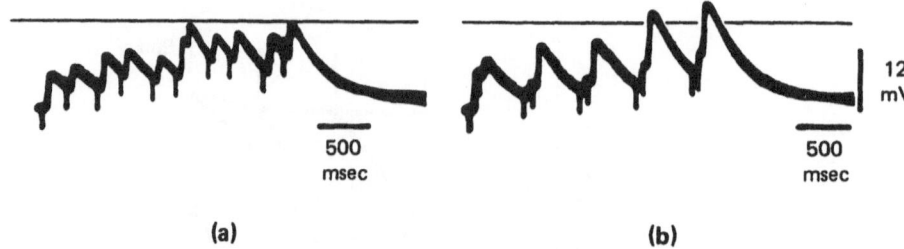

(a)   **(b)**

FIGURE 6.51 The effect of various degrees of irregularity within trains of stimuli on the EPSP. The pattern in (a) led to a response that more quickly arrived at the criterion level at which a spike was generated, while the pattern in (b) took a longer time but maintained high EPSP levels and thus a higher frequency of spike firing for a longer duration. Stimuli are indicated by the downward going lines—artifacts from the electrical stimulator (from Segundo, Moore, Stensaas, and Bullock, 1963).

The conclusions that have to be drawn from this interesting work are that the timing of the neural impulses and, particularly, the degree of interpulse irregularity are important variables in the determination of the efficacy of a presynaptic spike train. In fact, Segundo, Moore, Stensaas, and Bullock go even further, for they show that not only is the ability of a given presynaptic spike to modulate synaptic action dependent upon the timing of events that preceded it, but that even the recovery cycle following a *postsynaptic spike* is also a function of the preceding *presynaptic* activity. This means that even the explosive and regenerative spike action is not sufficient to obscure the prior influence of the temporal stimulus pattern that initiated that spike.

Segundo and his group suggest that the temporal effects they have observed in this simple preparation, while apparently complex, can at least, in part, be interpreted in terms of simple postsynaptic temporal summation. It should be remembered, however, in this context, that the overall timing of this invertebrate system is very slow. The three pulses used as stimuli to generate the sample data in Figure 6.50 had a total burst duration of 450 msec, and the long train of impulses with which these neurophysiologists worked had a total duration of about 4 or 5 sec. Compared to the vertebrate findings discussed in the next section, this is an extraordinarily long integration period, although not out of line with what we have observed so far in other comparable invertebrate experiments.

A good summary of related material can be found in Moore, Perkel, and Segundo's review (1966). For the purposes of our present discussion, this work plays an important role, for it does establish that interval variability, already demonstrated to be a theoretically possible candidate code and known to fluctuate as a function of stimulus intensity in biological systems, is capable of differentially affecting synaptic conductivity in at least certain preparations. This answers the second question in our model analysis, and it only remains to demonstrate some behavioral effect to accept this candidate code as a true code.

C. The Effect of Interval Irregularity on Psychophysical Judgments

In order to confirm interval irregularity or variability as a true code, as noted above, it is necessary to demonstrate that this neural dimension is also able to affect behavior. Conveniently, it turns out that there is a set of experimental conditions that allow this question to be answered by a psychophysical study of human sensitivity to spike action potential interval irregularity.

The main methodological feature of Segundo, Moore, Stensaas, and Bullock's experiment was electrical stimulation. This feature made it possible for them to produce a relevant and germane answer to the question of synaptic sensitivity to temporal pattern, because of the fact that pulse electrical stimulation, by virtue of the bypassing of the receptors, produces axonal action potentials on the basis of one spike for each stimulus pulse. This fact allows the experimenter to specify as his independent variable, the specific nerve action potential pattern evoked even in mixed nerves. Fortunately, there is an analogous situation with human subjects, in which this same relationship can be exploited. Though the sensory nerves for most of the senses are deeply imbedded in the bony portions of the skull, the human somatosensory system does have large and accessible nerves, which can be directly stimulated through the intact skin of the arms and legs. The median and ulnar nerves of the arm are particularly easy to use in this manner.

Dawson and Scott (1949) were among the first to discover not only that the great peripheral nerves of the somatosensory system could be stimulated through the skin, but, in addition, that the compound action potentials, so evoked, could also be detected and recorded percutaneously. In 1956, Dawson was able to distinguish between sensory and motor fibers and record sensory responses alone. Much additional work has been done with both surface and needle electrodes by the Danish team of Buchthal and Rosenfalck (1966) and reported in a major monograph, which describes the various factors involved in such stimulation and recording.

The ulnar and median nerves in the arm have, by an accident of anatomy, two points at which they become quite superficial, one at the wrist and one just above the elbow. The nature of the experiment, which must be carried out to test for the psychophysical effect of interpulse irregularity in man, is, thus, almost predefined by accidents of anatomy and available method. Thoughtful consideration suggests that the following conditions must be met.

1. Electrical pulse stimuli must be used to
   a. bypass the receptors
   b. give a one-for-one correspondence between stimuli and nerve action potentials.

2. The somatosensory system must be used because it is the only sensory modality in which the peripheral nerves are easily accessible.
3. Temporal or amplitude judgments must be used as the psycho-

physical test because the pulse electrical stimuli synchronize all of the responses of the constituent axons of the peripheral nerve. Thus, there is no phase or pattern information other than the overall stimulus determined one, and since it is probably the fine patterning of the timing of individual cell responses that encodes sensory quality, there is little qualitative variation. (See Chapter 11's summary.)

Condition 1b is especially critical, since the whole approach depends upon directly knowing (or experimentally manipulating) the spike pattern.

These conditions have been used in a series of psychophysical experiments (Uttal, 1960, and Uttal and Smith, 1967) to examine both a three-pulse and a prolonged burst situation analogous to the Segundo, Moore, Stensaas, and Bullock (1963) studies described in the previous section. It is important to note that the psychophysical response measures used in these two studies on human judgments differ not only from the electrophysiological measures used by Segundo and his co-workers, but also from each other. In the three-pulse psychophysical study (Uttal, 1960), a simple estimate of subjective amplitude was used as the dependent variable. In the psychophysical experiment with the prolonged burst (Uttal and Smith, 1967), the dependent measure is a little more difficult to define. The subjects were asked to tell which of two bursts was "irregular." Irregularity, as such, is not the subjective magnitude dimension with which we are mainly concerned, nor is it clear exactly what it means. The results of this latter experiment are, thus, indirect. They do not tell us exactly that sensory magnitude or, for that matter, any other sensory dimension is actually being encoded by interpulse irregularity (although we have a pretty good idea from our previous survey that it is). What they do tell us is that irregularity, *per se*, is discriminable on some basis and that, at least in a certain time region, irregularity is available as a sensory code.

The three-pulse study (Uttal, 1960) involved the presentation of triplets of constant current regulated electrical pulses spaced closely enough (all three occurred in less than 10 msec) so that the induced experience was a single unified event with no perceived microstructure. The triplet, in other words, was within the temporal acuity threshold duration. Thus, the only sensory dimension along which the experience varied was that of subjective intensity. Figure 6.52 shows both the stimulus pulses and the evoked peripheral nerve responses for a typical stimulus condition. The pattern of the triplet was varied in two ways. First, the interval between the first and the third pulses was varied in five different steps. Second, for each of these five steps of total triplet duration, the middle pulse was positioned at a set of different temporal locations in 1-msec steps between the first and third stimulus pulses, the number of positions depending upon the interval between the first and third stimulus pulses. Table 6.3 summarizes the various stimulus patterns used in this three-pulse experiment.

Two measures of the response produced by these stimulus patterns were used: the sum of the amplitudes of the evoked compound action potentials and a series of magnitude estimates of the subjective intensity

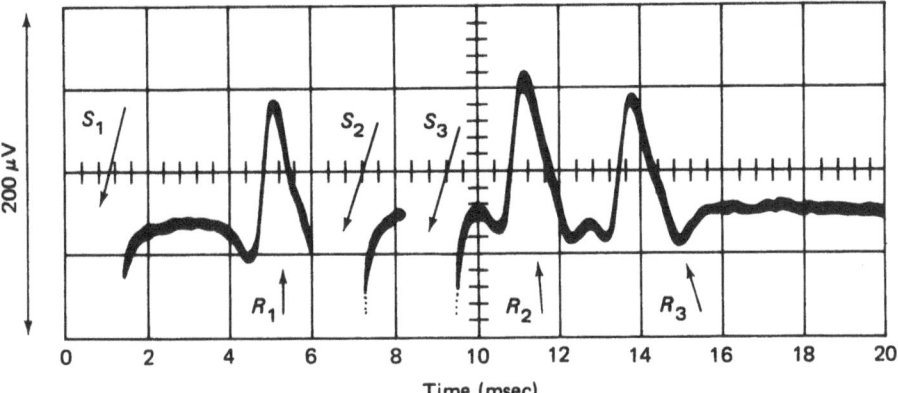

FIGURE 6.52 The three stimulus artifacts and the three neural responses in the experiment in which human psychophysical responses were compared with human peripheral compound nerve response magnitudes (from Uttal, 1960).

of the evoked experience. In this way direct comparisons could be made between the physiological and the psychophysical response.

Now let us consider the results of this experiment. It can be seen in Figure 6.53 that for four subjects the sums of the amplitude of the evoked nerve responses change in a relatively systematic way as these stimulus patterns vary. If the first two pulses are close together, then the second response will occur in the refractory period of the first, and it, the second response, will be of a lower amplitude than it might otherwise be. If, on the other hand, the second pulse is close to the third one, then the third response will be in the refractory period of the second, and it, the third response, will be smaller than it might otherwise be. Unfortunately, the oscillographic displays of the three stimulus artifacts (the deflections produced at zero latency by the stimulus pulses) and the three neural responses are overlapping to a considerable degree. Not all of the three response amplitudes can, therefore, be measured for all conditions. The three sets of curves in Figure 6.53 are thus necessarily incomplete. Fortunately, the sum of the amplitudes of these three neural responses can be predicted on the basis of what is known of the interaction between two pulses (Uttal, 1959). This has been done for a hypothetical "standard subject" and plotted in Figure 6.54. The result of this calculation is a family of dome-shaped curves with the maximum summed amplitude of the three responses occurring when the second stimulus is midway between the first and the third stimulus.

The data summarizing the psychophysical magnitude estimates obtained for this set of patterns is shown in Figure 6.55. They also exhibit the same domed shape. The important conclusion to be drawn from this experiment is that the two sets of data, the predicted sum of the neural response amplitudes (the validity of which was at least partially confirmed for those recordings in which the stimulus artifact did not obliterate neural responses) and the subjective magnitude of the sensation, agree quite well.

TABLE 6.3 STIMULUS CONFIGURATIONS IN THE THREE-
PULSE ELECTROCUTANEOUS EXPERIMENT (FROM UTTAL, 1960).

Config.	Delay in msec	
	P_2	P_3
1	1	8
2	2	8
3	3	8
4	4	8
5	5	8
6	6	8
7	7	8
8	1	7
9	2	7
10	3	7
11	4	7
12	5	7
13	6	7
14	1	6
15	2	6
16	3	6
17	4	6
18	5	6
19	1	5
20	2	5
21	3	5
22	4	5
23	1	4
24	2	4
25	3	4
26	1	3
27	2	3

In other words, for stimulus triplets, the interval irregularity does not appear to be carrying very much useful information, and the subjects seem to be insensitive to the temporal pattern of the stimuli. The main conclusion, therefore, is that the subjective magnitude of the sensation produced by the stimulus triplet is almost completely accounted for in terms of the summed amplitude of the neural response, when the three pulses occur within the temporal region in which the three stimuli feel to the subject like a unified sensation. Subjective magnitude in this time region (less than

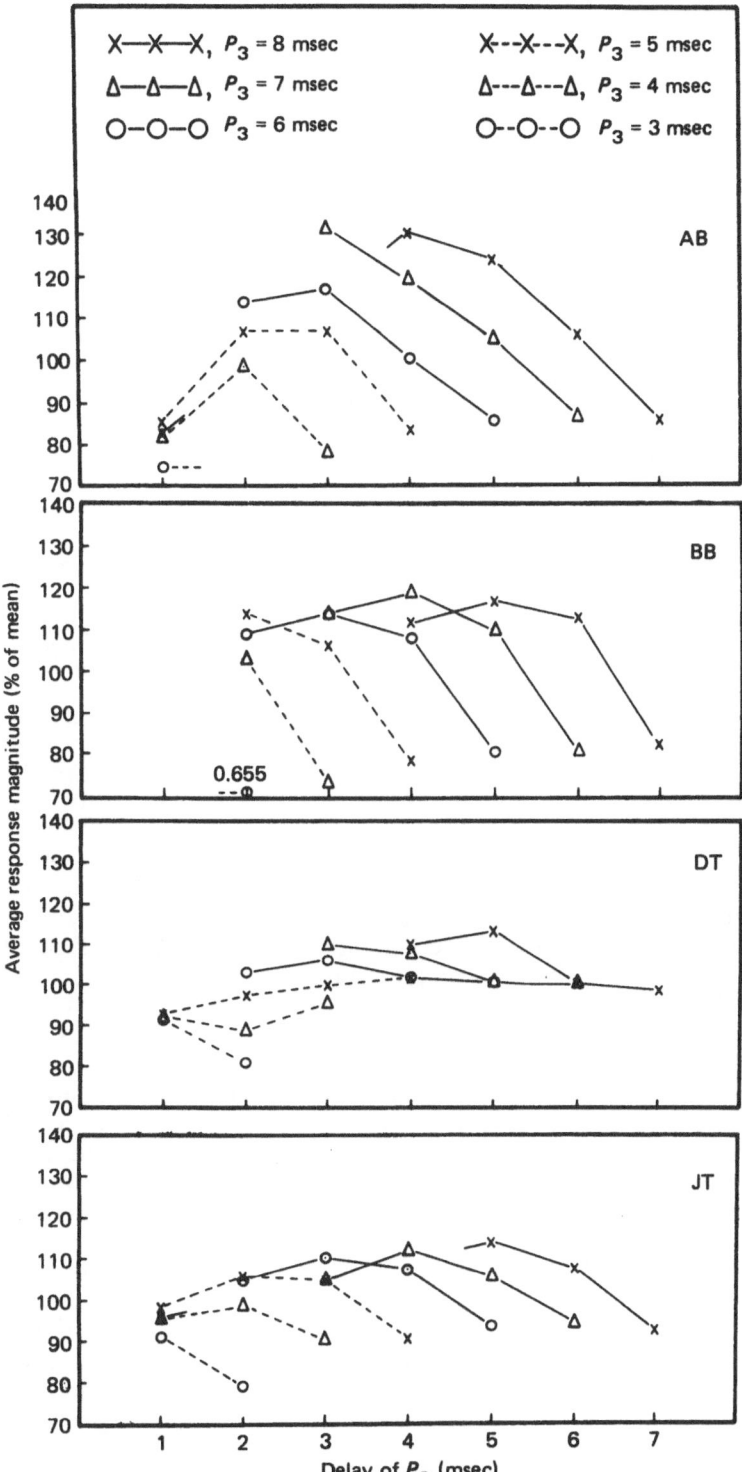

FIGURE 6.53 *The average summated neural response magnitude for the various stimulus conditions shown in Table 6.3. Data are pooled from four subjects. Not all values are present, because under certain conditions the stimulus artifacts obscured the neural responses (from Uttal, 1960).*

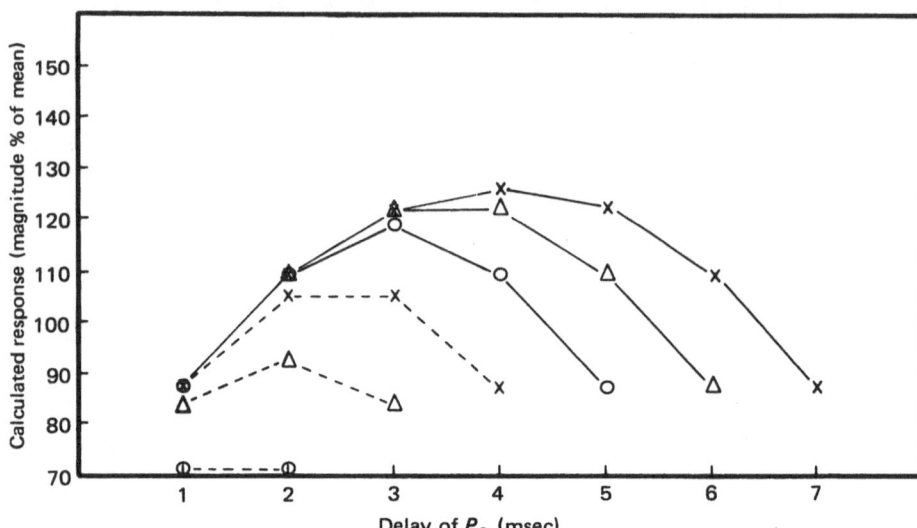

FIGURE 6.54 *Theoretically calculated summated response amplitudes of the neural responses to a stimulus triplet, assuming a standard form of the interaction between two pulses (from Uttal, 1960).*

about 10 msec) is, thus, apparently encoded by some counting procedure, which is sensitive only to the number of axonal responses that are reflected in the amplitude of the compound action potential, and not to the interval pattern. Interval seems only to exert its influence indirectly as it modulates the amplitude of the individual compound responses.

But this conclusion is valid only for the situation in which all of the responses occur within the region of temporal fusion. Does this same insensitivity to interpulse irregularity obtain with stimulus pulse patterns that are more prolonged and in which the individual pulses are greater than 8 or 10 msec apart? The answer to this question seems to be—no, this conclusion is not valid in the situation with longer bursts and with wider interpulse separations. The study (Uttal and Smith, 1967) that examined this question utilized much the same equipment and methodology as the three-pulse study just described, but asked the subject to make a judgment directly of irregularity. As we have mentioned, the general question that was being asked was, "Can the effects of interval irregularity as such be observed in psychophysical judgments?" Nevertheless, to answer this general question, the specific experimental question asked had to be: can a subject make use of the additional information in many irregular intervals to give a finer discrimination than that possible in a stimulus train with only one irregularity?

Figure 6.56 presents the results of two experiments in a way that allows this second comparison to be directly made. The upper curve plots the results of the first experiment, in which a series of pulse stimuli was used having only one irregularity—a single gap. A two-alternative forced

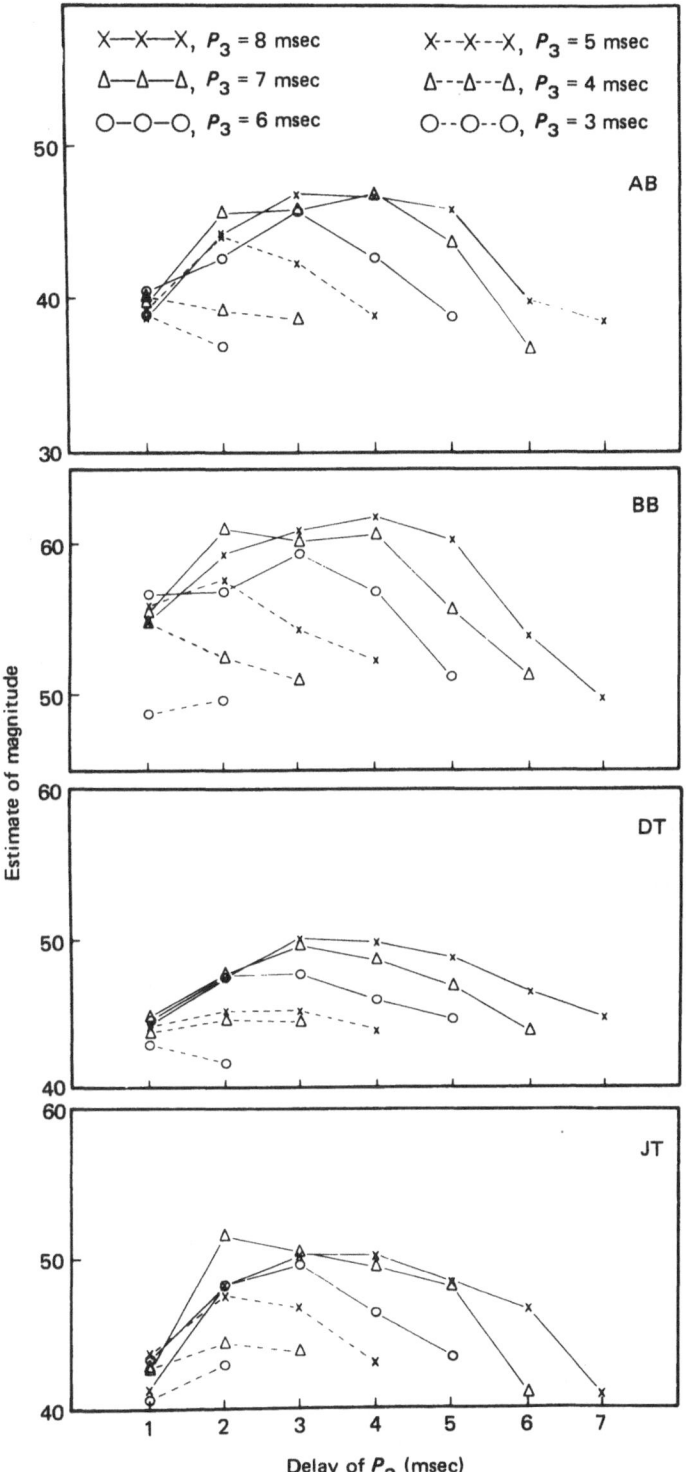

FIGURE 6.55 *The psychophysical data showing averaged magnitude estimates for the stimulus conditions shown in Table 6.3. Note the correspondence between this response pattern and the calculated neural response of Figure 6.54 (from Uttal, 1960).*

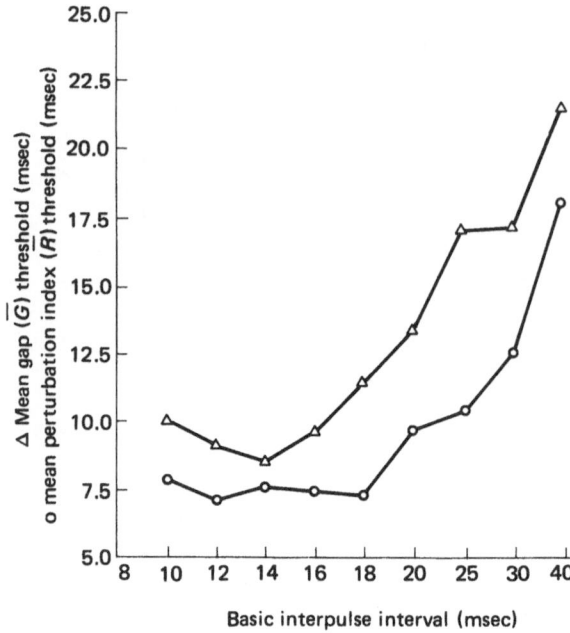

FIGURE 6.56 Psychophysical interval irregularity and gap detection experiments compared. Subjects do have a significantly better ability to detect overall irregularity as compared to the detection of a single gap in a stimulus train (from Uttal and Smith, 1967).

choice experimental procedure was used as the psychophysical method such that the subject was forced to say which one of two sequential bursts contained the single gap. The size of the gap was controlled by a contingent computer program, which reduced the gap size if it was detected, and enlarged it if it was not.

In the second experiment, the degree of interval irregularity of an entire stimulus train was controlled by a computer procedure, which was also contingent upon the subject's prior responses. In this case, rather than varying the size of a gap, the whole pattern of interpulse intervals varied according to a simple computational algorithm. Figure 6.47 (presented earlier in this chapter) illustrates the jittered stimulus pattern.

In this case, the subject's ability to discriminate the irregularities was considerably greater than the case in which only a single gap discontinuity was present. This result indicates that the subject is able to make use of the additional information contained in the statistics of the interval irregularity in this situation. This conclusion was further substantiated by looking at the effect of the number of gaps in an irregular train with varying numbers of pulses. If the subject is acting as a sort of statistical analyzer, we should expect his performance to improve as larger samples of intervals are presented to him. Figure 6.57 shows that this is exactly what happens. As the number of pulses in the stimulus train increases, his sensitivity to irregularity also increases, but only up to a limit of about 8 pulses.

Another important point concerns the general shape of the irregularity detection function of Figure 6.56 and the apparent discrepancy be-

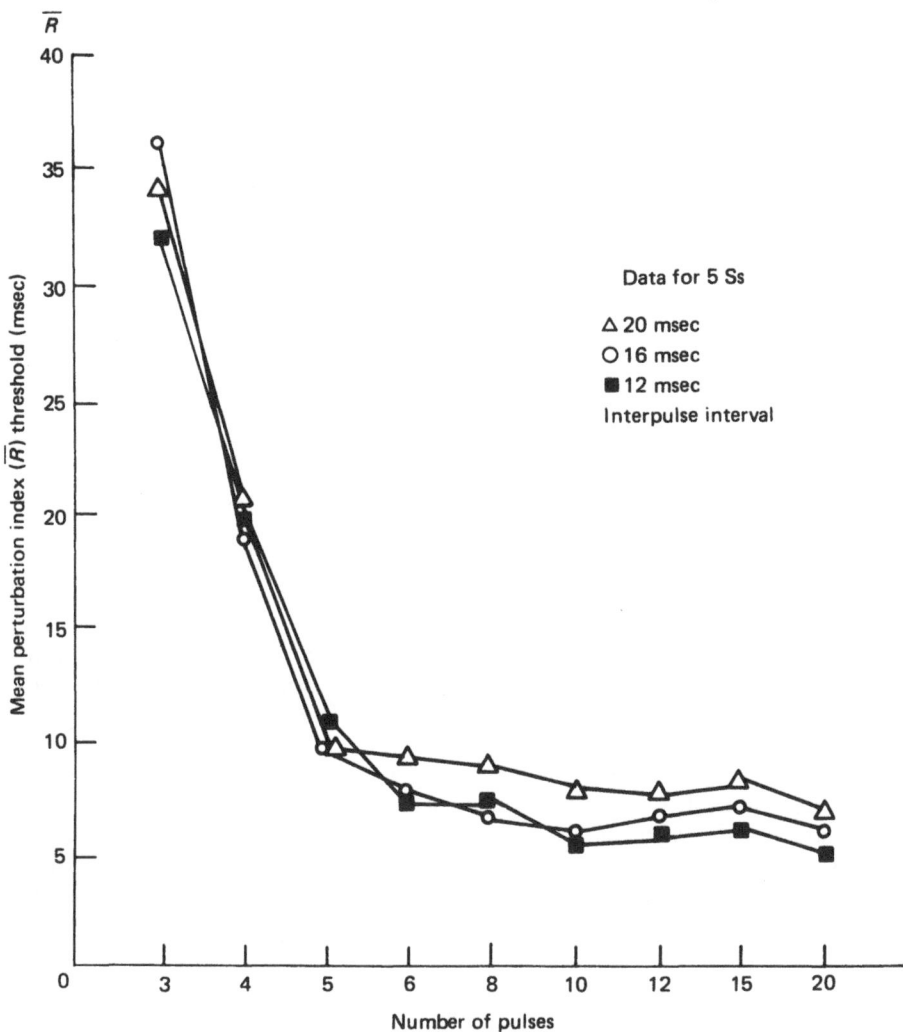

FIGURE 6.57 *The increase in the ability of subjects to detect irregularities as the number of pulses in the train increases. The fact that all three curves asymptote at the same point indicates that this is a counting process and not one dependent upon the overall timing of the trains (from Uttal and Smith, 1968).*

tween the data for the three-pulse situation (where interval was not important) and the longer burst situation (in which irregularity detection seems to be a well-developed capacity). The disagreement between the two situations is only superficial, for the three-pulse data deal solely with total intervals that are less than the temporal fusion threshold. Furthermore, an examination of the data obtained with irregular bursts suggests that there may even be three, rather than two, distinguishable regions of temporal response, each of which follows different rules; one region extending from 0 to 10 msec, one from 10 to 20 msec, and one for longer interpulse intervals.

This multiple branch characteristic of the response curve is very similar to one of the results reported by Mountcastle, Talbot, Darian-Smith, and Kornhuber (1967) for the detection of vibratory stimuli. They found that their response curve was made up of two segments with the point of inflection between the two, occurring at about the same inter-pulse interval, 20 msec, as the second break in Figure 6.56. They concluded from their results that there were two different somatosensory receptor systems operating in the detection of vibratory activity. The first was sensitive to low frequencies and was mediated by receptors located in the skin. The second was sensitive to higher frequencies and was mediated by receptors buried deep in the tissues of the hand. Which receptor system was activated, they suggested, was directly dependent upon the frequency of the mechanical vibration.

It is, however, possible that the two-segment curve obtained in their experiment was not a function of two different sets of nerve fibers, but rather two branches of a bipartite response curve of a single set of neurons. Considering the nature of the electrical pulse stimulus of the Uttal and Smith experiment, there is no reason to assume that the individual pulses affect different fibers or follow different current paths as their frequency of occurrence is increased. It is more likely that the segments of the response curve do not represent different groups of receptors or fibers, but rather represent a curve with multiple branches or characteristic responses for temporal processing by a single family of fibers.

Thus, the multiple arms of the response curves in both the Uttal and Smith and the Mountcastle *et al.* experiments may be alternatively explained by the following hypothesis. The temporal response of peripheral nerves exhibits a continuum of two or three regions of differing temporal processing capabilities as the frequency spectrum is scanned. Below inter-pulse intervals of 10 msec (100 Hz), there is a region of fusion in which there is generally a very low sensitivity to the temporal characteristics of the signal. In this time zone, the integrated number of impulses is more important than the interval pattern. Above 10 msec and below 20 msec, there is a region in which there is an independent sensitivity to the second-order statistics—the irregularity—of the interpulse intervals, and the mean frequency does not exhibit any substantial effect. Above 20 msec, one crosses into a region in which the mean interpulse interval is so large that the integrative powers of the nervous system are no longer capable of taking advantage of such higher-order statistical data, and judgments are made on the basis of mean interval or some other independent measure of the size of local intervals.

Do these data and conclusions correspond to those obtained in the experiments with *Aplysia*? In fact, and assuming that the differences in time scale of the invertebrate and vertebrate preparations can be ignored, the two sets of data do pretty well agree. Segundo, Moore, Stensaas, and Bullock (1963) point out that for "short durations and, thus, high frequencies . . . all trios of subthreshold shocks of moderate intensity evoke a spike, irrespective of timing"; that there is "an intermediate range of durations (for example, 500 msec) and frequencies in which different positions of S_2 are reflected by significantly different degrees of depolarization (to the third stimulus) and at higher frequencies, different spike probabilities." They conclude, "Consequently, it is justifiable to state that, under fixed conditions of nerve, cell, and EPSP size, there exists an intermediate input frequency range in which output is critically dependent on timing." No specific comment is made of even longer intervals, but with suprathreshold stimuli, the analogy can be easily made between the third branch of the Uttal and Cook response data and some gross frequency discrimination by *Aplysia*.

Thus, we have demonstrated in the course of our discussion that the variability of the intervals between spike action potentials:

1. is a natural consequent of stimulation with stimuli of varying intensity;
2. is a parameter which is capable of being transmitted across synaptic junctions; and
3. does differentially affect behavior in the form of psychophysical judgments.

In doing so, we have established that this candidate code is also available to be used as a code over at least part of the temporal domain, even though we have not finally established that interval variability is a code specifically for sensory magnitudes. The implication is that it is, but the analysis is admittedly not complete at this point.

V. AN INTERIM SUMMARY

This chapter has been an extended discussion of the factors involved in the neural coding of sensory magnitudes. We began our discussion by considering the contemporary view of the "threshold." Where once the threshold had been considered to be a sharp line of demarcation, it is now considered to be a region in which, at the very least, statistical processes operate and, at most, may possess no lower bound. We then discussed signal detection theory and showed how it could be advantageously applied to both psychophysical and neurophysiological data in the light of this new view.

We can summarize the material on the coding of the full range of stimulus and subjective magnitudes by noting that in neurophysiological experiments, almost all functions relating stimulus intensity and response tend to be compressed on the average. This compression holds true from the initial transduction and does not increase noticeably from the most peripheral signals recorded from the receptors to the highest levels of the central nervous system. This result directly leads us to the general idea that response compression is a feature of neural coding, which is primarily attributable to the transductive processes themselves. Further, the candidate codes, which seem most often to be used for the representation of intensive dimensions, include the number of responding cells, response amplitude (as measured either with the amplitude of a graded potential or with the integral of a pooled response), the mean frequency of spike action potentials, and the interpulse irregularity of the spike train.

Another important generalization, which we can draw from a comparison of the psychophysical data and even the central nervous system's neurophysiological data, is that there is no direct linear relationship between the two. The psychophysical functions are described by power functions, whose exponents range from 0.2 to 7.0, while the neurophysiological functions almost always seem to be compressed functions with averaged or integrated exponents that range only from 0.2 to at most 1.1. It seems fair to say, then, that the psychological exponents reflect something more complex than the simple sensory events evoked by the stimulus. Decision criterion, judgmental factors, and emotional overtone all seem to be words, which are probably descriptive of some of the processes involved in the psychophysical magnitude estimate processes, and thus far more complex systems of neurons are being assayed by the psychophysical procedures than by the neurophysiological ones.

We have also carried out an analysis of the acceptablity of a particular candidate code—spike interval irregularity—as a true code and have found that it can so be accepted, although it is not possible to specifically associate it yet with a particular common sensory dimension.

CHAPTER 7: THE NEURAL CODING OF SPACE AND TIME

In this chapter, we shall begin our discussion of a different set of dimensions and a different set of problems than the intensive ones emphasized in Chapter 6. The temporal and spatial dimensions we shall discuss are surprisingly closely linked in any psychobiological analysis, and often it is impossible to separate them without losing the meaningfulness of the data. It is the main purpose of this chapter to show how these two domains—the temporal and spatial—are linked and then to present both psychophysical and neurophysiological evidence that will help to establish the relationship between the perceptual and neurophysiological findings.

We shall first consider two ways in which fine discriminations become blunted. There is a loss in both temporal and spatial acuity as one ascends from the peripheral nerve response to the percept. This loss can be accounted for in terms of neural convergence and divergence, respectively, and we shall introduce and discuss each of these processes prior to the discussion of the psychophysical data themselves.

The next topic in spatial coding considered will be the emerging body of evidence that suggests that there is a marked interaction between nearby events at least at some peripheral levels of the afferent pathway. The important point being made is that signals do not, in general, travel along isolated and private lines, but do affect each other in numerous ways through a sort of parallel "cross talk" or interaction. We shall consider some of the psychophysical evidence that seems to reflect behavioral effects of this cross talk, and also the observed details of the neural nets that might mediate these interactions.

We, then, shall consider two related questions, the answers to which turn out to be surprisingly equivocal in the light of so much of what is taken for granted in today's psychobiological theorizing:

1. Does lateral interaction exist in other senses besides vision?
2. Does a similar form of lateral interaction exist centrally as well as peripherally?

We shall then discuss some of the mathematical nerve net theories of lateral interaction. These theories are very highly developed and play an important role in the formal modeling of both perceptual and neurophysiological findings in contemporary thinking. Next, we shall discuss the neural correlates and the psychophysics of purely temporal discriminations. Finally, we shall discuss the neural coding of spatial discriminations and show that in audition, in particular, perceptual space is best explained in terms of dynamic temporal and intensive codes, while in vision, static spatial codes seem to be most closely associated with spatial percepts.

I. INTRODUCTION

A. Some Complexities

We now consider the spatial and temporal aspects of perception, an area which is so broad and for which there is such an abundance of material that at the very best our coverage can be only partial. Therefore, almost any critical reader will find that some of the topics or studies in which he might have been interested are going to be missing from this chapter. The coverage of this material will necessarily be selective, and we shall survey only those aspects of spatial and temporal experience that may be reasonably subjected to some kind of neural coding analysis. This reservation is necessary because, while all sensory and perceptual phenomena, without doubt, are represented and encoded by patterns of neural activity, not all of these problems are equally amenable to study using the concepts and methodologies of our contemporary neurophysiology.

Unfortunately, however, there is no simple *a priori* way to separate those sensory and perceptual phenomena that we cannot treat in neurophysiological detail from those that we can. It is a matter of historical accident and *ad hoc* decision making. Some phenomena, such as the Mach band, for example, clearly have been prototypes for physiological analysis since their initial description, while other similar visual spatial illusions (for example, the Poggendorf illusion) have not yet been subject to a comparable analysis. In the next chapter we shall also deal with the problem of whether or not some of the current physiological theorizing has been, in fact, premature. This problem arises because some physiological processes are superficially similar in functional form to some perceptual phenomena, and thus analogues of functional form have often been mis-perceived as homologous neural mechanisms by some authors. Very often, properties initially explained by simple geometric neural net interactions are found later to depend upon very complex cognitive properties such as meaning or form similiarity. Neural net analyses are hard pressed, in spite of their superficial relevance, to handle such situations.

The point that is being made here is that interactions based upon the geometry of a stimulus pattern may not be satisfactory explanations when the stimulus information has been encoded and represented at some symbolic or semantic level, where a square is no longer a square geo-metrically but only in terms of certain cognitive implications. For example, where an entire object is masked as a total entity rather then only the por-tion of it that is close to a masking stimulus, it is hard to see how one can apply a theory of lateral interactions that is heavily dependent upon geometrical propinquity and well-defined distance functions.

We shall have little to say in this chapter about the spatial or tem-poral aspects of the chemical senses. Because of the difficulty of stimulus control, experiments involving spatial and temporal manipulations in these modalities are very hard to instrument. Moreover, one might also suspect, a priori, that these chemical modalities are not primarily designed to cope with the spatial and temporal dimensions. Those senses that have so evolved—hearing, vision, and to a lesser degree the somatosensory senses—will, therefore, be the main source of experimental information as we pursue our analysis.

Any generalization of the sort described in the previous paragraph is likely to fall victim to the inventions of some ingenious experimenter. Indeed, von Békésy (1964a) seems to have pushed the notions of lateral interaction and spatial localization to their extremes in his demonstrations of the ability of the olfactory and gustatory senses to localize chemical stimuli. This feat seems to be accomplished on the same basis (differences in time of arrival of the stimulus to different portions of the tongue or olfactory receptors) that underlies acoustic spatial localization. However, this occurs under some highly unusual laboratory conditions, which do not seem to obtain regularly in human experience. The general notion that the chemical senses are weak as discriminators of time and space still seems to be valid.

Another difficulty in organizing this chapter arises out of the fact that space and time interact so strongly and are traded off, one for the other, in many different situations. It is not always going to be satisfying to the reader that a particular topic has been suitably placed if it is con-sidered solely in terms of either spatial or temporal dimensions. Very often stimulus conditions that are varying in the temporal domain will be encoded by spatial parameters and, in fact, be perceived as varying along a spatial continuum. Similarly, we shall also often see instances in which spatial dimensions are encoded by signals varying in the temporal domain and examples of temporal neural response patterns critically dependent on spatial aspects of a stimulus. It is important, therefore, that we distinguish between a number of related notions. We must speak of the spatial or temporal pattern of the stimulus independently of the spatial or temporal pattern of the neural code. In some instances we must even keep these notions separate from the temporal and spatial dimensions of the perceived experience. To do so, of course, is to take advantage of the great strength of sensory-coding theory. It allows—in fact, emphasizes—that stimulus, neural and experiential patterns need not be isomorphic at their respective levels of representation.

B. Time and Space

What do we mean by time and temporal patterns? What do we mean by space and form? In considering the answers to these questions, we must first consider whether they really are two separate domains. A common sense answer is that they certainly are. We use rulers (rulers which, of course, may be as sophisticated as the wavelength of a certain kind of light) to measure distance and clocks to measure times. But this common sense answer is deceptive. The initial answer is common sense only in the terms of a particular physical model of reality—Newtonian physics and Euclidean geometry—which has been superseded among physical scientists for over half a century by constructs that are, at first glance, very much contrary to "common sense."

Classical Newtonian physics dealt with the three dimensions of space as if they were constant. The shape of the coordinate system did not depend upon the events going on in time in the system or the objects that were contained therein. Time was a separate factor, which could be measured or not in any given experiment. Yet, even in a timeless snapshot, the spatial coordinates remained rigid and fixed. Parallel lines were parallel (except for errors of measurement) out to infinity, and indeed the notion of infinity was axiomatic in this system, since no one could imagine what could lie on the other side of the end of the universe. Mass was constant and the laws of the conservation of mass and energy almost religiously adhered to.

The more modern relativistic theories, largely based on the contributions of that unique intellect Albert Einstein, have changed our perspective considerably. Not only has the notion of the interchangeability of mass and energy, along with the attendant enormous social consequences, been introduced, but even the parallel universe of Euclidean geometry has been replaced by one in which parallel lines meet somewhere "out there." Furthermore, and getting to the present point, the coordinate systems themselves came to be seen as depending upon the nature of the bodies contained within a volume and their states of motion.

Modern relativistic physics—the Einsteinian model of reality—further suggests that time and space are not as separate as our older common sense notions would suggest. The popular persistence of the "common sense" Newtonian notions of space and time is probably largely due to the fact that Einsteinian relativistic notions are primarily concepts that become relevant at levels of speed and size at which most people infrequently operate. The dimensions of our daily lives are well enough described by Newtonian ideas so that we never really deal with the discrepancies that physicists encounter when they are dealing with enormous or very small masses or great speeds.

In point of fact, even the idea that we use differing measuring instruments to measure time and space falls by the wayside in the illuminating light of the new clocks, which turn out to be the very same devices used as a ruler for the spatial dimensions. A modern clock is nothing more (or less) than a specific light emitted by some selected atomic substance. This is done by a process which, not too surprisingly, turns out to be the measurement with a spectroscope of the *wavelength* of the emitted line. The wavelength and the frequency of vibrations are then related by Equation (3.19) presented earlier in this book. The basic unit of time, then, is defined as the period it takes for a certain number of these vibrations to occur. In the world of atomic dimensions, space and time are no longer even separated by different measurement operations.

Thus, the major new contribution of Einsteinian relativistic physics may be viewed as the fact that space and time are now considered to be but alternate attributes of a multidimensional continuum, and neither can be considered independently of the other. Capek (1961) points out that this notion of the inseparability of space and time has often been misunderstood to mean that time has been reduced to simply another spatial dimension ("the fourth dimension"), but he emphasizes that in fact this is a misinterpretation of the real significance of the idea. He suggests, rather, that the new unity is "more accurately described as a temporalization or dynamization of space than a spatialization of time."

One of the advantages of the approach that considers time as not just another spatial dimension is that time need no longer be forced to fit the same set of characteristics exhibited by any of the other three spatial dimensions. It need not be required, for example, that time be bidirectional—a notion implicit in its assignment of the status of simply another spatial dimension. In bidirectional time, time machines and perpetual motion and a host of other science fiction ideas take on validity which still seems questionable. If Capek is right that we should dynamize or temporalize the three spatial dimensions rather than adding time as a fourth dimension, then we are able to hold on to a very important notion—the undirectionality of time.

In a notable modern consideration of the directionality of time, *Time's Arrow and Evolution*, Blum (1955) points out that there is a directionality imposed on time that is not imposed on a spatial dimension. That is the second law of thermodynamics—a physical law which he believes is time's "arrow," imparting a directionality to the sequence of events. The idea is that, on the whole, the universe must be running downhill to a state of greater and greater entropy or disorganization. In local regions, such as areas of time-space where ontogenetic or phylogenetic development is occurring, decreases in entropy (increasing order) can appear to occur, but this is at the expense of energy resources at other places in the universe. Thus, while organic evolution can produce an increasingly organized and more complex species, and while the individual grows from a state of minimum order to a greater degree of order, these local reversals of time's arrow represent anomalies, and the true overall state of the universe is one of increasing disorder.

The implications of modern relativistic theory linking time and space and of this notion of unidirectional time are enormous, and many philosopher-physicists have spent and will continue to spend a not inconsiderable sum of intellectual energy trying to fully interpret their significance. It is most important to note that psychobiological data and theory may also be impelling neurophysiologists and psychologists in exactly the same direction. If, as we have noted, temporal stimulus patterns are often represented by spatial neurophysiological patterns and spatial stimulus patterns by temporal neurophysiological patterns, then it is meaningless to talk about the spatial code independent of time. A simple spatial plot of the events involved in the neurophysiological representation of the localization of a sound source, for example, obscures the most critical information involved. Similarly, a "temporal snapshot" is not too unreasonable a description of the time function usually plotted as a result of single microelectrode experiments.

These ideas suggest the current emergence of a new sort of relativism in psychobiology, just as at the turn of the twentieth century, physics evolved a new concept of space and time in its domain. Time and space (as well as, to some degree, intensity and quality) should probably be looked at together rather than separately as we have in the past. Of course, this sort of a conceptual revolution is not going to come about immediately, and we shall have to depend upon the existing sorts of data until new methodologies, new equipment, and, perhaps most important, new perspectives evolve.

As for the questions of what is space, what is time, or even what is psychobiological space-time, we still are confronted with very much the same problem that we had when we tried to define the intensive dimension. There just are no adequately precise definitions possible. There are only conventions of general agreement and certain classes of operations that act as exemplars of what the concepts of time and space mean to experimenters. It is probably the case that a better picture of what is meant by time and space will emerge from the discussion that follows in this chapter than from any attempt to specifically define such abstruse concepts.

II. SPATIAL AND TEMPORAL ACUITY

Of all the neurophysiological correlates of perceptual phenomena, perhaps none is so simple to handle conceptually as is the problem of the loss of temporal and spatial acuity that occurs as one passes from the peripheral neural response to the psychophysical response. Yet, perhaps, no single concept is as fundamental and with such widespread implications. It is a fact that we are not able to separately feel or see two stimulus points that are closer than a certain minimum distance or to distinguish, as successive, two events that are closer than a certain minimum time interval. This is so in spite of the fact that the neural responses are quite distinct either spatially or temporally when one looks at the peripheral neural response. Yet centrally the neuronal response does display a corresponding loss in discriminability as it is distributed in both time and space far beyond the limits of the peripheral response.

We refer to the perceptual phenomena, which we shall discuss generally, as temporal and spatial acuity. The notion of spatial acuity includes, among other more restricted notions, the historic and fundamental ideas implicit in the measurement of the two-point threshold. The notion of temporal acuity has been generalized, on the other hand, into the more comprehensive concept of the "psychological moment." The moment is the indivisible period of time in which, at least, some workers thought subjects lost the ability to determine both simultaneity and successiveness. We shall discuss later the variations on the theme of the psychological moment that have emerged in recent years.

In the neurophysiological domain, psychophysical spatial acuity is embodied in the notion of the "receptive field." The receptive field is defined for some specific neurological structure, however, and this is sometimes forgotten in the psychophysical literature. A receptive field of a neuron, for example, is defined as that portion of the total receptive surface that is capable of eliciting a response from that neuron. It is important to remember that the fields of interaction, which are measured psychophysically, may not be identical to the receptive field of a specific and single neural unit. The psychophysical finding may, on the other hand, reflect the action of complex systems of overlapping neural receptive fields.

Nevertheless, there are conceptual, if not anatomical, correspondences between the two sets of data, which make a coding analysis such as the one that follows useful. Again the reader is reminded that the relation between the spatial extent of the percept and of the nerve is just as much as part of the coding problem as is the relation between subjective magnitude and action potential frequency with which he is more familiar.

The general problem of the loss of information as the signal ascends the nervous system is emphasized in the subsequent discussion of temporal and spatial acuity. Such data are critically important to our understanding of the rate and flow of information processing in the nervous system. Furthermore, the clear contrast between the acuity evidenced in the peripheral nervous response and that evidenced in the psychophysical response is one of the most obvious clues to the sort of pitfalls one can encounter when one attempts to explain psychophysics by referring to neurophysiological codes far removed from the central level at which the final decoding actually takes place. A model of coding based upon the characteristics and codes of the peripheral nervous response ignores the fact that a considerable amount of further processing, including the loss of information, has occurred between the two levels. It ignores the fact that information has, even at that level, already been encoded several different ways. It, thus, attributes a uniqueness to one level or one code, which is far from the reality of the situation.

A. Convergence and Divergence in Neural Nets

To begin our consideration of the neural coding of time and space, we shall consider two analogous concepts limiting sensory acuity. First, we must note the existence of the spatial receptive field, which tends to reduce spatial acuity in several sensory modalities. Because of the anatomical organization of many receptor surfaces, it is a general fact that stimuli applied to any portion of a relatively large area do not initiate activity solely in a single afferent neuron. Notwithstanding the presence of other neural processes which tend to sharpen the representations of stimulus patterns, the anatomical convergence of many inputs on a single output tends to make it less likely that the precise locus of incoming information can be identified.

Second, we should also note that there is a similar sort of diffusing effect limiting temporal acuity. Two stimuli that are separated from each other by less than some minimum interval cannot be resolved. This loss of acuity in the temporal domain is probably due to neural mechanisms, which are direct opposites of those responsible for the loss of spatial acuity. Spatial acuity is mainly lost because of the *convergence* of many input fibers onto a single output fiber. Temporal acuity, on the other hand, is lost primarily because of the great *divergence* of input fibers onto a far greater number of output fibers, the responses of which are extended over a considerable period of time. A single neural response in a peripheral somatosensory fiber, which may last for only about 1 msec, can lead to the activation of literally millions of central neurons, whose cumulative action lasts for 1 sec or more. The important physiological constructs of divergence and convergence that underlie these losses of temporal and spatial acuity were first described by Sherrington, a neurophysiologist who probably comes as close as anyone to playing the role for this science that Einstein did for physics.

Figure 7.1 (a) and (b) are simplified sketches of neural convergence and divergence, respectively. As shown in part (a) of this figure, the basic premise of convergence is that many input fibers from different locations synapse upon a single output fiber. In such a system, while information can be preserved concerning the pooled timing of the responses of the family of input cells, it is not possible to tell, by observing the activity of the output cell, whence the input signal came. This holds true not only for the electrophysiologist who might be observing the output of the cell with a microelectrode as well as the decoding mechanisms of some psychophysical subject's central nervous system. The different information needed to do so is simply no longer available, having been lost at the interface between the input and the output neurons.

Divergence, the opposing mechanism, is represented in Figure 7.1(b). Although divergence, as originally conceived by Sherrington, was a purely spatial concept (one input cell produces responses in a larger number of output cells), the notion as we shall use it is a more complex one. We shall be concerned with both spatial and temporal divergence such that both the number of cells involved in the response and the duration over which they are active are expanded. Spatial divergence is a simple notion and is explained fully by a single mechanism, but it should be noted that response duration can be expanded by two or more mechanisms. For example, a potent temporal extender would be a system of feedback loops, which maintain reverberatory activity. In such a network, a given cell would be reactivated either directly or indirectly by its own output. The reactivation might be mediated by a single synaptic relay or by the action of a highly complex neural net, but in each case the end result would be a prolongation

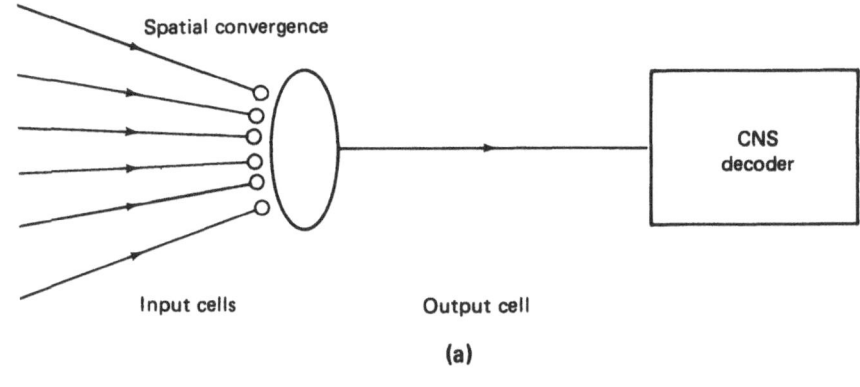

(a)

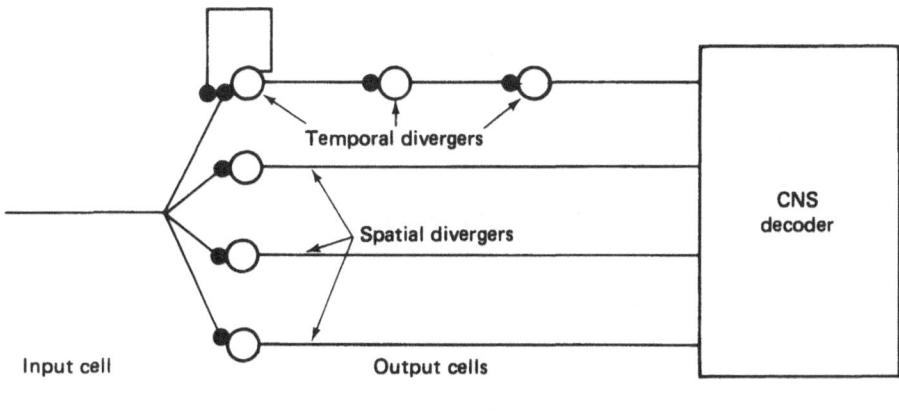

(b)

FIGURE 7.1 (a) *A schematic diagram of spatial convergence in neural systems.* (b) *A schematic diagram of spatial and temporal divergence in neural systems.*

of the time course of the original response. Another mechanism, which might also contribute to the prolongation of a neural response, is simply that chains of neurons of varying length may be involved. Though there are but a few (four or five) neurons in the typical direct sensory pathway, there is no assurance that very long sequences are not activated as responses course through the various levels of the central nervous system.

The end result of neural divergence, feedback, and the activation of chains of varying length is that a single spike action potential in a peripheral nerve can be extended into a central nervous system response that may last for many seconds. Information is certainly lost in this manner as the response is prolonged, for the ability to distinguish, when a stimulus occurred or if there were more than a single stimulus, is diminished as the response it evokes is extended over a long period of time. The loss of psychophysical temporal acuity [for example, two action potentials that are perfectly resolved at 1 or 2 msec in peripheral somatosensory nerves (Uttal, 1959; Rosner, 1961) can only be psychophysically resolved at 10 to 12 msec separation] is probably due to this sort of prolongation of the response duration at the level of the central nervous system.

In sum, neural divergence and convergence, while both necessary as integrating mechanisms, do tend to reduce the amount of available information—convergence by tending to establish a spatial receptive field in which differences in localization cannot be discriminated, and divergence by tending to establish a temporal period in which differences in time of occurrence cannot be discriminated. We shall now consider these two related notions in detail.

B. Spatial Acuity and Receptive Fields

1. The Two-Point Threshold—A Psychophysical Correlate of the Neural Receptive Field. The notion of the cutaneous two-point threshold, one kind of spatial acuity, was introduced into psychological research by Weber (1834). The classical two-point limen experiment involved the placement of the two points of a compass on the skin and the determination of the threshold separation required for the two stimuli to be discriminated as two rather than one point. One interesting early discovery was that the size of the two-point limen varies over the surface of the body. The most modern determination of these size differences at different locations on the surface of the body has been made by Weinstein (1968). His study was a modern replication of the classic work done over a century earlier by Weber. It was intended to extend the measurements of the two-point threshold by examining the effect of sex and of laterality in addition to the dimension of body part used by Weber. Weinstein used a group of 24 men and 24 women, all of whom were right-handed and the standard two-point compass as an aesthesiometer. Figure 7.2 presents the results of his work for men. An analysis of his data shows that as Weber observed, by far the strongest effect was produced by varying the part of the body examined. With regard to the parameters of sex and laterality, Weinstein found that few of the comparisons showed significant differences.

From the very beginning, Weber hypothesized that the two-point threshold was probably due to neural convergence. His notion was that the terminal arborizations of a given cutaneous afferent fiber spread over a relatively large area (clearly an antecedent of the modern idea of a receptive field) and that stimulation anywhere within this area led to indistinguishable sensations. The drawings of these areas, sensory circles in Weber's terminology, suggest however that he did not believe that they were overlapping. Overlap is a relatively modern concept and is now an integral part of the basic notion of the receptive field.

A further development, which has become apparent since Weber's early studies, has been the emerging realization that the sensory "circle" on the limbs is not a circle after all, but probably more generally has an oval outline. This is particularly noticeable when small electrical shocks are used rather than mechanical stimuli. Presumably the oval shape of receptive fields reflects the fact that the nervous system is organized such that

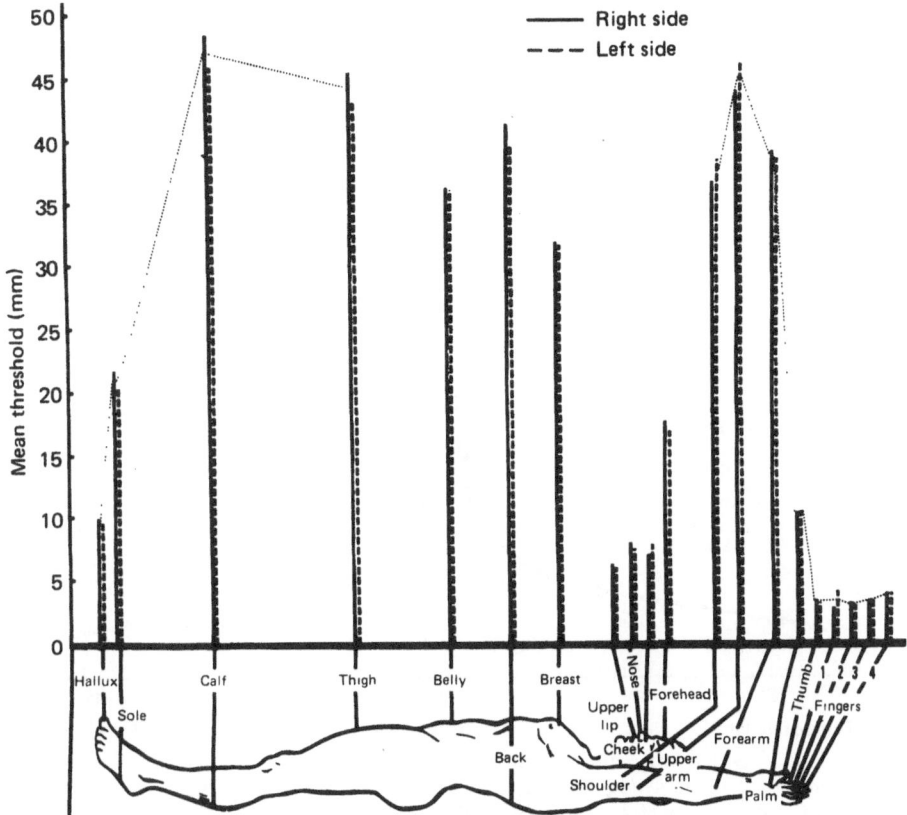

FIGURE 7.2 A drawing showing two-point discrimination values as a function
of body location for males (from Weinstein, 1968).

fibers run more along the limbs than across it. On the forearm particularly,
the difference in two-point thresholds can be as great as 10 to 1 when one
measures along rather than across the arm with electrical stimuli.

The visual analogue of the somatosensory two-point threshold is
acuity. The general problem here is to determine how close two photic
stimuli can be to each other and still be distinguished as separate entities.
A wide variety of acuity measuring tests have been developed over the
years including grids, letters, and broken circles. These devices usually indicate that the maximum visual acuity is about 1 min of visual angle. However, by far the most sensitive acuity measures seem to be obtained for the
"hanging wire." Thin lines, 2 or 3 sec of visual angle wide, a width which
is far smaller than the width of a single cone in the primate eye [which
according to Polyak (1941) varies from 12 to 18 sec of visual angle] can
be detected *if they are long enough!* The last phrase, "if they are long
enough," suggests that the limits on visual acuity are not solely determined by the dimensions of the retinal mosaic, or by receptive field size, but
that some sort of integrative or statistical processing associated with inter-

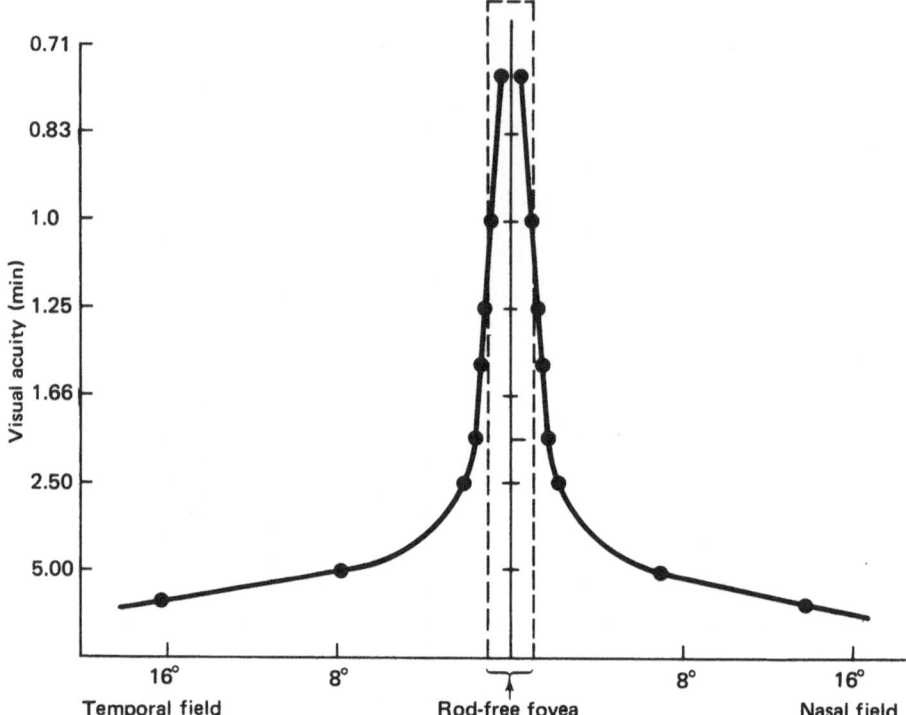

FIGURE 7.3 *Visual acuity plotted as a function of visual angle. Note that once away from the central 4-deg region, there is little further decline in acuity out to 16 deg of visual angle (from Alpern, 1969).*

action among adjacent regions is possible. Thus, a series of adjacent regions may each contribute to the collective process that detects the wire, even though no single region alone would have been able to elicit that response.

Visual acuity monotonically decreases as the stimulus moves further away from the fovea as shown in Figure 7.3, but most of the falloff occurs within the central 4 deg; after that the acuity function is relatively flat. Peripheral regions of the retina, where rods predominate, seem to have particularly poor acuity. This fact is probably attributable to the high ratio of convergence of rods on optic nerve ganglion cells, a number of which may be as high as several thousand to one. An excellent and complete discussion of many other of the psychophysical details of visual acuity and of the determining parameters is available in Rigg's chapter in Graham's (1965) important book on vision and visual perception.

Another means of formally specifying the ability of the eye to discriminate between adjacent objects involves the measurement of the subject's ability to tell whether a grating differs from a uniform field. The grating is generated either by means of photographic plates or on the face of a CRT in such a way that a time stable intensity pattern varies sinus-

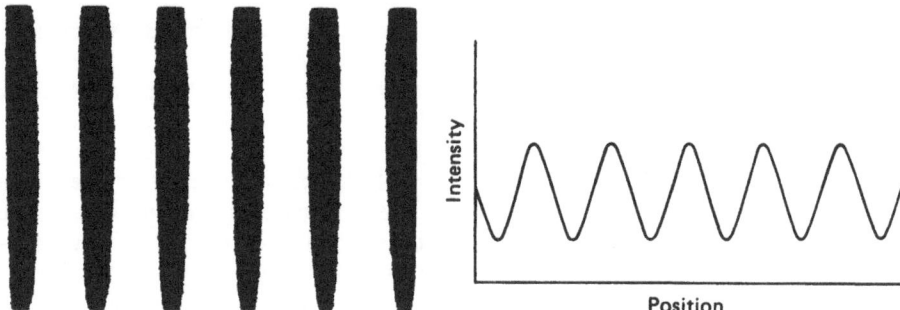

FIGURE 7.4 A spatial sine wave grating and a graph showing the brightness level across the grating (from Cornsweet, 1970).

oidally across the field of the image as shown in Figure 7.4. Schade (1956) was probably the first to use this type of modulation transfer function (MTF) or contrast sensitivity measure (CSM), but recently the notion has been further developed by Campbell and Green (1965), Green (1968), and by Davidson (1968). A particularly lucid and complete discussion of the technique has recently been given by Cornsweet (1970).

In brief, the contrast threshold of a sinusoidal grating of varying spatial frequencies (usually measured in cycles per degree of visual angle) is determined using the modulation ratio (the ratio of brightnesses of the darkest trough to the brightest peak) as a dependent variable. Figure 7.5 is a typical plot of the modulation ratio required for visual detection of the contrast of a green colored grating on a green background as a function of the spatial frequency of the grating. The ratio required is modest at low frequencies (broad bands); increases at intermediate frequencies (indicating that there is an optimal or resonant region), and then decreases steeply as

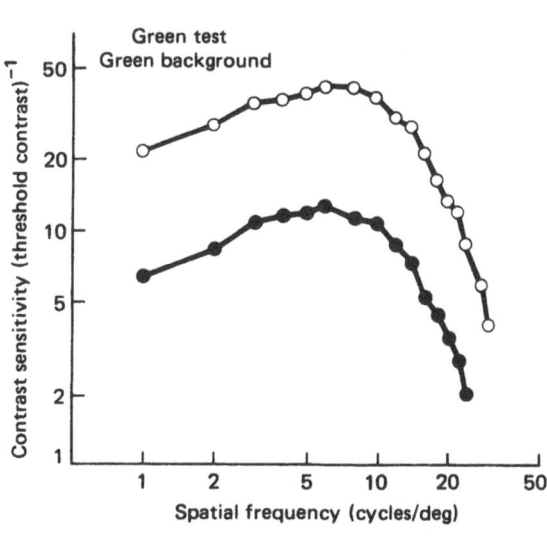

FIGURE 7.5 The results of an experiment in spatial sine wave detection. The subject's task was to detect a green grating against a bright green background. Data are presented for two different background brightnesses with the open circles being the results for the brighter of the two backgrounds (from Green, 1968).

the grid lines narrow and the spatial frequency increases beyond 10 cycles/ deg of visual angle.

Cornsweet has applied this notion to a far wider range of subject matters than just the notion of separable stimuli. His discussion also indicates how the simple modulation transfer function or contrast sensitivity measure can be used to predict the Mach band illusion. The reader is directed to that discussion for further details. However, it should also be noted that though the mathematical model of contrast sensitivity may adequately describe the phenomenon, this is not a necessary and sufficient proof that any particular neural interactive mechanism is in action. Several analogous mechanisms could produce similar results without showing any homologous structure.

Are there analogous phenomena in the auditory system? The answer to this question, which might initially come to mind, is the discrimination of differences in acoustical spatial localization, but as we have repeatedly pointed out, this phenomenon is probably not mediated by equivalent spatial neural mechanisms. Auditory spatial localization is a discrimination which, from a neural point of view, is quite unlike visual acuity—rather, it seems to be encoded by differences in the phase and intensity of the two transmitted dichotic signals. When considered from the perspective of the similarity of neural codes, the true analogue for spatial acuity on the skin or in the eye is auditory frequency discrimination itself. Two auditory stimuli produce different spatial patterns on the basilar membrane with maxima located at nearby points. This phenomenon is supposed to be the basis of pitch encoding and frequency (quality) discrimination and will, therefore, be discussed mainly in Chapter 10 when we consider theories of auditory quality coding. But the discrimination of similar tones must also be considered in the context of the present discussion, for this frequency discrimination appears to depend upon the ability to distinguish the patterns of stimulation on the cochlea in a way quite similar to that in which Weber's two-point limen was conceived to be operating on the skin. The corollary notion of receptive fields, namely, that they are overlapping, is also an especially important consideration in this auditory context, because the cochlear response patterns produced even by pure tonal stimuli are not highly localized, but rather are distributed across almost the entire surface of the cochlea.

Auditory frequency discrimination curves, which are the best analogues of the two-point threshold, can be measured in a number of different ways. All of the methods agree that the size of a just detectable change in frequency depends not only on the frequency of the stimulus, but also upon its intensity. The data, which are considered definitive in the description of auditory frequency discrimination, were obtained by Shower and Biddulph (1931) and have been replotted in an information packed fashion by Licklider (1951a). This chart is reproduced in Figure 7.6. This three-dimensional representation shows that frequency discrimination can be extremely fine; over a large region of the surface, the subject is able to distinguish frequency differences less than 4 cycles/sec. A first approximation to explaining these data may be obtained by also plotting in Figure 7.7 data adapted from von Békésy (1949), in which the locus of the maximum

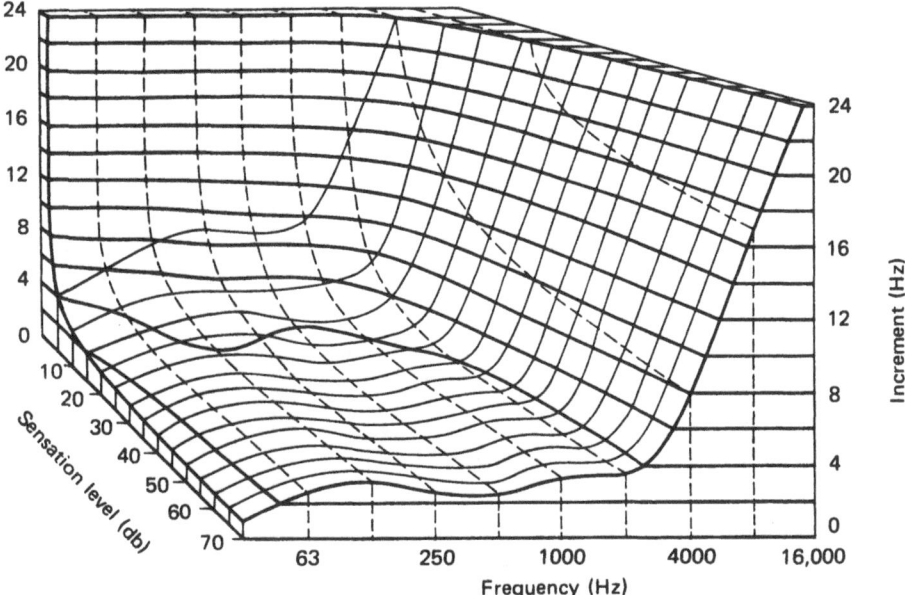

FIGURE 7.6 A plot of the surface representing auditory frequency discrimination as a function of acoustic stimulus frequency and amplitude. Auditory frequency discrimination is as good as 2 or 3 Hz in many parts of this space (from Licklider, 1951a, after Shower and Biddulph, 1931).

vibration of the cochlear partition is plotted as a function of the frequency of the vibrating tone. The function is roughly linear, and this could be used to explain the flattened portion of the frequency discrimination curve. Equal distances on the cochlea could, possibly, be associated with equal just noticeable differences in the psychophysical domain. Clearly, however, the notion of simple two-point discrimination cannot be pushed too far as a detailed explanatory model of auditory frequency discrimination.

Nevertheless, the general notion of spatial interactions as an explanatory mechanism for frequency discrimination has been furthered by the models developed by von Békésy. The difficulties of working directly at the microscopic level of the cochlea led him to develop a hydraulic model of the cochlea, upon which a subject could lay his arm. The arm played the role in this model of the array of hair cells aligned along the basilar membrane, while the fluid-filled rubber model (shown in Figure 7.8) modeled the fluid-filled cochlea. Vibratory patterns introduced at one end of the tube (just as they would have entered the oval window in the real cochlea) set up traveling wave patterns on the surface of the rubber "cochlea," which were then picked up and "processed" by the somatosensory system.

Von Békésy's notions of the significance of the various parts of the model system have been misunderstood in part by at least some observers. The actual physical localization of a band of maximum activity at a particular place on the rubber model was a function of the rubber tube, and not

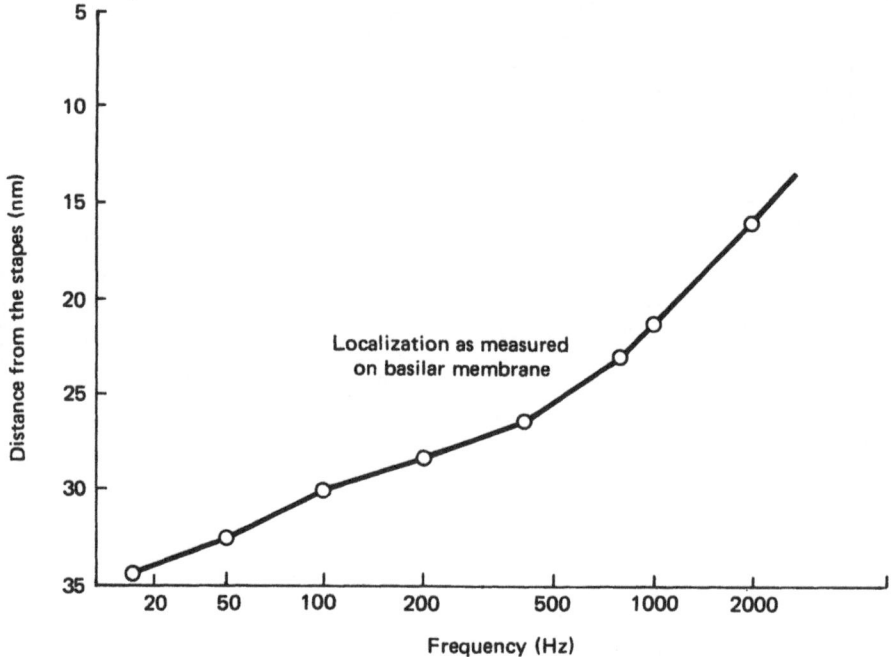

FIGURE 7.7 *A graph showing the location of the maximum amplitude of deflection on the basilar membrane as a function of the frequency of the stimulating stimulus (from von Békésy, 1949a).*

of any "neural interaction on the forearm." This point is well made by running one's finger along the tube. A maximum point of oscillation is clearly detectable at a particular place on the tube purely as a function of the frequency of stimulation and independently of whether the forearm is on the rubber tube or not. That maximum point is determined by the pattern of the traveling waves within the fluid-filled rubber chamber.

Von Békésy did, quite separately, emphasize the fact that there is further processing of this spatially localized information by the subject's nervous system. This sort of processing was assumed by him to be typified by a sharpening process, which tends to make the spatial experiences felt by the subject more precisely localized than the actual pattern of the stimulus transduced from the rubber tube would be expected to invoke. Such sharpening mechanisms were largely thought by him to be due to interactions among adjacent neural units, but as we shall see later, it is not completely clear that such neural sharpening really exists!

2. Neurophysiological Evidence for the Existence of Receptive Fields. Now that we have discussed the psychophysics of the two-point threshold and of some related perceptual phenomena, we shall turn our attention to those neurophysiological mechanisms that may possibly underlie or encode those experiences. Basic neuroanatomical evidence suggests that some sort of

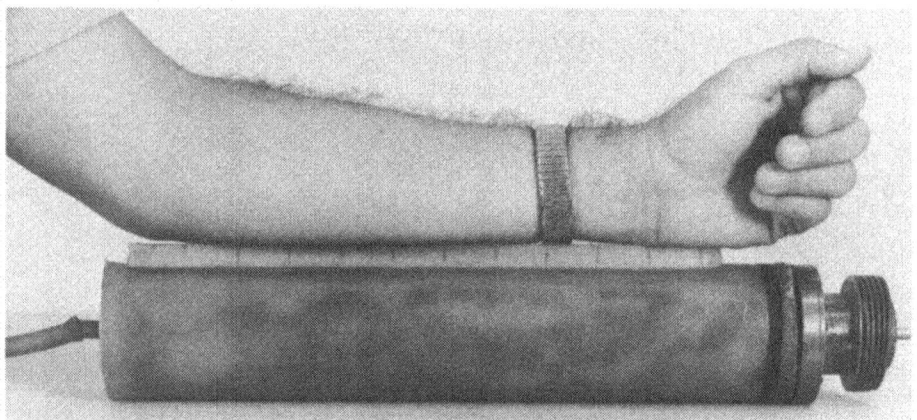

FIGURE 7.8 *Photograph showing von Békésy's water-filled rubber tube model of human cochlea. In this model, the arm is the model of the array of hair cells, and it is there that any lateral inhibitory interaction is analogized, but the tube does tend to spatially localize the different frequencies of different places independent of the presence of the arm (courtesy of Dr. Robert Cole, University of Hawaii).*

convergence is present in all sensory systems and that, therefore, the receptive field type of organization is ubiquitous. For example, in the retina Polyak (1941) has estimated that there are over 130 million rods and over 4 million cones, but that in the optic nerve there are probably few more than 1 million ganglion cell axons. On the average, then, the responses of multiple retinal locations must be signaled along single axons, and this is exactly what is meant by the notion of a receptive field. More recent evidence has indicated that perhaps a few foveal cones have private communication lines, but that virtually all rods share ganglion cell axons. At the periphery, the information from several hundred rods may all ultimately converge on a single ganglion cell fiber.

Similarly in the somatosensory system, although there are no synapses prior to the spinal cord, there are abundant ramifications of the cutaneous nerve fibers. This is also a sort of convergent mechanism for signals originating at different spatial locations. In this instance also, even though there are no many-to-one synapses, the information from the various branches is pooled along a single afferent nerve fiber.

The number of auditory nerve neurons has been placed at about 50,000 by Gacek and Rasmussen (1961) for many mammals (pig, cat, and monkey), while the number of receptor hair cells in their cochleas is only about 25,000. This is exceptional and, thus, once again points out the somewhat peculiar features of the auditory receptor mechanism. Nevertheless, as we saw earlier in the chapter on receptor anatomy, there is an overlapping sort of innervation which allows a specific region of the organ of Corti (a "receptive field"), including many hair cells, to be serviced by a single cochlear nerve axon. Furthermore, according to Stevens and Davis

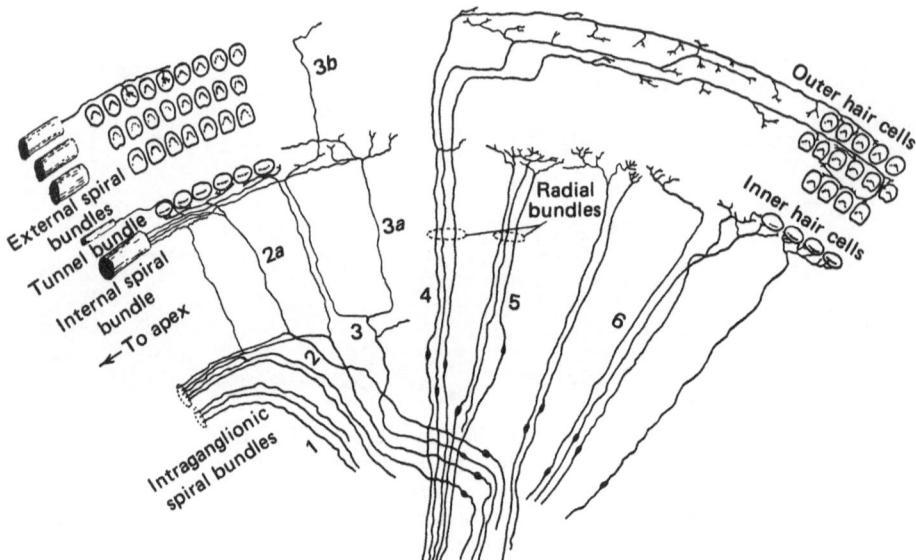

FIGURE 7.9 A schematic drawing of the arrangement of nerve fibers in the basilar membrane, showing the extensive opportunity for lateral inhibitory interaction and the convergence of the outputs of the receptors onto single auditory nerve fibers (from Wever, 1949).

(1938), single cochlea nerve fibers make contact with a very large number of external hair cells, although only two or three internal hair cells are connected to a single cochlear nerve neuron. Figure 7.9 shows the elaborate nature of this convergence.

It should be noted that the only way to determine the shape of the receptive field of a single neuron is to carry out an experiment with a particular and characteristic design. An appropriate stimulus is used to explore a region that might possibly be associated with the responses of a certain cell. By observing the evoked activity of the single neuron as the stimulus is moved about in the potential receptive, field its actual receptive field can be very precisely determined and its extent plotted.

However, the first sensory modality, in which receptive fields were plotted, was the somatosensory receptive system, and single neuron responses were not the physiological indicators used. Sherrington conceived of the idea of using reflex action as a means of mapping the "dermatomes" of whole somatosensory nerves. Dermatomes were clearly precursors of the modern notions of receptive fields. In a volume of his collected works, Sherrington (1940) describes the techniques for mapping the dermatomes on the limbs of Macaque monkeys, using blood pressure or the response of antagonistic muscle groups as the indicator of a response. His drawings, one example of which is given in Figure 7.10, illustrate how precise these techniques were for the definition of the field of action of an entire nerve. The technique typically involved the surgical isolation of a single spinal

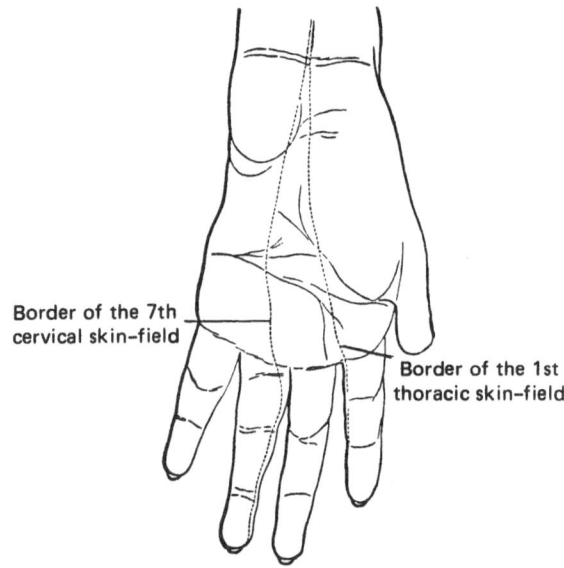

Border of the 7th
cervical skin-field

Border of the 1st
thoracic skin-field

FIGURE 7.10 A drawing of the hand of a monkey, showing the distinct borders between the regions serviced by different sensory nerves (from Sherrington, 1940).

nerve trunk, whose activation would give rise to the specific reflex. The skin was then probed and stimulated and a map prepared of the regions that would give the reflex. The area within which a response could be evoked was considered to be served by the single remaining nerve trunk.

This work was done in the late 1800s and antedated the development of the modern electrophysiological techniques for single cell analysis. In more recent times, electronic microtechnique has been applied to the same problem, and some important new insights into the degree of convergence (and, as we shall also see, the degree of divergence) have been obtained.

A most graphic representation of the size and shape of peripheral receptive fields in single neurons is given in Figure 7.11, which shows photographs of the hand of a monkey with two types of receptive fields drawn in. This picture (from Talbot, Darian-Smith, Kornhuber, and Mountcastle, 1968) shows the details of receptive fields of neurons in the median nerve of a Macaque monkey. Mountcastle (1961) also points out that the receptive fields for somatosensory cortical cells are up to 100 times larger than the peripheral neuron ones, indicating further spatial convergence at higher levels of the nervous system.

Perhaps the most extensive set of measurements and precise specification of receptive fields have been obtained in experiments on the visual system. While a number of relatively conventional recording systems have been used by numerous investigators, one of the most modern and most interesting is the computerized system developed by Spinelli (1967) to plot the receptive fields of the cat's optic nerve fibers. Figure 7.12 displays his complete system. Stimuli were presented on a 25 deg by 25 deg field by positioning a spot (either black on white or white on black) by means of an x-y coordinate servosystem, controlled by the output of a small digital

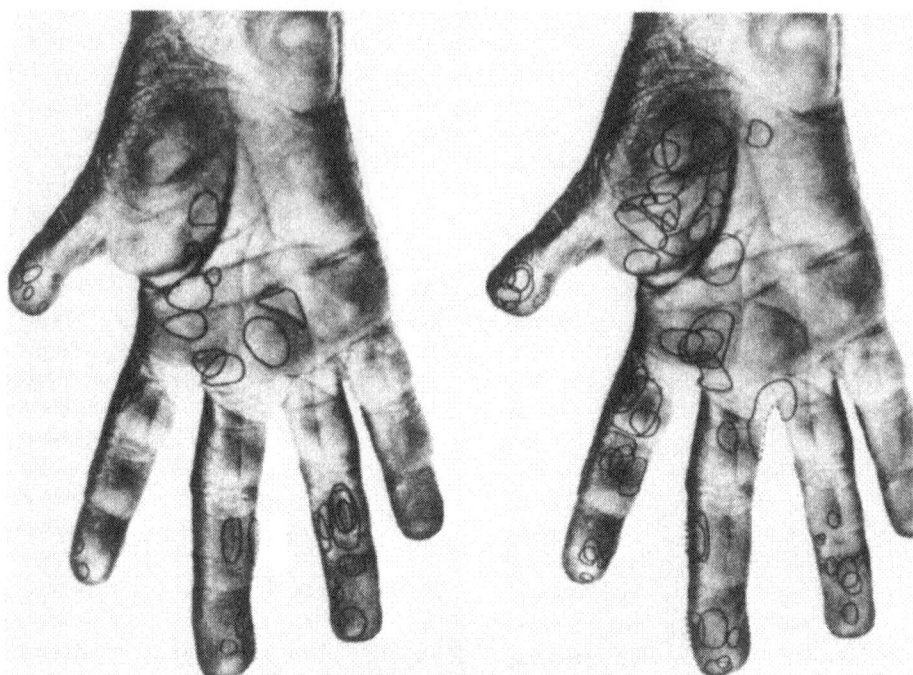

FIGURE 7.11 Drawings, superimposed on photographs of the monkey's hand, showing the shape and extent of the receptive fields of single afferent fibers (from Talbot, Darian-Smith, Kornhuber, and Mountcastle, 1968).

computer. The computer also picked up spike potential activity with micro-electrodes inserted into the optic nerve and counted the number of spike action potentials occurring when the stimulus was positioned at a particular location. To determine the extent and shape of the receptive field of a given optic nerve neuron, Spinelli programmed the computer to move the spot along 50 horizontal lines, each ½ deg apart and each 25 deg long. Counts were made of the amount of activity evoked at each ½-deg separation in both directions. The data were then plotted on a two-dimensional CRT display in the following manner. A spot of light was plotted in each of the 50 × 50 regions defined by the scanning procedure only if the number of nerve action potentials exceeded some criterion.

Figure 7.13 is a sample of this sort of plot. The two displays in this figure result from an experiment in which the direction of scan [(a) horizontal, (b) vertical] was varied, while all other dimensions were held constant to determine if direction of motion of the stimulus spot was an important parameter in defining receptive field shape. The similarity in shape and distribution of the dots in each case illustrates the relative indifference of the shape of the cat's optic nerve receptive field to the direction of movement of a stimulus. It should be noted, at this point, that this result

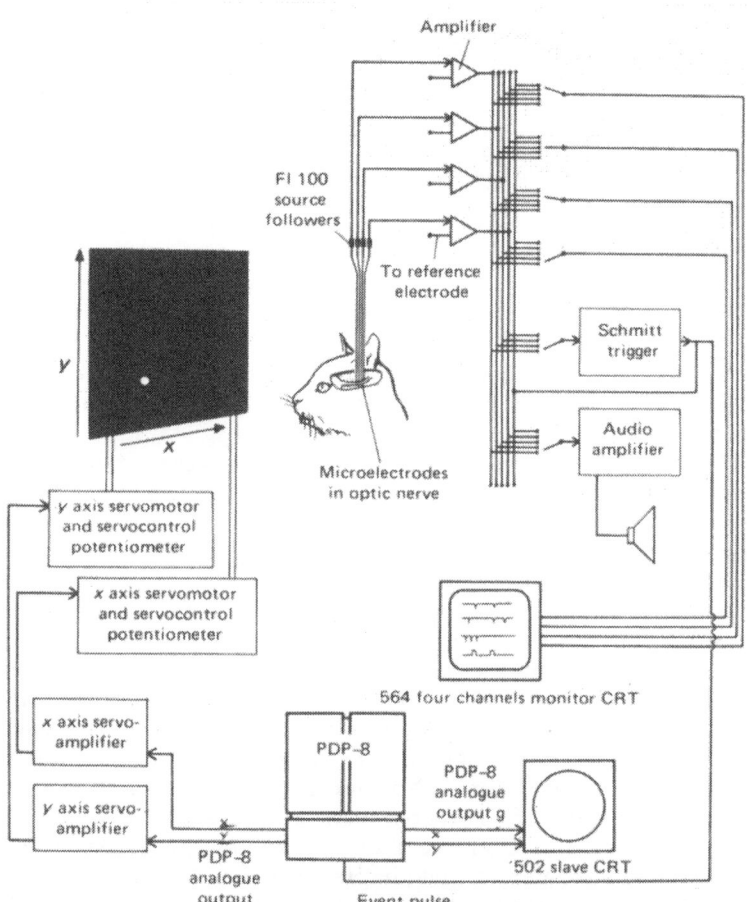

FIGURE 7.12 A diagram of the experimental apparatus used by Spinelli to automatically plot out the receptive field of visual system neurons. Note the PDP-8 computer, which automatically controls the presentation and location of the stimuli as well as tabulating the pulse modulated data generated by the Schmitt trigger—a device that emits a standard pulse whenever a nerve impulse crosses a criterion amplitude (from Spinelli, 1967).

is species specific and that we shall discuss later in this chapter retinal directional sensitivity in both the rabbit and the frog.

This sort of plot also begins to give us an idea of the complexity of the visual receptive field. The particular field shown is not uniformly excitatory, but in this case there is a central region in which a stimulus seems to inhibit the response to a level below spontaneous activity. Spinelli found this concentric organization to be very common, thus confirming Kuffler's (1953) earlier work. Other cells, particularly those with oval receptive fields, were organized in just the opposite fashion. An active central region

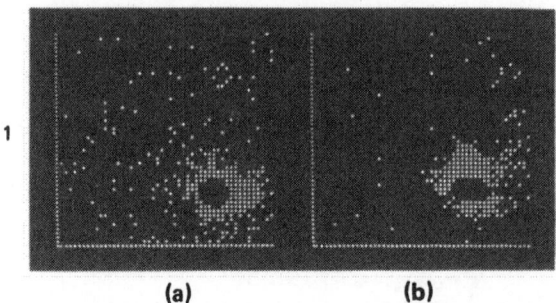

1

(a)   (b)

FIGURE 7.13 Two plots (a) and (b) of the same receptive field of a ganglion cell from the cat's retina. The two figures were plotted with horizontal and vertical scanning, respectively. Slight difference between the two indicates a modest directional sensitivity of this particular ganglion cell (from Spinelli, 1967).

was surrounded by an annular region of inhibition, in which the activity, rather than being evoked by stimulation, was actually depressed below spontaneous levels.

Spinelli's work, as well as illustrating a new computer technique that is an important advance over the usual single cell microelectrode time function paradigm, also illustrates, once again, the possible complexities of receptive field organization. In the cat's retina, at least, receptive fields appear not to be either simply shaped or monopolar. Regions of increased excitation or inhibition of ongoing activity may be enclosed by regions of the opposite polarity. Furthermore, Spinelli's attempt to determine if any directional sensitivity was present reflects the most important fact that the shapes of the receptive fields in some animals are determined by other features of the stimulus than simple position. Thus, a stationary spot might define one sort of receptive field for a given neuron, while a moving slit might give an entirely different shape and size for the receptive field of the same cell. Independent of artifacts, such as scattered light, the intensity of the stimulus may also alter the shape or size of the measured receptive field. As we shall see later in this chapter, this sort of data has been generalized to a very important notion—namely, that some specific features of a stimulus may lead to activation of a given cell, but in the absence of that feature, the cell may be totally unresponsive to any sort of stimulation. The emergence of the notion that the receptive field structure of a given neuron is not rigid, but labile, and may also depend upon the space-time pattern of the stimulus has been one of the most important neurophysiological conceptual developments in the last decade.

The receptive field structure of neurons of the visual cortex has been studied by Spinelli and Barrett (1969); Baumgartner, Brown, and Schultz (1964); and by Hubel and Wiesel (1962). Unfortunately, the three sets of data do not always agree—probably due to differences in technique.

For example, Hubel and Wiesel (1962)—work that we shall discuss in greater detail later in this chapter—reported that all neurons in the cat's visual cortex (area 17) had elongated receptive fields, whose axis symmetry was a line. As we shall more fully develop later, they also thought this to be associated with the fact that these cells were selectively sensitive to elongated "bar"like stimuli. Many of their receptive fields were arranged in a side-by-side arrangement with adjacent inhibitory and excitatory regions.

On the other hand, Spinelli and Barrett (1969) found that very large numbers (at least 44 percent) of their recorded units had circular receptive fields with the concentric and antagonistic arrangement of inhibitory and excitatory regions with which we have already become familiar in the retina. Baumgartner, Brown, and Schultz (1964) found that fewer than 20 percent of the cells in the cortex had the characteristics described by Hubel and Wiesel and provided substantive support for the notion that large numbers of cells in the cortex had circular or disk-shaped rather than linearly organized receptive fields.

It is thus clear that the last word has not yet been heard on this problem of the shape of the cortical receptive field. The possibility that shape changes under different dynamic conditions of stimulation remains with us. What is clear, though, is that neurons at all levels of the nervous system do exhibit receptive field organization resulting from the convergence of large numbers of receptor unit outputs onto the inputs of single more central cells.

Is there an auditory analogue of the neural receptive field? Coding considerations have already led us to the conclusion that auditory frequency discrimination is the analogue of the two-point acuity threshold in somatosensation and vision. Similarly, we might also argue that the receptive field notion is perhaps best represented in audition by the tuning curves of individual auditory neurons. Galambos and Davis (1943) had shown that each neuron in the cochlear nerve is characteristically activated by a band of frequencies that is progressively wider as the intensity of the stimulus increased. This leads to a V-shaped response area when threshold is plotted as a function of frequency and intensity for each neuron. Though we shall have much more to say of this phenomenon when we discuss neural quality coding, we can briefly introduce the idea here. Figure 7.14 shows the general pattern of these response areas for a few cochlear nerve cells. The V-shape of the response areas once again emphasizes the fact that the response area or receptive field extent is not fixed, but varies in width as a function of the amplitude of the signal. The shape of the typical response area was thought to vary as a function of the level of the auditory pathway at which neurons are being examined. Katsuki (1961) had suggested that the width of the response curves decreases the higher one gets in the nervous system until one reaches the level of the cortex. At the cortex—as in somatosensation, but unlike vision—there appears, however, to be additional further convergent interaction, which once again broadens the receptive field, and so some workers now feel that the hypothetical sharpening does not exist (Simmons, 1970).

This brief introduction to the concept of receptive fields has been intended to emphasize a number of points. First, the general ubiquitousness of receptive field organization excludes the primitive idea of private line signaling from each point on a receptive surface to a set of corresponding points in the central nervous system. A more modern statistical notion of pattern interaction and average or relative neural activity then emerges. Second, the notion of the receptive field is essentially one that emphasizes the sequential loss of information. Two spatial points, though perfectly resolvable in terms of the stimulus or early neural response, cannot always

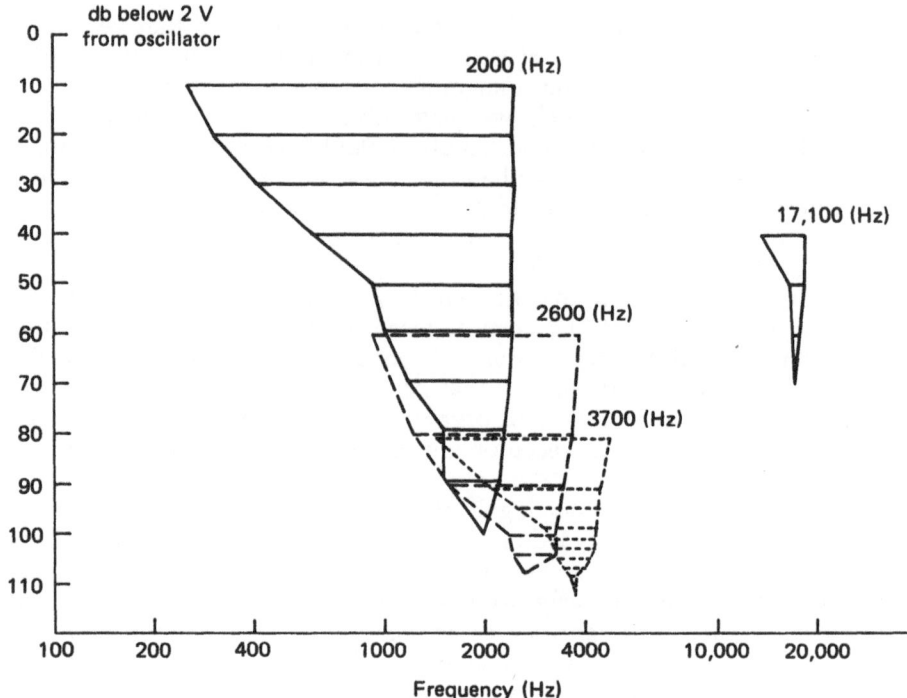

FIGURE 7.14 *The classic representation of the response areas of auditory nerve fibers (from Galambos and Davis, 1943).*

be discriminated in terms of either the later neurophysiological or psychophysical responses.

As we shall see, the notion of a uniform receptive field independent of activity in its neighbors is, however, also a gross oversimplification. We also have to consider the fact that there are very important neural interactions occurring among the neurons both within and between receptive fields. Before we discuss these spatial interactions, however, we must consider another way in which sensory information is lost. In this case we shall not be concerned with the problems of spatial acuity and spatial receptive fields, but rather with the fusion of temporally discrete stimulus events into events that appear to be perceptually simultaneous.

C. Temporal Acuity and the Psychological Moment

1. Masking and the Psychological Moment. Two sequential stimuli may be fused into a single sensory experience with no perceived temporal microstructure if they are separated by less than a certain minimum interval. The particular size of this minimum interval varies from one modality to another. These psychophysical data seem generally to be a function of the fact that very prolonged cortical responses are elicited by even the briefest of impulsive stimuli. As we have noted, a 1-msec spike can evoke a 1-sec-long cortical response. The ability to distinguish between two sequential temporal events, a notion we might refer to as temporal acuity, is analogous to the spatial two-point threshold acuity measure. Is there also a temporal analogue to the notion of the spatial receptive field? The answer to this question is yes, and an extensive literature has grown in the last decade concerned with the problem of what has been called the psychological moment or quantum. The psychological moment is conceived of as a period within which there is an inability to either distinguish simultaneous from sequential events or the order in which events occurred. In the following discussion, we shall concentrate mainly on the visual system, but it is clear that the lack of temporal acuity illustrated in this discussion is also a common feature of the other senses, although perhaps with different time constants. The interested reader is referred to Piéron (1952) for a comprehensive and comparative statement of the temporal acuity of the various senses.[1]

It should be noted first that studies of the loss of temporal separateness, that is, of perceptual simultaneity (Lichtenstein, 1961; Fraisse, 1966) or of short-term visual storage (Averbach and Coriell, 1961; Eriksen and Collins, 1965) or of the psychological moment (Stroud, 1955; Allport, 1968) all essentially deal with a similar general problem: how are the finely divided moments of real time transduced into the far less highly resolved temporal units within our perceptual system?

The studies just mentioned and a host of other similar ones make it clear that the ability to deal with time, as time, is also successively reduced in all sensory systems as one passes from the stimulus to the percept. We do not yet know the complete details of this loss; however, a central hypothesis, which may help explain experimental findings concerning simultaneity, sequential masking, and the psychological moment, is that there is a temporal dispersion of brief stimulus events into longer neural and subjective events due to the neural divergent mechanisms described above. There is ample direct and indirect evidence that this temporal defocusing or slurring does occur, and that micromoments of real time in the world of the stimulus are extended into much more prolonged psychological and neurophysiological phenomena.

The slurring of temporal distinctiveness and the dimensions of the psychological moment are often measured in an experiment in which the masking effects of a subsequent or preceding stimulus on a test signal are assayed with some sort of a masking procedure. Masking experiments are of several different kinds, and each seems to assay the effects of one or more different kinds of physiological mechanism. For example, one of the earliest forms of masking was that in which a very bright flash followed and masked a dimmer one (Crawford, 1947). This sort of masking occurs only monoptically and is thus thought to reflect the effects of some peripheral mechanism. Masking with random dotted noise (which we shall discuss in greater detail later) is dichoptic (the mask may be presented to the eye opposite to that receiving the signal with little diminution in the masking effect), suggesting a central locus. Metacontrast masking does not require overlap of stimulus and mask; the other types do.

---

[1] Much of the material in the following section is adapted from Uttal (1971a).

The general result is that there is some sort of a functional relationship between the degree of masking and the interval between the two stimuli. This period of interaction is, at least in part, identified with the psychological moment and the prolongation of the stimulus event into a longer lasting perceptual event. Similar moments, but with different time courses, can be measured in the other senses too. The interested reader may want to look at Kahneman (1968) for one of the most comprehensive and thoughtful discussions of the methods, findings, and theories of the visual masking literature.

Most important, it is clear that during the prolongation of the stimulus event, there is no *a priori* reason to assume that each successive portion of the prolonged event is weighted equally with regard to its perceptual efficiency. Experiments on visual masking of the several different kinds (Kinsbourne and Warrington, 1962a, 1962b; Schiller and Smith, 1965; Kahneman, 1968; Uttal, 1969c) suggest that there is, quite to the contrary, a weighting of the efficiency of any given masking stimulus, depending upon how close it is to the masked stimulus.

Herein lies the critical issue of the controversy surrounding the notions of psychological moments and perceptual simultaneity. The integrative mathematics, which is often used to analyze these events, is generally unable to distinguish the phase relations of the integrating period or moments (or whatever other name has been applied to the period of interaction surrounding the stimulus). Thus, like almost any correlation technique, the consolidation of experimental data into a simple statistical measure means a loss of some of the original information. Unfortunately, the phase information, which is lost when one pools data or performs a correlation, is the critical dimension in the controversy over discrete discontinuous moments and continuously sliding moments. From this point of view, all experiments that pool data over many trials must be considered ill-equipped to resolve the controversy.

What is meant by these two terms—the discrete discontinuous moment and the continuous sliding moment? Both refer to an integrating period, in which information about the temporal order of stimuli is lost. This term "moment" was probably first used by Stroud (1955), when he described his ideas of a discrete and discontinuous interval in which order information is lost, but the general notion of an integrating period has been used by many other authors. The term is used here in the more general sense, denoting the temporal interval between two sequential stimuli in which they interact in one way or another. Simply stated, the two kinds of moments describe different ways in which the degree of interaction may be weighted as a function of the size of the interval between the two stimuli. The notion of the continuously sliding moment is characterized by the assumption that a region in which interaction occurs surrounds every stimulus. This region is weighted differentially so that the closer one stimulus is to another, the greater will be the interaction. This idea is an analogue of the weighting function of the lateral inhibitory interaction described by Hartline, Wagner, and Ratliff (1956), but it operates in time rather than space. It might well be called the sliding window hypothesis.

It should be noted that the sliding window hypothesis is very similar to the notions of the temporal summation model of masking proposed by Eriksen and Hoffman (1963) and Kinsbourne and Warrington (1962a and 1962b), and further developed by Kahneman (1967), although the notion that weighted effectiveness of interaction is a function of the temporal distance from the stimulus is an added parameter not considered by some of these workers. The sliding window notion also has great similarity to the term "spread function" suggested by Baron and Krantz (1970);[2] one occasionally also hears the related terms "temporal receptive field," "psychological time quantum," and "sensory trace." Sperling and Sondhi's (1968) "impulse function" and Shallice's (1967) "moving average" also seem to denote similar ideas.

Another important consideration is that while we shall often refer to the window as a region surrounding the stimulus, implying that it occurs both prior to and following the stimulus, and while we often measure the function in this manner, the interaction is not truly bilateral. A period follows a stimulus event in which the trace of that event is capable of interacting with another stimulus event. Thus, a leading mask appears as a region of interaction preceding a test stimulus, if the criterion is the effect on the test stimulus; yet clearly what is really meant is the persistent effect of the leading mask on the trailing stimulus. The region of interaction surrounding a stimulus is, therefore, the period following it plus the period following any other stimulus that may have preceded it. This simplistic notion is weakened by the fact that even those masking situations that exhibit both leading and trailing masking (not all do) do not produce identical behavior in the forward and backward directions (Schiller and Smith, 1965; and Uttal, 1969a). This discrepancy is yet to be explained.

The usual alternative formulation, the discontinuous discrete moment notion, assumes that the weighting function is not differentially weighted and sliding with the stimulus, but is, rather, rectangular and not time-locked to the stimulus. From this point of view, any two events that occur within the same rectangular summation period would interact equally strongly, regardless of the interval between the two. The continuous functions of interval obtained in the several experiments mentioned above would, therefore, be produced by the statistics of the results of randomly placed periods of interaction over the many trials of any given experiment.

As we have said, the main criterion that distinguishes the continuously sliding moment from the discrete discontinuous moment is whether the period of interaction is rectangular and unrelated to the stimulus or whether it is a continuous differentially weighted function surrounding and time-locked to the stimulus event. Both of these possibilities are schematically illustrated in Figure 7.15. There is only one experiment (Allport, 1968), with which the author is familiar, that specifically tests this issue; all others, to the best of our present knowledge, are ambiguous. This elegant work of Allport is necessarily in the form of a demonstration rather than a statistical study using pooled data.

Allport's display was a series of 12 horizontal lines, which were plotted on the face of an oscilloscope in ascending or descending order.

---

[2] J. Baron and D. Krantz, personal communication, 1970.

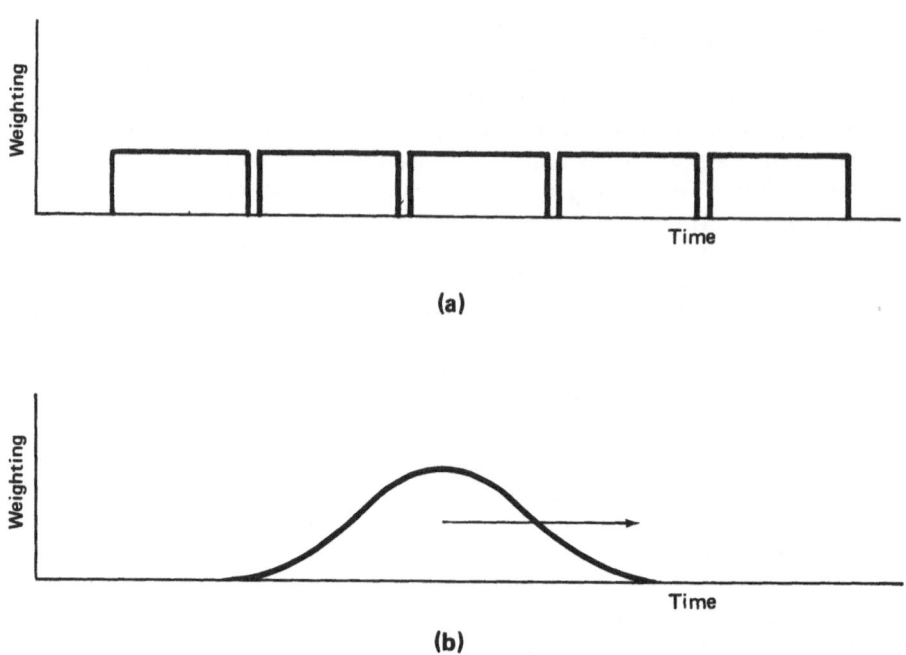

FIGURE 7.15 *Two drawings suggestive of the alternative models of the psychological moment. (a) The discrete, nonoverlapping, rectangular nonstimulus related moment. (b) The sliding and weighted moving window closely linked to stimulus events.*

Once the topmost or bottommost line was drawn, the display recycled starting at the lowest or highest line. The subject's task was to observe this pattern of moving lines when certain ones were omitted, thus producing a moving dark band. Allport's analysis involved the timing of the omitted bands. If psychological moments were randomly placed, then the dark band would appear to move in a direction opposite to its real physical movement. If, on the other hand, the psychological moment were continuous and "traveling" or "sliding," then it should move in the same direction as its real physical movement. All subjects participating in the demonstration reported the dark band to move in the direction of the real physical movement. Allport concludes, therefore, that there is no support for the latter of the two alternatives mentioned above, which he refers to as the "Discrete Moment Hypothesis" (following Stroud, 1955). He believes that his results support the notion that he calls the "Continuous or Traveling Moment Hypothesis."

It is now believed that the perspective of modern neurophysiology also renders implausible the notion of the randomly placed, rectangular, and discrete moment. Allport's carefully conceived experiments add further credence to the alternative point of view—that each stimulus event, no matter how brief, is surrounded by a temporal region in which it can interact with other stimuli. The work of many investigators in the field suggests further that this region of interaction is weighted by a function, which is dependent upon the interval between the two stimuli. We further assume, although this is subject to doubt, that this region of interaction slides continuously along the real-world time line. Questions of simultaneity arise because of indiscriminably small differences in the weights of sequential events.

Recently, Ross[3] has pointed out that while the moments may be continuous and traveling or sliding, it is also possible that they may not be constant in duration in different experimental contexts. It may be that the duration of the moment can be affected by the duration of the stimulus event, for example; if so, this would add a great deal of complexity to the problem as we know it today. It also would tend to emphasize the central nature of short-term sensory storage at the expense of peripheral explanations.

If, indeed, moments are continuous and sliding, some possible experimental questions become nonsensical, while others become empirical issues eminently susceptible to quantitative measurement. The search for the phase relationships of rectangular and discrete moments, in this light, is a vain search for a nebulous chimera. At the very best, we shall always be bounded by the problems of data pooling; at the very worst, discrete moments may simply not exist. On the other hand, if we accept the notion of the sliding moment as a conceptual model and as an initial axiom, we can make meaningful statistical measurements of temporal interaction.

2. *An Experimental Analysis of the Moment.* While it is not, by any means, yet clear what the specific neurophysiological mechanisms are, other than the general notion of divergence, which have to be invoked to explain the psychological moment, it is possible to measure its dimensions. Perhaps one of the most direct ways is to use a computer controlled display and data acquisition procedure. In the following section, we shall discuss a relatively novel experimental masking approach to the problem of the psychological moment, which will help to concretize some of the preceding discussion.

The author (Uttal, 1969c, 1971a) has studied the duration of the psychological moment by a masking test, which involved the discrimination of a set of dots making up a test pattern (like an alphabetical character) from bursts of random noise dots presented at some interval following the pattern. The general idea of this procedure is that the perceptual events initiated even by the very brief stimulus presentations are prolonged, and the responses initiated by the dots of the stimulus and the dots of the mask will interact to a degree dependent upon this prolongation. Presumably the subject's discrimination is based upon an ability to discriminate between different levels of the residual brightness of the fading sensory trace associated with each of the two stimuli.

This computer controlled experimental procedure is capable of giving especially precise control over stimulus presentation because all of the stimulus materials were generated on the face of an oscilloscope. The oscil-

[3] J. Ross, University of Western Australia, personal communication, 1971.

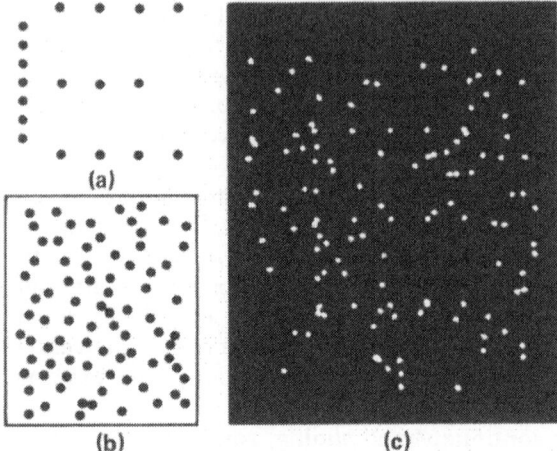

(a)

(b)   (c)

FIGURE 7.16 (a) An exam-
ple of the dotted characters
used in the dot masking experiments. (b) An example
of the dotted noise used in
the dot masking experiment.
(c) An actual photograph
taken from the oscilloscope
of the letter E embedded in
100 random noise dots. This
character can be seen better
in tachistoscopic exposure
than when viewed continu-
ously.

loscope had a special phosphor, the light output of which decayed in less
than 50 μsec to imperceptibly low levels. The interaction between the two
stimuli measured by the masking technique was, therefore, purely a function of temporal dispersion introduced by the various parts of the nervous
system. Figure 7.16(a) shows a typical dotted alphabetical character. Figure
7.16(b) shows a typical random masking dot pattern of intermediate density. This random dotted noise may either be presented in a single burst or
as a series of dots distributed over an extended period of time. In the
latter case, it is referred to as dynamic visual noise or DVN. Depending
upon the interval between the individual dots in the DVN, the eye is
capable of integrating or slurring a certain number so that many appear
to be simultaneously present.

Figure 7.16(c) shows the mixture of the dotted character and the
random noise. Only Figure 7.16(a) and (b) are really physical entities. The
mixture in Figure 7.16(c) is produced by the same temporal slurring we
have spoken about. Depending upon numbers in the mixture of signal
and noise dots, the alphabetic character will be more or less recognizable.

It should be noted that this technique will tend to underestimate the
duration of the persistence of the visual image. Most certainly there will be
some interval between the two stimuli at which the subject will be able to
completely discriminate the dots of the character from those of the noise
(the residual brightness will be sufficiently different), even though both
may still appear to be present to some degree at that and longer durations.
Nevertheless, with this caveat in mind, a good idea of the minimum duration
of the interaction between sequential visual stimuli can be obtained with
this technique. Figure 7.17 presents the results of a typical masking experiment (Uttal, 1969c), in which the interval between the stimulus and a mask
consisting of a series of randomly positioned DVN dots was varied in both
the leading and trailing configuration in separate experiments. As the
interval increased in either case, there is a corresponding increase in the

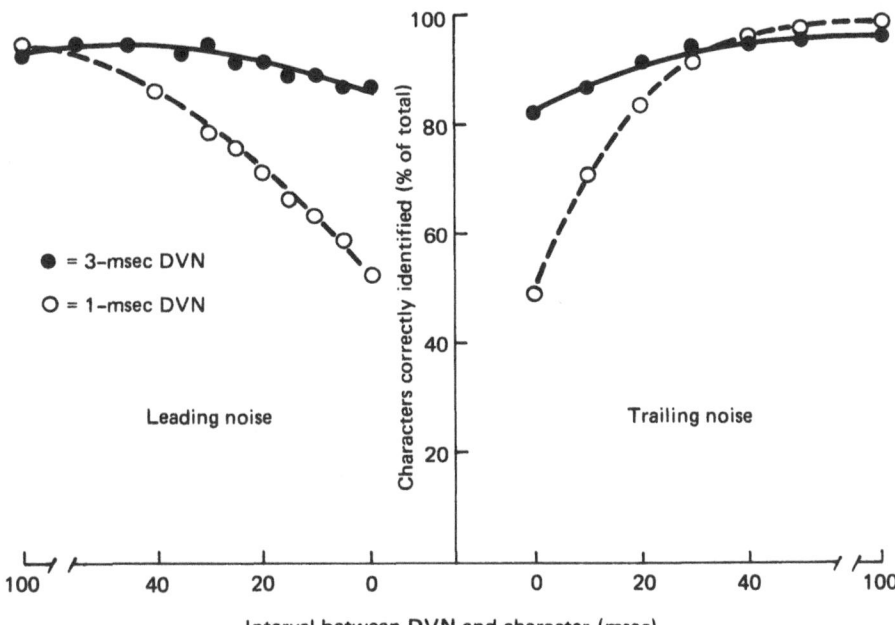

FIGURE 7.17 *The degree of masking as a function of the interval between lead-ing and trailing dynamic visual noise (DVN) of two different densities. Leading masking is seen to have a slightly more persistent effect than trailing (from Uttal, 1969c).*

proportion of the number of presented characters that are correctly identi-fied. Though the results are not exactly symmetrical, it does appear that there is nearly perfect identification at about a 30-msec interval when the mask trails the character and at about a 40-msec interval when the mask precedes the character. This is necessarily an estimate of the duration of the period of interaction between the character and the interfering noise that must be on the low side for the reasons mentioned above.

When the masking dots are all presented in a very brief burst follow-ing the signal character, there is also a period of interaction measured, which is almost identical to that measured with the distributed DVN mask-ing noise. Figure 7.18 shows this result only for the backward case, but a comparison of these data with those of the right-hand side of Figure 7.17 confirms the near identity of the duration of the period of interaction measured with either of these two methods.

Perhaps a better estimate of the true duration of the moment can be obtained in an experiment in which the signal character is both followed and preceded by a masking train of dots (see Figure 7.19). The character in this case will be in a temporal hole between the two masking DVN trains. In this case, the period of interaction is not simply the sum of the periods obtained for the forward and backward cases, but a much longer period (about 150 msec) as shown in Figure 7.20. Thus, hole size is much more

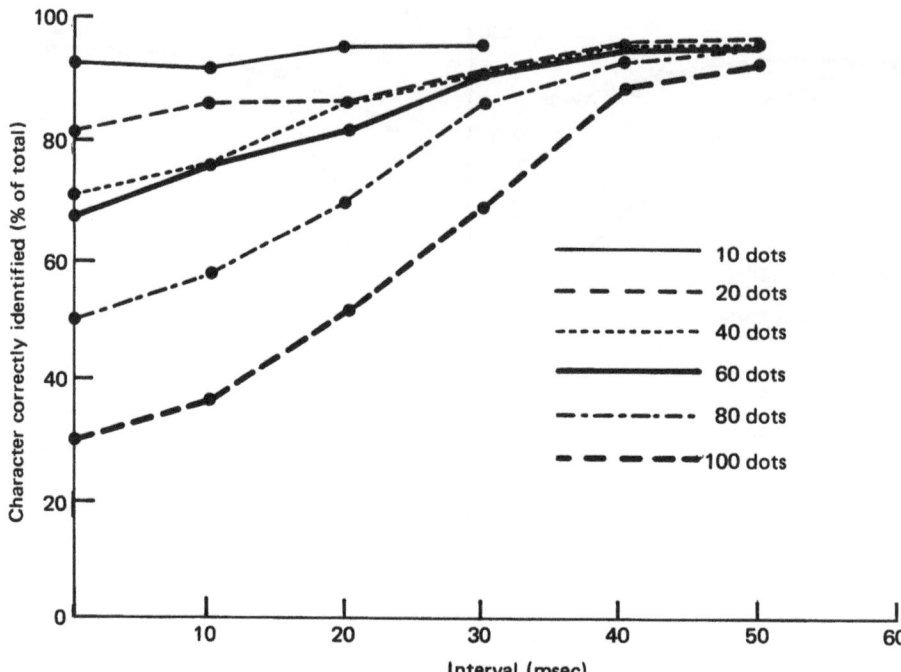

FIGURE 7.18 *The effects of variation of the number of masking dots and the interval between the character and the burst of masking dots on the recognizability of alphabetic character (from Uttal, 1971a).*

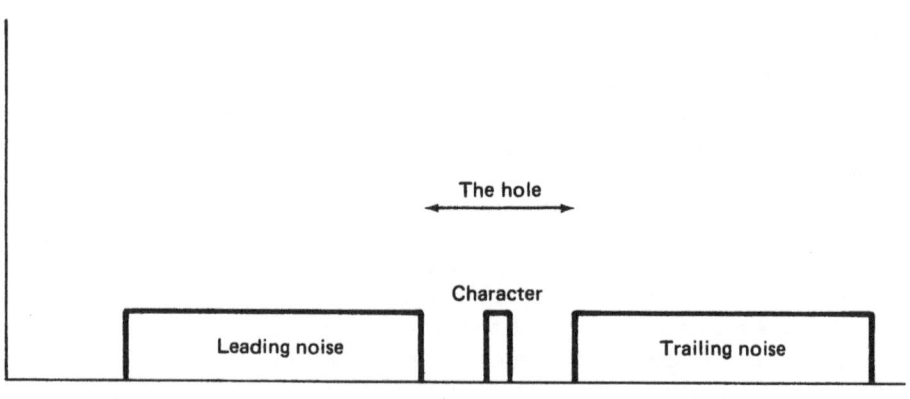

FIGURE 7.19 *The design of the "character in the hole" experiment, in which an alphabetic character was inserted in the temporal gap between a train of leading and trailing dynamic visual noise.*

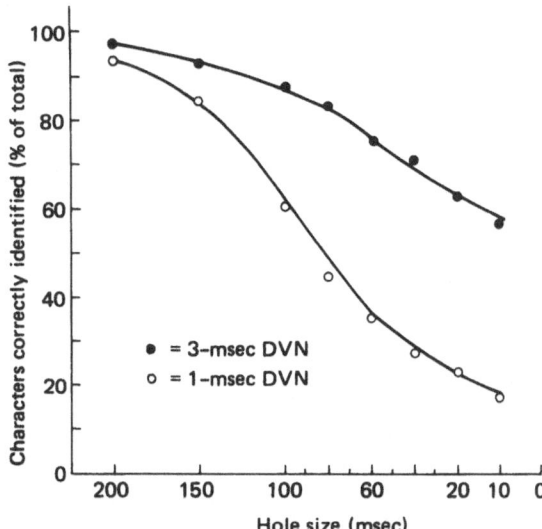

FIGURE 7.20 Results of the "character in the hole experiment" for two DVN densities (from Uttal, 1969a).

than twice the sum of the durations of the forward and backward effects separately.

In summary, there is a loss of both spatial and temporal acuity because of both convergent and divergent organization of the sensory pathways and central sensory structures. The notions of receptive fields and psychological moments, however, only begin to suggest the full complexity of the spatial and temporal interactions that occur among neurons at various levels of the sensory pathways. A major recent development in neurophysiological thinking has been the development of ideas concerning the spatial interaction of adjacent spatial stimuli in a way that transcends the simple fusion of the receptive field. Similarly, integration of or interaction among stimuli arriving at different times also has emerged as a major new concept related to a large number of psychological phenomena, especially those that have to do with the localization of some stimulus in space. As we discuss these processes, we shall see further examples of situations in which spatial aspects of stimuli are encoded by time, as well as ones in which temporally fluctuating stimuli are encoded by spatial patterns. The general problem that we now face is to describe and analyze these interactive processes and to draw from them the general principles that will be most instructive in helping the reader understand the operation of all sensory systems, regardless of the modality in which the observation was initially made. We shall turn first to an extensive consideration of studies of spatial interactions; then we shall briefly mention temporal interactions.

III. SPATIAL INTERACTIONS

It has probably been implicitly known for millenia by artists that their works must be slightly different from pure pictographic representation to give a realistic view of the world. The use of linear perspective, a mathe-

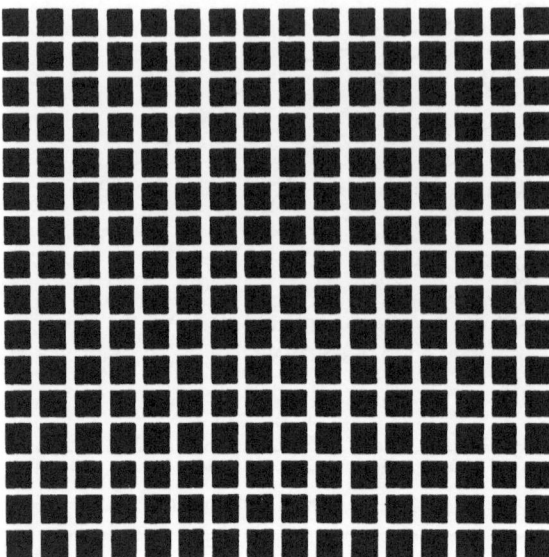

FIGURE 7.21 The Hermann grid illusion, demonstrating the grey areas at the intersection of the white grid lines.

matical notion formalized by Brunelleschi in the early days of the renaissance, for example, was introduced into drawing by Masaccio in the early fifteenth century, thus adding a third dimension to an art form, which had been mainly two-dimensional up to that time. Even earlier, many artists had realized that the apparent colors and brightnesses of a given area were dependent not only upon the constituent pigments, but also upon the spatial relationships of the area to its surroundings. This was an implicit, if not an overt, expression of the fact that nearby areas interacted to give different perceptual effects than would otherwise have been expected.

A simple display, which illustrates this sort of spatial interaction, is the famous Hermann Grid illusion reproduced in Figure 7.21. At the intersections of the white grid lines, there appear to be greyish patches everywhere except at the point of fixation. The effect is more pronounced for smaller grids than for more broad ones. The most important characteristic of this sort of "illusion" is that it is very strongly influenced by the geometry of the stimulus pattern. Other visual illusions seem not to be so strikingly dependent upon the local geometry, but rather vary in a uniform way over large regions. The classic simultaneous contrast illusions are of this sort, and later we shall discuss why it is believed that these two sets of phenomena may not be as closely connected as they have been thought to be by many current writers.

In the following material, we shall concern ourselves with the class of effects that are dependent primarily upon local geometry and that, therefore, seem amenable to a neural coding analysis. To do so, we must first consider the nature of the perceptual phenomena, for which we shall seek a physiological explanation.

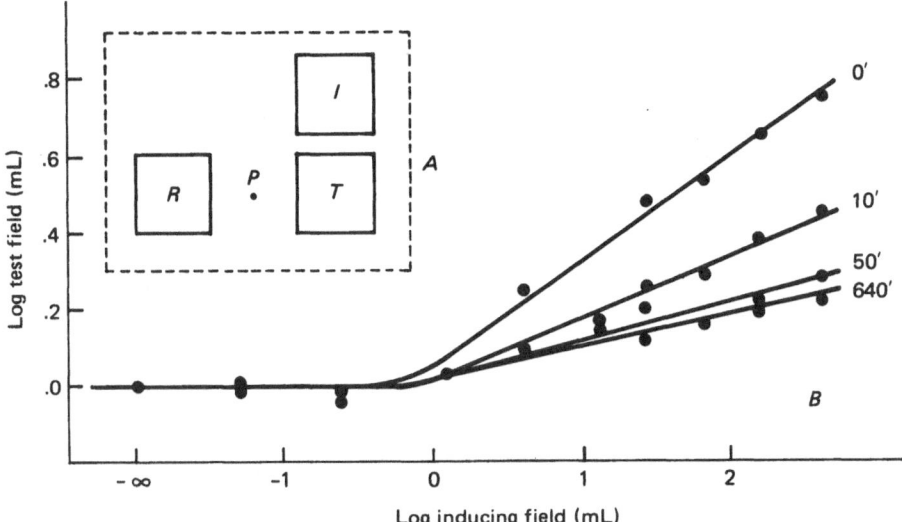

FIGURE 7.22 *A graph showing the lateral inhibitory interaction (B), which can be observed in a human visual psychophysical experiment using a stimulus as shown in (A) as a function of the spatial separation between the test (T) and "inducing stimuli" (I) and the brightness of the inducing field measured with a reference field (R) as a function of angular separation and brightness. P is a fixation point (from Leibowitz, Mote, and Thurlow, 1953).*

A. Perceptual Phenomena Related to Spatial Interactions

As noted, it is believed that the types of perceptual spatial interaction that do seem amenable to explanation by a simple nerve net interaction model are characterized by some functional relationship to the local geometry of the interacting stimuli. Two alternative experimental paradigms may be used to elucidate these geometrical functions. Inspections may be made of the interactions at regions of high information content, such as the boundary between large adjacent fields of different brightness or color. Alternatively, measurements may be made of the variation in the degree of interaction between two small regions that are placed at various differences from each other on the receptive surface.

This latter category of experiment has often been used to establish the distances over which interactive forces can be exerted in visual experiments; for example, Leibowitz, Mote, and Thurlow (1953) used a pattern of rectangles arranged as shown in Figure 7.22 to measure the distance function in human vision. The task of the subject was to match a "reference field" in brightness to a "test field," which was in close proximity to an "inducing field." As the experimenter decreased the separation between the inducing field and the test field, the inducing field became more effective in lowering the subjective brightness of the test field of constant illuminance. Thus, the brightness of the test field had to be increased for the match. A measurable decrease in the subjective brightness of the test field could be

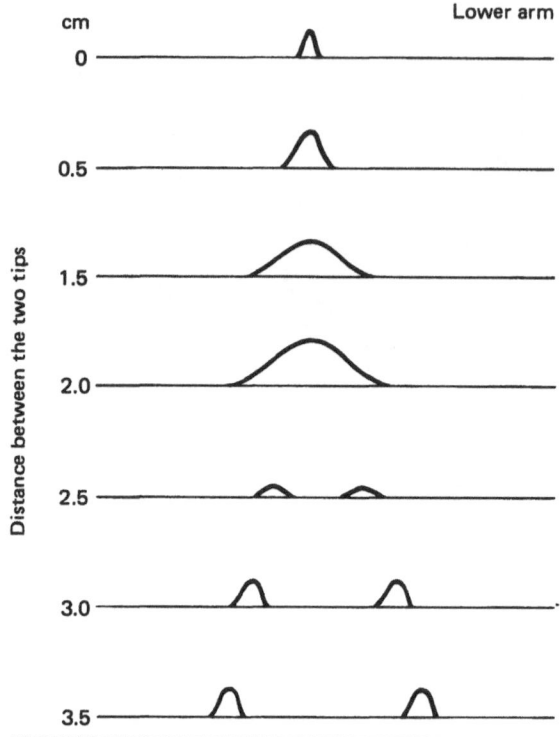

FIGURE 7.23 A graphic presentation of the perceptual effect produced by two mechanical stimuli applied to skin. When the two stimuli are presented close together, only a single fused sensation of low intensity and narrow spatial extent is felt, but when the two stimuli are separated by a somewhat greater distance, both the amplitude and the spatial extent appear to increase. At even larger separations, the sensation is no longer fused, and the subject feels two points of modest amplitude (from von Békésy, 1957).

measured even though the separations were as great as 9 deg between the test and inducing fields. As the illuminance of the inducing field increased, the perceived brightness of the test field also decreased. These findings are also shown in Figure 7.22.

MacKavey, Bartley, and Casella (1962) in a related study showed a similar inhibitory interaction in human vision and also discovered that the effects of the first inducing field could be reduced if it, in turn, was inhibited by a second one. This latter finding is analogous to the physiological disinhibition phenomenon to be discussed below.

Von Békésy (1957) has carried out a series of studies on the skin, which demonstrate phenomena very similar to those functional relationships obtained in visual studies. His findings are very important in furthering the notion of complex interaction in receptive fields, an idea that he has used as the theme of an entire book (von Békésy, 1967). The experimental paradigm in this study involved the use of two-point stimuli applied to the skin, but von Békésy, instead of using the conventional two-point threshold as a dependent variable, chose to draw what was the subject's impression of the magnitude and shape of the resulting sensation as a function of the separation of the two points. Though only quantitative in a limited graphical sense, this sort of data presentation can present an enormous amount of information in a clear and interesting manner. The results of this particular experiment, for example, are shown in Figure 7.23. Von Békésy noted that there appears to be systematic variation in the magnitude of the single sensation produced by two stimuli (within the two-point threshold) as they were moved closer and closer together. However, when the single percept separated into two distinguishable points (when the two stimuli were separated by a distance greater than the two-point threshold), the sensory magnitude of each point dropped substantially and did not increase again until the two points were quite far apart. This waxing and waning of the cutaneous magnitudes suggests that the notion of a purely convergent receptive field is probably a considerable oversimplification. Rather, there are further spatial integrations and interactions, which are superimposed upon the basic idea of convergent pooling.

If there is any single idea that has most captured the fancy of neurophysiologists in the last two decades, it may be said to be the notion of mutual lateral interaction among adjacent neural units. The interaction is said to be mutual because each unit seems to be depressed (or, less frequently, enhanced) reciprocally by the neighbor it inhibits. The polarity of the interaction, whether it is inhibitory or excitatory, is another issue of paramount importance. Some of the earlier studies suggest that the interaction is mainly inhibitory, but one of the important results emerging from von Békésy's psychophysical experiments on human subjects is that the interaction often reverses polarity at different separations. These data suggest the notion of a central field, in which the two stimulus intensities can be summated to produce a sensory magnitude greater than that produced by either alone. This central region, it is further suggested, may be surrounded by an inhibitory annular field, in which a stimulus would produce a response which, in turn, might tend to actually diminish the magnitude of the response produced by a second stimulus. As we shall see, there is substantial neurophysiological evidence to confirm this idea of concentric rings of opposite polarity in the vertebrate nervous system. To anticipate a bit, such an organization has become known as an antagonistic center-surround receptive field.

One of the most interesting, and nowadays familiar, perceptual phenomena associated with the interaction of spatial stimuli is the enhancement of contours—a phenomenon which was first described in detail by E. Mach (1865) and which is now known in his honor as the "Mach band." Recently, a very important book reviewing Mach's contributions to our understanding of the general problem of spatial interactions as well as his specific description of the contour enhancement effects has been published by Ratliff (1965). It would be hard to exceed the competent level or the sensitive and perceptive commentary that characterizes Ratliff's book, and the interested reader is, therefore, directed to that source for his full treatment. In the brief section that follows, we shall simply summarize the nature of the Mach band phenomenon as one compelling example of a psychophysical observation, which is probably mediated by simple lateral interactions among neurons.

In brief, if a stimulus pattern is presented across a retinal field such that a cross section of the physical light distribution can be represented by the solid line in Figure 7.24, the perceptual experience does not exactly follow the stimulus. Rather, a plot of the induced subjective magnitude would look more like the dotted curve in that figure. At the region joining

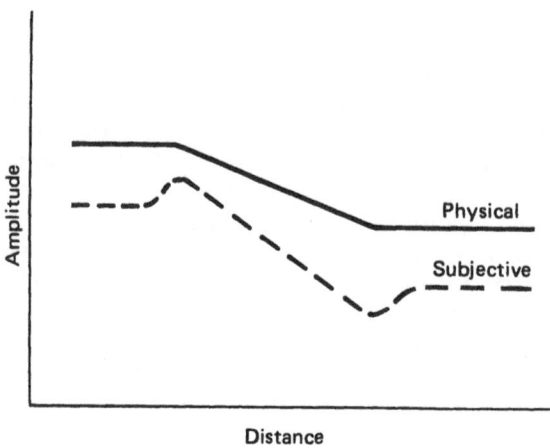

FIGURE 7.24 A drawing il-
lustrating the basic phenomena of the Mach band. A
physical stimulus, which is
simply a gradiant, is seen (or
heard or felt) as if there were
a more intense band at the
upper end of the gradient.
The contour intensifications
so illustrated are now believed by many psychobio-
logists to be mainly a function of lateral interactions in
the nervous system.

the area of constant low-level light with the beginning of the upward-going
gradient, there is a depressed apparent brightness level, and a dark band
thus appears. At the other end of the gradient where the gradient borders
on the constant bright area, an apparent bright band occurs. Just how
"real" these apparent bright and dark Mach bands can be is best illustrated
by some of the anecdotes related by Ratliff in his book. He tells how
astronomers, artists, and weavers, as well as psychologists, have all had to
deal with some curious problems of credibility as a result of these illusory
bands.

The important point in the demonstration of Mach bands is that the
function representing the perceived brightness distribution varies considerably from the function describing the physical stimulus luminance
distribution. It is sometimes difficult to get this notion across, for even in
photographs the effect can come streaming through in a way that makes it
difficult to convince an observer that the effect is mainly perceptual. This
is so for two reasons. The first reason is that the photographic film like the
human eye often has its own contrast enhancement mechanisms, not neural
but chemical. The second reason is that the stimulus conditions, which are
necessary for the evocation of the Mach band enhancement, are maintained
even in a photograph.

Many auditory phenomena, which appear to be analogous, may also
be cited, at least in part, to these visual spatial interaction phenomena. For
example, the general masking of one tone by another is probably due to
spatial interactions along the cochlea comparable to those producing the
Mach bands. Figure 7.25 is Licklider's adaptation of Fletcher's interpretation of Wegel and Lane's (1924) now classic summary graph of the tonal
interactions that occur between a 1200-Hz tone and a "secondary tone" of
varying frequency. In this drawing, the secondary tone is masked most
effectively when its frequency is higher than that of the masking tone. On
the other hand, when the masking tone is of a higher frequency than the
secondary tone, then the masking is relatively ineffective.

A wide range of other auditory interactions, probably also attributable

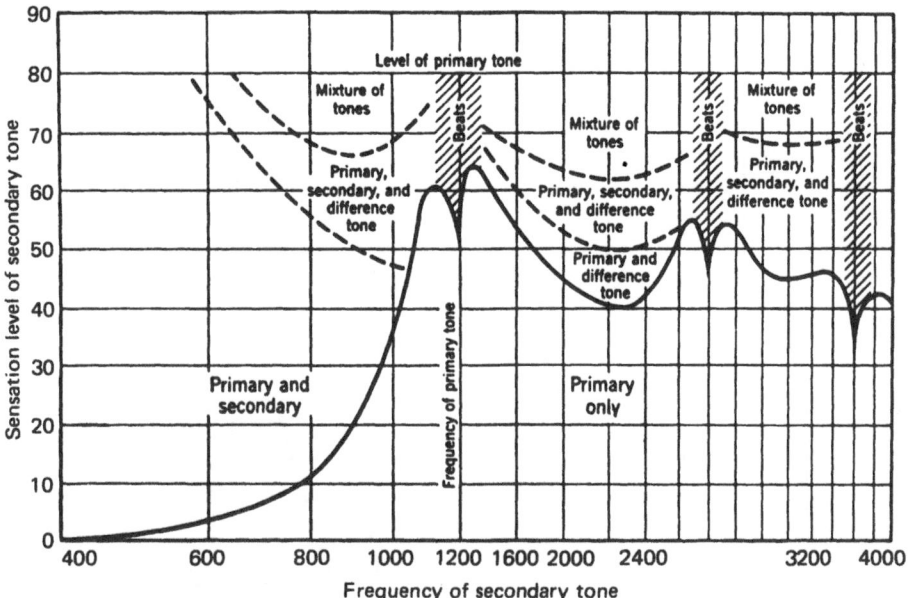

FIGURE 7.25 *The classic masking curve, showing the variety of interactions that can occur between two acoustic stimuli. When the two tones are close in frequency, beating occurs. (In some instances, combination, difference or summation tones can occur). In other instances, one tone tends to mask the other, requiring a larger-than-normal masked tone before it can be detected in the presence of the masker. Many of these interactions can be best understood in terms of spatial interactions on the basilar membrane (from Licklider, 1951b, after Fletcher, 1929, and Wegel and Lane, 1924).*

to spatial interactions along the cochlea, is also represented on this figure. At some frequency combination difference and mixture tones, as well as beats, occur.

One of the most interesting elaborations of the auditory masking paradigm as an analogue of visual spatial interactions is Carterette, Friedman, and Lovell's (1969) demonstration of what they believe to be auditory "Mach bands." These workers demonstrated that there was a heightened masking between a narrow band of white noise and a pure tone when the frequency of the test tone was at either border of the band of masking white noise. The noise in their experiment was generated by a computer technique, which produced a stimulus that had very sharp cutoffs at the upper and lower limits (edges) of a 100-Hz bandwidth. The general technique involved the measurement of the increase in loudness, which was required to compensate for the masking as one scanned a frequency domain varying from 0.4 to 0.8 kHz.

Figure 7.26 is a sample of their data, showing the gradual increase in loudness required for the detection of the test tone as its frequency is increased toward the lower edge of the noise band. In many cases, a decrease in the masking effect is observed when the tone is in the middle regions of

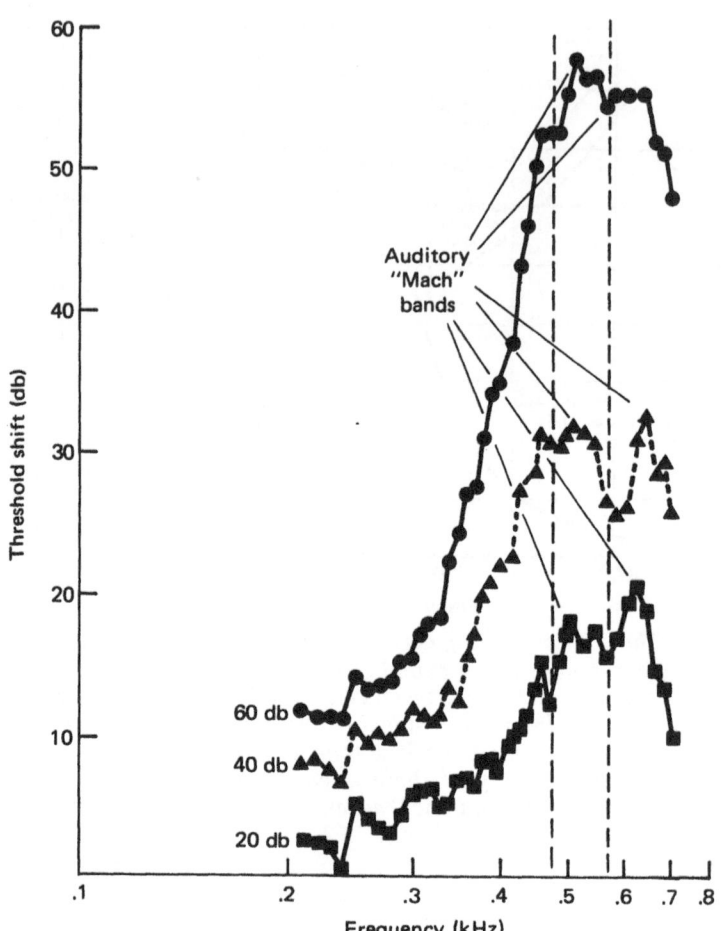

FIGURE 7.26 *An auditory phenomena that may be analogous to visual Mach bands. There is a peak in the masking function for tones near the edge of a band of masking white noise—the width of which is indicated by the two vertical dotted lines (from Carterette, Friedman, and Lovell, 1969).*

the noise band. Subsequently, there often appears another increase in the required amplitude of the test tone for detection as the test tone passes over the high-frequency edge of the noise band. It is the increases in the test tone level required for absolute detection at the edges of the noise band that Carterette and his colleagues believe to be analogues of the Mach band edge effects in vision.

In sum, there is a reasonably large number of spatially interacting processes observable in the various senses that are characterized by a dependence upon the local geometry of adjacent stimulus spaces. There are also, on the other hand, overall pattern effects such as simultaneous contrast, in which the entire stimulus object seems to be uniformly affected by its surround without any differentiation as a function of propinquity. It is possible that these two sets of data represent two completely different classes of phenomena, the latter possibly mediated by central mechanisms and the former by peripheral ones. In the following sections, we shall concern ourselves only with those neurophysiological data that clearly display distance and propinquity functions and that, therefore, appear to be plausible models of the former class of geometry sensitive illusions.

B. The Neurophysiological Data

1. Lateral Inhibitory Interaction in the Horseshoe Crab Eye. From his earliest observations on the Mach band and related visual phenomena, Mach stressed the point that the subjectively bright and dark bands were produced by neural interactions in the retina. His insights, interestingly enough, were based almost exclusively on the psychophysical data, yet they sound quite modern and familiar in the light of contemporary neurophysiological findings. A sentence from one of Mach's original papers reads: "Two retinal points stand in a reciprocal relation which is determined by a function of their separation."

Mach's mathematical model of perceived contour enhancement was founded mainly on continuous second-order differential equations, which described the process thought to be transforming the stimulus distribution into the perceived brightness distribution. Although, he frequently speaks of the reciprocal interaction of retinal points (in fact, one of the papers reproduced in Ratliff's book is specifically entitled "On the Dependence of Retinal Points on One Another"), the neurophysiology of his time did not allow him to be more specific about the anatomical or physiological nature of the interdependence.

Nevertheless, his writing suggests that he was fully aware of the necessity for postulating neural interactions on a very local basis. For example, on page 267 of Ratliff (1965), Mach is quoted as saying: "It appears to me that the phenomena discussed can only be explained on the basis of a reciprocal action of neighboring areas of the retina."

Most modern physiological theories of sensory lateral interaction, however, are founded upon the pioneering neurophysiological findings originally obtained by H. Keefer Hartline and his colleagues from their studies of the compound visual eye of the horseshoe crab *Limulus polyphemus*. Hartline and a number of his associates, most notably F. Ratliff and, more recently, B. Knight and F. Dodge, have used this remarkable animal as a model preparation in one of the most genuinely germinal and stimulating experimental programs ever to have come from any biological laboratory. As we shall see below, their findings have had widespread ramifications, not only in explaining the sort of spatial effects in perception that enchanted Mach so thoroughly, but also as a possible explanation of some other more recently discovered spatio-temporal interactions. While not all of these newer theories or microtheories will probably hold up under continued scrutiny, it is certainly a clear indication of the very great impact that Hartline's work has had to observe in how many different contexts other researchers have tried to use it as an explanation of their own data.

The anatomy of an individual ommatidium is presented in detail in

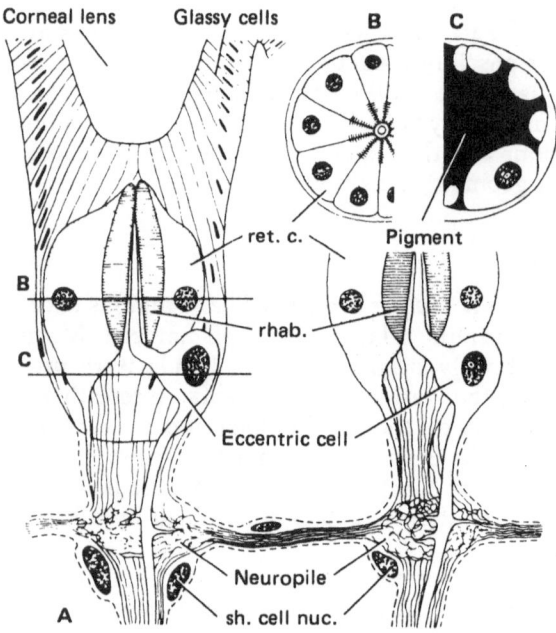

Corneal lens   Glassy cells   B   C

ret. c.   Pigment

B

rhab.

C

Eccentric cell

Neuropile

A   sh. cell nuc.

FIGURE 7.27 A drawing (A) of the neural connections at the base of a horseshoe crab ommatidium, showing two types of cross connectives. One connective type includes collateral fibers from the eccentric cell axon, and one includes collaterals of retinula cell axons: ret. = retinula, rhab. = rhabdom, sh. cell nuc. = sheath cell nucleus. (B) and (C) are cross sections viewed at the level of the lines labeled B and C (from Bullock and Horridge, 1965, after MacNichol, 1956).

Figure 7.27. For the purposes of the present discussion, all that is really required now is that we consider each ommatidium as a unitary receptor unit, interconnected with other similar units by the relatively simple linear collaterals shown in the figure. The lateral interconnectives between the ommatidia are now known to be made up of collaterals from both the axons of the retinula cells and of the eccentric cell. A peculiar feature of this network of interconnecting fibers is that whatever synaptic connections exist between them appear to be unpolarized. Granular material, apparently transmitter substance, is found on both sides of the possible synaptic connectives, and this means that either cell can be the presynaptic or, for that matter, the postsynaptic partner.

An important caveat, which should be remembered in this discussion, is that while the limulus eye is a most instructive experimental paradigm for the analysis of visual processes, it exhibits only inhibitory interactions. As we shall see, the data for both physiological and psychophysical experiments in the vertebrate eye seem better explained by networks in which both inhibitory and excitatory influences occur.

The work of Hartline's group was originally reported in four very important papers in the *Journal of General Physiology* (Hartline, Wagner, and Ratliff, 1956; Hartline and Ratliff, 1957, 1958; Ratliff and Hartline, 1959).

The general procedure used throughout the experiments was described in the first paper in this series. Photic stimulation was accomplished by appropriately shuttered light sources that were focused by an optical system that consisted mainly of an inverted microscope. In this manner, a controlled demagnification, which allowed a very small stimulus spot to be sharply focused on a single ommatidium, could be achieved. Individual unit records were usually obtained, not with microelectrodes, but by recording from single axons of eccentric cells dissected out of the optic nerve and laid across a wick electrode soaked with electrolyte solution. Occasionally, Hartline and his colleagues did use microelectrodes, but this technology was not really necessary for this preparation because of the ease with which single fibers could be isolated. Similarly, the significance of the information picked up from the single optic nerve fiber was very straightforward. This fiber was the direct extension of one eccentric cell to one ommatidium and reflected the activity solely of that single cell modulated only by the stimulus intensity and any inhibitory influences exerted by its neighbors. The interaction between two stimulated ommatidia could then be observed by stimulating each with a separate beam of light and observing the mutual effects.

Hartline, Wagner, and Ratliff have described the general nature of the response that was evoked when two cells were stimulated in words which can hardly be bettered.

> *Illumination of regions of a Limulus lateral eye in the vicinity of any particular ommatidium reduces the ability of that receptor unit to discharge impulses in response to light. During such illumination, the threshold of the receptor unit is raised, the number of impulses it discharges in response to a suprathreshold flash of light is diminished, and the frequency with which it discharges impulses during steady illumination is reduced.*
>
> (HARTLINE, WAGNER, and RATLIFF, 1956, p. 655.)

Another important aspect of their initial discovery was that the interactive effects were reciprocal or mutual. The inhibition exerted by one ommatidium on a nearby one was paralleled by an inhibition of the first by the nearby one. Thus, when two cells were simultaneously activated, the resulting level of activity in each was less than would have been obtained if only that one had been stimulated.

The nature of the anatomical mechanism underlying these inhibitory interactions was then explored by Hartline and his associates by a direct and definitive method. The interconnecting plexus, which hung between the responding ommatidia, was carefully dissected away. As increasing amounts of the tissue were severed, there was a corresponding decrease in the amount of inhibition, and the cell increased its rate of firing until finally all traces of the inhibition disappeared and the cell responded as it did originally without the inhibiting stimulus. The gradual diminution of the response weakly suggests that the effect is probably not mediated by propagated spike activity, but rather by graded potentials electronically conducted along the connectives between the ommatidia.

Having established the general nature of the phenomenon, Hartline, Wagner, and Ratliff went on to vary several of the critical parameters that defined the magnitude of the inhibitory effect. We can best summarize their results by again quoting from the 1956 paper directly:

1. *The degree to which the activity of an ommatidium is inhibited by illumination of regions of the eye is greater the higher the intensity of that illumination. (p. 659)*
2. *The more intense the inhibiting illumination, the deeper and longer lasting was the initial depression of the frequency of the discharge and the greater was the depression of the steady level that was reached after the inhibiting light had been shining for a second or more. (p. 660)*
3. *The larger the area of the eye illuminated by the inhibiting beam, the greater is the slowing of the rate at which the ommatidium discharges nerve impulses. (p. 662)*
4. *The response of an ommatidium is most effectively inhibited by illumination of other ommatidia located close to it; the effectiveness decreases with diminishing distance. Usually however, some degree of inhibition can be produced by illumination anywhere within a region surrounding it that may cover as much as one half of the total area of the eye. (p. 662)*

With regard to the shape of the inhibitory receptive field, they also found that the regions were not perfectly circular, but were oval like the eye itself. Hartline, Wagner, and Ratliff were able to map a typical inhibitory field around a given ommatidium for two different light intensities. These results from their work are shown in Figure 7.28 and indicate clearly that the size of the inhibitory field is also a function of stimulus intensity.

In the next paper in their series (Hartline and Ratliff, 1957), two additional important points were made. First, Hartline and Ratliff determined that the degree of inhibition of one ommatidium on another was a linear function of the acivity in the inhibitor. They also established the existence of an important indirect form of interaction, which they called disinhibition. If a stimulus situation with three aligned points A, B, and C is set up and the test activity recorded from point A, the following sequence of effects can be obtained. If point A is stimulated in isolation, there will be an amount of activity induced that is purely dependent upon the intensity of the stimulating light. If, in addition, point B is stimulated, then the activity at point A will be reduced in the manner we have seen, due to the lateral inhibitory interaction of B on A. If, however, point C is subsequently stimulated with a similar light source, the activity at point A will, quite to the contrary, increase. This will be so in spite of the fact that separate stimulation of only point C and point A will often show that the two are so far apart as to be outside of the area of mutual interaction. Hartline and Ratliff's explanation of the disinhibition phenomenon was that point C acted to inhibit point B. As B's activity was reduced, the effective inhibitory forces exerted by point B on point A were correspondingly reduced. In this manner a facilitory or summative effect could be simulated even though all of the interactions were, in reality, inhibitory.

The important point to be made here is that disinhibition exists and can mimic an excitatory interaction. Thus, it represents the prototype of a very important class of neural interactions, which includes superficially

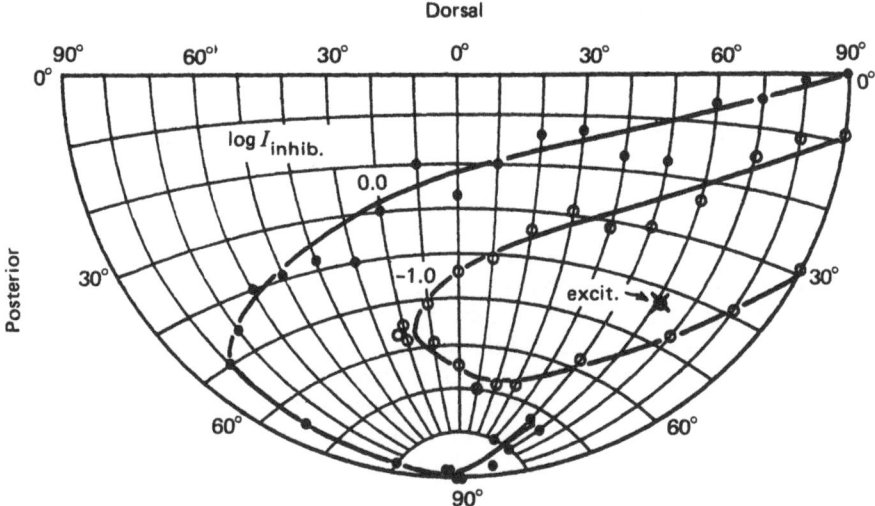

FIGURE 7.28 A drawing of the horseshoe crab eye, showing the isometric lines of constant amount of inhibitory effect for two different light intensities on a single excited ommatidium located at X. This figure tells us that the distance function of inhibition is not constant in all directions (from Hartline, Wagner, and Ratliff, 1956).

complicated processes that turn out to be synthesizable from neural processes of a much simpler kind. For example, Ratliff and Mueller (1957) have shown how simple lateral inhibitory interactions can give rise to such phenomenon as the "on," "off," and "on-off" responses in visual fibers.

In the light of this sort of emergent complexity when only a few cells with simple properties are combined, it is quite clear why Hartline's work has had such a fundamental impact and why lateral inhibitory interaction is a potentially powerful construct in expanding our understanding of neural interactions. This point was further emphasized in the third of their series of papers. Hartline and Ratliff (1958) considered the problem of the sort of interactions that occur in a situation that was a simple but very significant modification of the three stimulus disinhibition paradigm described above. In this modified experiment, point C was brought close enough to point A (from which the recordings are made) to exert its own inhibitory influence.

The question is then: how do the inhibitory influences of both point C and point B combine to jointly reduce the responses elicited by a given stimulus presented to point A? Hartline and Ratliff determined that these inhibitory influences combined in a simple and direct manner—they were simply cumulative. Though Hartline and Ratliff use the word additive, the situation, as they describe it, is a bit more complicated than a simple algebraic addition of the inhibitory effects of point B or point C acting alone. The additional complication, of course, is due to the fact that the two inhibiting points are not always independent of each other in this situation, but may also mutually inhibit the response of each other as well as the test point. Thus, the effect of both is less than the effect of the sum of each presented individually.

Nevertheless, the combined effect is the sum of the inhibitory effects of each, but as established after the level of activity of the inhibitor has been set by the combination of excitatory and inhibitory forces exerted on it. The effect is still simple—merely a summation—and in no way invokes mysterious or separate processes or the magical emergence of totally novel mechanisms, even though this additional consideration must be taken into account. Perhaps there is some insight to be gained here for later consideration of the more impressive processes of cognition, awareness, and intelligence, each of which also may be assumed to be a concatenation of essentially simple processes. While they are quantitatively large in number, there is no necessity for assuming that there is anything involved that is qualitatively different from the basic processes even at the more complex cognitive level. It is just this sort of pregnant possibility that is the basis of the wide acclaim the Hartline work has so richly earned.

In their fourth paper, Ratliff and Hartline (1959) took two very important further steps. First, they established the details of the distance function and demonstrated that both the threshold of the inhibitory effect and its magnitude (once the lower threshold was crossed) decreased the further away the inhibiting site was from the test site. Most excitingly, in this paper they also ingeniously simulated the perceptual Mach band and thus presented one of the most singularly compelling of the few direct pieces of evidence confirming a neurological model of a perceptual process. The ideal procedure would have involved the presentation of the classic stimulus gradient of stimulus intensity used in the psychophysical Mach band experiment (see Figure 7.24) and then a measurement of the amount of neural activity at a large number of different points across the surface of the horseshoe crab eye. Obviously, this is one of those places where the logistic limitations of the single microelectrode technique forces the experimenter to deviate from the ideal. To use a spatial array of microelectrodes would either involve a very large amount of equipment or a very large amount of electrode manipulation.

Ratliff and Hartline ingeniously suggested, as an alternative, a technique, which substituted time for space. They set up a single cell preparation, as usual, and then moved the stimulus gradient across the eye at a rather slow pace so that transient effects would be minimized. In this manner, they were able to observe the response of that single cell in what was effectively many different positions with reference to the stimulus pattern. Thus, it was as if they had moved their electrode sequentially from one receptor to another across the whole pattern.

Figure 7.29 is a plot of the three important parts of their findings. The insert shows the typical energy gradient of the physical stimulus. The curve indicated with triangles shows the amount of activity induced when the

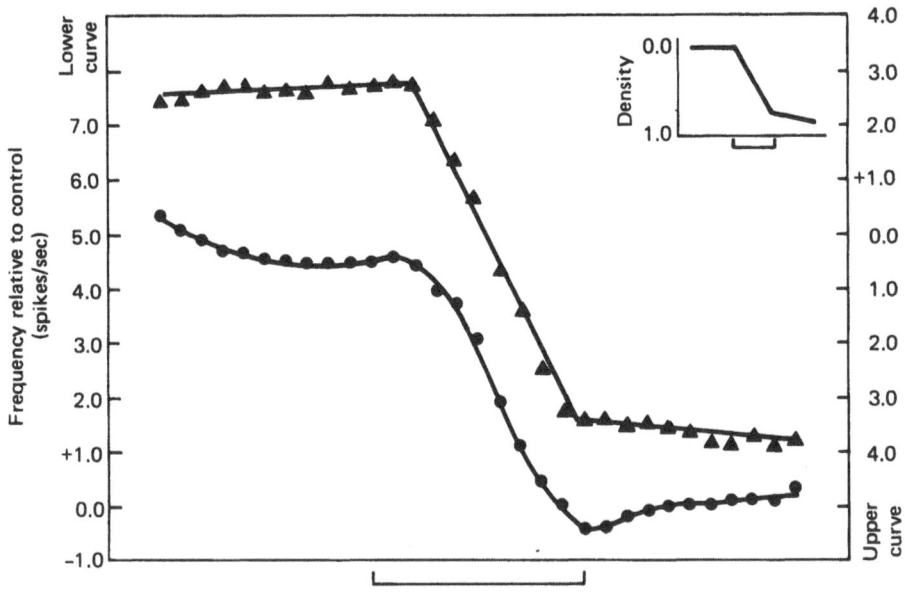

FIGURE 7.29 *An analogue of the Mach band experiment set up in the horseshoe crab eye. The insert shows the physical stimulus intensity pattern. The curve marked with triangles is the response obtained if all except the single ommatidium, from which the neural response is recorded, are shielded from the stimulus as it is moved across the eye. The curve marked with small circles shows the typical "Mach band" contour enhancement, which occurs when the whole eye is illuminated with the moving pattern. It is important to remember in this experiment that the recording is from only one ommatidium and that it is the stimulus that is being moved from place to place rather than the electrode (from Ratliff and Hartline, 1959).*

illumination was restricted solely to the region of the test receptor. In this case there is no activity elicited in the area surrounding the test ommatidium, and the response, predictably, simply reproduces the pattern of the stimulus intensity. However, when the entire stimulus pattern is allowed to fall on the horseshoe crab eye, then quite a different situation obtains. First, the overall amount of activity is decreased, thus confirming the general nature of the inhibitory interaction among the receptors of the limulus eye. More significantly, at the points of inflection of the stimulus gradient, there now appears a local increase or decrease in the amount of induced neural activity corresponding to the subjective reports of the bright and dark bands in the human psychophysical experiment.

It would be nice if we could at this point say "QED" and assume that the issue is completely resolved and that in fact a compelling theoretical model of the Mach band and related phenomena has been given. But it is still important to remember that this is a model system. The horseshoe crab has told us nothing of what he is "perceiving," and up to this point there has been no discussion of similar mechanisms in the vertebrate retina. It is to this matter we shall now turn and discover that, not unexpectedly, there is more to be said about the situation in higher animals.

2. *Lateral Interaction in the Vertebrate Retina.* The key data, which began to answer some of the questions of lateral neurophysiological interaction in the vertebrate retina, were first reported by Kuffler (1952, 1953) and were obtained from experiments carried out in the cat's eye. Prior to his studies of the interaction effects, Kuffler had been exploring the organization of receptive fields in the eye of this animal, using glass insulated metal microelectrodes. These tiny electrodes were inserted into the retina and were able to pick up, extracellularly, spike action potentials from ganglion cells and their axons. Thus, the data obtained by Kuffler were based upon a flow of information, which had already passed through at least two levels of synaptic interaction and had been already subject to considerable processing and integration. (The reader may want to refer back to Figure 3.17 in our section on retinal anatomy to reflect upon the diversity of neural connectives in and about the inner and outer plexiform layers of the retina at this point and consider the possible interactions suggested by such a net.) Clearly, the anatomy of the situation is considerably more complicated than that of the limulus eye, and correspondingly, the physiological behavior of the system was also found to be far more complex.

Kuffler made a number of important observations concerning receptive field organization. He had, for example, discovered that the receptive fields, while averaging 1 to 2 mm in diameter on the retina, varied considerably in size as the stimulus intensity changed—a fact reminiscent of Hartline's observations that the size of the field of inhibitory interaction in the limulus eye also varied with stimulus intensity. Kuffler further discovered that not only did the size of the field change, but the general organization and polarity of the interactions within the field could also vary with stimulus intensity or the size of the stimulus.

The receptive field of a typical ganglion cell was characteristically organized as shown in Figure 7.30. A series of three concentric regions could activate the ganglion cell in three different ways. Small stimuli applied to the central region would produce a pure "on" response; that is, spikes would be evoked only at the onset of the stimulus. Small stimuli applied to the outermost ring would produce a pure "off" response; that is, spikes would be evoked only at the offset of the stimulus, while stimuli applied to the intermediate ring would produce both "on" and "off" responses—spikes being evoked at both the onset and offset of the stimulus.

Given this type of receptive field organization, it is not surprising to learn that Kuffler discovered that the type of interaction observed between two stimuli was also more involved than that observed in the limulus eye. In fact, the best generalization of his results that can be made is that he found almost all possible forms of interaction that might have been hypothesized among the "on," "off," and "on-off" type of responses. It was possible, for example, to inhibit the "off" response of a test stimulus by the presence of a stimulus that produced an "on" response and vice versa, even

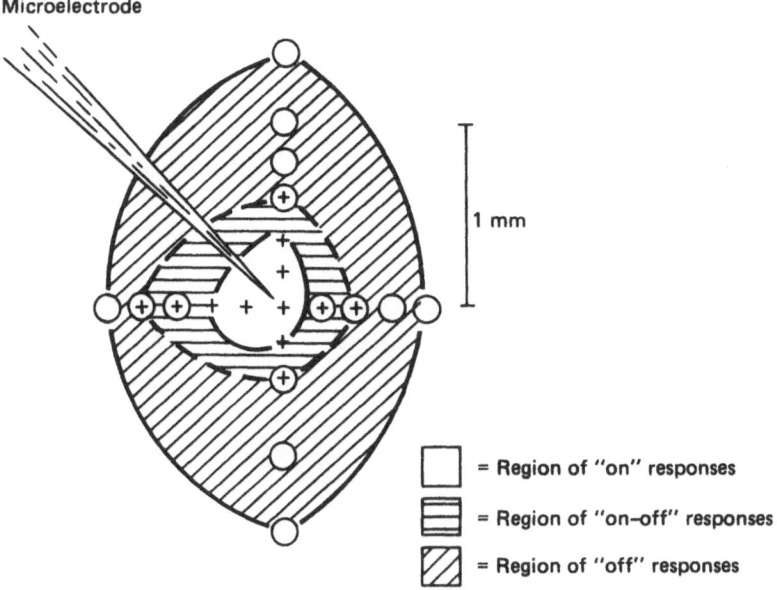

Microelectrode

1 mm

☐ = Region of "on" responses

▤ = Region of "on–off" responses

▨ = Region of "off" responses

FIGURE 7.30 Organization of a receptive field in the cat's retina. In this particular ganglion cell's receptive field, a center region capable of only producing "on" responses is surrounded by a middle ring of "on-off" sensitivity and then a larger annulus of purely "off" responses (from Kuffler, 1953).

though the results varied depending upon the intensity of the stimulating lights, and where the mask and test stimuli were located in the tripartite receptive field.

Figure 7.31 (adapted from Kuffler, 1953) shows the three different types of interaction patterns, which could be obtained by slight changes in the intensity of simultaneous stimuli in the same cell. In the first series of three plates (indicated as Series I), one stimulus is presented to a pure "on" region and another to a pure "off" region. If they are presented separately, the evoked responses are as shown in the two upper photographs. If the two stimuli are presented together, then the "off" responses can be inhibited if the intensity relations of the two stimuli are such that the stimulus evoking the "on" response is more intense, and the stimulus evoking the "off" response is less intense. The same cell will show an inhibition of the "on" response when the two stimuli are presented simultaneously, but the intensity relation reversed (Series II). Mutual inhibition of both the "on" and the "off" responses could occur if the two stimuli were both increased in intensity. The respective responses to both of the stimuli would be less than that to either alone (Series III). Kuffler also found that if the two stimuli were both inserted adjacent to each other in the part of the receptive field producing "on" responses, that "on" response could also inhibit other "on" responses. However, superimposing the two stimuli leads to a summation of their effects rather than a mutual inhibition.

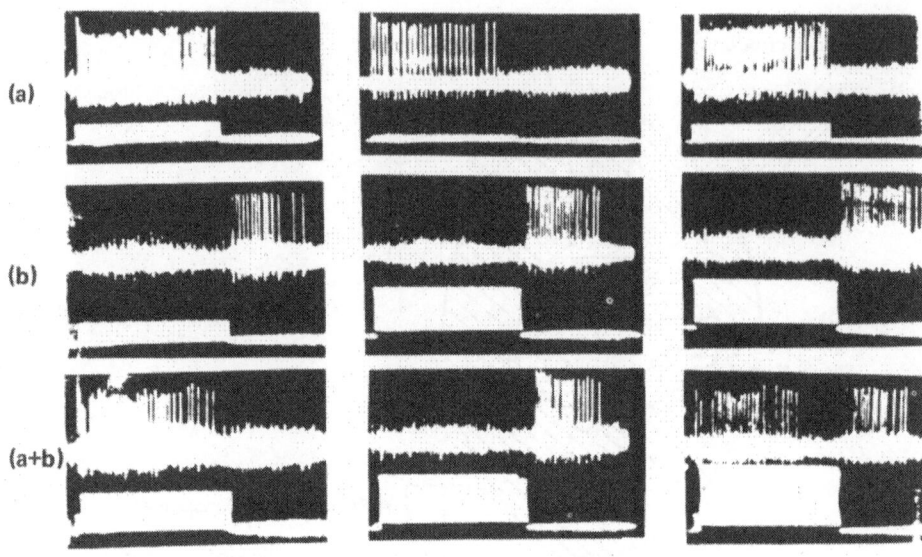

(a)

(b)

(a+b)

I   II   III

FIGURE 7.31 This set of pictures shows the complicated interactions that occur between space and intensity in the ganglion cell response of the cat's retina. Spot a was placed in the center of the receptive field and produced a pure "on" response. Spot b was placed in that portion of the periphery of the receptive field, which produced a pure "off" response. Depending upon the relative intensities of the two spots, the combined response might be either "on," "off," or a combined "on-off" response as shown in the three columns labeled I, II, and III (from Kuffler, 1953).

Perhaps the most important result of this work was the emergence of the notion of the center-surround antagonistic receptive field organization. While Kuffler observed center "on" and surround "off" organization, other investigators have also observed cells that are organized in just the opposite way; an inner region that, when stimulated, produces only "off" responses surrounded by an outer region which produces only "on" responses. This sort of organization has been referred to as an "off center" field just as the former arrangement Kuffler originally observed is now known as an "on center" type of receptive field.

Rodieck and Stone (1965a, 1965b) have, in recent years, pursued the same problem of receptive field organization in the cat's retina pioneered by Kuffler, and their findings are generally in agreement with his older results. In addition, however, Rodieck and Stone have shown that the antagonistic center-surround receptive fields are most effectively activated by moving figures (although as we shall see later, there was no evidence of a specific directional preference in the cat). Dark spots on light fields and light spots on dark fields produced identical results when used to activate inhibitory center and excitatory center receptive fields, respectively, regardless of the direction of movement. Velocity specificity also seemed to be present, but no shape specific sensitivity was observed except for sensitivity to the width (in whatever the direction of movement) of the stimulus.

Perhaps their most important contribution in the present context was Rodieck and Stone's speculation that both "on," "off," and "on-off" mechanisms and the center-surround receptive field organization are produced by the summation of two dome-shaped processes, one inhibitory and one excitatory, overlapping each other in the receptive field as shown in Figure 7.32, in such a way that the weighted sum of their effects determined the response. Each process may actually cover large and overlapping areas of the receptive field. "On," "off," and "on-off" responses are produced, from their point of view, by the summation of relative magnitudes of the two opposing effects. Thus, the surround is only functionally an annulus, and, in fact, the underlying mechanisms are of the same sort of uniform dome shape as the inhibitory fields observed in the limulus eye. The more elaborate receptive field structure in the vertebrate eye is presumably imposed because of the pooled effects of a dome-shaped excitatory pattern of interaction and the equally monopolar inhibitory pattern similar to that found in the horseshoe crab eye.

3. Do Lateral Interaction Mechanisms Exist in the Other Senses? The case seems fairly conclusive that there is a wide variety of spatial interactions possible among laterally displaced stimuli in vision. These effects can be reflected in many different ways in the peripheral evoked neural responses. The question now arises: is a similar sort of lateral interaction possible in the other senses? Naturally, it is to hearing we must turn first to consider this issue, and it is in this modality that, second only to vision, the most is known about possible lateral interactive mechanisms. Figure 7.9 showed why the plexus underlying the hair cell receptors may provide the necessary anatomical substrate for this interaction. We have also considered the psychophysical evidence earlier in this chapter.

But what of the physiological evidence? Galambos and Davis (1943) demonstrated that the response pattern of single auditory nerve fibers could be well represented by a V-shaped response region on an intensity-frequency plot, within which a stimulus is capable of evoking a response in that neuron. We have already discussed this point briefly in the section on receptive fields and shall present a fuller discussion in the next chapter on quality coding.

Galambos (1944), with the collaboration of Davis, subsequently discovered that tones with frequencies and intensities outside of the V-shaped response area could also have an effect on the response of these auditory nerve fibers. Generally, the effect was manifested by an inhibition of the spontaneous noise level in these fibers. All combinations of inhibitory arrangements were found with some cells inhibited by frequencies higher than those included in their response areas, some by tones lower and some by tones both higher and lower.

Recently some important additions to this notion of lateral inhibition of tones by other tones have been made by Greenwood and Maruyama (1965). They were also interested in the induced effects of stimuli that fell

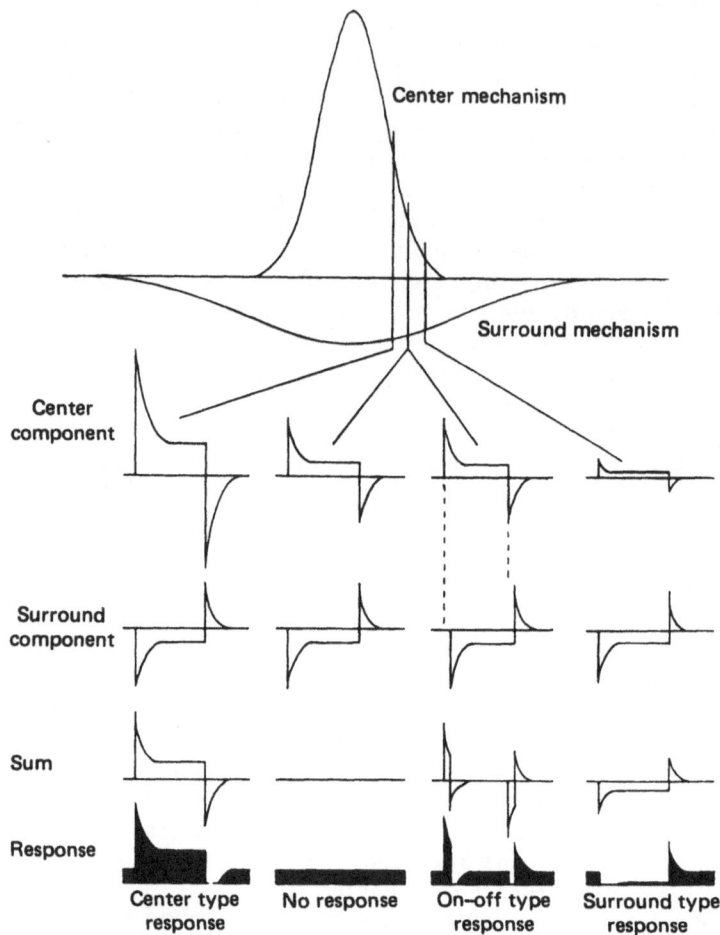

FIGURE 7.32 *A further demonstration of the complex effect of stimulus location and receptive field geometry on the response that may be obtained from even a simple type of field. The top figure shows Rodieck and Stone's interpretation of the concentric center-surround antagonistic receptive field as being the result of two dome shaped and monophasic areas of inhibition and excitation. Depending upon where a stimulus was placed in the field, it might produce different degrees of "on" and "off" responses as indicated by the second and third row of drawings. The sum of the two, directly a function of the spatial location of the stimulus, determines the nature of the output (from Rodieck and Stone, 1965a).*

outside of the response area of a given cell on the activity of that cell. As we have seen, Galambos, as well as defining the response area in collaboration with Davis, had also found that there were inhibitory effects of stimuli outside the response area. Greenwood and Maruyama have refined this preliminary observation and shown that if spatial coding analogies are kept in mind, the type of interaction that occurs is very similar to that found in the vertebrate retina. Indium-filled microelectrodes were inserted

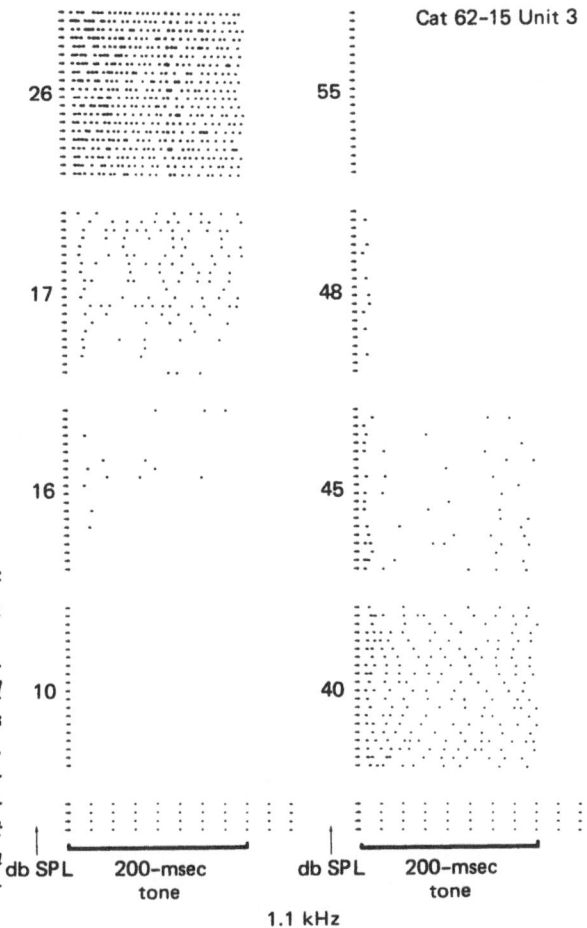

FIGURE 7.33 The pattern of response of a cochlear nerve neuron to a 1.1 kHz stimulus at several different intensities. The response is plotted horizontally for many runs at each stimulus intensity. Increasing the stimulus intensity first increases the response, but after 40 db it begins to decrease again (from Greenwood and Maruyama, 1965).

into single cells of the cochlear nucleus of the upper medulla, and the acoustically evoked spike responses plotted as a series of dot patterns. Each dot represented the occurrence of a single spike action potential. These response records were plotted on an oscilloscope with the horizontal axis representing the time after stimulation. Each time a new stimulus was presented, the oscilloscopic trace was lowered a small amount, and in this manner a full account of the activity following each of a series of stimuli could be recorded. If the dotted line is very dense, then the spike activity was also great; if it is sparse, then, so was the neural activity. Changes in the pattern of activity could then be observed as a function of other conditions as demonstrated in Figure 7.33, a sample record. Greenwood and Maruyama usually replotted their data to display the relationships between the inhibitory and excitatory response areas of the individual cochlear nucleus cell (see, for example, Figure 7.34, below). In this case, the horizontal axis on their figures has a dual meaning. First, it indicates the frequency of the stimulating signal, and second, it indicates the approximate

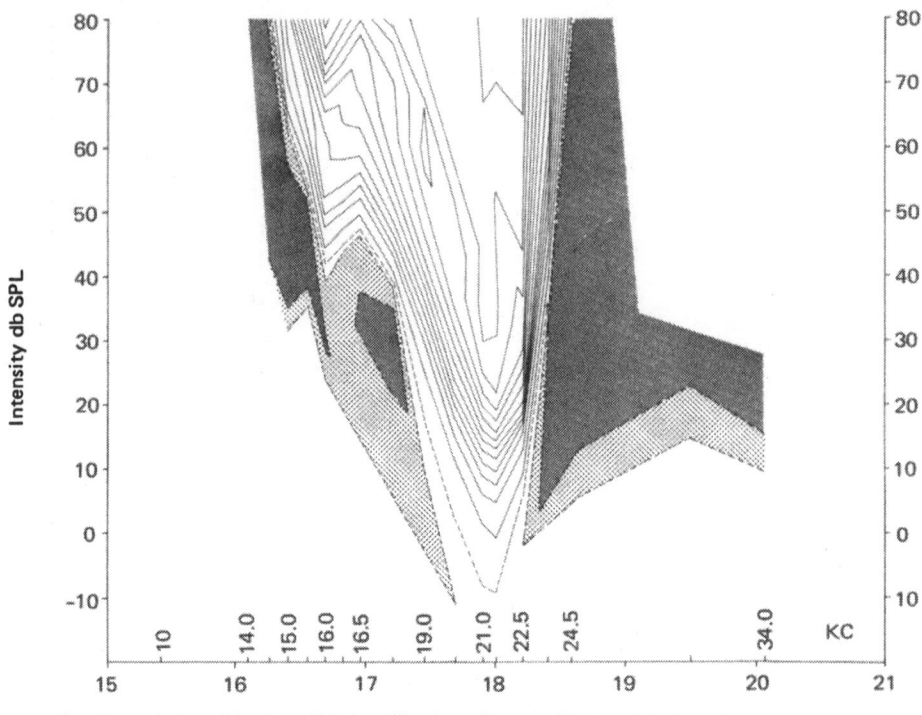

FIGURE 7.34 The response area of a single cochlear nucleus neuron with a center frequency of 21.5 kHz. The isometric lines in the middle define equal regions of excitation. The crosshatched regions indicate points in the intensity-frequency space that inhibited the spontaneous activity of this cell by at least three standard deviations below spontaneous activity. The stippled area indicates inhibitory regions in which there was somewhat less inhibition—between one and three standard deviations below spontaneous activity (from Greenwood and Maruyama, 1965).

point on the cochlea at which it is thought the maximum deflection occurs for that stimulus frequency.

A wide variety of cellular response types was observed by Greenwood and Maruyama, and the significance of the response patterns is not always immediately obvious. Not the least difficulty was caused by the fact that stimuli often exerted both inhibitory and excitatory influences sequentially as the stimulus intensity or frequency was varied. Nevertheless, there was a general or, perhaps it would be better to say, a prototypical form of response found in many cells that does seem to emphasize the basic form of the interaction. As measured by their influence on the amount of spontaneous activity, stimuli with intensity and frequency outside of the excitatory response areas of a given cochlear nucleus cell usually inhibit if the difference is not too great, but when the frequencies differ greatly, they exert no influence. Figure 7.34 displays this sort of interaction for a high-frequency cell, in which the response pattern was of this prototypical type. This complex figure contains a wealth of information. First, all of the contour lines connect points of equal response amplitude and polarity. Thus, a 21.5-kHz stimulus with an intensity 10 db above the reference sound pressure level produces just as great a response as an 18-kHz tone 50 db above that reference.

More pertinent to our present discussion, however, is the fact that opposite effects can be produced by stimuli of identical frequency but different amplitudes. The middle unshaded region of Figure 7.34 is a reconstruction of the usual V-shaped response area as defined by Galambos and Davis (1943). On the other hand, there is also a surrounding region, as indicated in this figure with dots or cross-hatching in which an excitatory stimulus, when only slightly shifted in intensity, will begin to inhibit spontaneous activity or activity induced with some other tone. The potential intricacy of this type of interaction is profound, for a stimulus can also change from an excitatory to an inhibitory one merely by a small shift in its frequency, even though its intensity is held constant. Conversely, stimuli with constant frequency can be made to alter the polarity of their effect by a slight variation in their intensity. The complexities that such simple mechanisms can and probably do introduce into the coding of such auditory patterns as music, for example, are quite beyond the analytical powers of our science at the present time.

A further important generalization that can be drawn from this sort of data is that the cochlea exhibits the same sort of antagonistic center-surround organization observed in the retina. There is a central region, always excitatory in the case of this auditory response area, within an antagonistic surround that is always inhibitory. This antagonistic center-surround organization is observed through the medium of tonal (temporal) interactions, but, hopefully, it should be clear by now that auditory tone pattern discrimination is, in large part, mediated by spatial neural patterns as a result of the mechanical analyzing action of the cochlea.

A similar sort of antagonistic center-surround organization has been observed by Mountcastle and Powell (1959) in cells of the somatosensory area of the monkey's cerebral cortex. A microelectrode was inserted into the cortex near a cell, which was activated by a specific receptive field on the forearm of the experimental animal. The receptive field could be traced out in the usual fashion. When a second stimulus was applied to a region surrounding that receptive field, the neural activity in the cortical cell was drastically reduced. Figure 7.35 shows the general shape and size of the antagonistic excitatory and inhibitory receptive fields on the monkey's arm of that cortical cell.

As usual, the process seemed to be quite reciprocal. Mountcastle and Powell's extracellular technique of recording also picked up the responses of other nearby cells, and in some records they were able to observe other cells activated by the same stimulus that inhibited the action of the test neuron. For these cells, the "inhibitory stimulus was an excitatory one." Furthermore, these cells could be seen to decrease their activity during the time the original excitatory stimulus was on. Figure 7.36 shows the effects

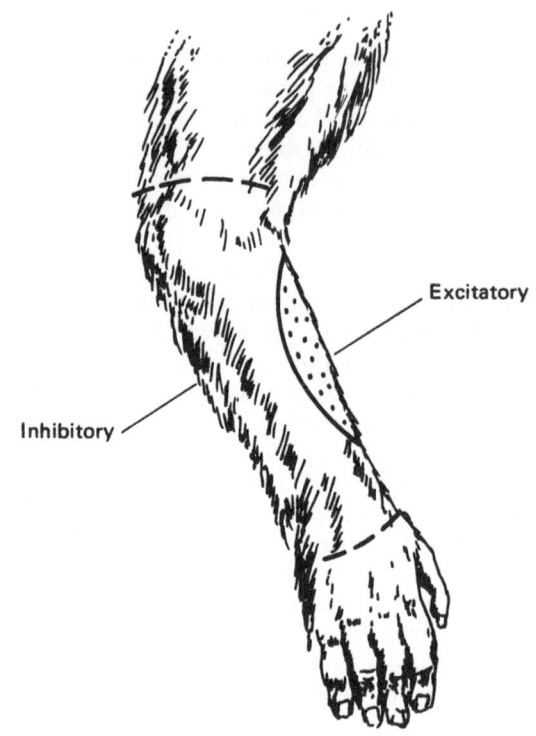

FIGURE 7.35 The antagonistic center-surround receptive field arrangement of a somatosensory corticall cell on the monkey's arm (from Mountcastle and Powell, 1959).

of the two stimuli on the responses of both cells. The interaction between the two is seen to be reciprocal in very much the same sense as the mutual inhibitory interaction in the limulus eye.

The general conclusions that may be drawn from all of this work is that there is interaction of spatially separated stimuli in vertebrate receptor systems just as there was in invertebrates. Although the pattern of interaction is far more complicated than the simple lateral inhibition found in the limulus eye, it is clear that some sort of lateral interaction is present at least peripherally and that it represents a very important mechanism, which must be taken into account in all accounts of vertebrate information processing.

In sum, the vertebrate lateral interaction seems to be characterized by an important geographic property. There usually seems to be some sort of an antagonistic center-surround organization such that a central region, in which stimuli may either excite or inhibit, is surrounded by a region of the opposite polarity. These receptive regions are defined, as we have noted, only in terms of a given input channel (an axon or a nerve). The same retinal locus may be inhibitory for one channel, but excitatory for some other one. Furthermore, it should be appreciated that the general result of simultaneous stimulation of the center and the surround is to reduce the effect of either stimulus presented alone.

FIGURE 7.36 *The response patterns of two somatosensory cortical cells that are linked in an antagonistic pattern. The excitatory stimulus turns on the cell whose response is marked with the dotted line. While the excitatory stimulus was on another, stimulus applied to the annular inhibitory region shown in Figure 7.35 excited an "inhibitory cell" and inhibited an "excitatory cell" whose response is marked with the solid line. This pattern of interaction is quite similar to the concentric center-surround antagonistic receptive field found in the eye and the ear (from Mountcastle and Powell, 1959).*

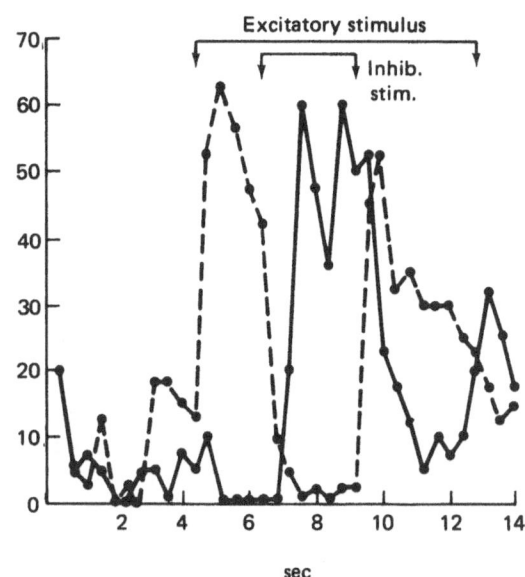

4. Do Central Lateral Interaction Mechanisms Exist? A very important point, usually neglected but of the utmost importance as attempts are made to utilize the lateral interaction mechanisms as a neurophysiological model of various perceptual phenomena, concerns whether or not such interaction occurs among central neurons or groups of neurons. Although there is satisfactory and sufficient evidence of peripheral lateral interaction, this same sort of study does not, unfortunately, directly confirm the existence of central interaction. Although central cells often reflect the results of simple geometrical lateral interaction, this finding does not tell us that such interaction necessarily occurred centrally. As with any other analysis of a closed input-output system, it is not possible to tell at what stage in the system a given transformation occurred by simply observing the relationship between the input and the output. To reduce the argument to its most extreme form (and one which we do not necessarily wish to champion at the moment), it may, on the other hand, have been that reciprocal lateral interaction is a geometrical process, which is only really possible within the limits of a simple neural plexus in the periphery. It may be, in other words, that this form of neural integration is meaningful only in the initial portion of the communication process, which conveys information from the periphery to the CNS. The question is not, it must be emphasized, simply a matter of whether or not inhibitory synapses occur in the central nervous system, but rather whether mutual lateral inhibition exists centrally in a way that is analogous to the geometrical relations that have been established for the periphery.

Because the type of experiment that is necessary to definitively answer this question is difficult to do, central reciprocal lateral inhibition has been only very infrequently discussed in a critical manner. The ideal experiment would require some way to separately stimulate, for example, cortical regions that were close enough to interact but that were sufficiently independent to avoid simultaneous activation when a stimulus was applied. Stimulus effects would have to be produced on the cortex, for example, with the same sort of topological relations as they are presented to the retina and mutual interaction observed in the absence of peripheral lateral interaction. But central structures are well known to be very heavily cross-connected, and this sort of experiment may, in fact, be impossible to perform.

A thought experiment, which might provide some possible approaches toward an answer to this question, may be proposed. Hubel and Wiesel (1963) have demonstrated that the ends of the cortical columns are laid out across the surface of the cortex in an irregular mosaic pattern. It should be possible to locate two adjacent areas that are preferentially activated by stimuli moving in opposite or perpendicular directions. In this manner, neither would be activated by the effective stimulus for the other area, and the change, if any, observed in the response pattern of one region when the second stimulus evoked activity in the adjacent region would be a true indication of the possible interactions. A corollary experiment would be to observe the interactions of columns that are not adjacent physically, but that are stimulated by stimuli moving in only slightly different preferential directions. Without evidence of interactions in either of these cases, the notion of lateral interaction among cortical columns, a hypothesis frequently invoked by some psychophysiologists in their models of such phenomena as metacontrast or sequential blanking, becomes equivocal.

Von Békésy (1967), in his most insightful and interesting book on sensory inhibition, has also considered this question of whether lateral interactions occur centrally. He also was faced with a paucity of direct experimental evidence of interactions at higher levels of the nervous system and was able to refer only to demonstrations of interactive effects recorded at the higher levels, but induced with natural peripheral stimuli. As noted, we do not believe that the question can be answered with this type of experimental paradigm.

Another way to demonstrate central lateral interaction, although somewhat indirectly, would be to show that there is an increased sharpening of the spatial spread of a particular patterned response at sequential levels. Indeed, it is the need for this sort of sharpening or "funneling" that is at the heart of von Békésy's expression of the fact that such central lateral inhibitory interaction "must" occur. However, as noted by Simmons (1970), there appears to be no such sharpening in the auditory system. He says, "In fact, most such tuning is already nearing completion in the cochlear nucleus" (Simmons, 1970, p. 359). We shall deal with this notion in greater detail in Chapter 12, when we discuss auditory neuron tuning curves and their relationship to quality coding.

A similar situation seems to obtain in the somatosensory system, according to Kenneth Casey of the University of Michigan. He notes (personal communication, 1971) that there is no reduction in the size of somatosensory receptive fields as one ascends the nervous chain. Iggo (1960) has shown that the receptive fields of C fibers are no more than about 2 × 2 to 5 × 5 mm at the periphery, and Winter (1965) has shown that peripheral A fibers have receptive field sizes that are usually no larger than 0.1 cm^2 for the cat's digits. In the dorsal column nuclei, Winter also describes the same receptive fields as being about 1 cm^2. In the monkey thalamus, they appear to be even larger; according to Poggio and Mountcastle (1963), they can be as large as 2 to 20 cm^2. In the monkey's cortex, Mountcastle and Powell (1959) describe receptive fields varying up to 35 cm^2. Clearly, rather than being funneled into smaller and smaller receptive fields, the receptive fields of the somatosensory system cells are generally becoming ever larger as one moves more centrally.

Another important finding in all of these reports was the relative rarity of center-surround organization. The center-surround organization appeared to be a very rare phenomenon with no more than 10 percent of the cells at any of the somatosensory levels exhibiting that now-familiar form of lateral inhibitory organization.

Similarly, visual receptive field size in the cortex seems not to be any smaller than those at the peripheral ganglion cell layer in the cat. (Compare the findings of Spinelli, 1967, with those of Spinelli and Barrett, 1969.) If anything, they are generally larger (and some diffuse types are quite a bit larger), suggesting that rather than sharpening, there has been an increase in the receptive field area due to the convergence of multiple inputs. It should be noted, on the other hand, that a few neurophysiologists have directly concerned themselves with the problem of central lateral inhibition and have what they consider to be positive evidence for such processes. Krnjevic, Randic, and Straughan (1964) specifically have shown a reduction in the responsiveness to stimulation with electrophoretically deposited L-glutamate when other nearby regions of the cortex were electrically stimulated. This is evidence for a sort of general inhibitory mechanism, some form of which would be necessary to keep brains from being in a constant state of activity or *status epilepticus*. Whether this generalized inhibition is analogous to the geometrical processes observed in the peripheral receptor net of limulus or the retina of a cat is, of course, moot.

More to the specific point is the work of Singer and Creutzfeldt (1970) concerning reciprocal lateral inhibition of neurons in the lateral geniculate body of the cat's visual system. They found that cells with center-surround antagonistic field arrangement did appear to be inhibited by nearby cells with the opposite polarity of organization. Thus, a center-surround unit with an excitatory center was inhibited, it seemed, by a nearby unit with an inhibitory center receptive field organization. However, these authors are also careful to note that the type of reciprocal inhibition they observe is not necessarily the same as the type we have already discussed. For example, they note:

> The organization of "reciprocal lateral inhibition" between the on- and the off-system will not improve spatial contrast like the classical type of lateral inhibition in Limulus and in the cat's retina.
> (SINGER and CREUTZFELDT, 1970, p. 329.)

Thus they clearly separate the mechanism they have studied from the simple geometrical sort of lateral interaction found in the periphery. They do, however, suggest that it might be a useful mechanism for sensitivity and successive contrast enhancement.

It is clear that this issue cannot be resolved at the present time. It seems that the receptive field and tuning curve data provide no support for continued lateral reciprocal interaction (of the peripheral sort) at higher levels, but it is also certain that there must be some sort of inhibitory process centrally to stabilize cortical activity. There is little evidence of further central sharpening in any sense modality, however, and that is the main point which this section is intended to make. (But, note the discussion of Gardner and Spencer's [1972a, 1972b] work below.)

C. Theories of Lateral Interaction

1. Ratliff's Summary. Ratliff's (1965) book has been especially useful, since it clearly points out the similarities among several theories that have been presented by different authors to explain lateral interactions in both the invertebrate and the vertebrate eye. Ratliff is careful to emphasize that while there are important differences between the simple inhibitory nets of the horseshoe crab eye and the combined excitatory and inhibitory interactions typical of the vertebrate retina or cochlea, all of the theories converge on a few common major ideas. The most important discrepancy among the different theories is, of course, the presence or absence of the central excitatory zone. Depending upon what particular mechanism in which particular species is being modeled, some of the authors ignore the presence of the central zone and assume that summation is a process that only occurs when two or more stimuli fall directly on a single receptor. In their models, summation, therefore, is only a reflection of the fact that the single receptor has spatial extent itself. On the other hand, other theorists, usually dealing with vertebrate receptors, assume that there is a network of excitatory interaction very much like the network of inhibition, which is the only sort of interaction found in the limulus eye. The nature of the differences and of the similarities has been best summed up by Ratliff in a chart which is reproduced in Table 7.1, showing both the assumed inhibition-excitation functions and the mathematical relations assumed in six of the most important theories.

Although Ratliff feels that the difference between Taylor's (1956) or Hartline and Ratliff's (1958) theories, on the one hand, and those of von Békésy or Huggins and Licklider (1951), on the other, can be minimized by simply assuming a blur function that spreads the stimulus, such a notion probably does not take into account a more fundamental difference between the two approaches. The theories that assume a very narrow excitatory region, corresponding only to the width of a single cell, do not necessarily assume that there is an excitatory plexus of interconnecting fibers. On the other hand, those with broad central regions always implicitly, if not explicitly, assume some sort of a central receptive field organization with neural interconnections organized such that the activation of many individual receptors can elecit a response in a single ganglion nerve fiber. From this latter perspective, excitatory neural nets are assumed to be present while from the former, they are not. It seems clear that this difference is fundamental and that the theories may be assumed to be of two clearly distinguishable types. The more general one includes both dispersed excitation and inhibition mediated by the appropriate neural nets, and the less general one involves only inhibitory neural interactions.

Ratliff further emphasizes that there are also some other differences among the several theories that are of note. The Hartline and Ratliff model (1958) and that of Taylor (1963) are the only two of the six theories described in Table 7.1, that are "recurrent"; that is, the inhibitory force exerted by each receptor is dependent upon both the stimulus applied to it and the inhibitory forces that are exerted on it by its neighbor. In this case, since the neighbor is presumably also recurrently affected by the response level of the first cell itself, the first cell's output is also indirectly a function of its own level of activity. A nonrecurrent system, on the other hand, is one in which the inhibitory action that is exerted by a cell is purely a function of the stimulus acting on that cell. The difference between the two has been graphically shown by Ratliff in a drawing, which is reproduced in Figure 7.37. Unfortunately, as Ratliff points out, it is difficult to determine from the overall response of the system whether the actual neural interaction, in the vertebrate retina, for example, is recurrent or nonrecurrent, since both single recurrent stages of lateral interaction or dual stages of nonrecurrent interaction can produce almost identical performance.

Since the models are nearly equivalent, if one disregards certain of the considerations we have mentioned, let us consider Hartline and Ratliff's own model as a simple example of the type of theory that is both plausible and useful in describing their important findings.

The basic equation of their model, which is, in fact, a system of simultaneous equation, can be expressed as follows:

$$r_p = e_p - \sum_{j=1}^{n} k_{p,j}(r_j - r_{p,j}^0) \tag{7.1}$$

This equation provides a means of computing the response of r_p of the pth axon, which is defined by this relation to be equal to the amount of excitation e_p produced by the stimulus falling on the receptor minus the sum of the inhibitory forces that are exerted on it by its j neighbors. The sum of the inhibitory forces is calculated by computing, for all of those j cells (from $j = 1$ to $j = n$) that inhibit the response of the pth cell, the term $k_{p,j}(r_j - r_{p,j}^0)$, where $k_{p,j}$ is a constant specifying the magnitude of the interaction between cell p and cell j; r_j is the response of the cell j; and $r_{p,j}^0$ is the threshold value of the response of the jth cell for any interaction between cells p and j. The constant $k_{p,j}$ is necessary because of the empirical fact (noted above) that the degree of interaction between any two cells varies considerably from one pair to another. It is a constant, fortunately for a given pair of cells and the interaction is linear over wide ranges. Otherwise, a very complicated system of nonlinear equations would be required to adequately model this system. The necessity to subtract a

TABLE 7.1 GEOMETRICAL AND MATHEMATICAL
CHARACTERISTICS OF SIX MODELS OF LATERAL INHIBITORY
INTERACTION (FROM RATLIFF, 1965)

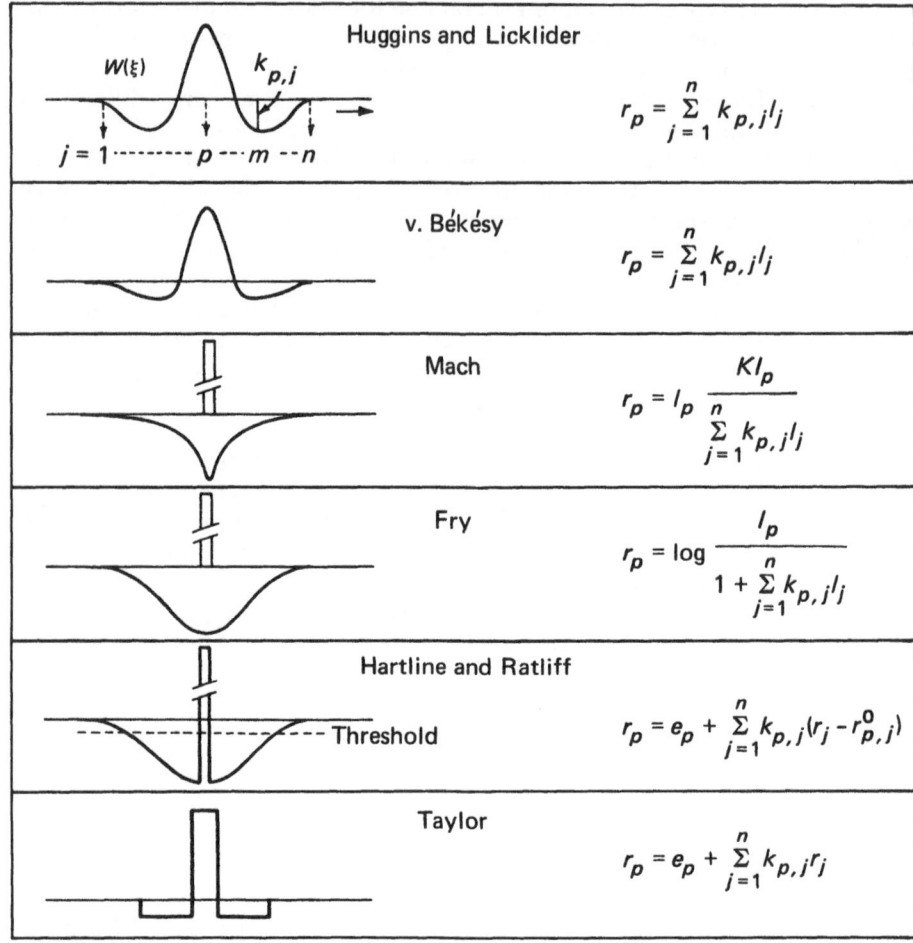

In this table $W(\xi)$ is the two dimensional inhibition-excitation function of which a cross section is shown; j is the parameter (that may assume values of p,m,n etc.) scanning the series of adjacent receptors; $k_{p,j}$ is the coefficient of inhibition between any point j and the central point p; r_p is the response of the central point p; I_p and I_j are the illuminations of points p and j respectively; $r_{p,j}^0$ is the threshold of interaction between points p and j; e_p is excitation produced by the stimulus on point p; r_j is the response of point j and K is a constant.

threshold term $r_{p,j}^0$ is also a direct result of the observed biology of the situation. Hartline and his colleagues had determined in their experiments that the threshold for the response of a cell to stimulation was generally lower than the level at which it could begin to exert inhibitory influence on another cell. Thus, there was a region in which the cell j could be responding to a stimulus without exerting any inhibitory influences on cell p.

Such a system of simultaneous equations can be solved by hand, but it is a laborious and difficult process. This is particularly so if the interaction

FIGURE 7.37 Two drawings that show the difference between (a) recurrent and (b) nonrecurrent lateral inhibitory interaction processes. The distinction is, simply, based upon whether or not the inhibitory action of a neighboring unit affects the excitatory process or impinges upon the cell beyond the point (marked x) at which the level of activity is defined (from Ratliff, Hartline and Miller, 1963).

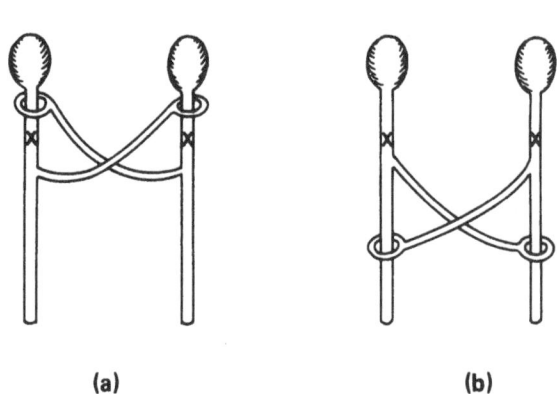

(a)   **(b)**

functions are assumed to be recurrent. In that case, a series of iterative steps approaching a stable solution to the problem must be used. A computer is, therefore, by far the superior means of solving the system of equations. Either digital or analogue processes can be used, but in this type of problem, in which simultaneous linear algebraic equations must be evaluated, there are considerable advantages to using a digital computer. Very rapid solutions are possible, but perhaps even more important, the ability to rapidly change the parameters of the equation or even the nature of the hypothesized neural interactions may help to facilitate the observations of a number of mathematical "experiments."

The present author had tried his hand at a computer simulation of the Hartline-Ratliff model some years ago. One important result that quickly emerged was that the distance function (that is, the set of $k_{p,j}$) that had to be used was of critical importance in determining the closeness of fit of the computed response to the observed response. If the distance function did not extend out far enough (for example, if cells were only inhibited by their immediate neighbors), then the Mach-band-like contour intensification oscillated in space, and rather than one dark band, a series of dark and light bands with successively diminishing amplitude appeared at both ends of the gradient of stimulation.

It should be emphasized here that the equations that we have presented here are descriptive only of the steady-state stable situation that obtains after the initial transients have disappeared. An entirely different formularization would be required to describe these transient responses, and there is little question that particularly in human vision they must play an important role in encoding dynamic visual stimulus patterns.

2. Von Békésy's Theory of Funneling. Though von Békésy's theory is one of the six models discussed in the previous section, his formulation of the notion is sufficiently unique that an additional comment on it is appropriate. It is particularly of interest in the context of this present book, because von Békésy has applied this notion to such a wide variety of different sensory phenomena. In one of his many important papers describing the similarity between cutaneous and acoustic sensations, von Békésy (1958) had coined the word "funneling" to describe the sharpening of diffuse stimulus patterns applied to a spatially extensive receptor surface within which there was lateral interaction. His model essentially involves a concentrically organized system, in which a central region of summative excitation is surrounded by a concentric ring-shaped area in which sensations are inhibited. Von Békésy clearly feels that this sort of organization is attributable to lateral interconnections at all levels of the nervous system. The important function of this funneling mechanism is to alter both the spatial distribution of a response and the intensity of the response. Stimuli that occur in the surrounding ring of suppression tend not to be felt, but are able to increase the amplitude of the sensation produced by stimuli in the central region, while stimuli presented in the central region summate and positively interact. Thus, a widely spread stimulus pattern tends to be channeled or funneled into a narrow region of sensation as indicated in Figure 7.38.

It should be noted that von Békésy's funneling model is not really a neural net model and is certainly not one that can be solely explained by peripheral mechanisms. Rather, funneling is a general statement of sensory phenomena based on his speculations of the kind of inhibitory and excitatory interactions at all levels of the nervous system that might account for them. This problem has recently been directly attacked by comparing neural responses from peripheral and central levels of the cat's somatosensory system to human psychophysical responses (Gardner and Spencer, 1972a, 1972b). These workers found that here were no peripheral neural interactions that mimicked the psychophysical phenomena of funneling. However, Gardner and Spencer did find that central neurons did exhibit an analogous funneling effect. They do state, nevertheless, that this central neural funneling is due entirely to excitatory summations and that there is no evidence in their data that lateral inhibitions occur centrally.

IV. THE NEURAL CODING OF TIME PATTERNS

A. A Comment

The study of time as an objective of psychophysical inquiry is a topic with many ramifications. Students of the subject like Fraisse (1963) or Frankenhaeuser (1959) have included within the rubric such topics as the perception of the duration of passed time, temporal order, effect of the environment, and even the threshold for the perception of duration. However, the neurophysiology of all of these topics is far beyond our current grasp, and thus they are irrelevant in a discussion of how time is neurally encoded. We have to turn to a much more circumscribed context to find a set of data that is meaningful in current neurophysiological terms. If there is any single topic that we might consider to fill this bill, it is the perception of rhythm or repetitive regularity. How are the rhythmic characteristics of a repeating stimulus perceived and encoded?

It is unusually important in this case that we establish what the limits of perception are before we attempt to find neural correlates, because it is quite evident that a good bit of the temporal information present in stimu-

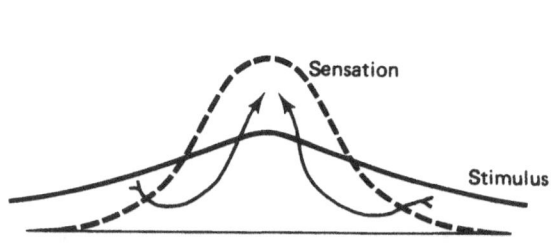

FIGURE 7.38 A sketch show-ing the funneling hypothesis according to von Békésy. An inhibitory region surround-ing an excitatory region has the effect of "funneling" the psychophysical experience into a narrower region than that defined by the physical extent of the stimulus. This is another way of expressing the lateral interaction process in which contours are en-hanced (from von Békésy, 1958).

lus patterns early in the encoding process is totally lost at higher nervous levels. We have already considered the problems of temporal acuity and simultaneity in our discussions of the psychological moment. In that case, the nervous system simply discards the details of the temporal pattern, and it would be pointless to attempt to find a central neural code for in-tervals less than those psychophysically detectable.

In other experimental paradigms, the same situation obtains, even though it may not be so obvious. Irregularities in the pattern of intervals between a repetitive stimulus train are often beyond the limits of detection. In some instances, however, even though the temporal pattern *per se* is lost, some other common sensory dimension may encode some of the temporal information contained in the stimulus pattern and thus allow a psycho-physical discrimination of two temporal patterns.

For example, Uttal (1970) has reported that the frequency of a flashing light can affect the ability to discriminate the presence of a temporal gap, even though the frequency of the train of flashes is far above critical fusion frequency. A small dot of light, lasting for about 30 μsec, was repetitively flashed on the face of an oscilloscope at frequencies of 1000 and 333 Hz. A gap (one irregularly large interval) inserted in the train of flashes was de-tected at significantly different threshold durations for these two repetition rates. Apparently, some vestige of the information contained in the high-frequency train was retained, even though each of the two trains was per-fectly fused. Probably, the subject was responding to differences in the average brightness of the train of light flashes that was a function of the total energy content of the stimulus. Thus, an intensive judgment was sub-stituted for a temporal one.

The detection of irregularities has already been discussed in the previ-ous chapter. In doing so, we bypassed, however, the problem of frequency discrimination itself, the first-order phenomenon of which interval irregu-larity is but a further perturbation. The ability to discriminate stimulus frequency varies considerably for the various senses for reasons that are fairly obvious. These are fundamental limits imposed on frequency dis-crimination in vision (and we are, of course, referring here to the frequency of a repetitive flash rather than to the frequency of the electromagnetic wave) by the physiological processes in the receptor and the rest of the retina that define the flicker fusion threshold. In audition, the high degree of frequency discrimination ability (and in this case we are speaking of the frequency of the acoustic signal), as we have seen, seems in large part to be mediated by a spatial recoding. When electrical stimuli are applied to the auditory nerve directly (Simmons, Epley, Lummis, Guttman, Frishkopf, Harmon, and Zwicker, 1965), then the frequency discrimination seems to be very much of the same order as that defined for electrical stimulation of the skin by Anderson and Munsen (1951). For low-frequency (50–300 Hz) electrical auditory stimulation (Simmons *et al.*), subjects required about a 30 pulse/sec difference before they could discriminate two stimuli. On the skin (Anderson and Munsen), the subjects also required a difference of 30 Hz below 100 Hz, but the threshold difference rapidly enlarged as the frequency increased.

If there is any generality that we might draw from these studies, it is that if one closely examines the purely temporal discriminative capabilities of the human observer, independent of recodings to intensive or spatial dimensions, they seem to be severely restricted. Presumably, the auditory system uses space as an additional code for frequency discrimination to achieve the high levels of performance obtained in psychophysical experiments. In the preceding, present, and following chapters, we have seen and shall see many other instances in which temporal codes are used to represent spatial, intensive, and even qualitative discrimination. We shall also note instances in which temporal differences are represented by spatial or intensive codes. This is a curious paradox, but entirely consistent with the basic premises of coding theory.

To illustrate the trade-offs among space, intensity, and time, we shall now turn to a discussion of an interesting set of studies concerning the experience of somatosensory flutter and vibration. In addition, these studies are a model of the useful contribution that can emerge from a combined psychobiological approach to the problems of sensory coding.

B. Mountcastle's Studies of the Physiological Basis of Flutter and Vibration Sensitivity

Workers in Mountcastle's laboratory at Johns Hopkins University have long been concerned with temporal coding in the somatosensory system. They have been making psychophysical and neurophysiological comparisons of the responses in a cutaneous modality, which they refer to as "flutter" at low frequencies and "vibration" at high frequencies. Psychophysical data obtained in human experiments and neurophysiological data obtained both at the level of peripheral nerves (Talbot, Darian-Smith, Kornhuber, and Mountcastle, 1968) and at the level of the cerebral cortex (Mountcastle, Talbot, Sakata, and Hyvärinen, 1969) in the monkey have been compared to determine how the stimulus pattern is represented as it is communicated up the ascending pathways.

The mechanical stimulus waveform with which they worked was a combination of a step or pedestal constant level displacement and a sinusoidally driven oscillation of displacement as shown in Figure 7.39. This

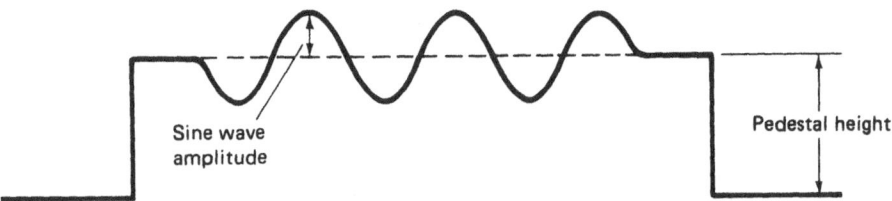

FIGURE 7.39 A sketch of the stimulus pattern used in the study of the neural correlates of flutter and vibration sensitivity. A pedestal of constant stimulus amplitude was used to raise the stimulus into an active portion of the intensity range. Superimposed on the intensity pedestal is a sinusoidal fluctuation of intensity which, although small in amplitude, selectively acts to produce wide ranges of neural and psychophysical responses (modified from Talbot, Darian-Smith, Kornhuber, and Mountcastle, 1968).

combination waveform was necessary to avoid the establishment of a high level of adaptation prior to the experimental stimulation, yet still allowed a reasonable absolute depression of the skin. The only other alternative would have been to use very massive oscillations, which could potentially damage the receptors and which were certainly far above thresholds. The pedestal stimulus also served to establish a base of background activity, against which the effects of the sinusoidal components could be evaluated. In this meticulous manner, typical of the great care that is characteristic of the work from Mountcastle's laboratory, single fibers were kept active for three or more hours. This same sort of stimulus was used in both psychophysical experiments on human subjects (in which the threshold of the sense of flutter-vibration was the main dependent variable) and neurophysiological studies on Macaque monkeys (in which several measures of the frequency pattern of the spike action potential response were the major dependent variables).

The psychophysical data recorded by Talbot, Darian-Smith, Kornhuber, and Mountcastle can be quickly summarized. The important part of their findings indicated that the threshold of detectability of the oscillating portion of the stimulus, as measured by the amplitude of the sine wave, varied monotonically, but usually with a point of inflection between two segments of the curve. Figure 7.40 shows typical results for two different locations on the hand: the finger and the thenar eminence (the root of the thumb). Talbot and his colleagues have interpreted the break in the curve of the data obtained from the thenar eminence as indicating that flutter-vibration sensitivity is mediated there by two sets of receptors. They also report corresponding neurophysiological evidence which, they believe, supports their notion of a dual somatosensory flutter-vibration system.[4] In fact, they found three different classes of peripheral neurons that responded in different ways to this kind of stimulus. The characteristics of the three different types are summarized in Table 7.2, which is reproduced here from their paper.

[4] But, note our earlier discussion on this matter in Chapter 6.

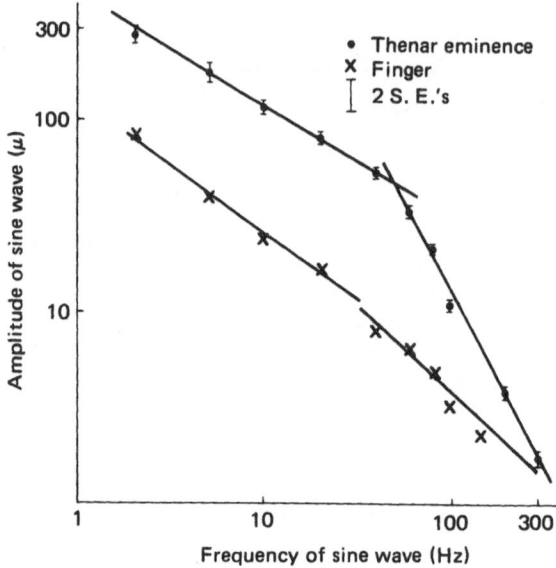

FIGURE 7.40 The relation between the psychophysical threshold of detection (as measured by the amplitude in micra of the sinusoidal component of the stimulus shown in Figure 7.39) and the frequency of the stimulus as measured at two different locations on the human hand (modified from Talbot, Darian-Smith, Kornhuber, and Mountcastle, 1968).

The first of these three types of peripheral somatosensory neurons observed by Talbot and his associates included slowly adapting cells, which tended to entrain with the peaks of the sinusoidal stimulus at low frequencies, but at intensities far below the human subjective threshold. Talbot and his colleagues conclude that this system, therefore, does "not contribute to the sense of flutter." In this manner, they may have demonstrated quite clearly what the present author has called a sign (see Chapter 5), for no sensory experience of any kind appears to be associated with these neural responses.

The other two systems were characterized by different anatomical locations and, as we shall see, also by different end-organ structure. The second system seemed to have its receptors along the ridges of glabrous skin, while the third system seemed to be associated with what were probably Pacinian corpuscles located deep in the skin.

Talbot and his colleagues conclude that the true codes for the flutter-vibration sense are generated by the second and third systems. Both of the systems are characterized by rather rapid adaptation to a constant stimulus. By the term "rapid adaptation," reference is made to the specific fact that both respond with but a single or, at most, a few spike action potentials at only the onset and at the offset of a stimulus. During the duration of a maintained stimulus, these two receptor systems, unlike the one described above, do not respond at all. However, with the sinusoidal component of the combined stimulus used in Talbot, Darian-Smith, Kornhuber, and Mountcastle's experiments, each cycle of the sine wave can act almost as a new stimulus and produce a response. Because of this characteristic, both of these systems are capable also of producing a train of spike responses that closely follows the frequency of the stimulating sinusoid. Figure 7.41

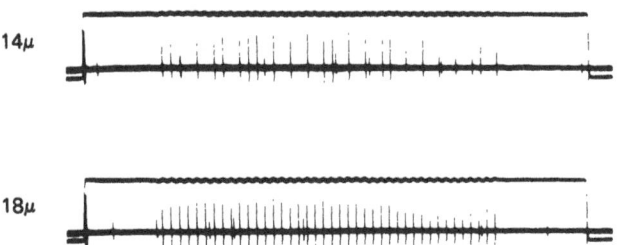

FIGURE 7.41 *Photograph of the stimulus and neural recording, showing the increase in entrainment as a function of a slight increase in the amplitude (from 14 to 18 μ) in the amplitude of the sinusoidal component of the stimulus for a quickly adapting afferent fiber in the monkey (from Talbot, Darian-Smith, Kornhuber, and Mountcastle, 1968).*

shows the increased accuracy of neural response entrainment as a result of a slight increase in stimulus intensity (the displacement was increased from 14 μ to 18 μ) for both of the two systems. Perhaps the most important characteristic distinguishing between these two systems is that the system with its receptors in the ridges of glabrous skin is characterized by best frequencies (that is, the frequencies at which the minimum amount of energy is required for threshold activation of one spike for each stimulus) between the range of 20 to 40 Hz. The characteristic curves for a set of these receptors are shown in Figure 7.42, while a similar set of characteristic curves has been plotted by Talbot and his colleagues for the Pacinian afferents and has been reproduced in Figure 7.43. In this case, the characteristic best frequencies can be seen to be mainly between 100 and 300 Hz.

Talbot, Darian-Smith, Kornhuber, and Mountcastle thus concluded that the combined sense of flutter and vibration is mediated by the two systems, each of which encodes a separate range of stimulus frequencies. They further conclude:

> *The perception of regular oscillatory movement depends upon the appearance in primary afferents of regular periodic trains of nerve impulses. . . . the discrimination between different frequencies depends upon a central mechanism sensitive to (which measures) the length of the periods in the input trains.*
>
> (*TALBOT* et al., *1968, p. 333.*)

Mountcastle's group (Mountcastle, Talbot, Sakata, and Hyvärinen, 1969) have gone on to consider the details of the central decoding mechanism in another closely related paper, which extends their results on temporal encoding to extracellular unit recordings from the cortex. Using glass-enclosed tungsten microelectrodes inserted into the postcentral somatosensory cortex, a set of three different types of cells was found similar in response characteristics to those found in peripheral nerves. Mountcastle and his col-

TABLE 7.2 CHARACTERISTICS OF THE THREE DIFFERENT KINDS
OF VIBRATION AND FLUTTER SENSITIVE NEURAL SYSTEMS IN THE
MONKEY'S HAND (FROM TALBOT, DARIAN-SMITH,
KORNHUBER, AND MOUNTCASTLE, 1968)

Class	Size (μ)	Peripheral Termination
Quickly adapting movement detectors	5-12	Dermal ridges of glabrous skin
Slowly adapting movement and intensity detectors	5-12	Dermal ridges of glabrous skin
Pacinian afferents movement detectors	5-12	Single or small cluster of Pacinian corpuscles, sub-dermal and deep tissues

leagues are very specific about this maintained distinctiveness of the three
systems:

> At the level of the primary somatic sensory cortex, we did not find
> evidence for cross set convergences upon cortical cells of [the] differ-
> ent sets of primary afferents.
>
> (MOUNTCASTLE et al., 1969, p. 461.)

Apparently, only a very small amount of integration of the afferent somatosensory signals occurs as the signals ascend through the various relay
points. Cells in the cortex seem to be reflecting the properties of the same
trio of slowly adapting afferents from glabrous skin, rapidly adapting
(low-frequency sensitive) afferents from glabrous skin and rapidly adapting
(high-frequency sensitive) afferents from Pacinian corpuscles.

However, the latter two systems, which played such an important
role for low- and high-frequency vibrations encoding, respectively, in the
periphery, did have one important difference in their cortical mechanisms.
On the one hand, the fast adapting glabrous skin system maintained its
ability to reproduce exactly the frequency of low-frequency stimuli all the
way up to and including the associated cortical neurons. Such a fact led

Table 7.2 (*cont.*)

Receptive Field	Adaptive Properties	Dynamic Sensitivity
Small, continuous graded. Activation by traveling waves limited to 5-mm surround	QA on–off type response to steady stimuli. Require liminal slope for activation	Exquisitely sensitive to oscillating stimuli in low-frequency range. Best tuning points *ca* 30 Hz
Small, continuous, graded. Precise detectors of variations of intensity	Onset transient a function of slope. Succeeding periodic discharge a function of intensity	Steady periodic discharge frequency modulated by sinusoidal stimuli in 2–10 Hz range
Point of greatest sensitivity, but field is unlimited. Activated by traveling waves from great distances	QA on–off type response to step stimuli. Require liminal slope for activation	Exquisitely sensitive to oscillating stimuli in the high-frequency range. Best tuning points *ca.* 250 Hz

Mountcastle and his colleagues to a most important conclusion, namely, that

> *Flutter* (*the correlate of low frequency stimuli*) *is the sensory experience which occurs* pari passu *with the appearance of periodicities in the discharge patterns of a certain set of post central neurons.*
> (*MOUNTCASTLE* et al., *1969, p. 477.*)

However, the other system, the one associated with the subcutaneous Pacinian corpuscles and high-frequency representation, did not maintain its ability to reproduce the temporal pattern of the peripheral message. Entrainment and frequency following up to 400 Hz, while still detectable as high as the level of the connectives between the thalamus and the cortex, were not discernible in any of the cortical cells identified as belonging to this group. In fact, these cells seemed not to be able to respond at frequencies higher than 100 Hz, and they quickly attained this rate of response at very low stimulus intensities. Indeed, upper limits on the frequency of firing of these cortical cells, while well below those upper limits found subcortically, were roughly of the same maximum frequency as those of the cortical system representing the fast adapting glabrous skin receptors. Thus, we may speculate that it is entirely possible that some sort of a recoding to a spatial dimension has occurred for this second system. While the coded represen-

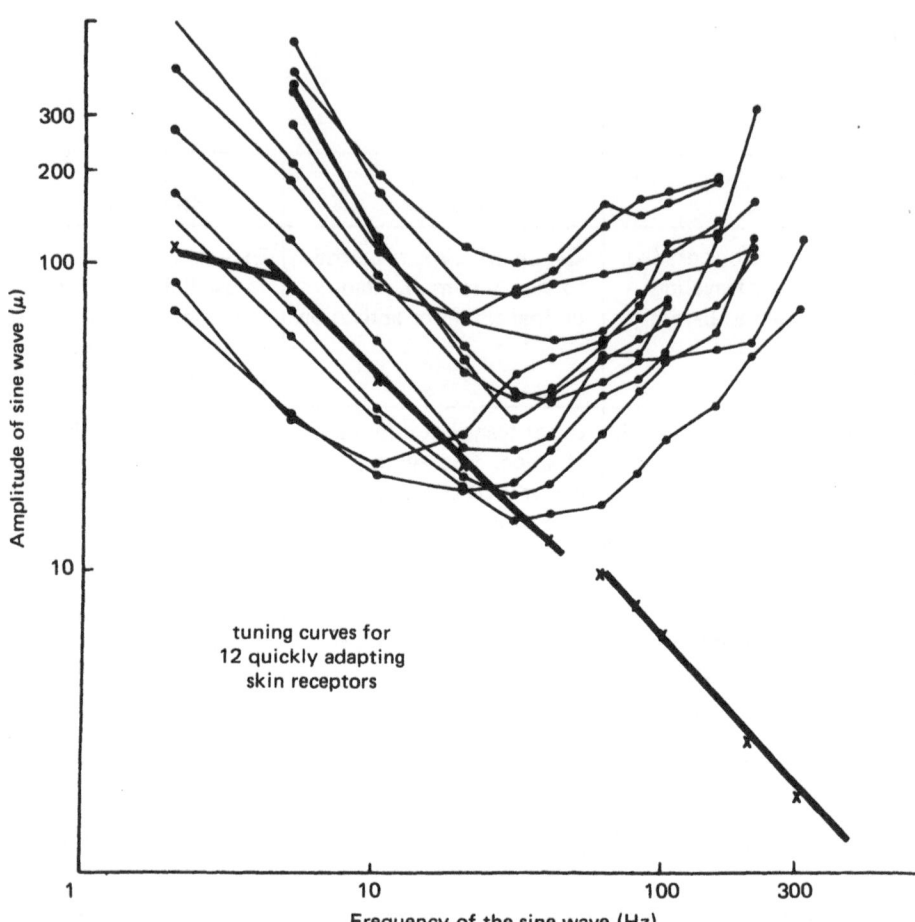

FIGURE 7.42 *Tuning curves for 12 quickly adapting fibers in glaborous portions of the monkey's hand. These curves are based on a criterion of the minimum amplitude of the sine wavé component of the stimulus required to produce one spike for each cycle of the stimulus. The dark line is a human psychophysical function for the finger similar to that shown in Figure 7.40 (from Talbot, Darian-Smith, Kornhuber, and Mountcastle, 1968).*

tation is no longer isomorphic with the stimulus dimension, space may now be encoding a temporal percept. We must remember that localized spatial activation is just as good a representation when viewed from the perspective of coding theory as temporally isomorphic code would be, and, therefore, it may not be inappropriate for us to paraphrase Mountcastle, Talbot, Sakata, and Hyvärinen in the following way:

> Vibration (*the correlate of high frequency stimuli*) *is the sensory experience which occurs* pari passu *with the appearance of activity at a particular location in a place coded set of post central neurons.*

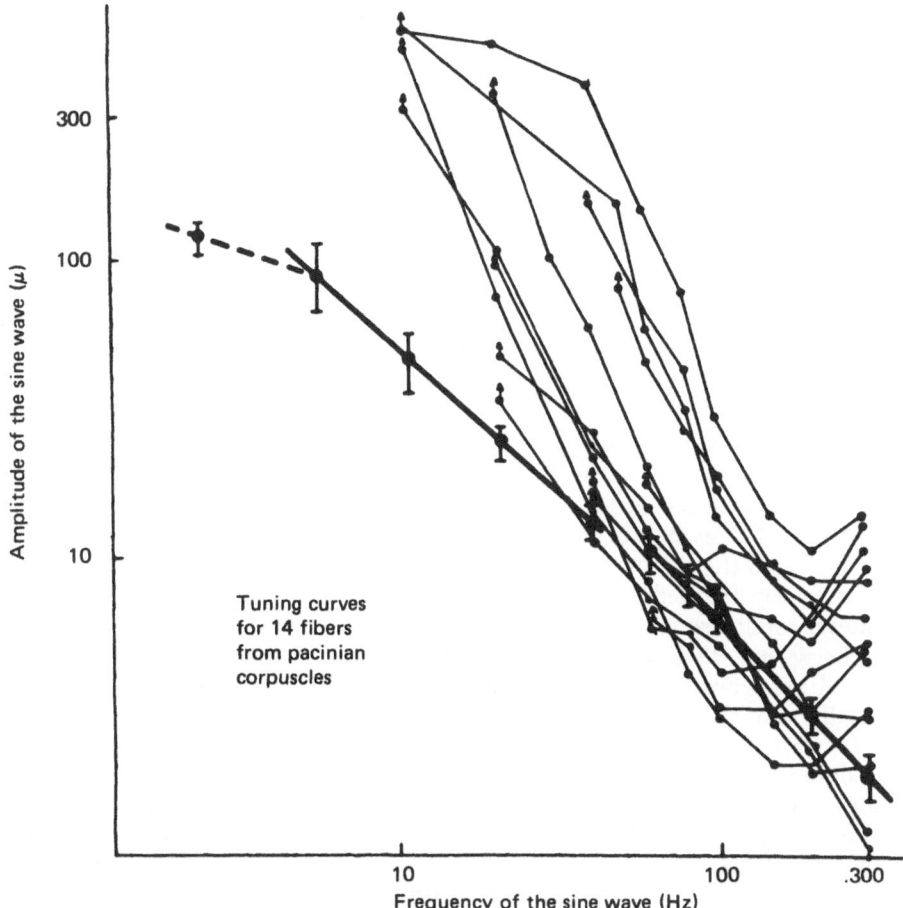

FIGURE 7.43 *Tuning curves for 14 afferent nerve fibers from Pacinian corpuscles in the monkey's hand. The dark curve is a psychophysical function from a human experiment. Note the difference in the center frequencies of these cells and those of Figure 7.42 despite the use of the same criterion (from Talbot, Darian-Smith, Kornhuber, and Mountcastle, 1968).*

While it is superficially easy to draw a conclusion about a coding relationship when stimulus and neural response are isomorphic, there, in fact, is no reason why equally vigorous conclusions cannot be made for nonisomorphic encodings. We may conclude that temporal stimulus patterns and the sensations associated with them may be represented in a number of different manners. The work of Mountcastle and his colleagues, in conjunction with similar temporal-to-spatial encoding studies in audition, makes it clear that time may be encoded in many different ways and that spatial representation of time patterns is a very frequent occurrence.

Another important summary point is that the sort of entrainment described by these investigators is also present in other senses and is, in fact, a relatively common phenomenon. The entrainment of neural impulses by sinusoidal varying signals has also been observed in the ganglion cell of the cat's retina by Hughes and Maffei (1966) for frequencies up to the flicker fusion threshold of about 50 Hz. Thus, the peripheral correlate of flicker fusion may be related to the detection of the intervals between sequential cycles of a periodic neural response. Furthermore, Rose, Brugge, Anderson, and Hind (1967) have studied entrainment in auditory neurons and believe that it may play an important role in acoustic frequency discrimination. We shall discuss this issue in greater detail in Chapter 9.

V. SPATIAL LOCALIZATION—REPRESENTATION BY TEMPORAL AS WELL AS SPATIAL CODES

A. The Psychophysical Data of Spatial Localization

In the previous sections, we mentioned a number of instances in which time patterns were re-encoded so that they were represented by spatial patterns. In the following section, we shall consider a topic—spatial localization—in which the converse effect obtains. In this case, spatial patterns are frequently represented by patterns of neural activity, in which the key parameter often seems to be time. In this situation, latency and phase differences between two signals play a key role in the representation of space. We shall first consider the problems of spatial location, as they have been classically investigated with psychophysical procedures.

It has been known for many years that localization of objects in the three-dimensional space surrounding our heads is a phenomenon that is, in large part, mediated by the combined action of the paired visual and auditory receptor organs. Visual three-dimensional space perception is cued by many different monocular cues such as interposition, motion parallax, relative size, areal perspective, and so on. The binocular cues of accommodation and convergence also play some role, but a lesser one than popular opinion conventionally suggests according to some recent work. The strongest and most compelling stereoscopic effects, however, seem to be due to disparate images projected on the corresponding points of the two retinas. A very large literature has grown up, describing the perception of depth that occurs when nearly identical images are projected on corresponding points, but this is a topic that we shall not consider in detail here. The interested reader is directed to the works of Ogle (1950), or to the very important recent contributions of Julesz (for example, 1960 and 1971), or to Graham's chapter on space perception in his encyclopedic review of vision (Graham, 1965) for a complete discussion of the geometry of three-dimensional space perception.

There is only one temporal phenomenon associated with three-dimensional space perception that we shall mention in this section to make a specific point. This is the famous Pulfrich phenomenon, a three-dimensional depth perception, which does seem, at first, to be mediated by a temporal difference in the signals being transmitted from each eye. However, as we shall see, these are temporal differences in the neural code, which seem to

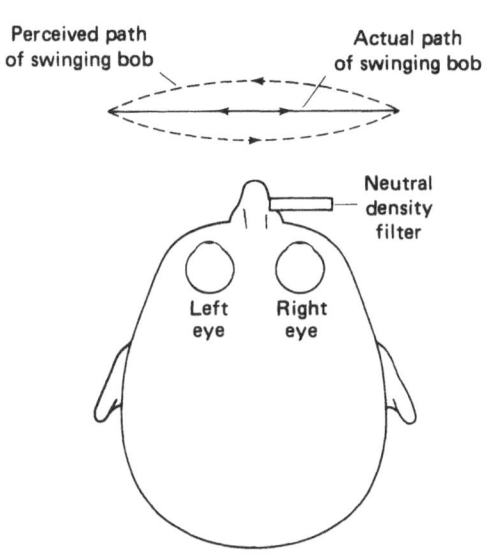

FIGURE 7.44 A schematic diagram showing the simple apparatus required to demonstrate the Pulfrich phenomenon. The solid line is the actual course of the swinging plum bob, and the dotted line is the apparent pathway. This phenomenon, though it at first glance appears to be due to a difference in temporal dimensions, actually is better considered as a result of spatial disparities.

be due mostly to intensity differences in the stimuli, and, furthermore, it all turns out to be an example of spatial coding anyhow. The basic paradigm of the Pulfrich phenomenon is presented in Figure 7.44. This view, from the top, is of a situation in which an observer is binoculary viewing a bob that is moving back and forth parallel to the plane of his face in simple harmonic motion along a path defined by the solid line. If a neutral density filter is inserted in the optical pathway of one eye, then the bob will appear to follow the path shown by the dotted lines, along a three-dimensional ellipsoidal path. The neurological model most often proposed to account for this illusion is that the dimmer light, which reaches the eye through the interposed filter, induces a neurological response that is of a considerably longer latency than that induced by the more intense stimulus to the other eye. This elongated latent period leads to an asynchrony between the responses of the two eyes, and the image to the filter occluded eye is retarded by a sufficient amount to produce a difference in which corresponding retinal points are "simultaneously" stimulated. Thus, when the bob is moving fast (as it would be at the center of its course), the corresponding retinal points, which are "simultaneously" stimulated, are relatively far apart and encode a displacement in depth in accord with the usual rules of corresponding points. In fact, therefore, even in this situation the critical cue seems to be one that is dependent upon simultaneous (or, more correctly, apparently simultaneous) responses. Temporal differences, thus, have been re-encoded into spatial disparities, albeit false ones, displaced from the true disparities of the retinal images.

Time, therefore, does not seem to really play a very important role in this aspect of visual localization. Time's role is only secondary, because it produces a difference in spatial localization due to the synchronous activation of false corresponding points by latency differences created by stimulus-intensity differences. Recently, Shipley and Rawlings (1971) have compared localization differences due to asynchronies in dichoptic stimulus presentations with those in the other senses (to be discussed in more detail below) and have found that psychophysical effects corresponding to those produced by 1- and 2-msec stimulus intervals in taste, touch, smell, and audition, require 70- and 80-msec intervals in vision. The discrepancy in the time scale suggests that fundamentally different processes may be in action in vision than in these other senses.

Neurophysiological and psychophysical data in both hearing and in somatosensation, quite to the contrary, indicate that timing differences are strong cues for the localization of an object in space. Consider the psychophysics of spatial localization in audition. It has long been known that both phase differences and the relative intensity of acoustic signals contributed to our perception of where an auditory stimulus was localized. Phase differences seemed to dominate at the lower frequencies under approximately 3000 Hz. At these lower frequencies, the existence of specific phase sensitive mechanisms is suggested. Intensive differences, on the other hand, seem to be most effective for the localization of stimuli with component frequencies higher than 3000 Hz. In fact, according to one of the classic studies in the field (Stevens and Newman, 1936), at about 3000 Hz the errors of localization are at their maximum, since neither mechanism seems to be operating at its maximum level of efficiency. Modern stereophonic recording techniques use both of these principles to provide a most effective illusion of different spatial localization of the instruments of an orchestra, even though only two speakers are in use. With stereophonic ear phones, it is possible to localize signals externally or even in different locations within the head.

If one moves from the domain of continuous tones, with the associated problems of correlating sequential cycles, to simple impulsive stimuli such as clicks, the precision of localization increases dramatically. In this case, it is possible to localize sounds that differ by no more than a few microseconds in their phase relations. Wallach, Newman, and Rosenzweig (1949), for example, have shown that with impulsive stimuli, the apparent source is always in the direction of the first stimulus and that the system is extremely sensitive even to differences in the range of a few microseconds. Figure 7.45 presents their findings for two subjects; their data indicate significantly different performance levels for intervals as small as 10 or 20 μsec.

Analogous spatial localization studies have been carried out by von Békésy (1957) on the skin. Von Békésy's experiments utilized an experimental paradigm quite similar to those in the classic auditory localization experiments. Two mechanical pulse stimuli (or, in some cases, electrical pulses) were applied to two nearby regions of the forearm with a variable interval of time also separating them. With an interval greater than some threshold value, the two stimuli were felt as separate events of moderate intensity at their separate locations. As the interval between the two pulses was decreased, the trailing stimulus slowly fades in perceived amplitude, and the leading one begins to assert itself as the sole perceived event. It not only changes in perceived amplitudes, but also moves in position. As the interval between the two stimuli becomes smaller and smaller,

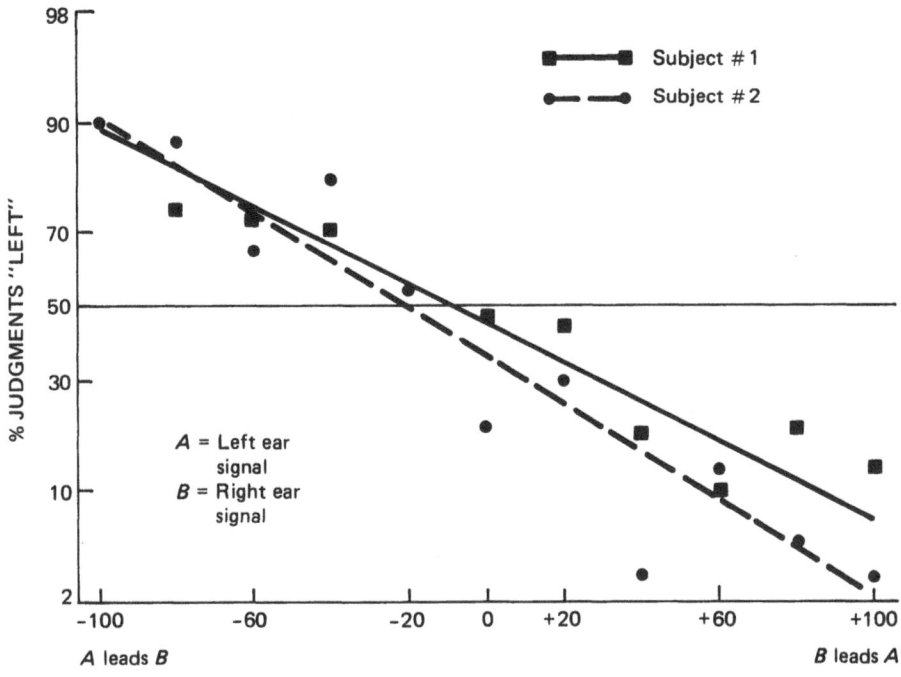

FIGURE 7.45 A chart showing the effect of the interval between two acoustic clicks on the spatial localization of the combined percept; data shown for two listeners (from Wallach, Newman, and Rosenzweig, 1949).

the subject's perception of the event, now a single entity, moves toward an apparent locus close to the point midway between the actual physical location of the two stimuli. At the same time, the perceived event generally becomes spatially more diffuse and less intense until it is finally centered between the stimulators—a situation that occurs when the two stimuli are exactly synchronous. If the alternate stimulus is then allowed to lead, the experience seems to reverse itself. The percept moves toward the alternate stimulator, decreases in size, and increases in intensity until the threshold separation between the onset of the stimuli is reached and the two stimuli break apart into equally large and equally intense events. All of these apparent amplitude and intensity changes are due entirely to the temporal difference in the occurrence of the two stimuli.

A critical difference between these findings and those in audition is that the ear apparently has some sort of a compensatory mechanism built into it, such that the combined percept is always constant in amplitude. There is little variation in the perceived amplitude of two fused acoustic stimuli, no matter where the combined event is localized in space. Figure 7.46 (from von Békésy, 1957) compares these two situations and displays, in a most conveniently graphic form, the results of both the experiment just described and its auditory analogue.

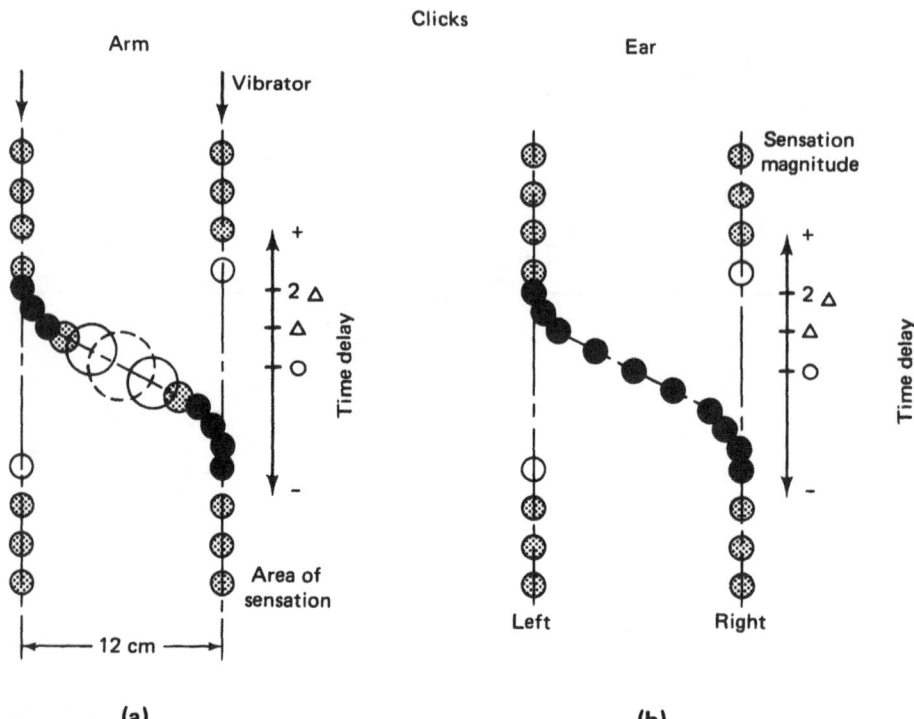

(a)   **(b)**

FIGURE 7.46 *A diagrammatic sketch of the difference in the spatial localization phenomena in hearing and on the skin. Part (b) is another way of plotting the data presented in Figure 7.45. When the two stimuli occur close enough together in time, they are fused into a single sensation, which is differentially located in space depending upon the interval between the two stimuli. In hearing, unlike its cutaneous analogue, there is some sort of an automatic gain control so that the subjective magnitude of the fused sensation always remains the same (from von Békésy, 1957).*

Von Békésy has also demonstrated an analogous spatial localization phenomenon in gustation. Using controlled streams of salt solutions asynchronously applied to two areas of the tongue, he was able to demonstrate that the two stimuli led to two sensations if they were very much separated in time, but to a single more diffuse, yet spatially localizable, single fused experience if they were separated by only a short interval. Figure 7.47 (reproduced from von Békésy, 1964b), using the same sort of chart as Figure 7.46, demonstrates that the precision of detection of intrastimulus interval in gustation, using spatial localization as an indicator, was on the order of 1 or 2 msec. Von Békésy (1964a) has also extended this work to the olfactory modality and shown similar results.

Thus, we can see that the precision of temporal measurements, which has been so poor when human subjects were asked to make purely temporal judgments, turns out to be greatly improved when spatial judgments are required of the subject. This finding illustrates once again that isomorphism

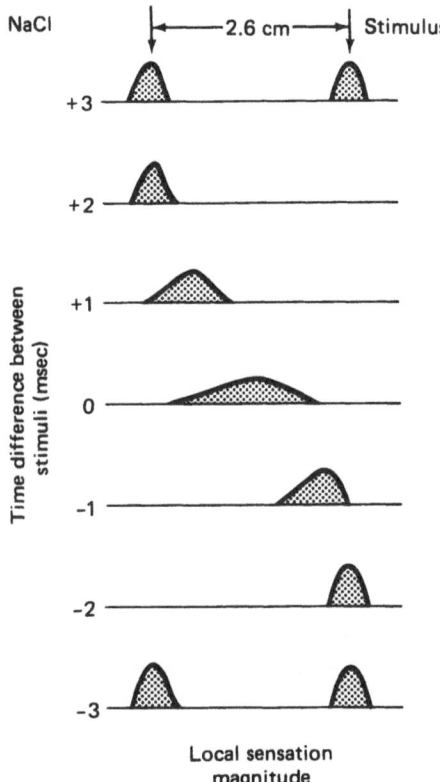

FIGURE 7.47 A plot (similar to Figure 7.46) of the localization of a gustatory stimulus on the tongue. Surprisingly, the temporal discriminability in this case is also very fine in spite of the absence of fine temporal experience in the gustatory modality (from von Békésy, 1964b).

of stimulus, neural code, and percept is not at all necessary. Freeing our perspectives from this particular trap can have some curious effects. Not only are we relieved of the constraints of the search for isomorphic codes for stimulus variables, but we also no longer find it quite so necessary to assume *a priori* that an isomorphic correlate is a more likely code for some stimulus dimension than a nonisomorphic one.

B. Neurophysiological Data of Relevance to Spatial Localization

As we have seen, the psychophysical data suggest that with the exception of visual depth perception, dynamic temporal dimensions play a preeminent role in the spatial localization of a stimulus. The neurophysiological data appear to correspond with these findings in all of the senses. The temporal relations of the nerve impulse pattern also appear to be preeminent everywhere except vision. In this latter modality, relatively static interactions of the retinally disparate images seem to play the key role.

In the following section, we shall consider some of the static properties of neural interaction underlying depth perception in the ascending visual pathways, and then review some of the highly significant contemporary neurophysiological data, which emphasize the temporal encoding of acoustic spatial perception.

1. *Static Visual Codes for Spatial Localization.* Because of the anatomy of the visual pathway, binocular stereopsis, the most powerful of the cues for visual depth perception, can only be mediated by mechanisms located at the very highest levels of the nervous system. It is generally agreed by most contemporary authorities that there is no neural binocular interaction at any level lower than the lateral geniculate body of the thalamus. In the lateral geniculate body, the presence of true binocularly sensitive cells has been disputed for many years. DeValois (1960) had been unable to detect any binocular interaction in the thalamus. His work supported a number of earlier studies, although there was at least one report (Bishop and Davis, 1953) that a few binocularly sensitive cells were occasionally observed in the cat's thalamus. In such a controversial situation, the reader may quite justifiably suspect that the phenomenon, if present, is rare.

A definitive study on the matter of lateral geniculate binocular interaction by Lindsley, Chow, and Gollender (1967) supports the notion that, though infrequent, binocular interaction is present in the cat's thalamus. Using stainless steel electrodes, they recorded extracellular spikes from a relatively large sample of lateral geniculate neurons and found that somewhat less than 20 percent of the cells were able to respond to some form of binocular or dichoptic stimulation. Interestingly, some of the cells behaved in a manner with which we have become quite familiar; stimulation of one eye would give rise to an increase in the activity of a particular cell, while stimulation of the other eye would reduce the activity of that cell. This antagonistic interaction is reminiscent of much of the data described earlier concerning receptive field structure and interaction. Nevertheless, it is to the cortex itself that we must turn for most of the detailed analyses of the possible mechanisms of binocular and dichoptic spatial perception.

Hubel and Wiesel (1962) had been among the first to look specifically at the problem of the representation of binocular depth perception in the cells of the visual cortex. However, Barlow, Blakemore, and Pettigrew (1967) have recently described some findings that update our current knowledge of this matter, and we shall concentrate upon these more recent data. Using microelectrodes inserted into the exposed primary visual cortex, they observed the response of single cells to combinations of binocularly presented visual stimuli. To obtain adequate responses, they had to use moving bars as visual stimuli, reflecting a preferential feature sensitivity described earlier by Hubel and Wiesel. The success of Barlow, Blakemore, and Pettigrew's studies depended upon the precise specification of the angular degrees of retinal disparity[5] of the visual stimuli applied to the two eyes. For many technical reasons, this was not an easy thing to do, but they were

---

[5] Retinal disparity is said to exist when the two retinal images fall on retinal points that will not produce fusion of the two images or, alternatively, fuse, but so as to produce a difference in the apparent depth of the stimulus.

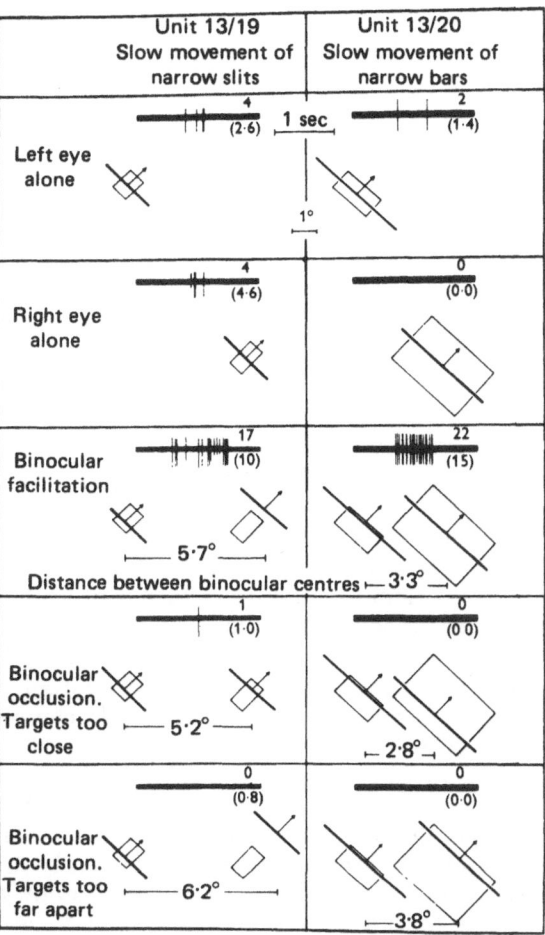

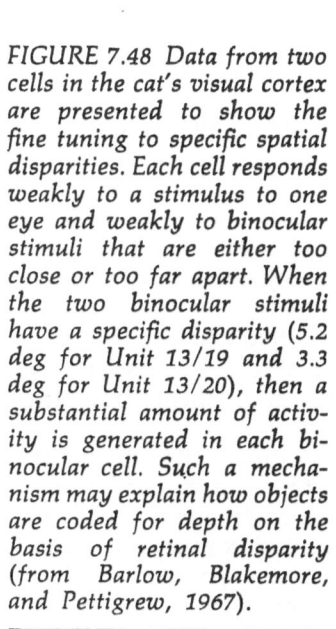

FIGURE 7.48 Data from two cells in the cat's visual cortex are presented to show the fine tuning to specific spatial disparities. Each cell responds weakly to a stimulus to one eye and weakly to binocular stimuli that are either too close or too far apart. When the two binocular stimuli have a specific disparity (5.2 deg for Unit 13/19 and 3.3 deg for Unit 13/20), then a substantial amount of activity is generated in each binocular cell. Such a mechanism may explain how objects are coded for depth on the basis of retinal disparity (from Barlow, Blakemore, and Pettigrew, 1967).

able to give a pretty good approximation of both the vertical and horizontal disparities by controlling eye position and by estimating the position of the nearly invisible fovea by physiological methods. The eye was immobilized by a continuous injection of Flaxedil, a muscle action depressant, as well as by a mechanical restraint. Estimates of the retinal disparity were based upon the assumption that the common point of view of the two foveas represented zero disparity.

The results of their experiments showed that binocularly activated single cells in the cat's visual cortex responded most vigorously when binocular stimuli were presented at a characteristic angular disparity. Individual cells responded weakly to monocular stimuli (to either eye) and even less strongly to stimuli that were either further apart or closer together than the characteristic optimum disparity for each cell. Figure 7.48 is a sample set of records for two cells with different optimum disparity angles, showing various combinations of stimulus conditions and the resulting neural activity.

Barlow, Blakemore, and Pettigrew conclude their paper with a suggestion that may be the basis of the key code in binocular depth perception. They point out that with a fixed convergence, the images of objects at different distances will have different disparities. Thus, a different population of cells sensitive to a different degree of disparity will be maximally activated for objects at different distances. In this manner, the phenomenal distance of an object (and the spatial stimulus dimension) may be encoded by a specific set of labeled cells (another quite distinct spatial dimension in the neural domain). Even though both dimensions are spatial, this situation represents still another form of coded representation, in which an information pattern has been transformed from one dimension to another while still maintaining the critical features of the stimuli. If this theoretical organization seems to be sketchy, we can, be fairly sure, considering the high level of the nervous system at which binocular stimuli first mix, that the primary neural mechanism for binocular depth perception is a spatial one located at the very highest cortical levels.

2. *Dynamic Auditory Codes for Spatial Localization.* In the visual system, as we have seen, there is no neural evidence of binocular interaction at levels below the thalamus, and little evidence of acute temporal sensitivities is evident in psychophysical findings. In the auditory system, however, the psychophysical data suggest a very high degree of sensitivity to the temporal dimensions of the stimulus, and the neurophysiological data consistently provide supporting evidence of possible convergent mechanisms from the two ears at the most peripheral levels.

The auditory system is anatomically organized quite differently than the visual system. As we have seen in Chapter 3, there appear to be anatomical possibilities for binaural synaptic interaction at very early levels of the ascending auditory pathway. This early anatomical convergence from the two ears might be vital to the detection of very fine asynchronies, since as signals ascend toward the central nervous system, they would be expected to increase their temporal dispersion, thus reducing the fidelity of reproduction of the stimulus timing. Galambos, Schwartzkopff, and Rupert (1959), for example, had originally established the fact that the superior olive contained cells that were capable of being binaurally activated. Cells in this nucleus were shown to be selectively sensitive to both the phase and the intensity differences of dichotic acoustic stimuli, the usual cues for spatial localization.

The complexity of the binaural interaction at this level has been further emphasized by a more recent study reported by Wernick and Starr (1968). They showed that such complex interaural interactions as the production of neurophysiological beats (equal to the difference frequency of the two dichotic signals) corresponding to human psychophysical phenomena could be obtained at this level. Gross evoked potentials, used as the electrophysiological indicator in their experiment, clearly showed slow modulations, which varied as a function of the stimulus frequency differences. The nature of the interaction was explored further by Boudreau and Tsuchitani (1968), who found that there were cells of the superior olive that were excited by stimuli to the ipsilateral ear and inhibited by stimuli to the contralateral ear—an antagonistic relationship, similar to the receptive field organization with which we have already become familiar. Interestingly, their analysis indicated that the inhibitory and excitatory response areas of a single cell were both of roughly the same shape, and both had approximately the same center frequency.

More recently, Goldberg and Brown (1969), also working in several of the olivary nuclei, have extended many of these findings and have found specifically that cells most sensitive to high-frequency stimuli (that is, with high-frequency centered response areas) were typically more sensitive to intensity differences than to phase differences. Those cells most sensitive to low-frequency signals (that is, with low-frequency centered response areas) were typically more sensitive to phase than to intensity differences. This finding is entirely congruent with the psychophysical data, which have also shown this same association. Within this dichotomy, however, they found that there were other important classifications of cellular behavior worthy of note. For example, cells sensitive to binaural intensity differences and presumably associated with high-frequency localizations could be excited by stimuli from either ear or inhibited by the stimulus from one ear while being excited by the other. However, only those cells that were inhibited by one ear seemed to be specifically sensitive to differences in the intensities of the binaural stimuli. Cells excited by both ears, by contrast, seemed to respond on the basis of the average sound level of the two stimuli. It is interesting to note that a comparison of the average or absolute sound level with interaural intensity differences would be an important means of providing additional information relevant to auditory localization. It possibly might also be the basis of the compensatory mechanism that maintains constant loudness as an auditory percept moves about in space.

The issue of whether or not analogous response patterns at the next level of the auditory pathway are specifically related to the problem of sound localization has been specifically considered in an important paper by Rose, Gross, Geisler, and Hind (1966). Recording spike action potential patterns from single cells in the inferior colliculus of a cat, they measured the effects of binaural stimuli, which differed in phase and intensity. They found that there were a number of different kind of cells present that were affected by differential binaural stimuli but in several different ways. Some cells turned out to be exquisite detectors of slight phase differences between two continuous tones. For example, Figure 7.49 shows the response rate of a cell that varied its frequency of firing from virtually zero to over a thousand spike action potentials per second as the phase angle of a 500-Hz tone presented to both ears shifted, even though the intensities of both the original and shifted tones remained constant. Rose and his colleagues found that the same cell, when stimulated with signals applied to either the right ear or the left ear alone, produced the nonmonotonic functions shown in the inset drawing of Figure 7.49. Both of these monaural responses, however, were at a level of activity that was considerably less than that produced by the combined stimulus.

A sampling of a wide variety of these phase sensitive cells by Rose and his associates showed that each cell has its own "characteristic delay time." Because of this individual characteristic, different cells would re-

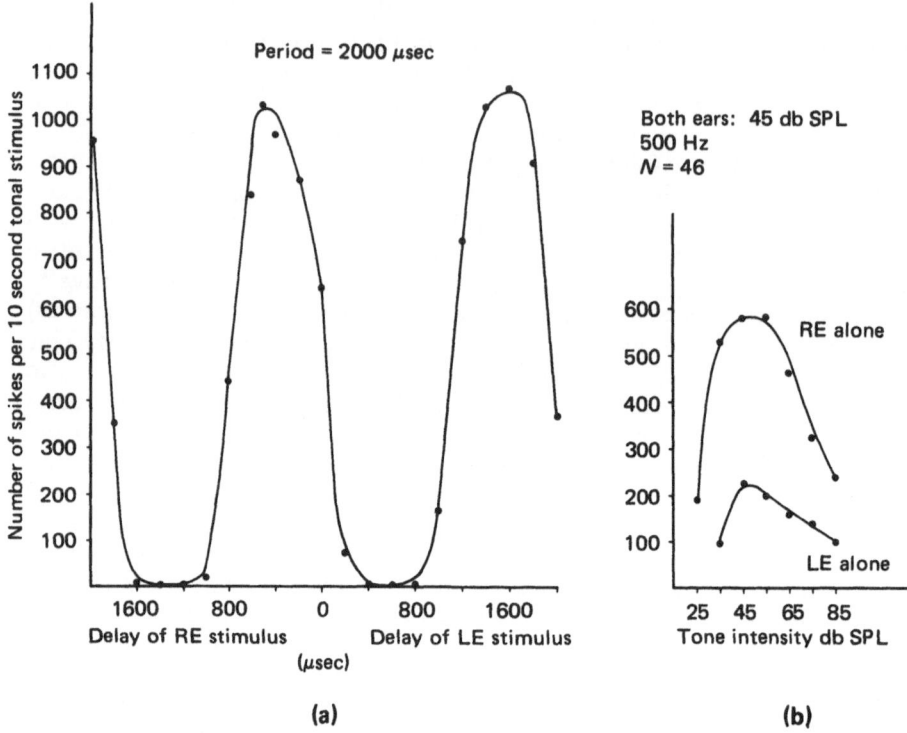

FIGURE 7.49 *Response of a cell in the inferior colliculus of a cat to phase differences in dichotic stimulation (b) Shows the negligible response, which is generated by stimuli presented only in one ear. When two stimuli are presented dichotically (a) the response over 10 sec is very much a function of the phase angle between the two. Properly phased dichotic stimuli can elicit a response magnitude that is very much larger than that produced by any monaural stimulus. Such a mechanism may be the basis of spatial localization in the auditory system (from Rose, Gross, Geisler, and Hind, 1966).*

spond maximally at different phase angles between the two stimuli. Once again, this is a clear example of a case in which the temporal differences have been re-encoded into a spatial representation. Spatial encoding of this sort is sensitive to time differences as small as a few microseconds, a value that once again corresponds to the known limits of psychophysically measured spatial localization.

Rose and his associates also observed another class of cells that were relatively insensitive to the phase difference between dichotic stimuli, but that were highly sensitive to their intensity differences. Sensitivities to intensity differences as fine as 1 or 2 db were observed in some of these cells. Unfortunately, one correlation, which one might have hoped to find, was not observed. These intensity sensitive cells were not solely those that responded at the higher center frequencies. Such a result would have been expected since, as we have seen, intensive differences seem to be more important for higher-frequency signals. In this case, intensity sensitive cells of this type seemed to be found across the entire range of the frequency spectrum.

Rose's group has also considered the issue of dichotic interactions of cells at the level of the cortex (Brugge, Dubrovsky, and Rose, 1964). These investigators found a small sample of cells that seemed to behave very much like the phase sensitive cells of the inferior colliculus. Small phase differences between dichotic stimuli led to substantial differences in both spike counts and the latent period before the initial response in these cells. Whether these cells were simply following the response of the cells at the lower centers or were truly responding to dichotic convergent inputs themselves is, of course, moot. The details of the anatomy suggest, however, that this may simply have been a following of an interactive process occurring at a lower level.

On the other hand, it is known that the presence of cortical cells is critical to the ability of an animal to detect phase differences and presumably also to the localization of sound sources. Masterson and Diamond (1964) have shown that extirpation of the acoustic cortical tissue, in which these types of cell occur, drastically reduced a cat's ability to discriminate intervals between clicks. Yet intensity discrimination *per se* seems to be very much unaffected by massive bilateral extirpations of the acoustic areas (see Neff, 1961, for a review of these topics).

In sum, then, we have seen that the encoding of spatial localization in vision and in hearing is done by mechanisms of fundamentally different organization. There is little anatomical opportunity for convergence of dichoptic stimuli in the visual system until the highest centers. On the other hand, the auditory system shows clear evidence of the mixing and interaction of dichotic signals at the lowest possible level (the second-order neuron). Nevertheless, both systems seem to be able to extract information about the environment and encode the perceptions of space and depth with a high degree of precision. This evidence for different levels of interaction and possibly different mechanisms for spatial localization in vision and audition does suggest that there may be limits to the generality of any unified theory of sensory coding.

CHAPTER 8: FEATURE DETECTION— NEUROPHYSIOLOGY AND PSYCHOPHYSICS

In this chapter, we continue our discussion of temporal and spatial coding by emphasizing a very important subtopic—the specific sensitivities that certain neurons seem to display to certain spatio-temporal features of the stimulus. The discussion is centered around the very important findings of two research groups that have been especially influential in recent years. While their empirical findings are very interesting in themselves, perhaps more important is the change in perspective that they have introduced into contemporary psychobiological thinking. We try to stress this theoretical contribution in the discussion. We, then, consider the issue of specific spatio-temporal sensitivity at several different levels of the nervous system, as well as the differences observed among species. Finally, we conclude the chapter with a discussion of the relevance of these data to human perception, the main purpose of which is to suggest that there are some limits on the applicability of the basic idea of neuronal feature detection to perceptual phenomena that seem to some to be identical but that, in fact, are only superficially analogous.

I. INTRODUCTION
Perhaps the most exciting development in the field of sensory psychobiology in the last decade has been the emergence of the important notion

of feature detection. The basic idea of feature detection is that very specific spatio-temporal patterns of stimuli are almost uniquely capable of initiating activity in particular cells. For example, a dot of light may be an effective stimulus for a particular visual cortex cell if, and only if, it is moving in a particular direction or expanding at a certain rate. An identically shaped stimulus will not be effective, unless its dynamics are appropriate, and a differently shaped object will not work even if it is moving at the appropriate rate. Both the spatial and temporal attributes of a stimulus must be right for it to do the job. As a further example, a particular sequence of tones may be able to activate a sequence-specific cell, while another quite similar one, perhaps even containing the same constituent notes but in a different order, may not be able to do so.

Single cell response specificity to particular patterns in time and space of this sort supports the notion of neurophysiological relativism discussed at the beginning of Chapter 7. It is often difficult to separate the temporal aspects of a stimulus from its spatial ones without losing everything. We are beginning to appreciate that the temporal and spatial codes are not simply summated, but are inseparable aspects of each other.

Unfortunately, the last decade, the period in which this notion of feature detection has been evolving, has not been a sufficiently long time for data to accumulate to equally describe all of the sensory modalities. We shall be mostly dependent upon the work of investigators who have been working in the field of vision for the subsequent discussion. There are only a few important references from auditory neurophysiology that can be considered to be relevant, and, sadly, there is little of interest to report from any of the other senses. Hopefully, this is a temporary state of affairs which will change soon, for psychophysical data make it almost certain that similar mechanisms must be operating in the other sensory modalities. The psychophysics of somatosensation, as von Békésy's work has so eloquently shown, exhibits much the same sort of response to spatio-temporal patterns that appear in vision and audition. Presumably, spatio-temporal patterns, which can key or trigger specific neural systems in olfaction or gustation, are also present. But the peculiarities of their stimulus environments suggest that it will be many years before we can reasonably expect knowledge to be available at the depth already obtained in vision.

It is very important for the reader to remember that in introducing this material on pattern detection, we are not introducing completely novel neural mechanisms. Most of the interpretations of specific feature sensitivities are based upon models involving simpler neural mechanisms of the sort we have already discussed. Edge detection is one form of feature detection and is certainly associated with the lateral inhibitory interactions previously mentioned. The detection of a spot or bar moving in a particular direction also, as we shall see, can be easily understood in terms of lateral interactions and neural delays. Thus, feature detection mechanisms sensitive to specific spatio-temporal patterns represent a somewhat more complex level of discourse, but one which is simply a direct derivation from the concatenations of simpler mechanisms.

The main point of this chapter will be to discuss the fact that sensory systems have evolved to be selectively sensitive to specific spatio-temporal features of the environment. A corollary of this general premise is that the features selected are those that have adaptive significance.

II. A GERMINAL STUDY—"WHAT THE FROG'S EYE TELLS THE FROG'S BRAIN"

Prior to the 1960s, the typical stimulus used in many neurophysiological experiments was an impulsive click or flash of light (or as H. L. Teuber put it, "bolts of lightning and flashes of thunder") with little complex structure and no temporal or spatial patterning. In 1959, Lettvin, Maturana, McCulloch, and Pitts published a very important paper that was to influence research for the next decade. The major impact of this paper lay in its suggestion that since the stimuli, with which the organism usually deals, are not simple impulsive stimuli, there was no reason to assume that the neural organization was evolved to deal with such stimuli either. Their paper concerned the responses recorded from single cells of the optic nerve and of the superior colliculus of the frog. Most insightfully, they entitled their paper "What the Frog's Eye Tells the Frog's Brain," a whimsically anthropomorphic title, which emphasizes the notion of complex processing in the periphery, rather than merely passive mosaic reproduction and transmission of the stimulus patterns. This work has stimulated a decade of research, in which the temporal and spatial pattern of a stimulus came to be considered to be as important, if not more important, than its intensity, extent, or its onset and offset times. There is no question of the fundamental importance of this new idea, and it would be well to quote specifically the sort of thinking that led these investigators to this most significant conceptual breakthrough:

> The assumption has been that the eye mainly senses light, whose local distribution is transmitted to the brain in a kind of copy by a mosaic of impulses. Suppose we held otherwise, that the nervous apparatus in the eye is itself devoted to detecting certain patterns of light and their changes, corresponding to particular relations in the visible world. If this should be the case, the laws found by using small spots of light on the retina may be true and yet, in a sense, be misleading.
> (LETTVIN, MATURANA, McCULLOCH, and PITTS, 1959, p. 1942.)

Their paper initiated an era in which neurophysiologists have begun to take into account a number of important facts. First, peripheral neurons are capable of responding differentially to complex stimulus patterns in a manner transcending simple registration and transmission. Second, complex stimulus patterns may produce responses that are not simply predictable from the notion of a mosaiclike replication of the spatial pattern. Third, the types of responses that are observed neurophysiologically in the frog's visual system at least, are associated in a meaningful way with the environmental tasks faced by the animal. The frog does not live in a world of static spots of light or of diffuse fields. It lives in a world of flies and dragon flies and, for that matter, snakes and hawks. These stimuli are better modeled by moving spot, or moving convex edges (in other words, by complex spatio-temporal patterns) than by dots or stationary forms briefly exposed. The surprising result that has emerged from their work and of other laboratories exploring similar processes is that this sort of specific pattern detection mechanism occurs as peripherally as the retina in at least some species.

Lettvin and his colleagues made other important conceptual contributions in that important and germinal paper. At the time it was published, it certainly seemed somewhat farfetched to make the statement that different anatomical types of retinal neurons could be associated with specific classes of behavioral responses. Yet, as we shall see below, evidence is accumulating that this is exactly the case. Specifically, and by way of completely clarifying this point, it should be noted that the key idea is that the different anatomical types are functionally different by virtue of the differing spatial distributions of their dendritic trees. Such differences in the extent and nature of the arborization allow various manners of interconnection to the more peripheral neural levels, and this means that each type can receive and emphasize a specific spatio-temporal distribution of excitation and inhibition.

Now that we have mentioned the fundamental changes of perspective stimulated by Lettvin, Maturana, McCulloch, and Pitts' paper, let us consider the specific findings. Their unique contribution, as we have said, depended upon the realization that the older stimulus paradigms were incomplete from both a behavioral adaptation and a neurophysiological point of view. To make more realistic visual stimuli, they hit upon the idea of using a 14-in. aluminum hemisphere upon which small dots, rectangles, and other stimulus shapes could be attached and moved by external magnets. Figure 8.1 is a drawing of the stimulus arrangement, showing the hemisphere upon which the stimulus was placed and the arrangement of the apparatus, which held the platinum black coated metal electrodes inserted into the optic nerve or the superior colliculus through a hole in the frog's skull.

By examining the effects of a variety of different kinds of stimulus patterns, four different classes of optic nerve fibers were found. First, a certain group of unmyelinated fibers, which was responsive to contrast, *per se* was found. A difference in the brightness of two portions of the visual field led to continuous firing of this type of cell. These "sustained contrast" cells had the additional properties of being able to maintain their activity for over a minute after the stimulus was removed. Furthermore, the output of these cells saturated at low stimulus intensity and did not vary with further increases in stimulus intensity.

The second type of unmyelinated cells, which Lettvin and his colleagues referred to as the "net convexity detectors," responded only to small moving spots (a fly?) but not to large moving objects, unless they entered the receptive field of the cell corner first. Dotted or checked patterns, even though containing small units, were not able to activate these

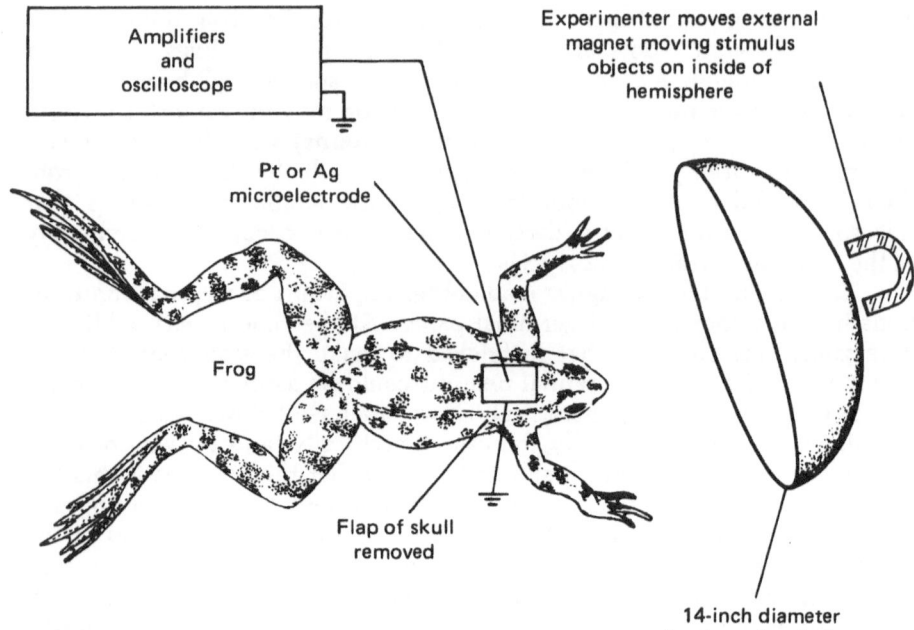

FIGURE 8.1 *The experimental arrangement used in the Lettvin, Maturana, Mc-Culloch, and Pitts (1959) experiment.*

---

cells. The adaptive utility of such a fiber can best be expressed in the author's words:

> A delightful exhibit uses a large color photograph of the natural habitat of a frog from a frog's eye view, flowers and grass. We can move this photograph through the receptive field of such a fiber, waving it around at a seven inch distance: there is no response. If we perch with a magnet a fly-sized object 1° large on the part of the picture seen by the receptive field and move only the object, we get an excellent response. If the object is fixed to the picture in about the same place and the whole moved about, then there is none.
>
> (LETTVIN, MATURANA, McCULLOCH, and PITTS, 1959, p. 1945.)

A third class, but in this case made up of myelinated neurons, was solely responsive to moving edges. A stationary edge, though of exactly the same shape, was totally ineffective in activating members of this third class of neuron. The fourth type included myelinated cells that responded to any overall dimming of the field. This cell type, with its characteristically large receptive field, also possessed the fastest conducting axons. It may be that this fourth cell type is behaviorally associated with the detection of predators. Whatever the evolutionary history of

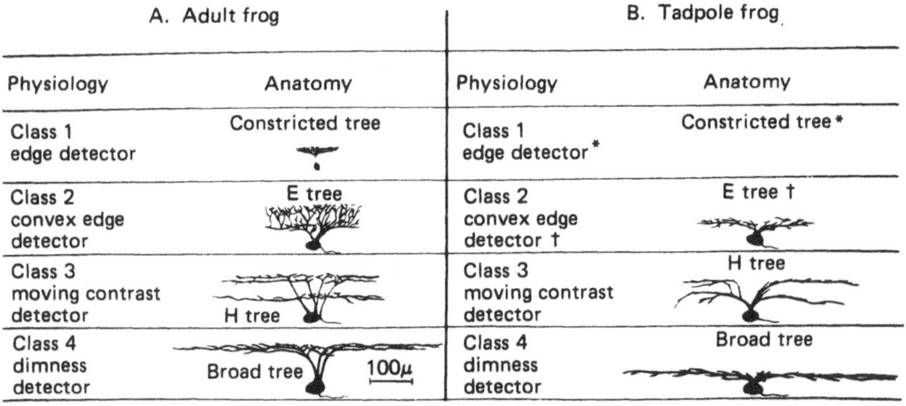

A. Adult frog		B. Tadpole frog	
Physiology	Anatomy	Physiology	Anatomy
Class 1 edge detector	Constricted tree	Class 1 edge detector*	Constricted tree*
Class 2 convex edge detector	E tree	Class 2 convex edge detector †	E tree †
Class 3 moving contrast detector	H tree	Class 3 moving contrast detector	H tree
Class 4 dimness detector	Broad tree 100μ	Class 4 dimness detector	Broad tree

FIGURE 8.2 *The four types of ganglion cell dendritic arborizations found in the adult frog and in the tadpole and the associated spatio-temporal specificities suggested by Lettvin and his colleagues. (*) Absent from tadpole; (†) absent from tadpoles retinal periphery (from Pomeranz and Chung, 1970).*

such a mechanism, it is a highly useful feature of the frog's neural mechanism, since this mechanism appears to be associated with some sort of an escape response—moving edges being typical of moving "hawks."

The four sets of fibers observed in the optic nerve by Lettvin, Maturana, McCulloch, and Pitts sort themselves out at the level of the superior colliculus. Each type projects to one of the four collicular layers, each of which seems to topologically represent the layout of the whole retinal mosaic. Thus, the retinal image is represented four different times, but in layers that are particularly responsive to four different features of the stimulus pattern.

Lettvin and his colleagues have suggested that the remarkable ability of the optic nerve (ganglion cell) fibers to respond to specific aspects of the spatio-temporal stimulus patterns is due to the fact that differently shaped dendritic trees of the four types of ganglion cells sample a variety of different inputs from the bipolar and receptor layers of the retina. Figure 8.2 shows the four types of ganglion cells that these investigators considered to be prototypical of the four-cell type cells of the frog's retina as classified by their neurophysiological behavior. Lettvin and his colleagues associated the sustained contrast detector with the constricted field ganglion cell, the convexity detector sensitive to small moving spots with the E type of ganglion cell, the moving edge detector with the H type, and the dimming detector with the broad tree. Recently, Pomeranz and Chung (1970) have carried out some developmental studies, which demonstrated that the four types of cells do not all appear at the same time in the metamorphic development of the tadpole. They further conclude that the associations suggested above by Lettvin and his colleagues are supported when one compares the presence or absence of a specific type of cell with the ability of the tadpole or adult frog's retina to produce one of the prototypical feature-specific responses. Pomeranz and Chung found, with microscopic examination, that during the tadpole stage of the frog's development, the restricted field ganglion cell is totally absent and that E tree ganglion cells are absent from the retinal periphery as summarized in Figure 8.2. Their electrophysiological recordings showed, correspondingly, that the sustained contrast type of response pattern was totally absent in the tadpole and that the small spot convexity detection process could not be observed in the tadpole's peripheral retina. This correlation adds substantial support to the earlier speculations of Lettvin's group, relating specific cellular anatomy and physiologic response pattern.

III. ANOTHER GERMINAL STUDY—HUBEL AND WIESEL'S MOVING BAR DETECTOR

About the same time that work was going on in Lettvin's laboratory at M.I.T., down the street at the Harvard Medical School a pair of researchers were beginning to report what was to be a most remarkable series of studies of the organization and specific sensitivities of visual cells in the mammalian nervous system. Hubel and Wiesel had quickly moved to take advantage of a very sturdy new tungsten electrode developed earlier by one of them (Hubel, 1957) that allowed very long and stable periods of observations from single cells in the central nervous system. The papers, which have been forthcoming from the continued collaboration of these two investigators, have been most compelling in establishing the fact that mammalian nerve cells also reflect coding mechanisms that are sensitive to the spatio-temporal pattern of visual stimuli rather than to simply the distribution of light on the retina. In the next part of this section, we shall trace the difference in response patterns at different levels of the ascending visual pathway. In this section, we shall, so to speak, start at the top to try to give a brief introduction to the type of electrophysiological techniques that formed the conceptual basis of much of Hubel and Wiesel's later work.

In the first application of the new electrode, Hubel (1959) observed specific sensitivity to spatio-temporal features of stimulus patterns in cells of the visual cortex of the cat similar to the response patterns Lettvin and his colleagues had discovered in the frog's optic nerve and tectum. Recording from the striate cortex of unrestrained cats, Hubel had found large numbers of cells that were unaffected by the general level of retinal illumination, but that produced large amounts of spike activity when a small spot of light was moved across the retina. Not only was the movement of the spot necessary, but those cells also seemed to have preferential directions of movements for maximal activation. In a later paper that year, Hubel and Wiesel (1959) mapped out the shape and polarity of the receptive fields of these cells and showed that these fields were organized somewhat differently than those observed in the retina by Kuffler (1953). Rather than concentric rings of inhibition and disinhibition, the antagonistic regions in the cortex seemed to be usually arranged in side-by-side patterns as shown in Figure 8.3. Although not all of the cortical cells mapped required movement to elicit responses, the responses were en-

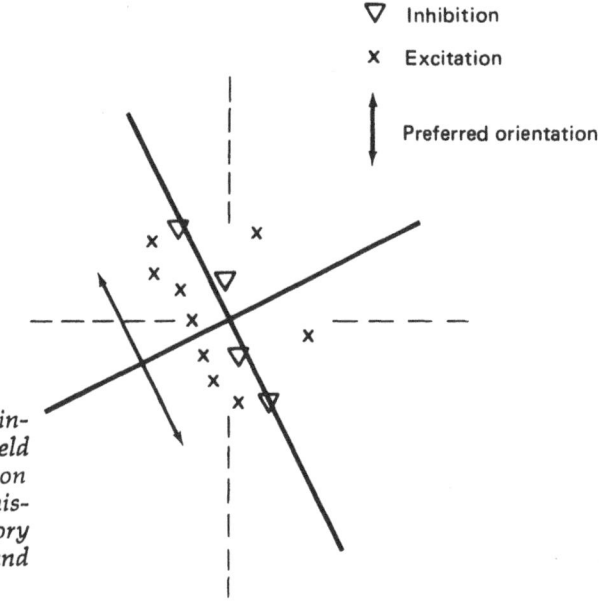

∇ Inhibition

x Excitation

↕ Preferred orientation

FIGURE 8.3 A typical linearly arranged receptive field of a cat's visual cortex neuron with side-by-side antagonistic excitatory and inhibitory regions (from Hubel and Wiesel, 1959).

hanced from almost all cells when the stimulus was moving in a particular direction. It should be noted that the response of many of these cells seemed to be dependent upon not only movement and a preferential direction, but also upon the shape of the moving stimulus. While bars of light were effective for some cells, dark bars or moving edges were found to be the best stimuli for other cells. Presumably, the effectiveness of these elongated stimuli is associated with the shape of the receptive field and the adjacent elongated regions of inhibition and excitation.

Shortly thereafter, Hubel and Wiesel (1962, 1963) made another important discovery about the cortical organization of the moving bar detectors. Suggestions had come from work in some of the other senses (for example, Mountcastle, 1957), as well as from anatomical studies showing vertical structural organization, that the cells of the cerebral cortex were araanged in functional, as well as structural, columns oriented normal to the surface of the brain. The notion was that these vertical columns, while not distinguishable by any anatomic boundaries from neighboring columns, did have functional properties that were quite different from column to column and that there would be abrupt changes as a microelectrode crossed the invisible boundaries separating them. Hubel and Wiesel showed that if a microelectrode was pushed into the cortex in such a way that it penetrated into the successive layers of a single vertical, cortical column, the experimenter would pick up spike trains from a succession of individual cells, all of which behaved in the same way. An important observation was that each cell in the penetration series was specifically sensitive to the same direction of movement of a bar-shaped visual stimulus. Of course, it was not always possible to keep the cell within one column in their experiments, but it was clear when the micro-

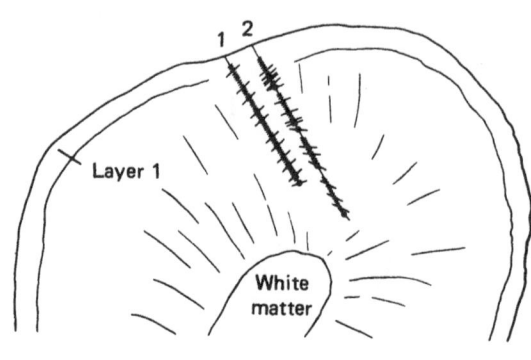

FIGURE 8.4 Two parallel pathways of microelectrodes into the cat's visual cortex. One of the tracks apparently has slid down a column, in which all of the cells have specific sensitivities in the same direction (1). The other track (2) crosses from column to column hitting many cells with different directional sensitivities (as indicated by the small cross lines) in sequence (from Hubel and Wiesel, 1963).

electrode emerged from one column and entered another, the preferential direction of activation would change to a new orientation and remain so oriented until the electrode entered another column. Figure 8.4 shows the results for two typical deep penetrations. One of the penetrations has fortuitously slipped down a single column, and all of the cells were maximally sensitive to stimuli moving in the same direction. The other penetration, however, crossed from one column to another several times as indicated by the succession of preferential orientation which was encountered.

From the surface of the cortex, another view obtains. Figure 8.5 shows the shape of the surface mosaic of the columns. The dotted lines outline the areas that Hubel and Wiesel believed to be associated with single columns. The preferential direction of the cells sampled in that column is shown by the small bars. Note carefully that the cross-sectional area of these columns is only 1 mm or so on the cortex and that adjacent regions seem not to have any special relation with regard to their preferential direction to that of their neighbors. The shape of the columns, furthermore, was quite irregular; some were round, and some more elongated. The major correlated anatomical fact is that the individual columns do appear to be organized along the direction of the fibers of the optic radiation, which extend from the white matter to the superficial grey matter of the cortex.

Hubel and Wiesel have made another anatomic point of considerable interest. The classic notions of cortical localization assumed some sort of topologically constant projection of the retinal mosaic. However, their new findings and the discovery of the orientation specific columns have made it quite clear that the retinal mosaic is, in fact, represented many different times over on the cortex. Each retinal point is represented in many different columns, each of which corresponds to a specific direction of movement of the barlike stimulus across the point. This multiple representation is in addition to the multiple representation of the retinal mosaic in several different regions of the cortex (for example, the three classic visual areas in the cortex regions known as 17, 18, and 19).

Hubel and Wiesel (1965) have also discovered that the spatio-tem-

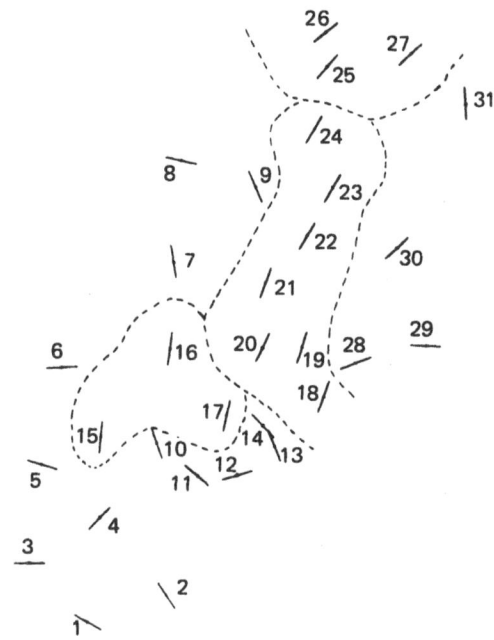

FIGURE 8.5 The organization of cortical columns as viewed on the surface of the brain. There is no apparent organization or relation between adjacent columns. The small lines indicate preferred directions. Numbers refer to the sequence of penetrations (from Hubel and Wiesel, 1963).

poral specificity of the cells in the cat's cortex involves more than a single type of response. In fact, they determined that there were at least four different kinds of cellular feature extractors present. Some cells displayed the simple shape and direction of movement specificity that we have already discussed. The three other classes, however, seemed to include cells that received multiple convergent inputs from this primitive type of cell. In fact, there appeared to be a hierarchy in which each successive class—simple, complex, lower-order hypercomplex and higher-order hypercomplex—produced responses, which presumably resulted from integration of the inputs from many cells of the next simpler type. Each had a specific stimulus geometry, which maximally activated it. Some (the simplest ones) responded only to stimuli in a particular location and at a particular orientation, while others (the more complicated ones) seemed to be able to respond to multiple positions and directions, but still requiring some sort of particular movement and shape for their optimal activation. The hierarchy and specific sensitivities of each of the four types are presented in Table 8.1, which has been summarized from Hubel and Wiesel (1965).

In recent years, this table of visual cortex cellular organization has been challenged by other workers. Spinelli and Barrett (1969), in particular, have challenged the notion that line-shaped stimuli are of particular importance, even when one is dealing with elongated receptive fields. In their study, they found that some of the cells, which Hubel and Wiesel had thought to be uniquely stimulatable with lines, could also be stimulated with moving spots or dots of light. Nevertheless, whatever the outcome of specific aspects of the controversy, it is clear that Hubel and Wiesel's

TABLE 8.1 CORTICAL CELL TYPES SENSITIVE TO SPECIFIC ASPECTS OF THE TEMPORAL-SPATIAL PATTERN OF VISUAL STIMULI (ADAPTED FROM THE DISCUSSION OF HUBEL AND WIESEL, 1965)

Cortical Cell Type	Best Stimulus Shape	Other Stimulus Conditions	Possible Mechanism
Simple	Edges, bars, slits, all with preferred orientation of movement	Critically dependent on location within receptive field	Interaction of inhibitory and excitatory influences of receptive fields
Complex	Edges, bars, slits, all with preferred orientation of movement	Independent of location within receptive field	Integration of the output of a number of simple cells
Lower-order hypercomplex	Edges, corners, tongues, and angles of particular sizes	Specific to length of stimulus. Some cells required a stimulus exactly the width of receptive field. Other required one which ended (a tongue) within the field. Stimulus must not extend beyond a certain point.	Integration of the output of both inhibitory and excitatory complex cells
Upper-order hypercomplex	Edges, corners, tongues, and angles of particular size	Similar to lower-order hypercomplex. But in addition, cells of this group responded in two preferred directions 90° apart.	Integration of the output of two or more lower-order hypercomplex cells

work has been of the greatest significance in opening the door to a new understanding of neuronal circuitry. By their emphasis of the specific sensitivity to spatio-temporal features of the stimulus, they have helped to reorient many of the basic premises of sensory-coding theory.

Another very important issue concerning these feature specific receptive fields has been emerging in recent years. How do these receptive fields change as a function of maturation and experience? Clearly a great deal of plasticity is possible in receptive field structure even to the point that environmental stimuli may be able to determine the shape of the field. Though this topic is not directly germane to the main concern of this book, it is clear that the subject will be extremely important to students of development.

IV. DIRECTIONAL SENSITIVITY IN THE SUBCORTICAL VISUAL CENTERS OF MAMMALS

The work of Lettvin, Maturana, McCulloch, and Pitts and that of Hubel and Wiesel have stimulated many other investigators to examine other centers of the ascending visual pathways for evidence of feature detectors. Subsequently, a number of investigators began to find evidence of similar directionally sensitive cells at all other levels of the visual system, although with some curious species differences.

Arden (1963) was examining the receptive fields of lateral geniculate cells of the rabbit when he, too, discovered that small spots of light, which were relatively ineffectual stimuli when immobile, became remarkably effective when they were moved about in the receptive field. Not only was the movement of the spot necessary for the effective elicitation of responses, but many cells seemed to exhibit preferential sensitivity to movement in a given direction.

Kozack, Rodieck, and Bishop (1965) reported a comprehensive study of the effect of moving stimuli in the lateral geniculate body of the cat. They found units that were directionally sensitive, but without the same narrow range of specificity reported by Hubel and Wiesel in the cat's cortex. However, when this work was extended to the cat's retina (Rodieck and Stone, 1965b), they found that, while the center-surround arrangement was present and the responses were sensitive to such factors as size, shape, contrast, and speed of movement of stimulus objects, retinal cells were, in fact, not directionally sensitive! This finding is in sharp contrast to the observation of directional sensitivity in the retina of the pigeon (Maturana and Frenk, 1963) or of the rabbit (Barlow and Hill, 1963), as well as many other animals.

How can directional sensitivity arise out of the interaction of simple neurons, which are not themselves directionally sensitive? Perhaps the most instructive example of such an analysis, using the rabbit retina as a model system, has been presented by Barlow, Hill, and Levick (1964). First, let us discuss the details of their experimental procedure and some of their findings, and then we shall consider their neural model of directional sensitivity.

Fine tungsten electrodes were inserted directly through the rabbit's sclera into the retina. Extracellular ganglion cell spikes are recorded in this manner, and this means, of course, that the responses observed reflect the integrative activity of at least two preceding synaptic levels and probably several other horizontal interactions. Barlow, Hill, and Levick report the presence of ganglion cells organized with antagonistic center-surround receptive fields, as well as ganglion cells that seemed to be activated solely on an "on" and "off" basis without the antagonistic surround arrangement. These latter cells, in particular, seemed to have specific sensitivities not only to the direction, but also to the speed of the moving spot. Figure 8.6 (adapted from Barlow, Hill, and Levick) shows the differential sensitivity to direction of movement of a particular center-surround type of cell. It can be clearly seen that this cell is maximally sensitive when the stimulus is moving upward and declines in sensitivity to virtually zero response levels when the stimulus is moving downward.

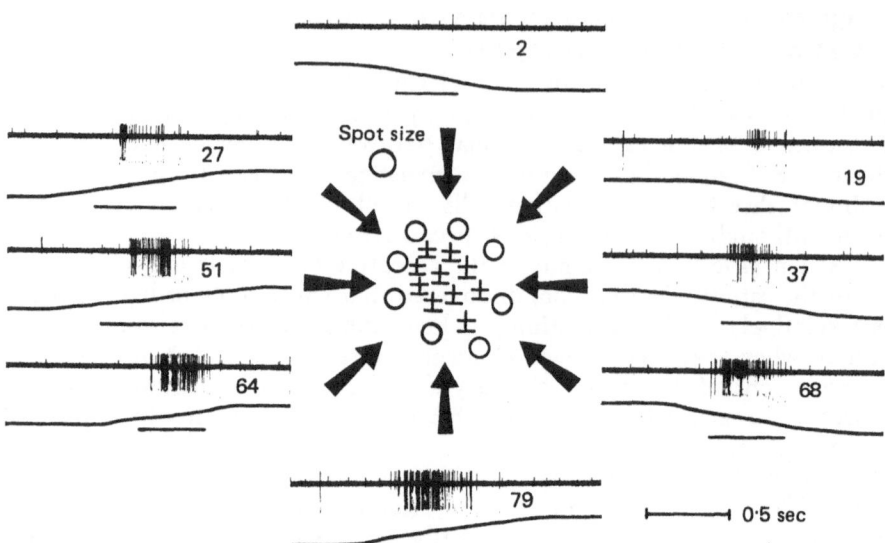

FIGURE 8.6 *Directional sensitivity in the ganglion cell of the rabbit retina, showing the response of a cell which is maximally sensitive to upward moving stimuli and minimally sensitive to downward moving ones. Numbers indicate spike count, and ± marks indicate the size of the receptive field in which both "on" and "off" responses were elicited by stationary spots curved lines indicate movement of stimulus; straight lines indicate periods of stimulus illumination (from Barlow, Hill, and Levick, 1964).*

Intermediate directions of movement produce intermediate numbers of spike action potentials.,

Barlow, Hill, and Levick also observed two other types of cells in the rabbit retina, in which the speed rather than the direction of a moving stimulus was critical in determining the amount of induced spike activity. One type had a rather large receptive field and proved to be maximally activated by stimuli that moved very rapidly. Figure 8.7 shows the pattern of response, indicating a greater sensitivity to rapidly moving stimuli. On the other hand, there were also ganglion cells present, which had very small fields and were maximally activated by very slow moving stimuli— a most unusual sort of specific sensitivity the adaptive utility of which is not immediately obvious. Figure 8.8 demonstrates the heightened sensitivity of this type of cell to slowly moving stimuli.

Barlow and Levick (1965) have also shown that retinal direction sensitivity in the rabbit is primarily due to the retinal differentiation of the response on the basis of the sequence in which various portions of the receptive field have been stimulated. If a sequence is presented in the opposite order, then the effect of the stimulus would be nil or, in some cases, it might even inhibit the level of spontaneous activity. They believe that some sort of inhibitory lateral interaction is the basis of the sequence

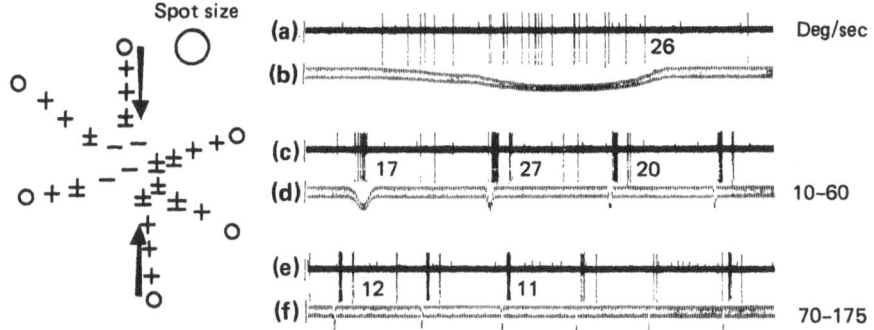

FIGURE 8.7 *Response of a cell with a large receptive field. This cell responds best to movements that are moderately rapid. (a), (c), and (e) are the spike responses resulting from the movement shown in (b), (d), and (f), which are photoelectric traces of the stimulating light (also showing considerable 50-Hz ripple from the power source). The small numbers indicate the number of spikes in the preceding burst. This cell obviously responds best to intermediate speeds of movement. Symbols as in Figure 8.6 (adapted from Barlow, Hill, and Levick, 1964).*

detection process. This is not a conclusion that can be drawn *a priori*, for there are two complementary mechanisms—one excitatory and one inhibitory—which could produce exactly the same sort of directional sensitivity. Other tests must be made to determine whether an excitatory or inhibitory process accounts for this particular feature detection process. Perhaps the distinction between the two possible mechanisms can be made more clearly by considering two possible logical systems, as Barlow and Levick have done, each of which is capable of producing a response only when the stimulus is moving in a preferred direction. Figure 8.9 (adapted from Barlow and Levick) shows the two hypothetical nerve nets. One operates on the basis of an excitatory interaction; the output indicative of movement in the preferred direction occurs only when the stimulus activates a given receptor *and* the receptor that preceded it in that order and at a particular interval. The other possible mechanism is based upon an inhibitory process; an output will occur if a stimulus activates a given receptor, but only if the prior receptor has not been activated in the period defined by the time delay. In this case, the directional sensitive mechanism is one based on the inhibition of a response that otherwise would have occurred. In the former case, a response can occur only if gated or allowed by an appropriately timed excitatory response.

Barlow and Levick carried out experiments that showed that two spatially disparate stimuli activated in sequence produced a smaller number of spike action potentials than when the two were presented separately. This suggested to them that the mechanism for the sequence detection, and thus the directional sensitivity, was, in fact, more likely to be an inhibitory mechanism than an excitatory one. To complete the story, some correlation must be shown between the hypothetical logical mecha-

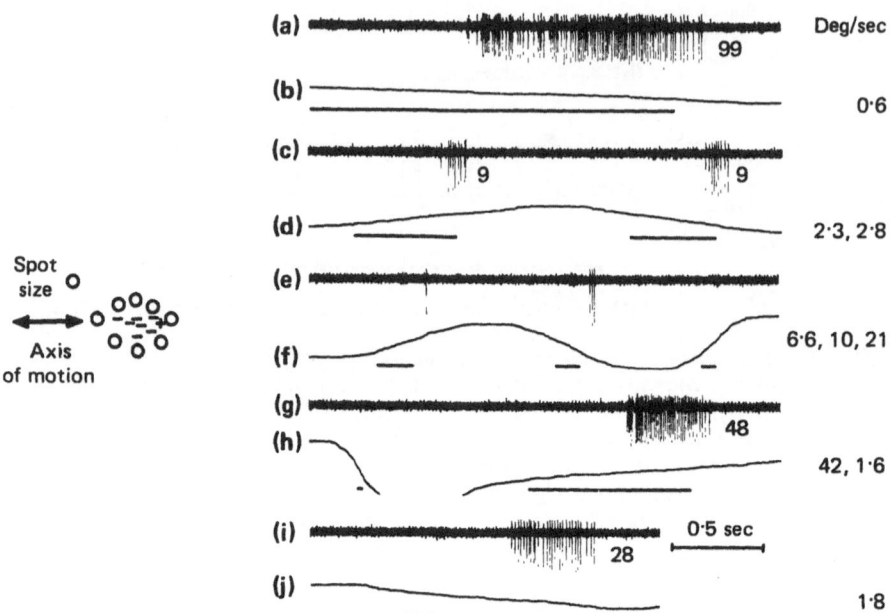

FIGURE 8.8 Response of a cell with a small receptive field. This cell type responds best, surprisingly, to very slowly moving stimuli as indicated by the small number of spikes to rapidly moving stimuli and the large number evoked by slowly moving stimuli. Symbols as in Figure 8.6 (from Barlow, Hill, and Levick, 1964).

nisms and the known anatomy of the rabbit's retina. Figure 8.10 is Barlow and Levick's schematic diagram of the anatomy of the rabbit retina. The function of the logical "and" (the gating or allowing function) units is performed by the bipolar cell, such that no output will occur unless both of the inputs are activated. Inputs from the horizontal cells are assumed to be mainly inhibitory and able to prevent the bipolars from firing if a group of cells has already been activated at an appropriate prior interval. The conduction time of the horizontal cells is supposed to be identifiable with the time delays indicated in Figure 8.9. As Barlow and Levick note:

> The strength of the proposed scheme arises from the fact that a function can naturally be assigned to the neural elements that are known to exist without making esoteric or revolutionary assumptions about how they work.

> (BARLOW and LEVICK, 1965, p. 497.)

For the purposes of our discussions, this model represents a sample of the sort of neural interaction that will probably have to be invoked to explain the action of feature sensitive cells of varying degrees of complexity and hypercomplexity at all levels of the nervous system.

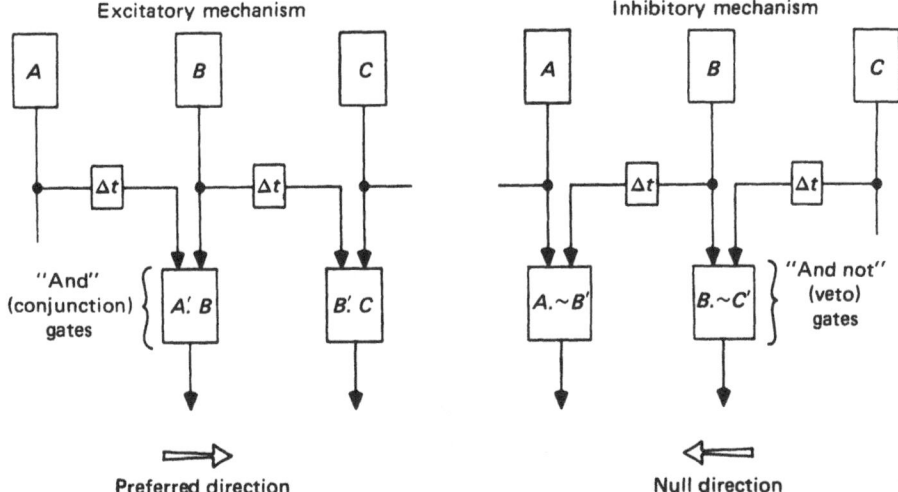

FIGURE 8.9 Two equivalent logical circuits, both of which may display directional sensitivity, but which are based on (a) summation and (b) inhibition
mechanisms, respectively. Δt is a time delay unit, which delays the signal from
a preceding receptor sufficiently to allow either synchrony (thus enabling the
"and" gate) or dysynchrony (thus enabling the "veto" gate) of inputs from
adjacent receptor units (from Barlow and Levick, 1965).

V. FEATURE DETECTION IN AUDITION

As we said in introducing this section, neurophysiological feature detection mechanisms in the other sensory modalities have been only infrequently reported. Nevertheless, there is at least one body of evidence
that suggests that mechanisms analogous to the spatio-temporal pattern
recognizers of the visual system are also present in the auditory system.
Whitfield and Evans (1965) obtained such data in a sampling of neurons
in the auditory cortex, which selectively responded to complex tonal patterns. Like Hubel and Wiesel, as well as Lettvin, Maturana, McCulloch,
and Pitts, they had become convinced that simple stimuli, either in the form
of impulsive clicks or constant tones, did not evoke the true diversity
of responses of which cortical cells were capable. Instead of constant
tones or impulsive clicks, Whitfield and Evans, therefore, used frequency
modulated tones as their stimuli. If we proceed under the assumption that
frequency is to cochlear locus what stimulus position is to retinal locus, it is
clear that these frequency modulated stimuli are close analogues of moving spots or slits in the visual domain. And, indeed, the data obtained did
seem to exhibit many of the properties we have already become familiar
with in the visual sense.

Figure 8.11 shows one of the typical records obtained in their experiments. The lower trace in this figure reflects the modulations of the
frequency of the stimulating tone. The early unmodulated flat portion
of the stimulus represents a period during which its frequency was held
constant. Clearly, the neuronal responses adapt very little. On the other

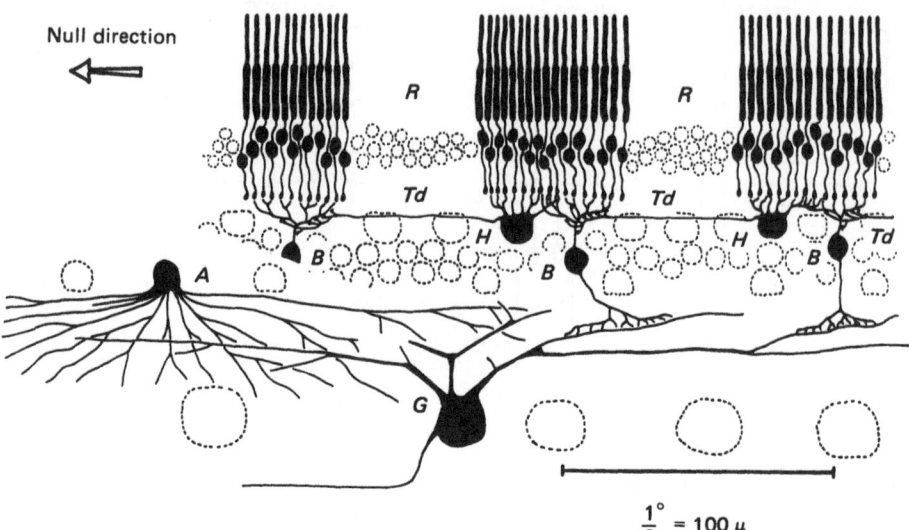

Null direction

$\frac{1}{2}^{\circ} = 100\,\mu$

FIGURE 8.10 A more anatomically reasonable model of the inhibitory circuit which, Barlow and Levick feel, shows how certain known structures could fill the role of the logical unit shown in Figure 8.9. (R) receptor layer, (Td) teleodendria of the horizontal cells, (H) bipolar cells, (A) amacrine cells, (G) ganglion cells. The ganglion cells act as the logical veto cells of Figure 8.9, and the horizontal cells serve to insert the time delay (from Barlow and Levick, 1965).

hand, it can be seen that elicited responses are almost in perfect synchrony with the later modulations of the frequency of the stimulating tone, a sort of entrainment that we will also see occurring with tonal stimuli of constant frequency (Rose et al., 1967) in Chapter 10.

In fact, Whitfield and Evans report that as many as 10 percent of the cells that they investigated were not capable of being stimulated by any constant tone under any conditions, but did vigorously respond when the frequency was modulated in some manner. A most interesting part of their data concerns a group of cells that were excited only when the stimulus tone was varying its frequency in a particular direction. The response areas and the preferential direction of frequency change of some of these cells are shown in Figure 8.12. As can be seen, some of the cells produce spike activity only when the frequency is increasing; others only when the frequency is decreasing; and others differ in their directional sensitivity, depending on whether the signal is in the high- or low-frequency region of the response area. The analogies between such auditory "directional" sensitivities and those of the visual system discussed in the earlier section are self evident.

On the other hand, there are newly discovered examples of feature sensitive cells in the nervous system that do not seem to be analogues of any other known process. Recently, for example, Thompson, Mayers, Robertson, and Patterson (1970) have encountered some curious cells in

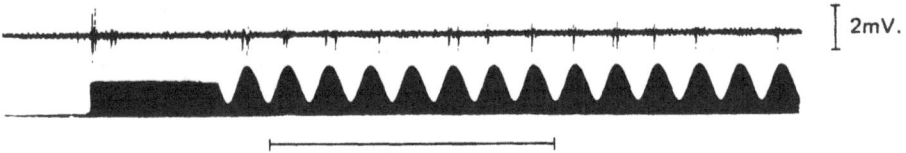

FIGURE 8.11 The response of an auditory cortex cell to a frequency modulated acoustic signal. The lower curve is the frequency envelope, not the signal itself. The response shown in the upper trace quickly adapts to a constant 11.6-kHz tone, but becomes responsive again when the frequency is modulated as shown (from Whitfield and Evans, 1965).

the association areas of the cat's brain that seem to be able to count a certain characteristic and specific number of input stimuli before emitting their own spike potential response. Interestingly enough, these highly specific counting responses were produced regardless of which sensory modality was used as an input, and the cells, therefore, are examples of polysensory neurons. Nor for that matter did the interstimulus interval seem to be important, a dimension which should have affected the counting behavior if it were due simply to some "charging up" sort of process. Whatever the mechanism, this is an example of another sort of feature sensitive process; in this case, the feature is the number of input stimuli.

VI. DO LATERAL INTERACTION AND FEATURE DETECTION MECHANISMS ADEQUATELY MODEL HUMAN PERCEPTUAL PHENOMENA?[1]

The purpose of the following section is a somewhat digressive one in light of the main theme of this book, but perhaps one of the most important parts of all that has to be said. The neurophysiological findings, which we have just discussed, have been remarkably effective in stimulating a considerable amount of psychobiological theorizing, particularly in regard to perceptual phenomena. However, not all of this theory, some believe, has been justified by adequate identifications of the neural and psychophysical mechanisms being compared. Often, it seems as if a sort of psychobiological "silly season" has taken hold of many would-be theorists and that they have fallen victim to what is just the most recent of a long history of reductionistic fads.

All of this, of course, is nothing new. From the earliest recorded notions up to contemporary theories, the prevailing technology has usually been the source of many of the basic premises. [See Brazier (1959) for a more complete history of the psychobiological thinking which permeates the history of physiology.] Thus, Aristotle and Galen turned to the circulatory system—the heart and blood—as the potential source of the various "vapors and spirits" (a hydraulic-gaseous model) for their very persistent views of mental life. The view that the blood was the basis of

[1] Much of the following material has been adapted from Uttal, 1971b.

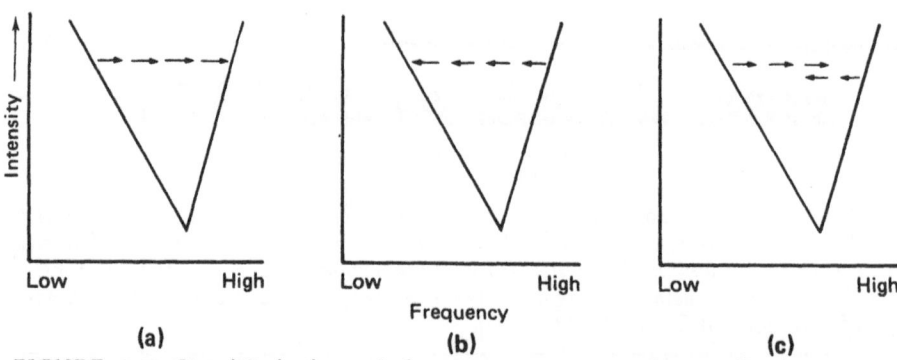

FIGURE 8.12 Simplified plots of the response area of three cells that respond only when the frequency of the input signals varies. (a) The response area of a cell that responds only when the frequency of the stimulus increases. (b) The response area of a cell that responds only when the frequency of the stimulus decreases. (c) The response area of a cell that responds to any frequency change (from Whitfield and Evans, 1965).

the mind lasted from their time up until the seventeenth century, and even such a genius as William Harvey still accepted it. His contemporary, Descartes, though taking a slightly different approach and assuming that the pineal body was the seat of man's mental life, thought that the mind operated on a hydraulic basis. An interesting twist to his theory was the supposition, however, that various fluids were pumped about through the then recently discovered to-be-tubular nerves.

During the latter part of the eighteenth century, scientific theorizing was dominated by Newtonian thinking. His postulation of an "ether" led many biologists to seek similar ethereal models as explanations of nervous function. In the nineteenth century, the emergence of electrical telephonic technology led some to speculate that a similar mechanism was the basis of nervous activity. The two decades following World War II saw the rise of conceptual models based upon similarities and analogies between the brain and the recently developed electronic digital computers.

In retrospect, these hydraulic, mechanical, ethereal, telephonic, and computer-based theories all seem relatively naive; from our current vantage point, it is quite easy to see how each generation of reductionistically oriented theorizers was so easily seduced into using the most current, exciting, interesting, and potentially useful technology as the basis for its ideas. This was natural enough, for what was past had already been tested and found wanting, and even in our currently advanced times, there is no way to build a theory on an unborn idea. But the fact to be emphasized is that each generation thought for a while, at least, that they had the answer denied to their predecessors, only to see it rejected later.

It is not quite so easy to realize that one's current fad may only be that—only one more link in a growing chain of interesting ideas, of which the most recent link is momentarily, if not ultimately, the terminal one. In each generation, the temptation becomes stronger. Each new technology *is* more powerful than its predecessor and explains more, and more tempting yet, it promises to explain still more. As a further inducement, it is certainly also true that, according to some measures, the technologies *are* converging in the right direction.

This brief history sets the stage for the thesis of this section, namely, that there is a current fad in neurophysiological explanation of perceptual phenomena that is not yet recognized as such and that also may be unjustified. Just as in recent years we have begun to be suspicious of simpleminded computer-based models of mental processes, we should begin to consider the possibility that perhaps *some* of the psychological models based upon neurophysiological data have been extended beyond reasonable explanatory limits.

In the following sections, we shall first consider some of the specific instances in which feature detection models have been, it is believed, applied inappropriately to perceptual phenomena, and then point out some of the psychophysical data that seem inconsistent with such an approach. A few discrepant neurophysiological data will then be considered. Perhaps the point of this section was best summed up by Charles Harris of the Bell Telephone Laboratories when he said:

> *Some people forget that when neurophysiological data are used as explanations for psychological phenomena, they become neurophysiological theories.*

A. The Psychobiological Theories

The impact of the compelling and exciting neurophysiological data concerning the feature specific mechanisms we have already described was to suggest to some psychologists that certain of the processes, which had been handled only descriptively at best by the qualitative theories of the previous decades, might be better explained by hypothesizing similar simple neurological nets in the human nervous system.

Some of the earliest examples of this sort of neurophysiological modeling were deceptively straightforward. McCullough (1965) found what appeared to be a near analogue of the directional sensitivity of the Hubel and Wiesel cortical columns when she reported color adaptation effects of hypothesized edge detectors. Whether or not the effects are peripheral (retinal) or central is still not clear, and the interested reader is directed to Blakemore and Campbell (1969) and Gilinsky and Doherty (1969), who considered this point in detail.

Andrews (1965), basing his conclusions mostly upon preferred perceived orientations in a psychophysical experiment, points out a number of similarities between his data and the Hubel and Wiesel results. Much to his credit, he does point out that "alternative hypotheses could be invoked."

Blakemore and Sutton (1969) reflect an analogous, though reverse, direction in their thinking when they say that grating adaptation experiments of this sort may allow a means for "the study of the trigger features of optimum stimuli of human sensory neurons."

Mayzner's group (for example, Mayzner, Tresselt, and Helfer, 1967; Buchsbaum and Mayzner, 1969; and Mayzner and Tresselt, 1970) has vigorously supported the notion that lateral inhibitory interaction between Hubel and Wiesel type cortical columns is responsible for the "sequential blanking" effects found in their experiments, using a computer controlled cathode-ray oscilloscope to produce stimulus patterns. They hypothesize a form of interaction between columns that are not only specific to direction of line movement (as reported by Hubel and Wiesel), but also to the number of sides in a stimulus polygon or even to word meaning.

Campbell and Kulikowski (1966), examining the effect of orientation on visual resolution, also link their data to Hubel and Wiesel type directional sensitivities. Noting that "it is, of course, not possible to argue convincingly from psychophysical data to neurophysiological descriptions of the visual system," they find that some of the characteristics of the Hubel and Wiesel data are very similar to some of the data obtained in their experiment, not only qualitatively, but in the details of the range of angles of sensitivity of the compared effects as well.

Dember and Purcell (1967) feel that the Hartline type of lateral inhibition is the most likely candidate to explain the psychophysical disinhibition effects they observed in a visual masking study. Perhaps the most sophisticated theoretical position in this area has been taken by Weisstein (1968). Pursuing her own earlier experimental work (Weisstein, 1966) and that of others, she has developed a very compelling mathematical model for metacontrast effects, based upon notions of lateral inhibitory interaction. Metacontrast is a phenomenon first observed by Stigler (1910) and later popularized by Alpern (1953), in which nonoverlapping stimuli, presented subsequent to a test stimulus, decrease the apparent brightness of that preceding test stimulus. The two classic stimulus patterns used in the metacontrast experiment are the concentric ring and central disk, and the three side-by-side rectangles as shown in Figure 8-13 (a) and (b), respectively. The central disk or central rectangle is, respectively, the test stimulus, which is suppressed under appropriate conditions in each case. Alpern (1953) discovered that the flanking rectangles, for example, were able to mask or diminish the brightness of the central rectangle only when they followed it. When the flanking rectangles preceded the central one, there was no inhibition. The metacontrast phenomenon has been closely linked with apparent movement by Kahneman (1967) and has been shown to be present when the test and masking stimuli were applied to opposite eyes (Kolers and Rosner, 1960).

Metacontrast is visual phenomenon, which has been beset with controversy since Alpern's original studies. There is considerable argument concerning whether or not the response curves relating the metacontrast phenomena are U-shaped or monotonic (see Eriksen, Becker, and Hoffman, 1970) as well as with regard to their physiological basis. Recently, Weisstein (1969) published a most provocative paper dealing with the same general problem discussed in this section of this chapter. In it, she spoke rather more hopefully of psychophysical techniques as a means of exploring single cell mechanisms than some other investigators would be willing to accept. While Weisstein does appreciate the difficulties involved in go-

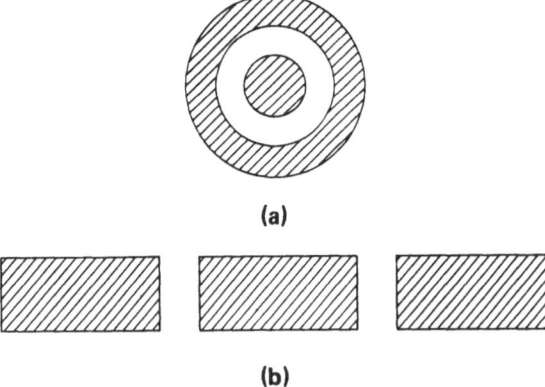

FIGURE 8.13 Two standard stimulus patterns that can be used to produce metacontrast effects. (a) Concentric disk and annular ring. (b) Three side by side rectangles.

ing from a behavioral description to a neuronal analysis, she seems willing to assume that many behavioral tests do reflect the operation of simple neural networks. Rothberg (1968) has also used Weisstein's data to develop a computer model based upon similar notions of lateral inhibitory interaction.

Pantle and Sekuler (1968) postulated the existence of a hierarchy of size-detecting feature filters in an attempt to explain the results of some experiments in which only some grating line widths inhibit the detection of subsequently presented gratings of similar size. An abundance of other recent data using sinusoidal stimuli has been accumulated in the past few years by an increasing number of investigators. Many of them also assume that spatial frequency analyses are made by neural units in the brain sensitive to specific frequency features.

In sum, we can see that the idea that psychophysical data directly reflect the operation of simple feature filters has gained wide currency in the psychological literature.

B. Some Discrepancies

But consider that, in fact, there have been no actual identifications of physiological nets underlying any of these results in other than invertebrate preparations. The mode of argument of all the papers cited above is always based upon analogous forms of response. Nevertheless, all have strongly suggested that the observed results are largely due to very specific neural micromechanisms. From a general epistemological point of view, such assumptions are based upon the most treacherous grounds. The main idea behind analogue computers, for example, is based upon the fact that certain systems, which are organized in similar manners, may exhibit comparable behavior even though they are made of completely different components. The typical electrostatic office copier, for example, displays behavior that is very much like the Mach band observed in human vision. In the copier, however, this contour intensification is due to the lateral inhibitory interaction of powders and electric fields, rather than to neural interaction. Yet the conclusion drawn by the cited physiological psychologists is not one of process or analogue similarity, but specifically one of structural identity.

Earlier in this book, attention was called to the fact that there must necessarily be a distinction made between the neural signals that are identifiable with behavioral processes (true *codes*) and those that, while they may correlate with the stimulus, actually are only irrelevant concomitants (*signs*). Presently we are specifically concerned with the question of whether or not the effects of many of the fascinating and exciting single cell interactions we have already discussed are exhibited in psychophysical responses or whether the contemporary suggested correlations are spurious and misleading. In this discussion, attention has been concentrated on those papers that do not support the notion that single cell behavior is reflected in molar behavior to present the other side of the case. Once again, it must be emphasized, this is not meant to discredit the more general notion that some sort of neural activity underlies all behavior, but rather this approach represents a critique of the very special associations made between predominantly peripheral and relatively simple neural net interactions on the one hand, and some very special perceptual phenomena on the other. Our discussion is essentially a plea against premature oversimplification of what probably will turn out to be very complex physiological mechanisms of only superficially simple perceptual phenomena.

1. Missing Parts. A necessary axiom of the general thesis that the operations of simple feature-filtering networks are reflected in molar behavior is that the features to be detected must be present. This axiom might be said to be "syntactical," for it deals with the specific geometrical placement and structure of the parts of the pattern. From this point of view, the meaning or significance (semantic content) should not be an effective variable if a feature-filtering model is correct. However, some recent experiments, in which the critical stimulus material is actually missing, suggest that some kinds of form perception may be influenced more by general organization and context than by the presence or absence of specific features or the simple geometrical information content of the stimulus pattern.

Warren (1970) reports the results of a very interesting experiment, in which a masking sound (such as a cough or a tone) is used to completely replace a speech sound in a recorded sentence. Because of the sequential redundancy, as expected, listeners in this situation have no difficulty in reproducing the sentence, including the missing sound. However, surprisingly, they also report that they do hear the missing speech sound. The redundancy built into the recorded sentence is not only sufficient, therefore, to convey the meaning, but also to allow the listener to perceive the missing speech sound, even though it is not there. Interestingly enough, Warren also shows that if the missing speech sound is not replaced with an extraneous noise, but simply clipped out of the recording, it is easy to detect and locate the gap.

This auditory study is an analogue of a number of visual phenomena. Our inability to deal with lacunae, as lacunae, is a striking phenomenon, which has been too infrequently studied. The minimum thresholds for visual temporal gap detection (Uttal and Hieronymus, 1970), the inability to detect the "blind spot" of the eye, and other similar phenomena all speak to this point. Leeper's (1935) classic studies of the perception of fractured figures also clearly show that the perception of form is influenced by overall organizational factors other than specific features. The general significance of the remaining portions of partial figures becomes instantly clear when appropriate clues of meaning are given in a way that could hardly be conceived of as being due to the action of simple neural feature filters. Man's perceptual history is filled with many other instances in which missing parts are filled in or incongruous parts ignored by the perceiver. A whole vocabulary of such descriptive terms as "perceptual filling" had evolved to describe these perceptual phenomena in the tradition of Gestalt psychology.

The dot patterns used in some of the experiments mentioned earlier (Uttal, 1970, 1971a) also are forms with missing parts, for no continuous features are actually present—only arrangements of dots. Thus, the features are only suggested by the statistical relation of the dots, and any explanatory model of these phenomena based on feature analysis alone would have to involve higher level statistical or global evaluation of the cumulative response of individual local receptive areas.

One of the initial results of these studies (Uttal, 1969c) was that not all characters were identified with equal ease. At very high noise levels, at which most characters could not be detected with any greater success than chance levels, the four characters I, K, L, and X were still surprisingly recognizable. The character X was on this list because of a rather curious artifact. In the font used in that experiment, X, unlike all other characters of the special alphabet, had no long straight lines of dots (see Figure 8.14 for a complete set of the characters) and was, therefore, almost invisible even at moderate noise levels. The subjects learned quite early that when they saw nothing at all, they had probably been presented with an X and thus they reported that character. Quite artifactually, therefore, the "recognition score for X" was elevated. The characters I, K, and L, however, were recognized at supernormal levels for two different reasons. First, their confusion with other members of the alphabet stimulus set was lower than that of the other characters; second, they contained long straight dotted lines, which uniquely defined these three characters. Long lines of dots appeared to be more easily detected than the shorter fragments that provided the distinguishing criteria for many of the other characters. When other members of the character set containing long lines of dots received low recognition scores, it was usually due to the difficulty of detecting the shorter line segments that were critically necessary to define which of several confusable characters was actually presented.

The parameters of line detectability are thus of considerable interest in relation to the specific problem of geometric form recognition. In one study (Uttal, Bunnell, and Corwin, 1970), the parameters of line density, orientation, and dot numerosity were studied to determine what effect, if any, these parameters had on line detectability. Dynamic visual noise (DVN) as described earlier was used to degrade the dotted line stimulus, which otherwise would have been almost perfectly detectable at all brightness levels above the threshold for the individual dots.

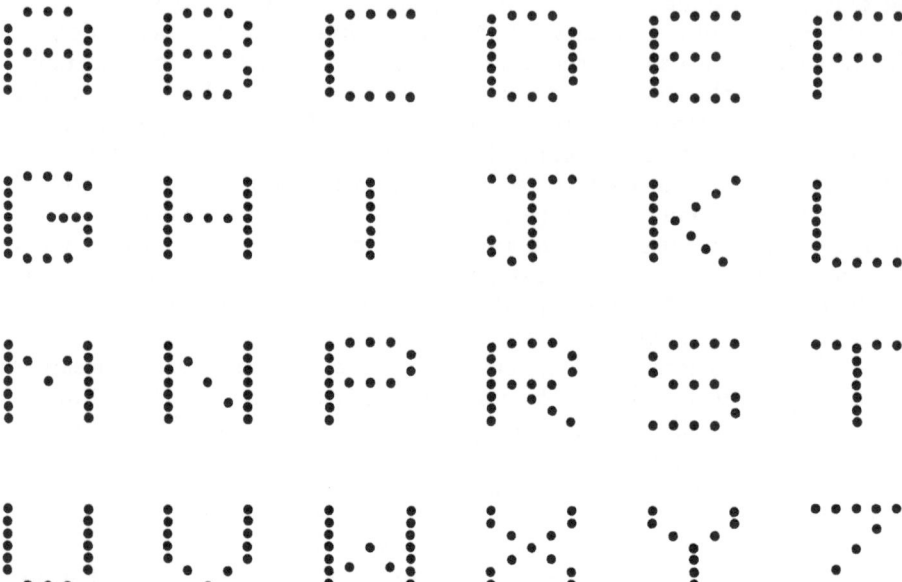

FIGURE ·8.14 A sample set of alphabetic characters that can be used as test stimuli in the dot masking experiment (from Uttal, 1969c).

The task of the S was to identify the orientation of a dotted line embedded at the center of a two-second-long burst of dotted visual noise of variable density. One of the main results of the experiment is shown in the curves plotted in Figure 8.15. The data have been separated into a family of four curves separated as a function of the spacing between the dots that make up the straight line. The variation in the recognizability of the various patterns is shown as an effect of various levels of masking DVN by plotting the percentage of the total number of dotted lines, which were correctly oriented against the noise level. It is clear from this rendition of the data that the spacing of the dots is a key factor in the detection and correct orientation of the straight lines. It was also shown that beyond four or five dots, dot numerosity had no effect on the recognition score.

The main impact of this experiment arises out of its requirement that the subject select, from a number of isolated point stimuli, a particular set that is aligned, in some statistical manner, along a common axis. The fact that the dots of the line are no more interconnected with one another than they are with the dots of the noise and are, actually, in some cases less so makes it hard to understand how a peripheral spatial filter or feature-extracting mechanism sensitive to this form or organization could operate at the noise densities used. On the contrary, we would have to hypothesize a very elaborate set of receptor signal analyzers, which would have to operate on statistical distributions in a way that comes very close to modern discussions of decision making and other cognitive interpretative functions, and is increasingly distant from the simple geometrical

FIGURE 8.15 Results of an experiment on the recognizability of dotted lines of various dot spacings. ■ = dot spacings of 17.5 min; ● = 35 min; ✕ = 52.5 min, and ▲ = 70 min. The horizontal axis indicates the interflash interval between dots in the DVN, while the vertical coordinate represents the percentage of the total number of lines presented that were correctly oriented by the S (from Uttal, Bunnell, and Corwin, 1970).

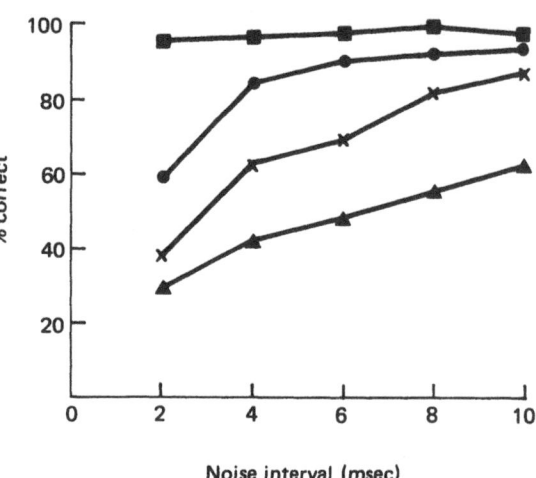

neural interactions that probably underlie such phenomena as Mach bands.

2. *Some Other Psychophysical Data.* The missing part experiments are only one subset of a much larger group of psychophysical experiments, which suggest that the obtained psychophysical results do not concur with microtheories based on the action of simple nerve nets.

Mayzner's support of the relevance of Hubel and Wiesel's data to sequential blanking has been noted above. However, it is not at all clear that his results have been interpreted appropriately. While Mayzner's notions are extremely stimulating, it is all too easy to see how they are contradicted by his own data. In a recent elaboration of his views (Mayzner and Tresselt, 1970), he points out that the meaning of the stimulus materials is very effective in defining the sequential masking effects he has observed in so many different forms. To quote his interpretation:

> The implication of these results seems clear. If the first five letters displayed form a word, the inhibitory field effects of the last five letters displayed prove almost totally ineffective in producing sequential blanking effects, while if the first five letters do not form a word, whether the second five letters form a word or not, inhibitory effects are very strong and sequential blanking occurs most readily. Thus, it would appear that not only can input content or geometry greatly modulate sequential blanking effects, but word meaning can also produce equally powerful modulating or attenuating effects on sequential blanking.

(MAYZNER and TRESSELT, 1970, p. 611.)

He then goes on to discuss how this means that the higher cortical centers must be deeply implicated in the sequential blanking effects. In this regard he is correct, for experiments in the present author's laboratory have shown that a sequential masking effect first observed by Schoenberg, Katz, and Mayzner (1970) with five simple dots is obtained very strongly if the three masking dots are viewed by the right eye and the two masked dots are viewed by the left eye. Since there is no possible neural interaction prior to the lateral geniculate body in this case, it is at this level or at the level of the cortex that the effects must be mediated.

Mayzner and Tresselt explain this sort of sequential blanking effect in terms of lateral inhibitory interaction between cortical columns of the sort described by Hubel and Wiesel. It seems that Mayzner's suggestion requires that columns be available which are selectively sensitive, not only, as observed, to line movement directionality, but also to meaning or polygonal geometry, in a way that had not been observed in the neurophysiological laboratory. These hypothetical columns go so far beyond the observed data that it seems more reasonable to talk about inhibitory interaction of quite a different kind. While there may be mutual inhibition, it is a sort of semantic inhibition based upon the activities of nervous mechanisms that are very, very complex and might indeed have little structural similarity to the highly delimited sensitivity of a column of cortical cells. The inhibitory interactions may be analogous in some limited sense, but are certainly not homologous.

An important related fact is that even in some of the quasi-geometrical masking paradigms such as metacontrast, it seems unlikely that lateral inhibitory interaction works in the simple way hypothesized by some theorists. For example, form similarity appears to be necessary for simple metacontrast. It is sometimes forgotten that when this particular kind of backward masking was discovered, it was extremely difficult to find stimuli that exhibited the classical metacontrast described by Alpern (1953) or Kolers (1962). The many studies done with disks and concentric rings or with the three adjacent rectangles in the last few years obscure the fact that the effect is not ubiquitous. In fact, metacontrast is a somewhat rare phenomenon, which occurs only in a few highly specific situations, all of which necessitate form similarity. Figure 8.16 is a set of masking figures, which have been used in the author's laboratory (Uttal, 1970) to test for metacontrast effects. Only the combinations labeled (a), (k), and (m) produced substantial masking of the central figure. Thus, prior form recognition seems to be very important in this type of masking situation, again suggesting that very-high-level cognitive functions may be more important than simple geometrical propinquity in the understanding of these effects.

In that same paper (Uttal, 1970), specific attention was given to whether or not three specific characteristics of peripheral lateral inhibition, which are usually reported, were obtained in backward masking with dot patterns. Though this stimulus material is quite special, it is of some interest to note that none of the three conditions led to the usual results. Stimuli interacted only when they were overlapping in the same visual space; disinhibition was not obtained when a second masking pattern followed the first; and dichoptic masking was nearly as strong as under monoptic and binocular conditions. Other higher cognitive mechanisms, such as limitations on the information-processing capacity of the nervous system (pattern confusion), were thus implicated, but hardly the simple sort of lateral inhibitory interaction found in the eye of *Limulus polyphemus*.

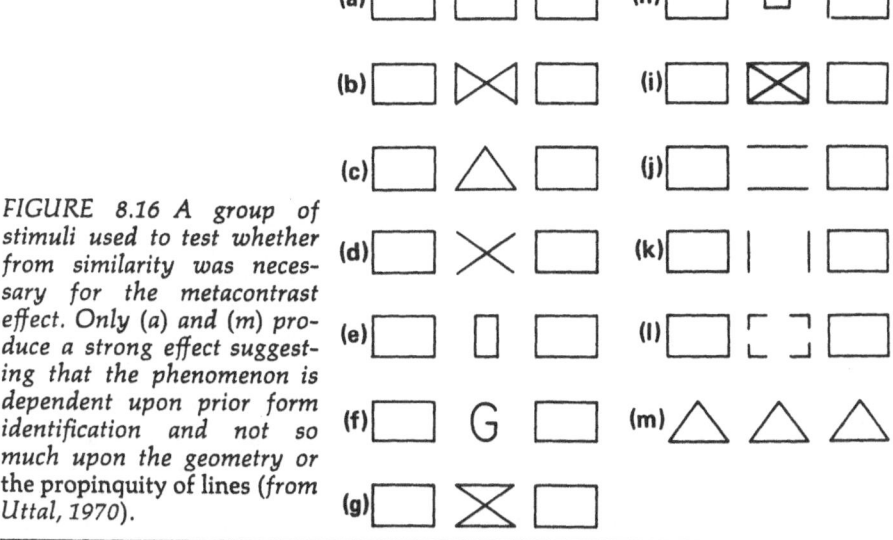

FIGURE 8.16 A group of stimuli used to test whether from similarity was necessary for the metacontrast effect. Only (a) and (m) produce a strong effect suggesting that the phenomenon is dependent upon prior form identification and not so much upon the geometry or the propinquity of lines (from Uttal, 1970).

Kahneman (1967) has called attention to the fact that the metacontrast type of masking and apparent movement are very closely related. Implicit in his suggestion is also the notion that many of these masking effects are mediated at the highest levels of the nervous sytem through mechanisms of the utmost complexity, rather than through relatively simple peripheral interaction. Metacontrast, he suggests, may be more a difficulty in the interpretation of "impossible" apparent motion than a lateral interaction process.

Furthermore, Julesz and Hesse (1970) have performed an interesting experiment, in which areas of rotating short line segments (best described by their term "needles") were plotted by a computer for a motion picture display. They discovered that differences in speed of rotation of the needles in a circular central test patch and a surrounding annular region of similar line segments would lead to the perception of the test patch as a distinct subunit. However, if the test region differed from the surround only in the direction of rotation of the line segments, subjects were not able to perceive it as a separate entity. Julesz and Hesse had designed their experiment specifically to test whether or not the directional sensitivity of single cells observed in the Hubel and Wiesel, and Barlow and Hill work could exhibit a molar psychological effect. Their final paragraph is most interestingly stated:

> The finding that clusters of locally rotating line segments which are seemingly well matched to the neurophysiological feature extractors do not yield a global psychological percept may be of some interest. It outlines for the neurophysiologist some of the limitations of the human visual system.

> (JULESZ and HESSE, 1970, p. 244.)

Their work is of the utmost importance to the argument being presented here. Julesz and Hesse argue that their results indicate the absence of "integrating mechanisms that can extract the directionality of a set of similarly moving edges." It might be further suggested that these studies outline not so much limitations of the human visual system as of that brand of physiological theorizing that originally linked such simple physiological mechanisms to such complex perceptions. Their findings suggest that the microscopic characteristics of single cells may not, contrary to the suggestions of the workers to which we referred earlier, be simply or directly reflected in certain kinds of molar perceptual behavior.

From another perspective, we might consider observations on perceptual illusions. Weintraub and Krantz (1971), for example, have conducted some experiments on the directionality of the Poggendorf illusion. When the two parallel lines are either horizontal or vertical, the illusion is maximal, but tilting the entire display away from these axes leads to a precipitous drop in the strength of the illusion. Although some acuity measures have been shown to be axis-sensitive to a slight degree (Taylor, 1963), it is hard to conceive of some simple cellular axial sensitivity of the visual system that could lead to the very gross effects that Weintraub and Krantz observed. These effects must be a function of much more complicated cognitive mechanisms. Similarly, the Zolner and Hering illusions are examples of phenomena in which the overall pattern dominates the geometry and leads to the perceptual distortion of straight lines into curved lines. While one could postulate relatively simple neural net mechanisms exhibiting analogous behavior to explain these illusions, it seems far more likely that very complicated central neural mechanisms mediate such field effects.

Another relevant psychophysical datum, which seems to have been often overlooked, was obtained by Nachmias (1967). He showed that visual contrast sensitivity effects, thought to be typical of lateral inhibitory interaction, generally do not occur when very brief exposures are used. This finding is a behavioral analogue and confirmation of neurophysiological data obtained earlier by Barlow, Fitzhugh, and Kuffler (1957). In the brief tachistoscopic light of the experimental design of most of the masking experiments, it becomes increasingly difficult to understand how lateral inhibitory interaction can serve as a model for some of these spatiotemporal perceptual phenomena.

Another discordant note is struck by the classic simultaneous contrast experiment with either monochrome or colored stimuli. These phenomena have been frequently cited as effects of lateral neural interactions. For example, Ratliff (1965) has linked the classic simultaneous contrast stimulus (as shown in Figure 8.17) with Mach bands and has suggested that ". . . all must share some underlying physiological mechanisms in common." But it should also be noted that there are very substantial differences between the contour effects and the broad field effect. The Mach band is clearly affected by the details of the geometry of the stimulus situation. The brightness at any point is specifically a function of the distance the various components are from one another. On the other hand, the simultaneous contrast phenomenon, like the metacontrast one de-

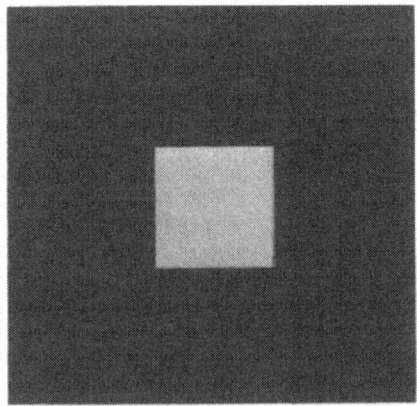

FIGURE 8.17 The classic simultaneous contrast stimulus. The lower grey square
should appear darker (be-
cause of the lighter background) than the upper grey
square.

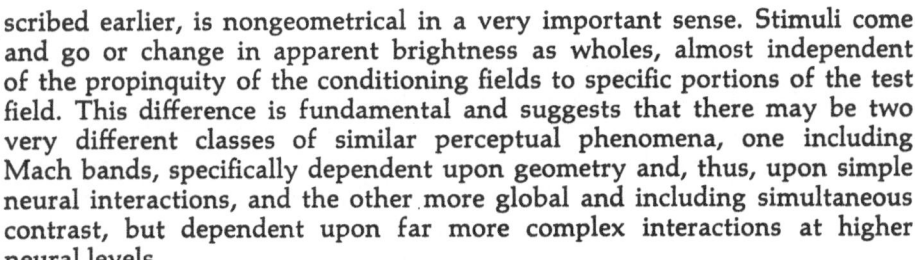

scribed earlier, is nongeometrical in a very important sense. Stimuli come
and go or change in apparent brightness as wholes, almost independent
of the propinquity of the conditioning fields to specific portions of the test
field. This difference is fundamental and suggests that there may be two
very different classes of similar perceptual phenomena, one including
Mach bands, specifically dependent upon geometry and, thus, upon simple
neural interactions, and the other more global and including simultaneous
contrast, but dependent upon far more complex interactions at higher
neural levels.

Koppitz (1957), for example, has shown that Mach bands cannot be
produced by dichoptic mixing of two stimulus patterns which, if presented
jointly to either or both eyes, would produce the Mach band effect. Fig.
8.18 shows his experimental paradigm. A ramp or gradient of visual intensity is presented to one eye and a level plateau of visual intensity to
another. When the two are brought together in the dichoptic field so that
their edges touch, the conditions for the appearance of a bright Mach band

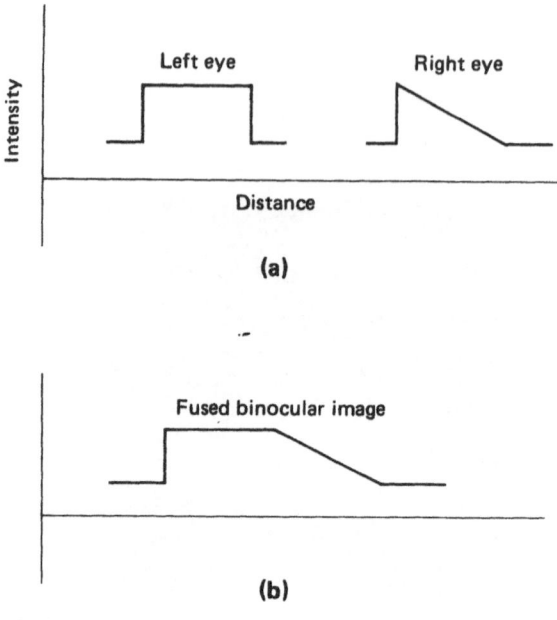

FIGURE 8.18 The design of if Mach bands could be produced binocularly. When the Koppitz' stimuli to determine two upper monocular stimuli are combined in binocular fusion to produce the usual gradient, there is no observable enhancement indicating that the Mach band effect is mediated by neuronal interactions in the peripheral retina (courtesy of Dr. Werner Koppitz, Mt. Kisco, New York).

would be satisfied. However, no Mach band appears. The visual system apparently is not able to carry out the same interactions centrally that are performed in the retina to produce the Mach band.

A closely related contour effect is the famous Hermann grid experiment reproduced earlier in Figure 7.22. If a similar attempt is made to reproduce this phenomenon by dichoptic presentation of the two parts of the stereoscopic slide shown in Figure 8.19, there is no evidence of the grey spots at the intersection of the white lines, which were so evident at all locations (except at the fixation point) in the monocular presentation. This latter stereoscopic slide, incidentally, is quite hard to keep stably fused, and a considerable amount of rivalry occurs. After some practice, however, there are periods of stable fusion, and it is within these time periods that the absence of the grey spots is noted.

On the other hand, Figure 8.20 is a drawing of a picture pair which, when presented in a stereoscope, produces a simultaneous contrast effect even though the stimuli presented to each eye do not and cannot produce any such effect individually. When the two figures are jointly presented, the upper square formed from the mixing of the grey square from the left-hand picture and the black square from the right-hand picture is apparently darker than its counterpart below. This difference is attributed to the difference in the mixed brightnesses of the background fields. A similar demonstration has been made by Levelt (1965), who feels that the effect is due to the difference in contours presented to each of the eyes. Nevertheless, he, too, agrees that the effect is central—the main point being made by this demonstration. Julesz (1971) has also shown similar effects with random dot stereograms.

In sum, there appear to be many differences between the simultane-

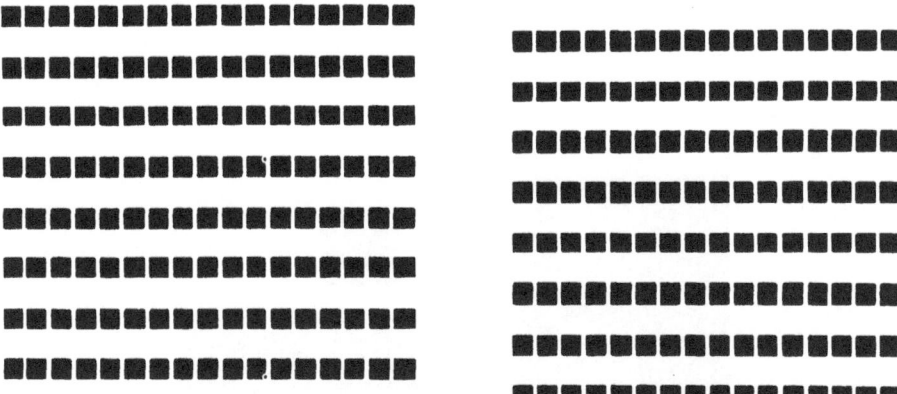

FIGURE 8.19 A stereoscopic slide prepared to determine if the Hermann grid effect can be produced dichoptically. Although this slide is difficult to fuse because of a strong retinal rivalry effect, during the stable periods there is no evidence of the grey spots. The suggestion, therefore, is that the Hermann grid, like the Mach band, is mediated by neuronal interactions in the periphery.

ous contrast and contour enhancement phenomena, which suggest that they are mediated by mechanisms at vastly different levels of the nervous system. Contour enhancement does appear to be peripheral and dependent upon local geometry, while the simultaneous contrast mechanism appears to be central and global rather than local.

As we have noted, metacontrast and apparent motion also can be obtained under dichoptic presentation conditions. Therefore, since we know that binocular representation does not occur below the level of the thalamus, these phenomena must be mediated by mechanisms well up in the central nervous system. All of this seems to support the notion of two classes of phenomena: one, geometrical and peripheral and the other, non-geometrical and central. It should also be noted that analogies based on the Hartline data often tend to confuse the spatial notions of lateral interaction, that is, simultaneous presentation for prolonged periods of spatially disparate stimuli with sequential presentation of overlapping visual form without regard to some of the major differences between these two experimental paradigms.

Another difference between the Mach band and simultaneous contrast phenomena relates to the additivity of two or more inducing fields or of increases in the area of a single contrast field. Hartline and Ratliff (1958) had shown that in Limulus, the inhibitory effects of the two stimuli are linearly additive, although one must take into account the reciprocal interaction between them to arrive at a correct numerical value. Hartline's group has also shown (Hartline, Wagner, and Ratliff, 1956) that as the area of the inhibiting field increases, the inhibitory effect also increases. In fact, all of the lateral inhibitory interaction models that Ratliff (1965) discusses exhibit this sort of additivity. By contrast, Cole and Diamond (1971) have shown that the proportion of the total area of the surrounding

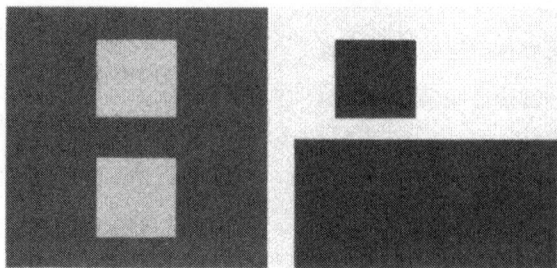

FIGURE 8.20 A stereoscopic slide prepared to determine if the simultaneous contrast illusion can be produced dichoptically. This slide does give rise to a simultaneous contrast effect in spite of the fact that neither monocular view could possibly produce any brightness difference. See text for complete discussion.

contrast field used in a simultaneous contrast situation does not affect the magnitude of the contrast. Diamond's (1960) theory of brightness enhancement, it should also be noted, was only able to describe adjacent rectangle interaction and not the contrast effect of a surrounding circular inducing field on a circle. This difference in mathematical description also suggests that different neural processes may underlie each of these phenomena.

Simultaneous contrast, though, displays another important effect, which suggests that simple geometry is not the basis of the phenomenon. Gogel and Mershon (1969) and Mershon and Gogel (1970) have shown that the contrasting effect of a surround on a target is diminished if the two appear not to lie in the same stereoscopic plane, even though the lateral relations hold. Their interpretation is that this finding argues against any theory that places the contrast effect in the periphery. Simultaneous contrast, thus, according to their view, as well as the other arguments already cited, must occur at a level at or above that mediating stereoscopic depth perception.

We may also refer to a recent paper by Weisstein (1970) herself for additional evidence that simplistic physiological models do not apply to some of the very complex perceptual experiences. In this most intriguing paper, she has shown that the masking effects of a grating on a subsequently displayed test pattern occur even if the region of the grating, in which the test patch is shown, is obscured by a cubelike drawing as shown in Figure 8.21. Weisstein claims that this result means that there probably is a neural mechanism, which encodes the information "in back of" in this stimulus situation. It is almost certainly true that she is correct in this

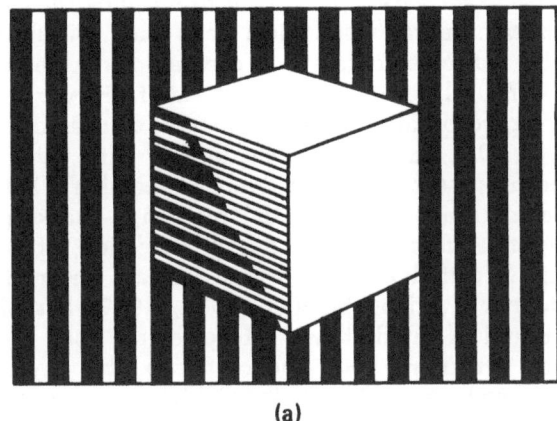

(a)

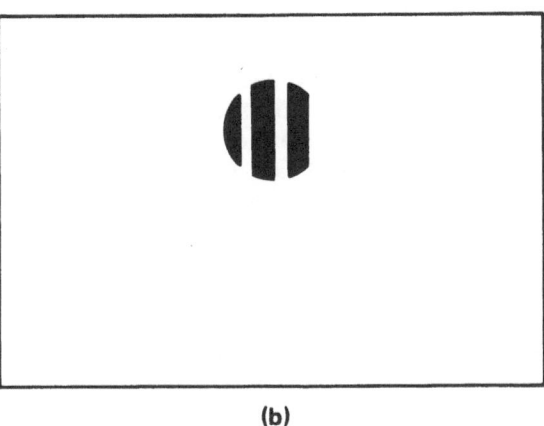

FIGURE 8.21 An adaptation field (a) and a test stimulus (b) which can be used to show that the grating adaptation effects do not require that the grating specifically stimulate the tested region. The perception of the grating is still interfered with to some degree even if it is placed in the region obscured by the cube (from Weisstein, 1970).

(b)

assumption, but it is probably also true that this hypothetical mechanism is also far more complex than the simplistic notions of neuron interaction or columnar structure that Weisstein, among others, has invoked to explain some of the masking effects found in this and related masking paradigms. She is careful to note that these observations are related to higher level "symbolic" mechanisms in coding the concept "in back of" but, in doing so, fails to note that many of the simpler correlations observed between other perceptual phenomena and neural mechanisms also might be mediated by such symbolic mechanisms. Rather than adaptation of directionally sensitive receptors, the symbolic value of "similarity" may be the key issue. Just as she has had to extend the existing theoretical structure to include highly complex "in back of" coding mechanisms, other results superficially analogous to known physiological mechanisms may also require "symbolic mechanisms" that go far beyond the observed neural data.

3. A Few Discrepant Neurophysiological Data. Attempts to correlate specific neurophysiological data with specific perceptual phenomena have also led to some data that contradict the notion that the operation of simple neural net mechanisms is satisfactory explanatory models for some of the perceptual phenomena we have discussed.

One line of research dealing with visual sequential interference has been pursued very effectively by Schiller. Distinguishing among three different kinds of sequential masking—masking in which a bright diffuse light reduces the likelihood of detection, of a dimmer smaller light masking of complex patterns that overlap, and metacontrast, where the stimuli do not overlap—Schiller (1968, 1969) has shown that it is only when stimuli of the first two categories are used that the single cells of the lateral geniculate body and cortex exhibit any analogous interactive effects. The metacontrast situation, which has so often been subject to this quasiphysiological kind of theorizing, shows no lateral geniculate cellular response analogues that might be correlated. Schiller goes on to say, ". . . metacontrast is a complex phenomenon, which may depend on levels in the visual system above the LGN [lateral geniculate nucleus]." (Schiller, 1968, p. 865.)

In related work, Fehmi, Adkins, and Lindsley (1969) find very peripheral suppression of the neural response, but only when the stimuli overlap in the same manner as in the Schiller experiments.

DeValois and Pease (1971) have shown, furthermore, that single cell responses from lateral geniculate neurons definitely separate simultaneous contrast and the border effects leading to such phenomenon as the Mach band into two separate and distinct processes just as suggested by the psychophysical data. Comparable lateral interactions among these cells were observed when stimuli, which led to psychophysical contour enhancement, were used. However, there was no evidence of any suppression of the neural response when the stimulus was similar to that producing the simultaneaous contrast effect described earlier. DeValois and Pease conclude that these latter data are compelling arguments for much more complicated and more central cortical mechanisms for simultaneous contrast. The implication is that the geometry of the situation is not critical, and therefore mechanisms such as lateral inhibitory interaction and center-surround organization probably play a small, if any, role in such phenomena.

C. Conclusions

It is important to clearly express a significant caveat at this point. The following concluding comment is not intended to suggest that the entire monistic philosophy underlying modern psychobiology should be rejected or that the neurophysiological data are, in any way, less than fully valid within their own realm. Rather, it is intended to stress the idea that neurophysiological reductionism for the particular aspects of visual perception discussed in this section may have been somewhat premature. The general question of whether or not aspects of single cell activity can be detected at the molar psychological level is critically important. But this section attempts to raise the more specific question of whether or not these very particular perceptual phenomena can be meaningfully ascribed to lateral inhibitory interaction, feature filtering, or cortical columns in the light of some of this recent psychological and physiological evidence.

Someday, future psychobiologists may consider this current trend in "explanations" exactly as we now look upon the computer models, the telephonic models, or the even more ancient hydraulic and pneumatic models of brain function, as simply the subsequent stage in a series of reductionistic fads. It is entirely possible that they will also make some judgments about reductionism itself, which may not differ too drastically from those judgments made by physicists in the field of gas dynamics. Few physicists would consider a microscopic analysis of the dynamics of individual gas atoms as a possible and practical means of predicting the overall behavior of a container of gas. Instead, they use the external metrics of pressure, volume, and temperature—statistical estimates of the central tendencies of the individual particles.

Psychologists may, in the not-too-distant future, also come to the same sort of conclusion—that complex mental activities, though admittedly based on the pooled statistical properties of ensembles of individual cells, still cannot, in any practical sense, all be explained in terms of the individual behavior of these microscopic structural units.

This may be more obvious in some aspects of psychology than in others. The communication of information patterns through the ascending pathways does seem amenable to some types of single cell analysis. The explanation of complex perceptual phenomona, however, may lie at a level of complexity with which no current neurophysiology can deal. It may also be true that we shall have a difficult time distinguishing between processes which, superficially, seem closely related by experimental designs, but which may have quite different underlying mechanisms.

For example, it is probably true that retinal lateral inhibitory interaction does, in fact, operate in some ways that can be detected behaviorally, as in the perception of Mach bands on the Hermann grid. Nevertheless, other mutual inhibitory mechanisms, which are superficially quite similar, may be based on far more complex mechanisms. It is for this reason that the taxonomies that Schiller (1969) and, similarly, Fitzgerald (1970) developed to distinguish the several different kinds of masking are so important in helping us understand these phenomena.

It is also important to note differences in the meaning of the terms *feature extraction* and *coding* at the cellular level and at the operational or psychological level. Feature-extraction theories of visual perception may deal with greatly mediated representations of visual forms. Words, for example, are wonderful mediators for the coding and subsequent recognition of visual forms. The word *square*, for example, is a nongeometrical code for a certain geometric form, as in *a,a,a,a,* or even 四角 . Once appropriately coded, the features (for example, corner, side corner, and so on) that make up any particular geometric form can be stored and retrieved, or allowed to interact with one another in ways that are not directly related to the spatial location of the parts or overall geometry of the stimulus. Mutually antagonistic processes could be present, although not based on the classical geometrical lateral inhibitory interaction. Thus, recognition schema operating on coded features are entirely possible and might even exhibit processes and dimensions analogous to many neuro-geometric effects, although the schema may be mediated by entirely different neural mechanisms of, for all practical purposes, infinite complexity. Psychobiology may yet have to face the probability-determinism schism that physics faced a few decades ago and, like physics, finally come to the conclusion that there can be little fruitful outcome from dealing deterministically with the microscopic elements of a complex ensemble.

VII. AN INTERIM SUMMARY

We have now completed our discussion of the psychophysical and neuro-physiological topics, which revolve around the many issues of spatial and temporal coding in the various sensory modalities. One of the most important summary points, which should be self-evident at this point, is that it is very difficult to unravel the spatial and temporal dimensions from each other. Space and time seem to be, in many instances, interconvertible one into the other, or linked in such a way that a temporal or spatial snapshot alone loses the most critical parameters of the sensory code. Sensory-coding theory may, therefore, be required to postulate some sort of a relativism axiom concerning the temporalization of spatial dimensions in much the same way as has happened in physics.

In the last two chapters, we have considered a number of special problems, such as the neurological basis of depth perception in vision and spatial localization in audition, which emphasize the fact that isomorphy is not necessary in a neural coding schema. It seems in the nervous system as if time often represents spatial dimensions. For example, auditory space is coded in large part along a temporal continuum. Auditory pitch, a correlate of the temporal frequency of the stimulus, seems to be transformed, on the other hand, into spatial relationships by nonneural preprocessing. It is these sorts of findings that have made it impossible to separate the material in this chapter into two separate categories.

Another general outcome, which must be noted here, is that spatial and temporal discriminative abilities as expressed in psychophysical experiments usually are quite imprecise in relation to the fineness of the stimulus world. The general neural properties, which appear to account for this loss of discriminative ability, are the divergent and convergent network processes of the nervous system. Convergence of many sensory receptor inputs into a few transmission neurons leads to a loss of spatial acuity—a general property which is reflected in the ubiquitous presence of "receptive fields" for almost all neurons more central than the receptor itself. Divergent mechanisms, on the other hand, account for the elongation of brief real-time micromoments into psychophysical macromoments. A 1-msec nerve response in the periphery may give rise to central neural activity that lasts for seconds. With this elongation comes a loss in the ability to discriminate between both the order and simultaneity of successive stimuli. Thus is introduced the notion of the psychological moment, the temporal analogue of the spatial receptive field.

Clearly, one of the most important sets of notions that have emerged from the last two decades of neurophysiological research is that the overall spatio-temporal pattern of the stimulus is important, probably far more important than the simpler dimensions of occurrence of an impulse stimulus in defining the neural response. Lateral interactions between adjacent receptors and the time sequence of these interactions allow a number of highly specific feature detection properties to emerge in neural response patterns. Contour sensitive mechanisms, critical time-space patterns capable of elicting activity where generalized stimulation is not, and special sensitivity to moving objects of specific shapes all emerge as fundamental mechanisms of the nervous system. The elucidation of the physiological mechanisms and of related psychophysical phenomena has been one of the most important emerging traditions of this period.

However, there are a number of caveats that must also be observed. It is not yet certain that some of the more superficial process analogies between behavior and neurology are truly structurally related. Some processes, only superficially similar, have been misassumed by some workers to be identical. In this chapter, we considered whether this is a valid approach.

We turn now to another area—those problems that concern the representation of the quality of a stimulus and consider both the basic psychophysical evidence, which has to be explained, and the neurophysiological findings, which are relevant to the specification of a coding schema for quality.

CHAPTER 9: THE NEURAL CODING OF SENSORY QUALITY—VISION

I. INTRODUCTION

We now turn to the other great experiential domain—sensory quality. As in the previous chapters, we would like to begin our discussion with some attempt to define what is meant by sensory quality. Disappointingly, we are in no better shape than when we attempted to define quantity or to unravel the often intermingled temporal and spatial dimensions of sensory experiences. Sensory qualities also seem to be elusive entities which, although everyone seems to have reached common agreement concerning their nature, evade a precise and rigorous definition. We are tempted to add to the circularity of the definitions we have already given and say that if one holds the sensory magnitude constant and fixes the perceptual temporal and spatial pattern, any further differences that can be discriminated by subjects are by exclusion qualitative in nature. But this sort of definition, of course, adds little to our understanding beyond the generally accepted popular definitions.

It is equally unsatisfying to attempt a definition in terms of the nature of the physical stimulus, but it is probably necessary. Each of the sense organs has evolved to display a maximum sensitivity to a particular kind of physical energy. Perhaps the best we can do is to define qualities for each of the senses individually in terms of the stimulus. For example, visual quality is defined as the range of experiences that are produced by stimulating the eye with photic energy varying over the wavelength range of 400 to 780 nm. To the degree that different stimuli can be distinguished from one another on the basis of wavelength alone, each visual stimulus wavelength or indiscriminably narrow band of wavelengths is associated with a particular visual quality. Equivalent definitions can be made for some of the other senses, although such definitions break down when there is no single dimension of stimulus variation. The cutaneous and chemical senses respond to multidimensional stimuli, and the experiences produced in each case are not so simply classified.

Another major distinction, which must be kept in mind during our discussion of the neural coding of quality, is that there are probably two separate ways in which the term quality is used. In some gross manner, we must distinguish among the macroqualities of sensory experience—the great sensory modalities—vision, touch, smell, taste, and hearing. On the other hand, within each one of these modalities, we also have to deal with microqualitative differences among experiences—a domain in which we would use such terms as distinguishable hues or pitches.

The distinction between macro- and micromodalities, of course, becomes less clear when we talk about mixed experiences such as that collectively referred to as cutaneous sensation. In this context, it is not always clear whether there are many macromodalities or a set of micromodalities. The different cutaneous experiences, such as heat, touch, pressure, tickle, and itch, do not seem to be neatly analyzable or synthesizable one from the other. Similarly, the classic but probably incorrect qualitative descriptions of the olfactory and gustatory modalities usually involve the classification of these senses into "fundamentals" such as sweeet, sour, bitter, and salty or a set of fundamental odors, but not all would agree that these "fundamentals" play the same role as the primary colors of vision. In olfaction and gustation, each of the "basic" smells and tastes appears, from some points of view, to be more comparable to color vision *in toto* than to individual hues. One olfactory or gustatory quality does not continuously grade into another as do the colors or pitches. It seems, in general then, that our definition of quality is not only less than precise with regard to macromodalities, but also with regard to what actually constitutes a micromodality in somatosensation, gustation, and olfaction.

It is probably also true that there is a closer relationship between the language we use to describe sensory quality and our analyses of what constitutes a fundamental or primary experience than some solely physiological or psychophysical sensory scientists would be willing to admit. It is still moot whether the language reflects the biology, or the theoretical models of sensory quality merely reflect the language. Amoore's analysis of basic smells, for example, is based upon commonly accepted linguistic usage —the words people use to describe smells—and although, hopefully, there is in this language some reflection of the basic biology and chemistry of olfactory receptors, it is difficult to say with certainty that the number "seven" has any special significance. Furthermore, there are two issues involved, even in this statement that should be separated and that have interacting physiological, psychophysical, and semantic overtones. First, are the seven basics that Amoore identifies really fundamentals? Second, even if they are, are they the only ones or are there more? The familiar anecdote about the many names for the different kinds of snow that exist in the Eskimo language is relevant here. As we shall see, the number of "primary" smells one accepts may be more a matter of the precision of the decision criteria applied by the experimenter than the biology of the subject.

The point being made is that the search for primaries in the somatosensory, gustatory, and olfactory senses may be quite artificial and stimulated only by the success of the notion of primaries in color vision. In fact, however, there may be very little to support the notion of primaries in the sense that a small number of basic smells, touches, or tastes can be used to synthesize all other possible experiences. Certainly such an idea is not a part of auditory theorizing, where analysis rather than synthesis is more often the framework of discussion.

The interaction between the biology and the descriptive models of sensory quality coding has been a basic issue for many centuries. In the material of the next three chapters, we shall try to present and discuss those alternative theories of sensory quality coding that have a specific neurophysiological or anatomical point to make. In doing so, we shall pass over without mention those theories of sensory quality coding that are merely descriptive. Since most of the theories of sensory coding, even those with a specific physiological or anatomical premise, were inspired by certain aspects of the psychophysical data, we shall attempt to make explicit both what the specific psychophysical data are and what its neural implications are.

In the last 20 or 30 years, a very important revolution has occurred in sensory quality theories. Electrophysiological and anatomical techniques have been used to provide explicit and direct criteria for the selection of which of several previously suggested and equally plausible alternative theories is, in fact, the most useful one. The indirect speculations and deductions from behavioral data in the past have thus been augmented by these new approaches in a way that has lifted a veil of confusion or speculation from many important problems. The direct observation of the spectral absorption of human cone pigments, for example, has made it possible for us now to be absolutely explicit about which of an infinitely large set of potential trichromatic fundamentals, each perfectly plausible from some mathematical or psychophysical point of view, actually is valid. All theories must now conform with regard to the absorption spectra of the photochemicals from now on.

Another important generalization, which has become increasingly evident, is that the classical models were not, in fact, mutually inconsistent. We now know, for example, that alternative theories of color vision both seem to be correct, but each at a different level of the afferent visual pathway. Similarly, alternative theories of pitch encoding seem to hold in audition, but at different regions of the acoustic spectrum.

The fact that alternative theories are correct in alternative domains once again reminds us of the basic tenet of neural coding theory—namely, that information may be represented by entirely different coding mechanisms in different situations, yet all such representations are equivalent with regard to the message content.

The prime axiom of quality coding has traditionally been Müller's law of specific nerve energies. This statement referred to the fact that regardless of what stimulus was applied to a sensory nerve, the sensation so induced was of a quality specific to that nerve. Müller's law does seem to be correct when we discuss coding at the level of macroquality. There appears to be no way to stimulate the cochlear mechanism so that a visual impression is produced, or the retina so that an auditory experience obtains. Electricity, the universal stimulus, always seems to produce sensations specific to the particular nerve being stimulated. However, no matter how comprehensive Müller's law is in terms of the macromodalities, it seems as if it is completely inadequate in explaining the coding mechanisms, which account for our ability to distinguish between micromodalities within one of the great senses. In the rest of this chapter, we shall see that all sensory neurons at all levels of the ascending nervous systems are, to a greater or lesser degree, broadly tuned. That is, all sensory neurons respond not to a single narrowly defined stimulus, but rather to a range of stimuli, each of which is able to invoke widely differing microqualities. Obviously, in this case the neurons are not specific in the sense Müller meant. Activity in a given visual neuron, for example, can be interpreted as red, green, or blue by the central nervous system, depending upon the relations between its activity, and those of other associated neurons. In the subsequent sections of this chapter, one of the main generalities we shall be able to draw will be of this sort of broad tuning at all levels of the nervous system and in all of the sensory modalities.

The general plan of our discussion in the next three chapters will be to deal with each sensory modality individually. We shall first consider the principal psychophysical data for each modality that must be explained by a reductive theory. We shall then discuss the classic theories of quality coding themselves and then the modern neurophysiological contributions that bear specifically on the problem of that modality's quality representation. Finally, we shall present what is, in our view, the most up-to-date contemporary theory of quality coding for each of the senses. In Chapter 13, we shall sum up what appear to be the generalities common to all of the quality coding premises.

II. THE KEY PSYCHOPHYSICAL DATA

A. The Duplex Retina and Its Psychophysical Correlates

A large number of different pieces of anatomical, biochemical, and behavioral data present convincing evidence that the retina contains two different kinds of receptor cells. This finding is referred to as the theory of the duplex retina. From the earliest recorded times, we have evidence that men were aware that their daytime vision was different in some critical ways from their nightime vision. Thus, the earliest evidence for the duplex retina theory was behavioral. Early microscopic investigations showed an anatomic basis for this behavioral differentiation. There were two distinct forms of retinal receptors present, which could be seen to be either cylindrical or conical in form. This observation confirmed earlier speculations that there might, in fact, be two distinct photoreceptor systems simultaneously resident in the human eye. One, now known to be mediated by the rods, is monochromatic and able to operate at lower light intensities, while the other, mediated by three kinds of foveal cones, operates best at higher levels of illumination.

In Chapter 4, when we discussed visual transduction, we also noted that the most widely accepted theory of photoreception asserted that four different kinds of retinal photopigments were to be found in certain kinds of vertebrate eyes. Direct observations of the effects of these photopigments have been made in two closely related teleosts (the carp and the goldfish) as well as in primates. The outer segments of the rods of the fishes were loaded with a substance, which Wald has referred to as porphyropsin, a derivative of retinal$_2$, while the rods of the primate contain a substance known as rhodopsin derived from retinal$_1$. In each animal, each of three types of cone apparently contains one of three other pigments, the absorption spectra of which are assumed to underlie trichromatic vision.

There are many different psychophysical indications that support the notion of a duplex retina. For example, during the adaptation process in the dark following exposure to a brief light, the threshold sensitivity undergoes a gradual change so that dimmer and dimmer lights can be seen as time passes. Repeated measurements over the years have shown that under certain conditions, the increase in sensitivity during this dark adaptation process is a two-limbed curve with a noticeable break occurring after about 7 min in the dark. These conditions include:

1. that a sufficiently bright adapating light is used;
2. that the area of the retina illuminated includes both rods and cones;
3. that a broad spectral band is used to light-adapt the eye prior to the dark adaptation; and
4. that a normal observer is used without any form of color blindness that might obscure the break.

Figure 9.1 shows a typical decrease in threshold intensity (known as dark adaptation) as a function of time in the dark under these conditions. The first part of the curve is assumed to be due to a rather rapid increase in the low sensitivity cone system, while the second part of the graph is attributable to the increasing sensitivity of the slower adapting but far more sensitive rod system. The break in the dark adaptation curve is assumed to be caused by the crossover of the dark adaptation curves of the rods and the cones, respectively. Such assumptions are based, in part, on data obtained from subjects who suffer from a congenital absence of all three kinds of cones (rod monochromats) and who thus exhibit only the slow segment attributed to rod dark adaptation or from peripheral regions of normal retinae. Foveal dark adaptation curves, on the other hand, are almost pure cone responses and display only the more rapid but less sensitive portion. Similarly, if red light is used prior to dark adaptation, the dark adaptation curve is almost solely the product of the more rapid cone response. Both of these latter observations also support the idea of the duplex retina.

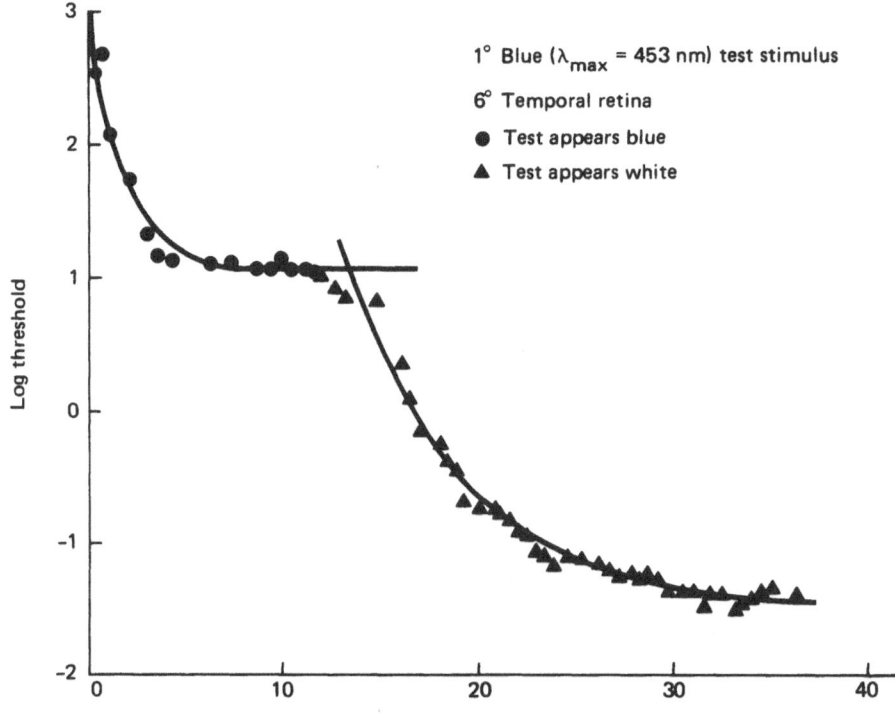

FIGURE 9.1 A typical two segment dark adaptation curve clearly showing the rod-cone break (courtesy of Dr. Matthew Alpern, University of Michigan).

Another type of data that reflects the duplex nature of the retina concerns the wavelength function of absolute sensitivity under conditions of high illumination and under conditions of low illumination. If one determines the relative spectral sensitivity of human vision at high illuminances, it is the spectral sensitivities of the cones that predominate. Such a spectral sensitivity curve is referred to as the photopic luminosity curve. If, on the other hand, the spectral sensitivity is determined in a dark-adapted subject at low light intensities, then the data, referred to as the scotopic luminosity curve, exclusively reflect the spectral absorption characteristics of the rods.

There are two ways in which these two curves can be plotted. If both the photopic and scotopic data are normalized on a graph in such a way that full scale represents the maximum response for the optimum stimulating wavelength of each, then the curves appear as shown in Figure 9.2. This representation, however, is often quite misleading, for although it emphasizes the difference in peak spectral sensitivity, it ignores the fact that the absolute sensitivity of the scotopic curve is so much greater (that is, so much less light is needed) than the photopic one. A somewhat better way of plotting these same data that avoids this difficulty

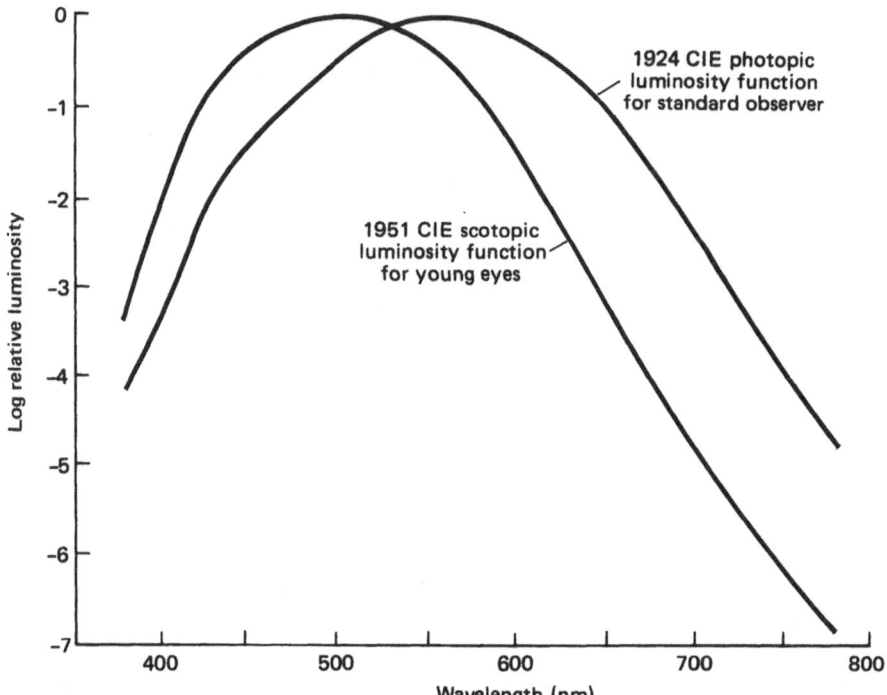

FIGURE 9.2 *The CIE relative luminosity curves for scotopic and photopic vision normalized by assuming equal maximum sensitivities for rods and cones and plotted as a logarithmic attenuation from that reference level. But see also Figure 9.3 (from Graham, 1965).*

is to utilize an absolute radiant energy scale. This was done by Wald (1945), for example, and his version has been replotted in our Figure 9.3. In this plot, the difference in absolute levels of sensitivity is much more clearly shown, and thus the true relationship between the two curves is made clear. It should be noted that these two curves reflect two different photochemical situations. The scotopic curve is a psychophysical correlate mainly of the absorption spectrum of a single substance—rhodopsin. On the other hand, the photopic curve is the cumulative effect of the absorption spectra of three different photochemicals—those that we have already referred to in Chapter 4 as erythrolabe, chlorolabe, and cyanolabe —the three cone pigments.

The photopic luminosity curve can be seen to peak at about 560 nm and the scotopic curve about 500 nm. This difference in the peak absorption of the rhodopsin, on the one hand, and the mixture of the three cone pigments, on the other, leads to several other important effects in addition to the break in the dark adaptation curve already mentioned. There is, in addition to the increasing absolute sensitivity of the retina as it dark-adapts, a shift in the wavelength—the Purkinje shift—to which the eye is relatively most sensitive. A light-adapted eye is most sensitive to lights

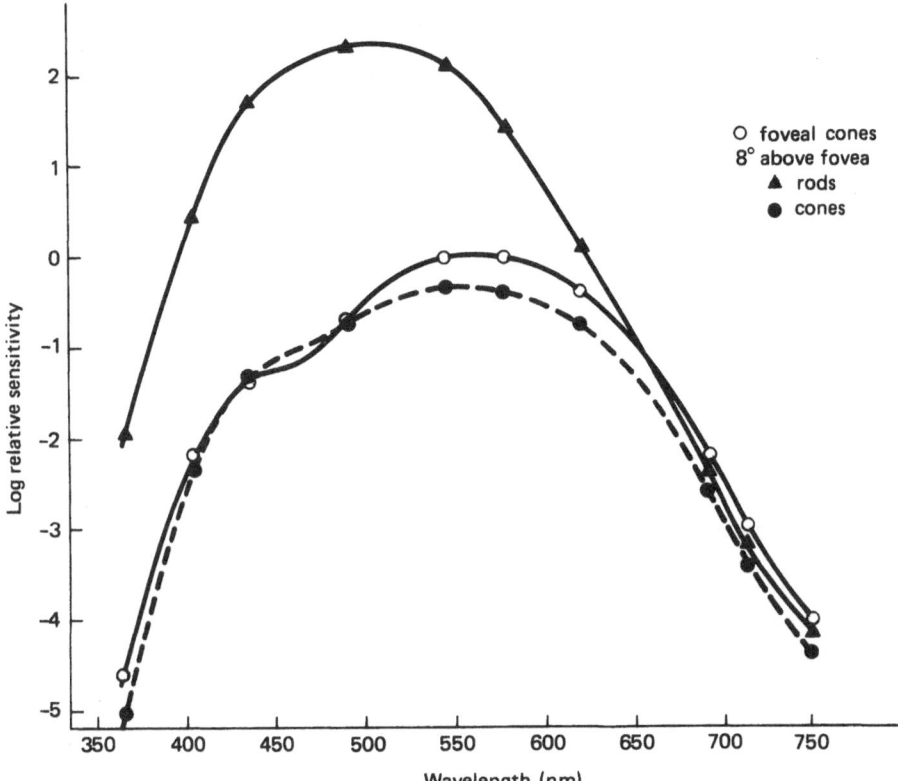

FIGURE 9.3 The same data shown in Figure 9.2 but not normalized. This means of graphing the scotopic and photopic curve emphasizes the fact that cone vision is three log units less sensitive than rod vision. Data for cones at the fovea and at 8 deg from the fovea are shown. Rod measurements are taken 8 deg from the fovea (from Wald, 1945).

in the yellow region of the visual spectrum, while a dark-adapted eye is most sensitive to blue or green lights. The effects of this shift as one gradually dark-adapts can be remarkable. If red and blue stimuli are matched for equal brightness in intense light, the blue will become subjectively brighter than the red under scotopic conditions.

Whereas lights containing only monochromatic wavelengths remain relatively constant in their chromaticity as the intensity of the light changes, lights composed of mixed wavelengths tend to change colors as their intensity changes because of this shift in peak sensitivity. Mixed colors, such as combinations of yellow, orange, and red, tend to be yellowish at high intensities, but to take on definite blue and green tones at low intensities. This phenomenon is known as the Bezold-Brucke phenomenon (or shift) and may be related to the shift in the relative contribution of each of the four retinal photopigments to the luminous function at differing levels of light adaptation.

Differences in critical flicker fusion characteristics as a function of the level of light adaptation have also been noted. At high light intensities, all color lights seem to exhibit the same flicker fusion frequencies, while at lower intensities, each spectral color seems to follow its own characteristic flicker fusion curve as shown in Figure 9.4 from Hecht and Schlaer (1936). The implication of this finding is that at high levels of light, the cones all have the same flicker fusion characteristics. In fact, however, this can be shown not to be true. Brindley, Du Croz, and Rushton (1966), for example, were able to show that the portion of the chromatic system that responds to blue has a lower critical flicker fusion frequency than those portions responding to the longer wavelengths. To bring out this difference, however, they had to preadapt the eye with red and green lights to selectively desensitize these receptors. It was only in this way that the blue system with its lower absolute level of sensitivity could be studied in isolation.

The technique of preadapting the retina with a given colored light to reduce the sensitivity of one of the three chromatic receptor classes was invented by Stiles (1949).

In sum, the retina exhibits a wide variety of psychophysical functions that are dependent upon the fact that the retina is a duplex system of one type of rod and three types of cones. The generality of this duplexity theory is well established and in large part explicable on the basis of the photochemical differences between these two types of retinal photoreceptors.

B. Trichromatic Color Mixture

It is a fact that a person with normal color vision can match or reproduce any color or color combination by manipulating a color mixer with only three controls. This is the basic fact of trichromaticity and is the basis for much of the theorizing about the neurological mechanisms that underlie this most important quality dimension. This notion can be expressed mathematically in the following way:

$$C \equiv aC_1 + bC_2 + cC_3 \tag{9.1}$$

where C is the color to be matched, and $\equiv$ represents the notion of "can be matched by" rather than any notion of numerical equality. In this equation, the coefficients a, b and c represent (to a first approximation) the percentage of each of the three colors C_1, C_2, and C_3, which are used for the color mixing.

The terms C_1, C_2, and C_3 refer to a set of three "fundamentals" or "primary" colors that can be used to achieve the match. In theory, any set of three colors can be used as the fundamentals, and the basic notion of trichromaticity has often been phrased in the following manner: *any color can be matched by appropriate amounts of any fixed set of three colors.* The only restriction is that the set be orthogonal; that is, no one of the three matching colors may be a mixture of the other two. The choice of what the triad of primary colors is to be, therefore, is theoretically arbitrary. Indeed, they need not be monochromatic or even equal in

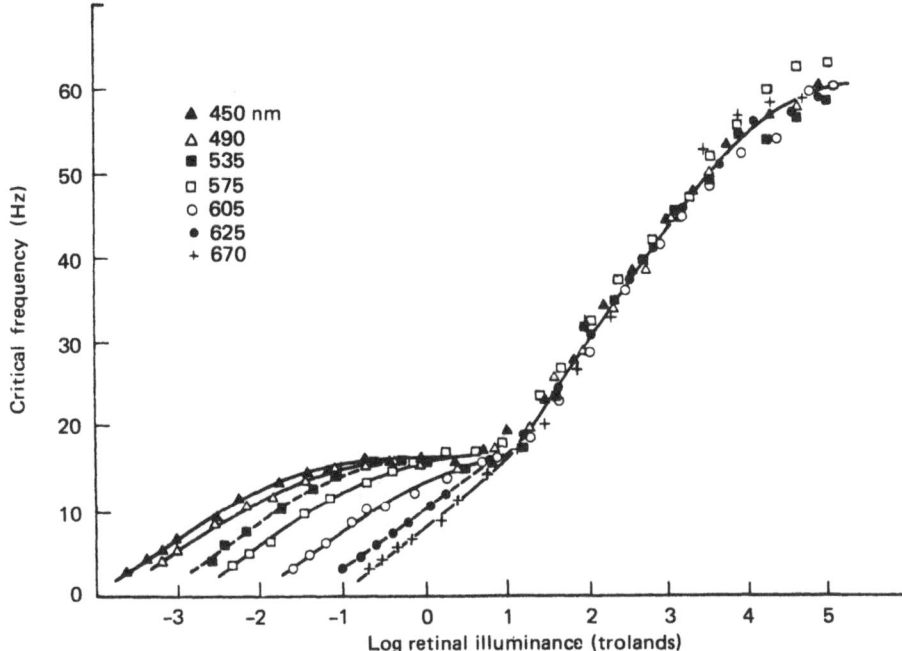

FIGURE 9.4 *A graph showing the relationship between critical flicker fusion frequencies for different colored lights and the intensity of the stimulating lights. Above a certain threshold, there is no differential effect of color, while at low light intensities, each color displays its own characteristic flicker fusion curve (from Brown, 1965, after Hecht and Schlaer, 1936).*

brightness. However, certain practical considerations (and empirical data, as we shall see below) compel us to choose triads of primaries that are somewhat restricted. For example, if three primaries are chosen, all of which are in the long wavelength end of the visual spectrum, then one of the coefficients *a*, *b*, or *c* will have to be negative. A negative coefficient means that that particular one of the triad of fundamentals has to be added to the color that is being matched rather than to the other two members of the triad. Negative coefficients may also be necessary when monochromatic primaries are used in some instances, but the existence of a negative coefficient does not diminish the basic notion of the fact of trichromaticity, namely, that three and only three variable light sources must be manipulated to match all other colors.

The choice of the triad of primaries, as we have said, is completely arbitrary. The triad may consist of any three monochromatic colors, any three bandwidths of the visual spectrum, or any combination of monochromatic wavelengths and extended bandwidths. Not only is the spectral composition of the triad arbitrary, but so too is its intensity or luminosity. However, the choice of a particular triad will determine the magnitude of the set of coefficients *a*, *b*, and *c*.

The coefficients a, b, and c, defining the characteristics of a color match of some unknown, may be considered from a number of different points of view. Given a certain triad of primaries, they may be defined as nondimensional ratios by the following three equations:

$$a = \frac{C_1}{C_1 + C_2 + C_3} \tag{9.2}$$

$$b = \frac{C_2}{C_1 + C_2 + C_3} \tag{9.3}$$

$$c = \frac{C_3}{C_1 + C_2 + C_3} \tag{9.4}$$

where C_1, C_2, and C_3 reflect, in this case, the absolute amounts of the three primaries in a given color mixture. Since each of the coefficients is defined in terms of the proportion of one colored light to the sum of all three, it is immediately clear that the sum of the coefficients must be equal to 1 when defined in this manner. Thus,

$$a + b + c = 1 \tag{9.5}$$

Another way in which the same information may be represented has been recently developed by Cornsweet (1970). Rather than using a formula that is specified in terms of the relative proportion of the three primaries, he defines a system of color matching, which is specified in terms of the quantal absorption of three retinal pigments. His model is based upon the notion that a mixture of three primaries will match some other color if the number of quanta absorbed by each member of the set of three photosensitive pigments is the same for the matched and the matching stimuli. Or expressed formally,

$$N_{a0} = N_{a1} + N_{a2} + N_{a3} \tag{9.6}$$

$$N_{b0} = N_{b1} + N_{b2} + N_{b3} \tag{9.7}$$

$$N_{c0} = N_{c1} + N_{c2} + N_{c3} \tag{9.8}$$

where N, in general, refers to the number of quanta of light absorbed by one of the three photopigments. Each of the three pigments (subscripted a, b, and c) will absorb a certain number of quanta from each of the four involved lights: the unknown (subscripted 0) and the three primary colors used in the color match (each of which is subscripted 1, 2, or 3, respectively). Thus, the number of quanta absorbed by the b photoreceptor when stimulated by the first of the primaries would be indicated N_{b1}. A light will be matched by adjusting the intensities of a set of primaries until the quantal absorption in each of the three photopigments is equal for the unknown and the combined effect of the three matching colors.

Both of these formulations, one in terms of the ratio coefficients and one in terms of quantal absorption, are, of course, equivalent, and it is possible to go from one to the other easily. Each is an expression of the basic fact that we wish to emphasize here, namely, that trichromacy is the basic characteristic of normal color vision. This means that when color matching and color mixing psychophysical experiments are carried out, only three degrees of freedom are required.

The tridimensionality of color space allows us to represent it in a three-dimensional spatial plot in a compressed and simple manner. There are two ways in which this can be done, one based upon the ratio coefficients, and one based upon Cornsweet's quantum absorption notions.

The method based upon ratio coefficients allows us to display in a two-dimensional plot many of the three-dimensional features of color mixing and trichromatic vision. One form of this plot, usually known as the CIE [Commission Internationale de L'Eclairage (International Lighting Commission)] chromaticity diagram is illustrated in Figure 9.5. This particular chromaticity diagram is one based upon a set of monochromatic primaries with wavelengths of 460, 530, and 650 nm. A different set of primaries would produce a chromaticity diagram, which differs in shape from this one to the degree that the primaries differ from this standard set. An important practical criterion for the choice of a set of primaries is that when they are mixed in equal proportions, the mixture will produce a relatively good white. On this CIE chromaticity diagram, the horizontal coordinate represents one of the coefficients of the trichromatic equation [Equation 9.1], which specifies how much of the long radiation color (usually red) is present. The vertical coordinate, in turn, represents the coefficient of the intermediate wavelength (usually green) primary. Knowing these two numbers, the coefficient of the third short wavelength component (actually a blue) is uniquely specified, since $a + b + c = 1$ and no third dimension need be specified.

The CIE chromaticity diagram is packed with an astounding variety of information. One of the most important subsets of data contained within it is the definition of the required combinations of the three primaries that must be used to match the spectral colors. Spectral colors, of course, are the sensations produced by the spectrum of visible monochromatic stimuli. The continuous curve shown in Figure 9.5 is the locus of the triads required to reproduce each of the spectral colors ranging from the near infrared to the near ultraviolet. This locus of points also essentially represents the outer limits of the color world, for each spectral color represents the purest or most saturated color possible. Under some conditions, such as those following chromatic adaptation, combinations of coefficients, which seemingly produce colors that lie outside of the spectral locus, can be obtained. Such combinations of color coefficients represent supersaturated colors, but the interpretation of such phenomena is equivocal.

As one moves along any line connecting the locus of spectral points and the center of the chromaticity diagram, one is approaching the other end of the saturation continuum—the purest white in which no color

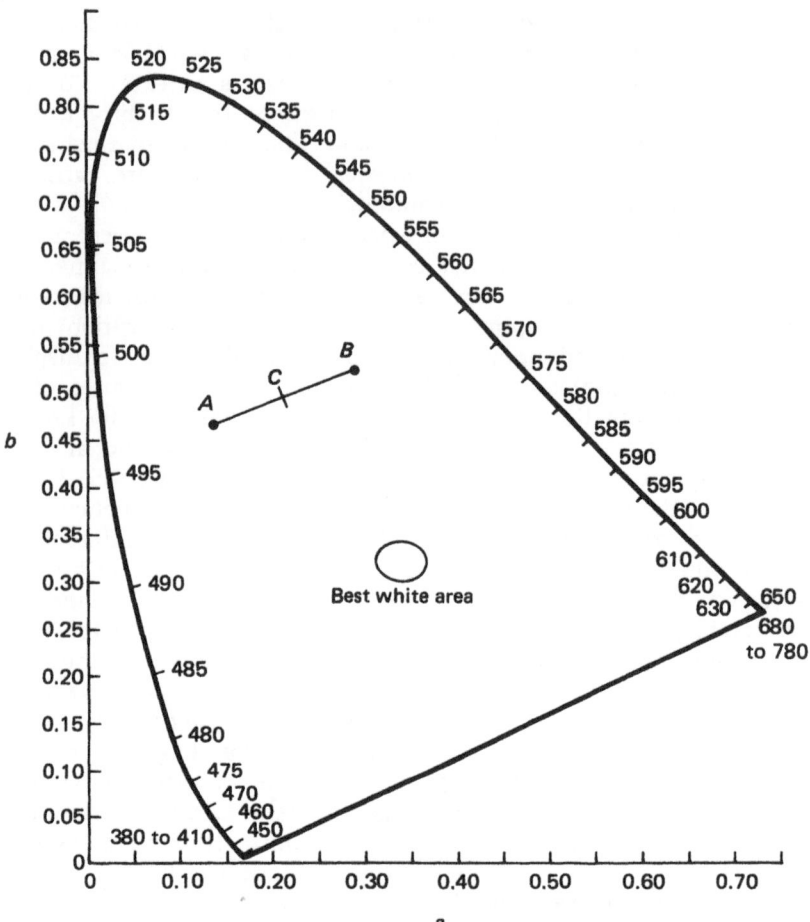

FIGURE 9.5 *The standard 1931 CIE chromaticity diagram plotting the a coeffi-*
cient against the b coefficient. Since a + b + c = 1, c is also thus uniquely de-
fined. The circled center region approximates the most white of the whites
obtained in a three-color mixture experiment. The straight line shows a means
of calculating the chromatic resultant C of the mixture of two colors, A and B
(adapted from Optical Society of America, 1953).

tones are observable. Thus, one is moving from the most saturated
chromatic stimulus to the most desaturated chromatic stimulus, and points
lying along this line represent increasing degrees of desaturation.

Two-color mixing is also simply represented on the chromaticity
diagram shown in Figure 9.5. For any two colors lying anywhere within
the spectral locus, the center of gravity of a straight line joining the
points that represent each color is representative of the color of their
combination. For these special cases, in which the two colors lie at the
ends of a straight line that passes through and is centered in the central
white region, the two colors are said to be complements of each other.

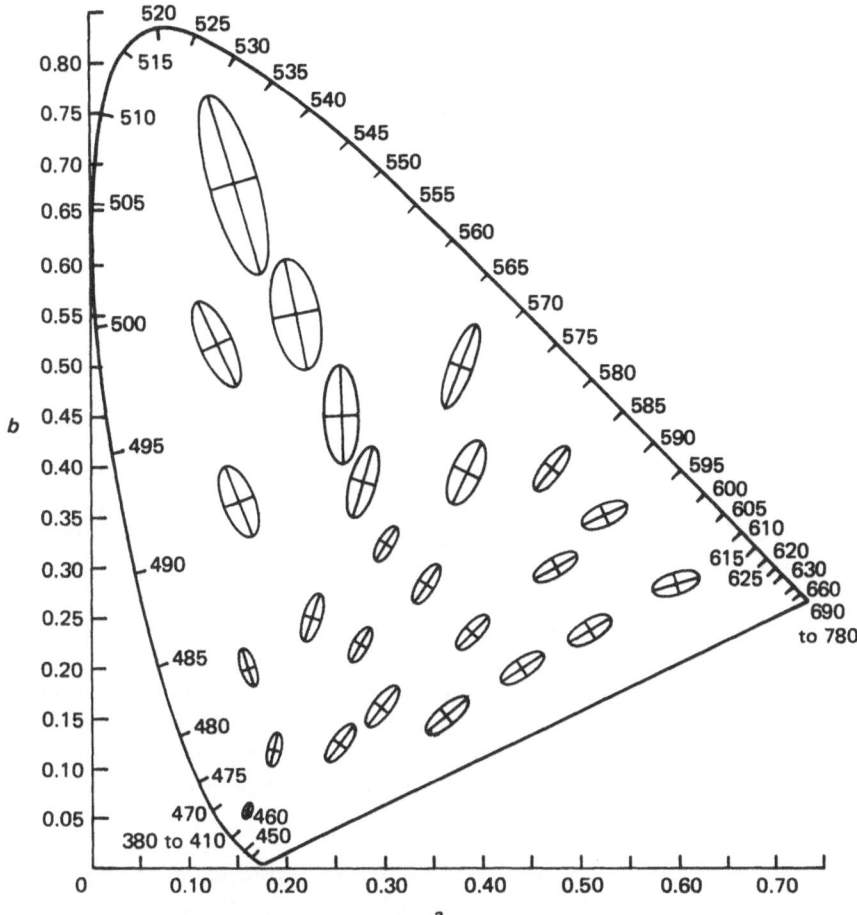

FIGURE 9.6 *The system of MacAdam ellipses, which show the regions in which colors are not differentiated from one another. The dimensions of the ellipses are defined by a measure of the standard deviation of the wavelength of indiscriminable colors in a two-color discrimination experiment (from MacAdam, 1942).*

In other words, when these two colors are mixed in appropriate amounts, the resultant is a white.

Another interesting set of data, which is included on some drawings of the chromaticity diagram, is the set of MacAdam ellipses. MacAdam (1942) had shown that there were areas on the chromaticity diagram within which the normal human observer could not distinguish any difference between the set of color mixtures that were so defined. MacAdam demonstrated that these areas were in the form of ellipses, in which the orientation of the major axis varied systematically depending upon where, in the chromaticity diagram, one was working. Figure 9.6 shows one plot of a system of MacAdam ellipses. The small size of the ellipse in the lower left-hand corner of the curve suggests a very great sensitivity to color differences when the slightest changes are made in the amount of red or green light. On the other hand, at the top of the chromaticity diagram, the very large ellipses suggest that, in the yellow-green region, there is a reduced sensitivity to the effects of changes in the amount of red, and even less effect on the perceived color when very substantial changes are made in the amount of green in the color mixture. In the lower right-hand corner of the chromaticity diagram are ellipses of intermediate size, indicating that the observer's sensitivity to changes in either two or three of the triads of fundamentals is intermediate.

The chromaticity diagram can also be used as a starting point for discussing many other detailed rules of color mixture. It is quite obvious that any given point on the diagram can be produced by a number of different color combinations. For example, any given point on the CIE chromaticity diagram can be produced by the combination of any of the pairs of colors at the ends of any of the family of straight lines that pass through and have their center of gravity at that point. Yet, regardless of the colors of the pair of component colors that are used to produce the color represented by that point, all of the mixtures are indistinguishable. Such combination colors, of equal chromaticity, but produced by even the most widely varying components, are called metameric matches.

The experiments and data concerning color mixture are varied and extensive. Much of the data has been summarized in a set of rules generally known as Grassman's laws, and over the years, the rules have been extended and rephrased to reflect current theory and experiment. Perhaps the best modern statement of these rules has been summarized by Graham (1965, p. 372):

1. *Any mixed color, no matter how it is composed, must have the same appearance as the mixture of a certain saturated color with white (Helmholtz, 1866, 1924–25, vol. 2). (The wavelength corresponding to the saturated color is called the dominant wavelength.)*

2. *When one of the two kinds of light that are to be mixed together changes continuously, the appearance of the mixture changes continuously also (Helmholtz, 1866, 1924–25), vol. 2).*
   a. For every color there can be found another complementary or antagonistic color which, if mixed with it in the right proportion, gives white or gray, and if mixed in any other proportion, an unsaturated color of the hue of the stronger component (Titchener, 1924).
   b. The mixture of any two colors that are not complementaries gives an intermediate color, varying in hue with the relative amounts of the two original colors and varying in saturation with their nearness or remoteness in the color series (Titchener, 1924).

3. *The mixture of any two combinations which match will itself match either of the original combinations, provided that the*

> *illumination of the colors remains approximately the same* *(Titchener, 1924).*
> 4. *The total intensity of the mixture is the sum of the intensities of the light mixed (Grassman, 1854).*

While the CIE chromaticity diagram has been the standard spatial representation of the data of color mixture, Cornsweet's (1970) tridimensional representation presents a new alternative, which may prove to have considerable advantages in years to come. As we noted previously, Cornsweet plotted his three-dimensional graphs in terms of the number of quanta absorbed. The basic assumption underlying this approach is that all quanta that are absorbed by any of the three possible cone pigments have an equal physiological effect, regardless of the wavelength of the illuminating light. Since it uses absolute quantal absorptions, the Cornsweet plot must be a true three-dimensional one, for the quasi-two-dimensionalization inherent in the equation, $a + b + c = 1$, is not present in this situation. Thus, the number of quanta absorbed by each of the three photopigments is not normalized and must be represented as independent degrees of freedom. Figure 9.7 shows an example of Cornsweet's method of plotting the chromatic trispace and also the locus of the spectral colors.

Although the curve representing the locus of spectral colors looks, at first glance, as if it were simply a two-dimensional plot, this is merely a consequence of the fact that the absorption coefficient of the short wavelength or blue receptor substance is quite small compared to the others. It is a general result that the blue light contributes less per incident quanta to the overall luminous experience than does the medium wavelength (yellow-green) or the longer wavelength (red) sensitive receptors.

Each point on the spectral locus on Cornsweet's chromaticity diagram (Figure 9.7) is plotted by determining the relative absorption of each spectral wavelength by the three photopigments. The three coefficients of absorption are thus defined. It is then assumed that a 1000 quanta/sec of that particular wavelength compose the incident signal. It is, therefore, a simple and direct calculation to specify the three coordinates. One simply multiplies each of the three determined coefficients by 1000 to determine the number of quanta absorbed by each of the three chromatic color pigments. In Cornsweet's words, this is the "effect on system" *A, B,* or *C.*

The locus of the spectral colors represents the same information as the locus of spectral colors on the CIE chromaticity diagram, and much of the other color mixture information is also inherent in Cornsweet's plot in more or less the same manner.

C. Stiles' and Wald's Increment Threshold Experiments

In spite of the fact that color mixing data provide the basis for a number of very useful models of color mixing, there is, in fact, little within that entire body of knowledge that speaks to the problem of the human color receptor spectral response characteristics. The fact that almost any triad of fundamentals can be used in a color mixing experiment to produce a match for an unknown color means that there is no way to determine from the color mixing data alone anything unique about the characteristics

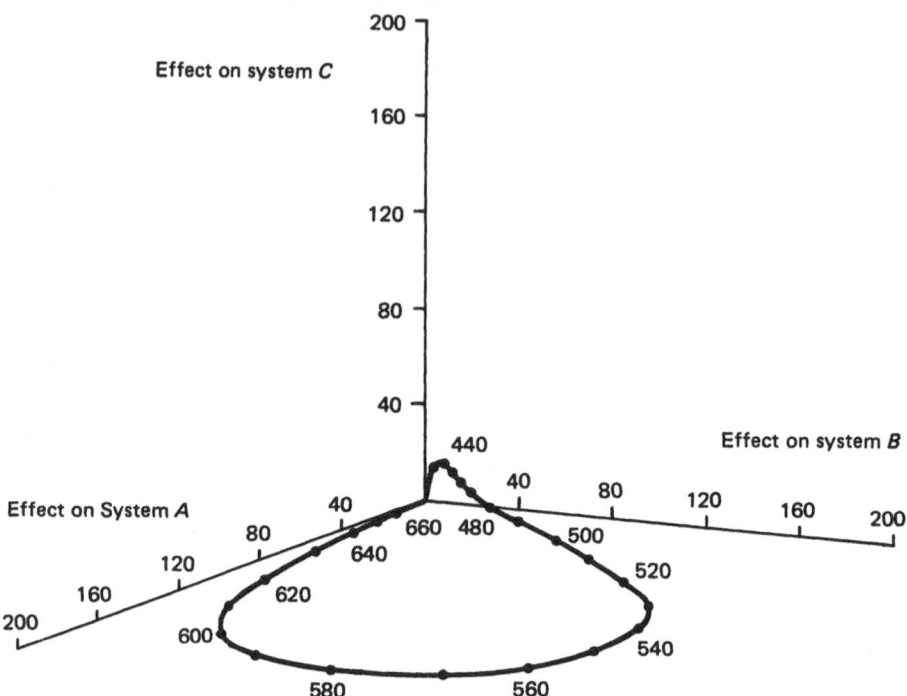

FIGURE 9.7 *An alternative means of plotting the chromaticity diagram in a three-dimensional space. The three coordinates indicate the proportion of 1000 quanta, which are absorbed by the three photochemicals, respectively. Though the curve appears to be primarily in the A-B (red-green) plane, it is truly three-dimensional. The distortion is due to the low level of absorbance of the blue (C) system (adapted from Cornsweet, 1970).*

of the basic absorption spectra of the three types of cones. There is, however, some psychophysical data that do suggest a possible solution of this problem. Stiles (1949, 1959) has used a technique of increment thresholds in a way that is analogous to the technique used in the usual dark adaptation experiment. In this way, he was able to demonstrate a multiple segment curve similar to the rod and cone segments of the conventional dark adaptation curve. He interprets these multiple segments as a reflection of differences in the absorption spectra of the three different cone photochemicals. From these multisegment curves, and assuming a certain mathematical relation between the energy of the adapting field and the energy of the just detectable test increment, Stiles has been able to predict a set of curves that, he believes, are specifically the spectral sensitivities of the three photoreceptors.

Let us consider Stiles' technique and findings in detail because of the almost unique role they play as psychophysical indicants of receptor photoabsorption characteristics. The general psychophysical technique was the detection of a small spot of light of one color on a background of another color. The stimulus consisted of a 10-deg background adapting field of wavelength μ and a briefly illuminated 1-deg test flash of wavelength λ. The technique is rather straightforward once these conditions have been established. The amount of energy of a just perceptible test stimulus is simply measured as a function of the intensity of the background. This can be done for many combinations of the test and background colors.

The constant background illumination performs an important additional function beyond merely setting the level of light adaptation. It also acts as a selective adaptor of the three photoreceptors. Thus, a red adapting light will tend to diminish the sensitivity of the red and green receptors, but leave the blue cone sensitivity relatively intact. Since the overall threshold response of the whole system is obviously a function of the pooled influences of the three receptor types, this selective adaptation will have the effect of enhancing the relative contribution of the blue in comparison to the red and green. The overall response will, thus, be biased more in the direction of the unadapted blue receptor than it was when none of the three was light-adapted. Thus, just as workers once obtained a break in the dark adaptation curve by using different levels of white light to selectively bias the response of the dark adaptation curve in a way that resulted in the rod-cone break, Stiles now does the same thing with chromatic adaptation and obtains the sort of curve that is shown in Figure 9.8a. In this particular case, a bluish test tight (476 nm) was superimposed on a yellowish green adapting light. The curve shows three distinct segments, which Stiles, in this case, has named π_4, π_1, and π_3 (π_2 and π_5 being additional segments, which occur under certain other experimental conditions). The π_1, π_2, and π_3 segments obtained in these and in other related experiments are all thought by Stiles to be due to the action of the blue cone. He attributes the π_4 segment to the action of a green cone and π_5 to the action of a red cone.

The critical next step is to go from the "adaptation" curves, of which Figure 9.8a is one example, to the individual spectral sensitivity curves of the photoreceptors. Unfortunately, this involved a number of mathematical considerations and some intervening functions. The full details of Stiles' derivation are beyond the scope of our present discussion, but fortunately he has summed them up graphically in Figure 9.8b. Assume that the three curves on the left-hand side of this figure are the three spectral absorption curves for the three photoreceptors. Assume also that there is another spectral function involved, which is displayed by the three curves in the lower right-hand corner. This second set of three curves represents the change in the background field intensity that has to be made to raise the threshold for a test flash by one log unit as a function of wavelength for each of these three receptor systems. These two spectral functions will, then, be related by the third set of "linking" functions in the right-hand quadrant of the figure. Due to the fact that this is a mixed system, the threshold in the increment experiment will be determined by the lowest value of any of these three linking functions. The bottommost envelope indicated by the combined dotted and solid line is the current example. The combined envelope is exactly the sort of curve that was obtained and displayed in Figure 9.8a.

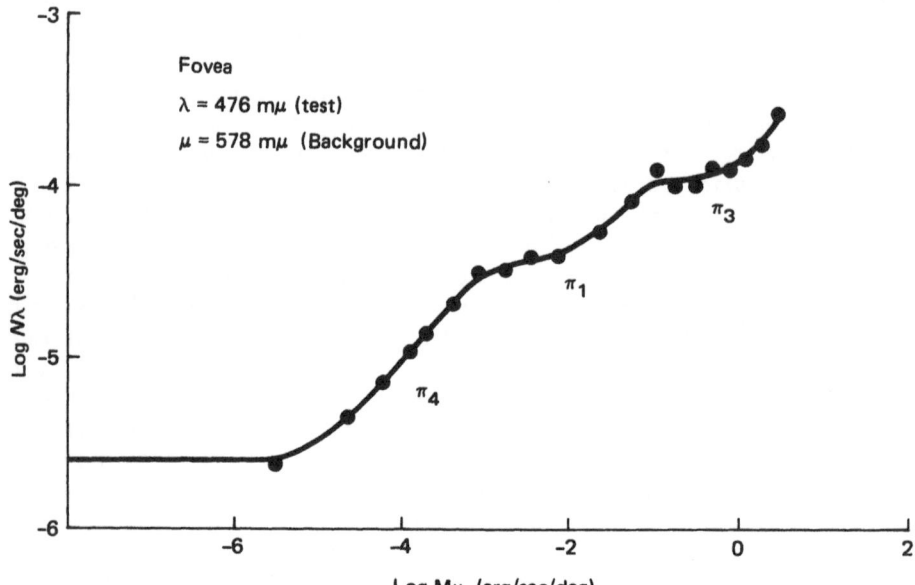

FIGURE 9.8(a) A plot of the threshold of the test stimulus as a function of the background illumination level. The curve obtained in this experiment is a multi-faceted one, in which each segment reflects some aspect of multiple receptor mechanisms. See text for full details (from Stiles, 1959).

By processing a large set of such adaptation threshold curves (typi-fied by the dotted curve of the present case), Stiles was able to reason backward to the shape of the three photoreceptor curves. Although we shall not go into the details of this analysis, we have tabulated his con-clusions in Table 9.1, which shows the general characteristics of the spec-tral response of the three cone types as well as the rod.

While it is most important to note that Stiles' π functions are not identified with the individual absorption curves, it is on the basis of these π functions that he was able to derive one of the few reasonable sets of cone spectral sensitivities based purely on psychophysical data. His three spectral sensitivity curves for the cones have peaks at 440 nm, 540 nm, and 575 nm. These values should be compared with the biological data presented later in this chapter.

On the other hand, Wald (1964, 1966) has used Stiles' preadaptation and increment threshold technique to produce what he believes are direct psychophysical correlates of the absorption curves of the three photopig-ments. His technique was very much like that used by Stiles, but by select-ing a set of adapting lights that included yellow (to reduce the sensitivity to long wavelength stimuli), purple (to reduce sensitivity to both long and short wavelength stimuli without affecting the middle of the spectrum to any great degree), and blue (to reduce sensitivity to short wavelength stimuli), he produced three curves that seemed to closely approximate the

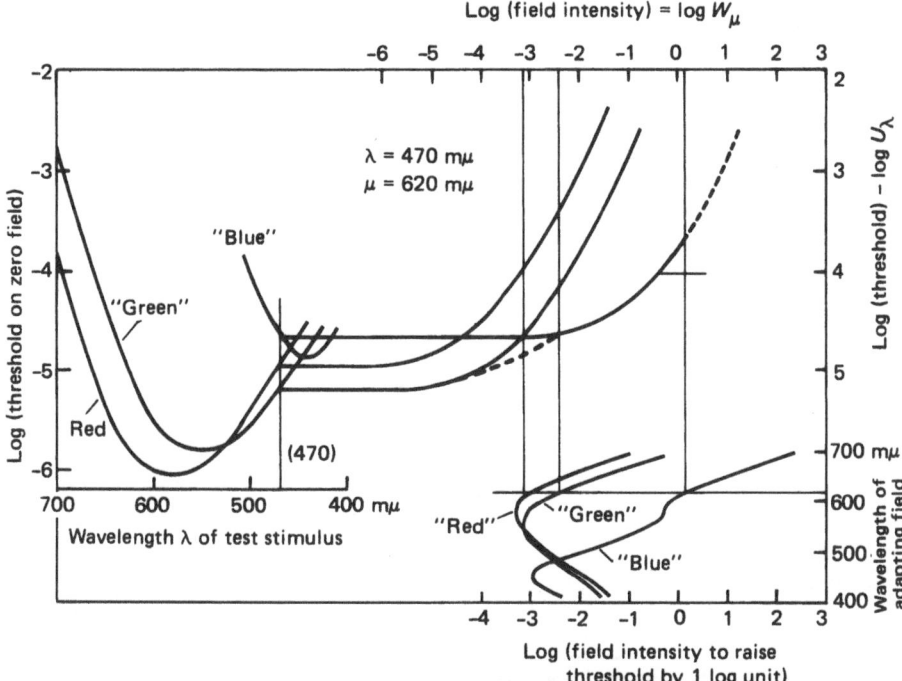

FIGURE 9.8(b) A graphical means of showing how the individual photoreceptor spectral absorbtion curves are derived from the increment threshold data shown in Figure 9.8(a) (from Stiles 1959, after Stiles 1949).

responses found with direct absorption type measurements (see below). The three response curves peaked at 430, 540, and 575, respectively, values in close agreement with the Stiles data.

This same procedure has also been used, more recently (Wooten and Wald, 1973) to show that the various types of cones are present in extremely peripheral portions of the retina, a surprising result in terms of the usually accepted notions of a color-blind retinal periphery.

D. Hue Discrimination and Color Blindness
One of the most basic of the psychophysical problems with which any theory of color vision must always deal is the basic nature of hue discrimination. How small is the difference in the wavelength of a given illuminant, which can be distinguished as a hue difference? The experiment necessary to answer this question is usually carried out using a device that allows side-by-side comparison of a test field and an adjustable comparison field. Experimental data pertaining to this problem have been repeatedly obtained over the years by several different investigators. The major interesting feature of the data is that it is a very irregularly shaped curve. Figure 9.9 presents what is now considered to be the classic plot of these data—a summary of several experiments by Judd (1932). The w-

TABLE 9.1 THE RELATIONSHIP BETWEEN STILES' "π" COMPONENTS OF
THE ADAPTATION CURVE AND THE FOUR PHOTORECEPTOR MECHANISMS*

Mechanism	Symbol	Remarks	Wavelength of Maximal Sensitivity (nm)
Rod	π_0	Absent at the fovea	503
"Blue" cone ...	π_1	at approx. 2.6 log units	440
	π_2	at approx. 1 log unit	? (Between 440 and 480 mμ)
	π_3	at approx. 4.0 log units	440
"Green" cone ..	π_4		540
"Red" cone ...	π_5		575 (very flat max.)

* This table also indicates the peak sensitivities of the spectral absorptions of the four photoreceptors in the human eye (adapted from Stiles, 1959).

shaped curve is seen to exhibit its highest sensitivity—a minimum detectable hue difference associated with a wavelength shift of less than 1 nm—at wavelengths of the incident light of about 480- and 580-nm.

The lack of an ability to discriminate colors in this normal manner is known as color blindness. A more precise definition, necessitated by the many different kinds of color blindness, is based on the number of degrees of freedom required by a subject to match all the colors in the space defined by either CIE or the Cornsweet chromaticity diagram. Normal trichromatic vision, as we have seen, requires the presence of three independently controllable primary colors in the color mixture for the perfect matching of all other colors. Various forms of weak or anomalous trichromatic color vision have been observed. Subjects may be protanomalous (with a lowered sensitivity to long or red wavelengths) or deuteranomalous (in which the subject appears to have lowered sensitivity to the median or yellow-green wavelengths). In both of these forms of anomalous trichromatism, the subject is still required to use three colors to match all samples of the chromatic visual space. Wide deviances are found, however, among the amounts of the three primaries, which are required for the matching of a given color by an anomalous and a normal trichromatic subject. A protanomalous trichromat will tend to use far more than normal amounts of red for his matches, for example. A deuteranomalous trichromat will use more yellow-green than normal for his color matches.

On the other hand, there also exists a group of people with deficient

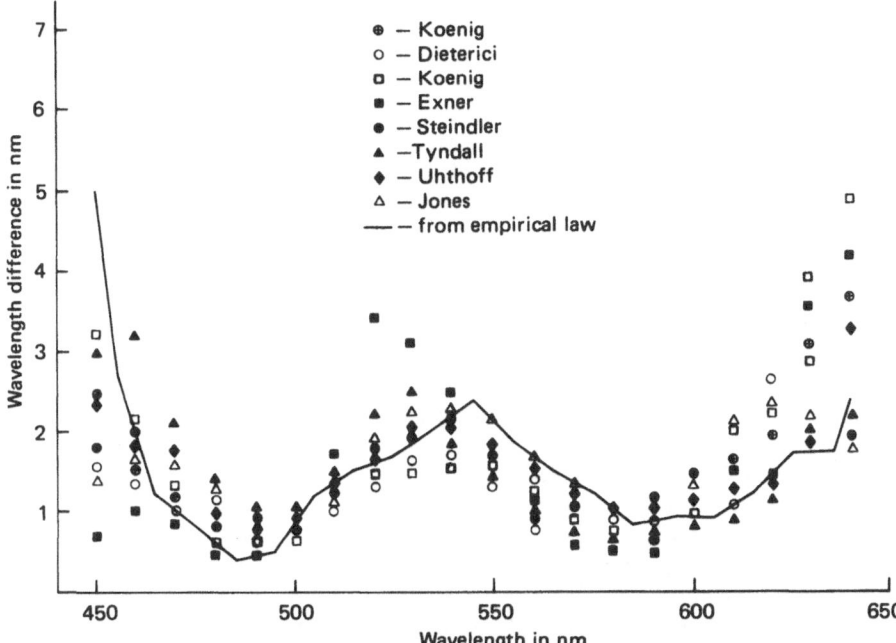

FIGURE 9.9 *A summary of several experiments measuring the differential threshold for changes in stimulus wavelength as a function of wavelength (from Judd, 1932).*

color vision such that only two primaries are required for matching any other color in the chromaticity space. People with such a deficiency are called dichromats. As was the case with anomalous trichromats, there are several distinguishable types of dichromatism. Subjects may exhibit behavior that classifies them either as persons suffering from dichromatic protanopia, deuteranopia, tritanopia. Protanopes are incapable of responding adequately to reds, deuteranopes to yellow-greens, and the very rare tritanopes to the blues. As with anomalous trichromats, deficiencies in other psychophysical tests such as hue discrimination are also exhibited by dichromats as well as the color mixing deficiencies. Hue discrimination in dichromats may be 10 times as insensitive as normal trichromats (that is, a difference in wavelength 10 times normal is required). This is an important factor in diagnosing the specific neural basis of each condition as well as the nature of the chromaticity confusion. On the other hand, the specific nature of the changes in the luminosity curves of dichromats has been a matter of considerable debate over the years. Protanopes seem to generally exhibit a diminished sensitivity at the red end of the spectrum, deuteranopes in the green region, and tritanopes seem to have a slight diminution in their luminosity curves at the blue end of the spectrum. However, the complexities of the changes in the luminosity curve, both in relative amplitude and in the degree to which the entire luminosity curve is shifted among dichromats, are very involved matters and will not be dealt with further in this chapter.

Sufferers from the most extreme form of color blindness, monochromats, are, for all practical purposes, incapable of discriminating among hues on any basis other than brightness difference. Thus, any single color can be used to match all other colors anywhere in the chromaticity space. There are two types of monochromat that can be distinguished on the basis of their luminosity curves. One type displays a photopic luminosity curve, which is indistinguishable from the scotopic luminosity curve. The other type displays a photopic luminosity curve, which is midway between the normal scotopic and the normal photopic luminosity curves. It has been suggested that the first type of luminosity curve is produced by a retina with no cones at all, while the second by a retina with only one of the three normal types of cones present. For this reason, the term rod-monochromat has been used as a descriptor of the former type, and the term cone-monochromat as a descriptor of the second type. For purposes of color mixture, both types still act as if a single color could match all other colors. Both kinds of monochromats also typically show many other kinds of visual difficulties related to their abnormal retinal. It is not known whether there are three different kinds of cone-monochromats—a possibility which is suggested by the fact that any one of the normal three types of cones might be present alone in this system. The relative rarity of this type of color blindness makes any such hypothesis extremely speculative, and we shall have to wait until a sufficiently large sample of monochromats have been studied to definitely answer that question.

E. "Fundamental Yellow," Complementary and Paired Colors, and Neutral Loci

As one scans the literature of color vision, there constantly recurs a most interesting statement. This statement is that there is something special about yellow, so that it is not "perceived" in psychological exepriments as a mixture of other colors as are such colors as greenish-blue or yellowish-red (orange). Rather, some workers in the field consider yellow to be "psychologically" just as primary as red, green, and blue. This statement is difficult to interpret, for at first glance it is not exactly clear why other color naming situations might not lead to a wide variety of other so-called psychologically fundamental colors. The idea of a "perceptual analysis" of mixed colors, such as yellowish-green into their constituent yellows and greens, is also a notion that is not completely clear in light of the general nature of synthetic color mixture and metameric matches. Many authors have used the idea of a "primary yellow" as the starting point in their arguments for opponent color theories of color vision (see below), but this point is probably a misunderstanding of the basic idea of the trichromatic data we have already discussed. The basic fact of color mixture is that any color can be produced by appropriate mixtures of three primaries, and at least from that phenomenological point of view, there is no *a priori* way to convincingly argue that any particular color is more fundamental than any other.

In spite of the confusion regarding the definition and existence of a "fundamental yellow," there is a certain amount of hard data that do suggest that there are links between certain color pairs such that they either operate together or in opposition. This sort of data is more compelling than the vaguely defined "fundamental yellow."

One of the most important of these pieces of evidence, suggestive of linked processes, is found on the chromaticity diagrams themselves. Complementary colors are defined as those pairs of colors which, when mixed in appropriate amounts, produce a completely colorless or unsaturated white light. Complementary colors are represented on the diagram as the colors at the ends of any straight line whose center of gravity lies in the central white region. Thus, there are many colors that tend to cancel out the chromaticity of a linked partner and that, therefore, presumably may be linked at some physiological or anatomical level.

A number of other ways in which pairs of colors seemed to be linked have been summarized by Hurvich and Jameson:

> How can this system of three independent processes be made to account, for example, for the apparent linkages that seem to occur between specific pairs of colors as either the stimulus conditions or the conditions of the human observer are varied? Why should the red and green hues in the spectrum predominate at low stimulus levels, and the yellow and blue hue components increase concomitantly as the spectrum is increased in luminance (von Bezold, 1873)? Why, as a stimulus size is greatly decreased, should discrimination between yellow and blue hues become progessively worse than that between red and green (Farnsworth, 1955; Hartridge, 1949)? Why should the hues drop out in pairs in instances of congenital color defect or when the visual system is impaired by disease (Judd, 1949; Kollner, 1912.)?
>
> (HURVICH and JAMESON, 1957, pp. 384–385)

It has also been noted (Linkz, 1964), as well as by Hurvich and Jameson (1957), that it is impossible to conceive of or to find words to describe a reddish-green hue or a yellowish-blue hue. The difficulty in finding a color for which we could use such color names, they believe, reflects the fact that the relationship between blue and yellow, on the one hand, is different than that between yellow and red, on the other. But this sort of data also suffers from the same difficulties as does the distinction of yellow as a primary color—color names are based on word usage and subjective judgments that are peculiarly elusive when one attempts to precisely define the operations involved in their elicitation.

A more compelling set of data has been developed by Jameson and Hurvich (1955) in their attempt to develop a quantitative opponent color theory. Noting that a relatively wide range of spectral hues produces a sensation of yellowishness, blueness, greenness, and redness, they attempted to determine the relative strength of each of these sensory experiences by mixing in with each hue-inducing wavelength varying amounts of a postulated opponent color until all traces of the original color disappeared. Thus, for example, a band of stimulus wavelengths varying from about 500 to 700 nm would produce color responses that were reported by the subject to have some amount of yellowish tone. Various amounts of blue light would then be mixed with each of a series of wavelengths within this band, and the amount of blue required to completely cancel any "yellowishness" measured as an indicator of the strength or chromatic valence of the yellow response at each wavelength.

Figure 9.10 shows a sample set of cancellation data for the visible spectrum, at various places in its course, that are capable of eliciting some red, yellow, green or blue experience. The data are plotted in terms of the amount of the opponent color that had to be added at each wavelength to eliminate any residual "redness, yellowness, greenness or blueness." On this graph, it can be seen that the maximum amount of blue required to cancel yellowishness from one band varying from 490 nm to 650 nm was at about 530 nm and that the function dropped off on both sides. A wavelength band varying from 480 nm to 580 nm elicited some green experience, which had to be neutralized with a red, the largest amount of which was required also at about 520 nm. The fact that a single wavelength should produce some green and some yellow should not be too surprising. There is a range of wavelengths whose color names include greenish-yellow and yellowish-green, for example. When adequate amounts of red had been introduced to completely neutralize the green, the residual color would be a yellow. When adequate amounts of blue had been introduced to completely neutralize the yellow, the residual color would be a green.

The curve also shows that the band of wavelengths that induces blue color tints runs from 430 nm to 480 nm. These colors had to be neutralized with yellows, and maximal amounts of yellow were required at about 450 nm. The red curve, on the other hand, is somewhat peculiar because reddishness is an experience that is introduced by both long and short wavelengths. At the shorter wavelengths, the experience of purple includes tints that most people describe as including some reddishness. At the longer wavelengths, the sensations are color named reds and oranges. To remove all of the reddishness from a short wavelength from about 400 to 470 nm, green light had to be added, peaking in the amount required for neutralization at about 440 nm. At the longer wavelengths, the range of red-inducing stimuli was about 580 to 700 nm, and the peak amount of green required for neutralization occurred at about 620 nm.

It should be noted that there are a number of behavioral difficulties with the Jameson and Hurvich neutralization procedure. First of all, it was both necessary and difficult to define, for each of these basic colors, exactly what the bandwidth of spectral wavelengths is that evokes the particular sensation. Secondly, upon mixing the postulated opponent color in with the chosen wavelength, it was not always the case that the mixture turned out to be white. It often became an unsaturated version of one of the other opponent pair. Thus, blue and a yellowish tone could be mixed together, and the observer might be faced with deciding whether there was any yellow in a resulting green or red field.

These, then, are a few of the psychophysical data of the sort on which the various theories of color quality coding are based. In the

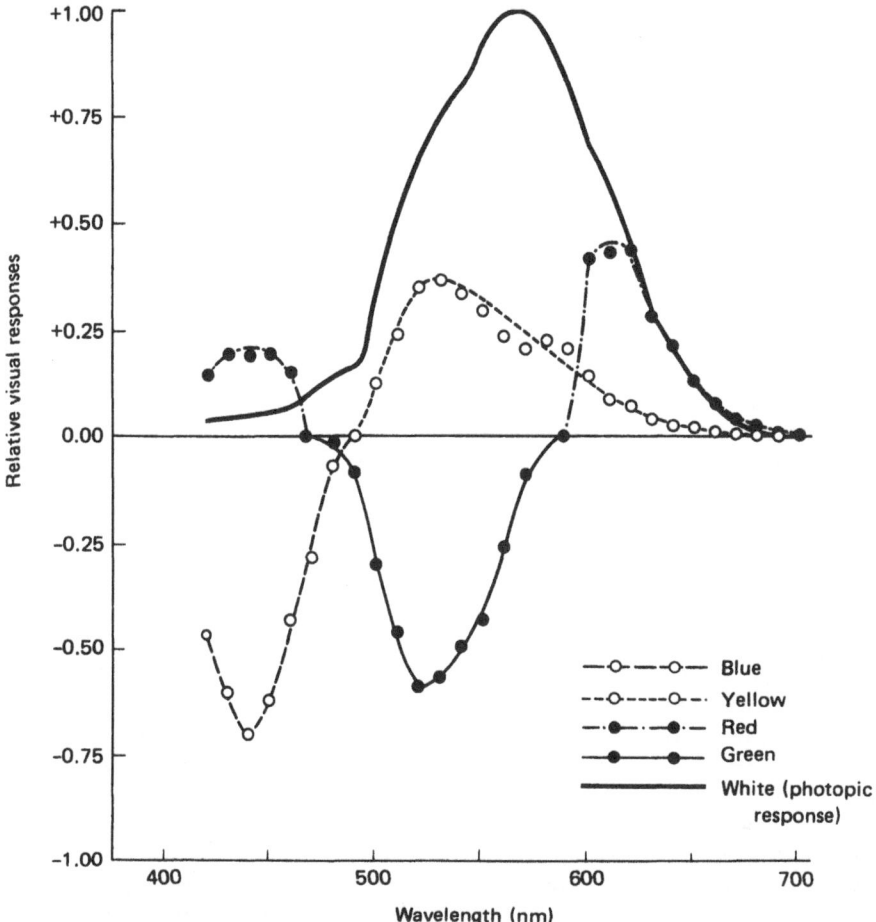

FIGURE 9.10 *Chromatic response functions for a single subject, indicating how much opponent color must be added to eliminate the residual chromatic effect of the colors indicated. The photopic luminosity curve is also shown for this subject (from Jameson and Hurvich, 1955).*

following sections, we shall discuss the alternative theories, the biological evidence that constrains these theories, and finally make a statement of what is believed to be the most widely accepted contemporary model.

III. THE COMPETITIVE THEORIES

As one reviews the enormous literature on color theory, it quickly becomes clear that no brief review or summary is going to be comprehensive enough to do justice to all of the distinguished workers who have contributed to this field. It is also clear, however, that much of the intellectual effort expended on the controversies in this field was aimed at models that were totally descriptive and unrelated to the coding problem. This was necessitated by the fact that, until the advent of modern neurophysiology, theorists were forced to argue only from the findings of psychophysical experiments to the underlying neural codes. As in so many other instances involving a "black box" approach, this is a procedure which has often been fruitless, since so many alternative proposed internal mechanisms can give rise to the same external behavior. In the following discussion, we shall concentrate our attention on those aspects of the competitive theories that contain specific neural hypotheses and ignore those that are formulated only in terms of mathematical theories of color space.

A major physiological issue has always been the nature of the trichromatic fundamentals and the ways in which they might be added together. In particular, the question was repeatedly asked: were the absorption spectra of the primaries closely spaced or widely dispersed? From the psychophysical data, many theorists attempted to reason back to the specific shape and number of the response curves of the group of primary colors. In the following section, this will be one of the main themes of our discussion.

A. The Trichromatic Theories

The basic nature of trichromatic color mixture was recognized relatively early, and by 1801 Young was able to state a visual theory, which postulated specifically that color vision is mediated by three retinal receptor systems. A major premise of his theory, which has proved to be most durable, is that the ratio of activation of the three systems is the key cue for the various color sensations. Young postulated specifically that there are three, and only three, different chromatic systems in the retina, and that each has a different spectral absorption curve. It is important to note, however, that there is nothing fixed in the various trichomatic theories about the nature of the absorption curves of the three systems. Young, Helmholtz, and a host of others who have followed, for many indirect and sometimes misleading reasons, suggested one after another triad of primaries that conceivably could serve to explain color vision effects. Indeed, the empirical fact that almost any triad allows color matching of any spectral hue (given the only exception that one be allowed to mix one of the three with the to-be-matched color) prohibited the direct specification of the nature of the triads from psychophysical evidence. Some workers, notably Young himself as well as Helmholtz (1924–25), König and Dieterici (1893), and Thomson and Wright (1953) among others, have suggested and developed theories on the basis of absorption spectra that are relatively broad and very widely spaced. Figure 9.11 (a) and (b) show two sets of fundamentals as proposed by some of these workers. On the other hand, over the years some investigators have suggested that the spectral absorption curves of the cones are very narrowly spaced. For example, Figure 9.11 (c) shows one of the sets used by Hecht (1934) in his theory of a mathematical color space.

An important conceptual point is that the trichromatic theory is, in fact, only a theory of the receptors. Few of the proponents of the trichromatic theory over the years have ever said anything about any higher level of neural coding. The sole biological assumption of all trichromatic theories concerns the absorption spectra of the receptor photochemicals.

What, then, are the basic ideas of trichromatic theory? First, it is postulated that color perception is mediated by the cones, specialized photoreceptors found mainly within or near the fovea of the retina. Second, it is asserted that there are specifically three kinds of cones, no more and no less. Third, the outer segment of each type of receptor cone is presumed to be filled with a photochemical that differs in its absorption spectrum from that of the other two. Fourth, on the basis of differences among the three receptors in absorption coefficients for the same wavelength, it is thought that relatively different amounts of neural activity are generated in each by different colored lights. Fifth and finally, there is a psychobiological coding assumption that on the basis of this difference in the relative rates of activity in different neural pathways or groups of afferent neurons, different chromatic sensations occur.

The important point to note in this brief summary of the trichromatic theories is that from their first formulation by Young to the most modern treatment, they have all been restricted to a very limited kind of physiolo-

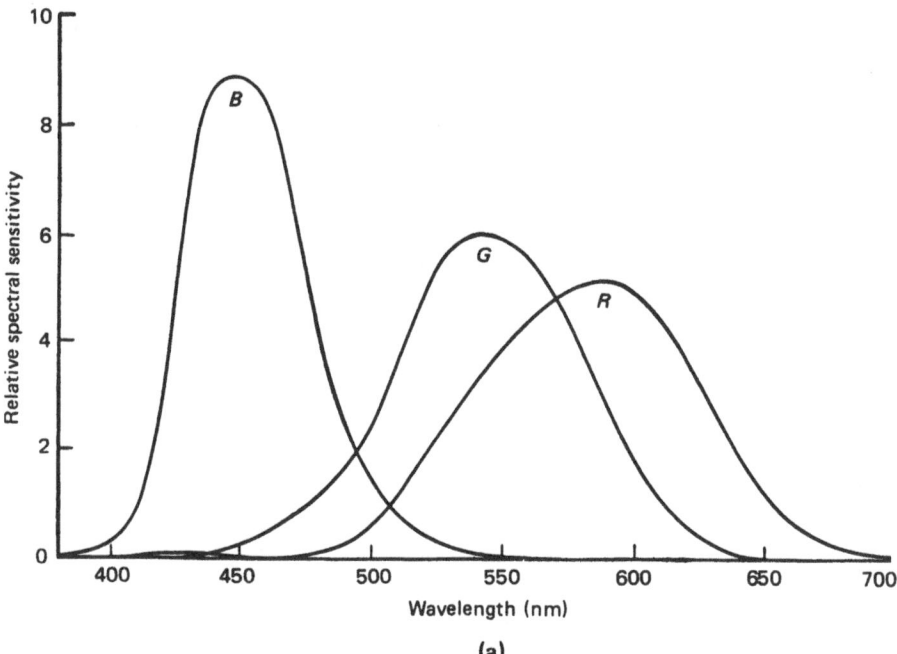

(a)

FIGURE 9.11 (a) The three fundamental spectral sensitivity curves according to the original Young and Helmholtz trichromatic theory (from Judd, 1951). (b) The three fundamental spectral sensitivity curves according to Koenig and Ladd-Franklin theories (from Judd, 1951). (c) The three fundamental spectral sensitivity curves according to Hecht (1934).

FIGURE 9.11 (Cont.)

9
8
7
6
5
4
3
2
1
0
Relative spectral sensitivity
B
G
R
400
450
500
550
600
650
700
Wavelength (nm)

(b)

Relative spectral sensitivity
B
G
R
400
500
600
700
Wavelength (nm)

(c)

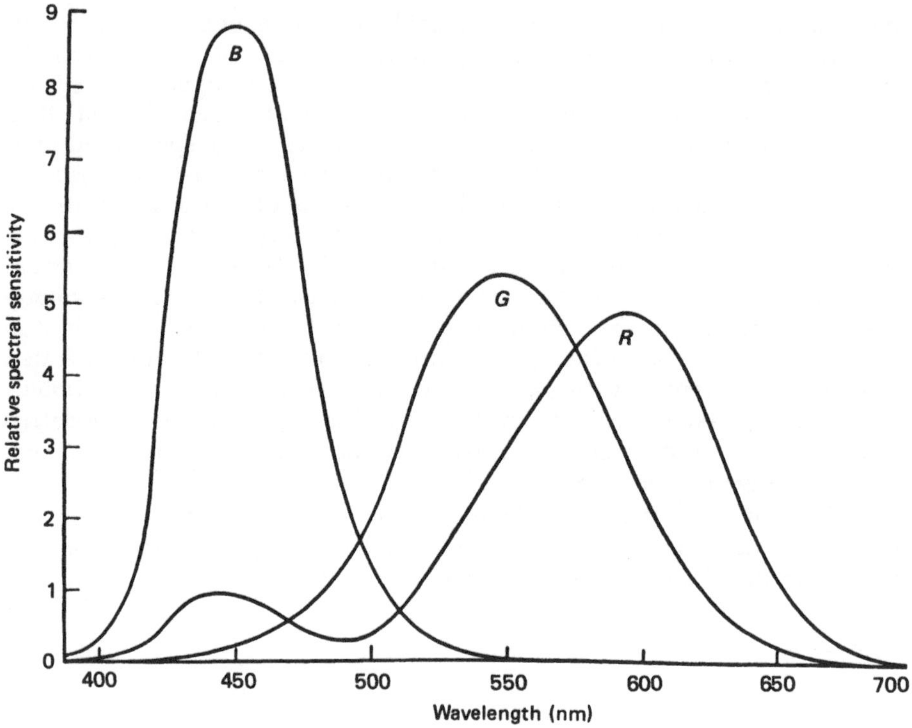

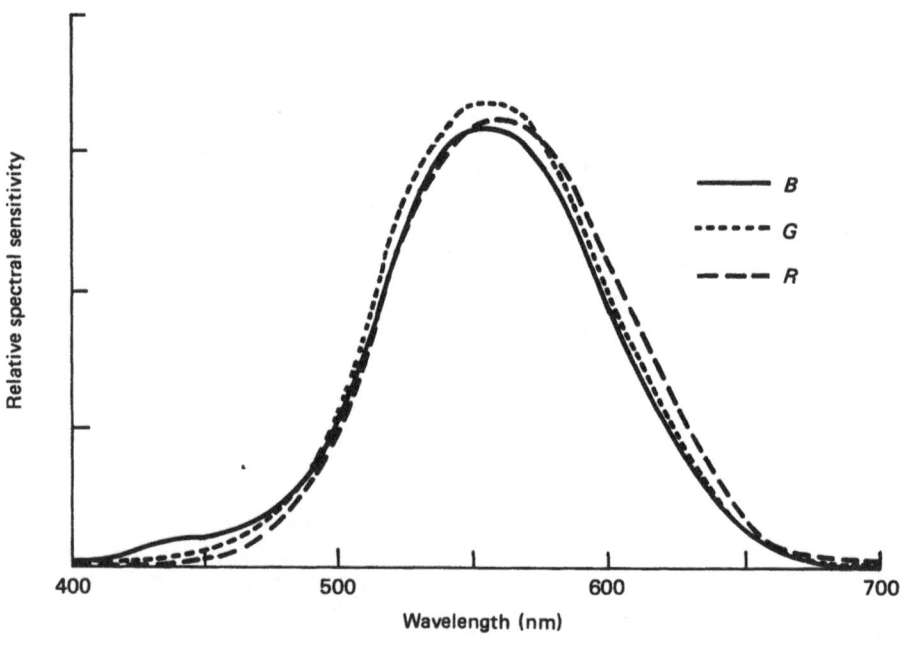

gizing. The main biological assumption, common to all of the theories, was that the retinal receptors were of three kinds. All theories imply that relative amounts of activity in adjacent neural pathways are the key code for quality, but the details are rarely spelled out. The major controversy among those who championed one or another form of the trichromatic theory was the breadth and overlap of the spectral absorption curves of the three primary colors, yet little empirical psychophysical evidence (see our previous discussion of Stiles' work as one extraordinary example) could be developed that uniquely supported any particular triad or degree of overlap. The empirical data only said that three independent manipulations of the color mixture were necessary to match any other color, but contributed nothing to the choice of any particular triad.

Thus, as one compares the various trichromatic theories of color vision that appeared over the years, it can be seen that, for the most part, they were nonphysiological, once having passed the assumption of a specific triad of absorption curves. Helmholtz's (1892) original treatment of hue discrimination on the basis of trichromatic receptors introduced the notion of a mathematical color space—in other words, a mathematical description of the color that was perceived on the basis of activation of the presumed set of three primaries. This notion of a color space and the orientation toward a theory that was primarily a mathematical description of color vision, was continued by Hecht (1930) and by Stiles (1946), and both of their descriptions are also marked by a remarkable absence of physiological detail or speculation about what is going on beyond the receptors.

B. The Opponent Color Theory

Hering (1878), influenced mostly by considerations of the psychological nature of perceived primary colors, felt that the notion of three-color receptors, all of which were essentially dormant until stimulated, was an inadequate model. Noting the linkages of various kinds that seemed to occur among various colors, he proposed the first of what is now known as the opponent color theories. Unfortunately, controversy and debate over the years have obscured a very important fact, namely, that the original version of the Hering opponent color theory with its four primary sensory colors (red, green, blue, and yellow) was also a trichromatic theory at the retinal photochemical level, and if carefully analyzed, it can be seen that Hering's original formulation really represents nothing more than an alternative set of the three retinal receptor absorption curves. He assumed the existence of a blue-yellow receptor as well as a red-green one and a black-white one. An important difference in the details of his theory, however, was that he assumed that luminous stimulation could not only lead to an increase in the amount of neural activity elicited from visual receptors, but in some situations could lead to a reduction. For example, in his hypothetical red-green unit, red increased and green decreased the base level of neural activity.

In other words, Hering's theory deeply involves the notion of spontaneous ongoing neural activity in the absence of a stimulus, which could be inhibited by lights of particular wavelengths or enhanced by other wavelengths. Not withstanding this new twist, it is often overlooked that Hering's theory is also a trichromatic one in that it also assumes that there were only three different types of photoreceptor pigments in the retina. However, rather than receptors with maximal monophasic excitatory responses in the red, green, or blue portions of the spectrum, he assumed that two contained a substance that was capable of being either broken down or regenerated, depending upon the color of the incident light. He further assumed that one of the three photochemicals was generally sensitive to either darkness or light. Hering assumed that this substance was broken down by stimulation with any wavelength light stimulus and regenerated in the dark, thus, he thought, explaining some of the information about light and dark adaptation. Another substance was sensitive to both red and green lights. In red light the substance "degenerated," but it was regenerated in green light. The third member of the triad was regenerated by blue, but degenerated under the influence of yellow light. The breakdown and regeneration of the three photopigments meant that the absorption curves of at least two had to have both negative and positive values. Figure 9.12 shows the generation-degeneration absorption curve suggested by the Hering theory. It is important to note that where the curves cross the horizontal axis, it was assumed by Hering that there was no stimulated neural activity. Thus, a blue light of about 475 nm produced no action in the red-green system, even though it substantially increased the amount of neural activity in the blue-yellow system due to the breakdown of the blue-yellow receptor substance. Similarly, there is a point on the spectrum (about 500 nm) that strongly regenerates the red-green substance, producing, presumably, a sensation of pure green, but with no yellow or blue tones. Similarly, at 575 nm, it is assumed that a pure yellow is produced without any red or green tones. At intermediate points, the colors produced are mixtures of two of the four colors of the two opponent pairs. The similarity of these curves to the Hurvich and Jameson psychophysical data should be noted, but also the differences.

In sum, then, the original Hering opponent color model was also a theory whose main biological assumption concerned the nature of the photochemicals in the peripheral receptor. Like the classic trichromatic theories, it assumed three and only three photochemicals, but said nothing at all about the nature of coding at higher levels. Hering's great contribution was to introduce the notion of opponent mechanisms into color vision discussions.

IV. THE BIOLOGICAL DATA

There is only one way to resolve many of the controversial issues concerning the neural and photochemical basis of color vision, and this is to make direct measurements of the necessary parameters from the point of view of chemistry, physics, and physiology at the various levels in the ascending pathway. To determine the nature of the true primary absorption curves of the photochemicals as well as the actual number of different types, chemical and optical studies of the wavelength-dependent response of each must be carried out. To determine whether the trichromatic notion of three overlapping excitatory response systems or the opponent hypothesis with both

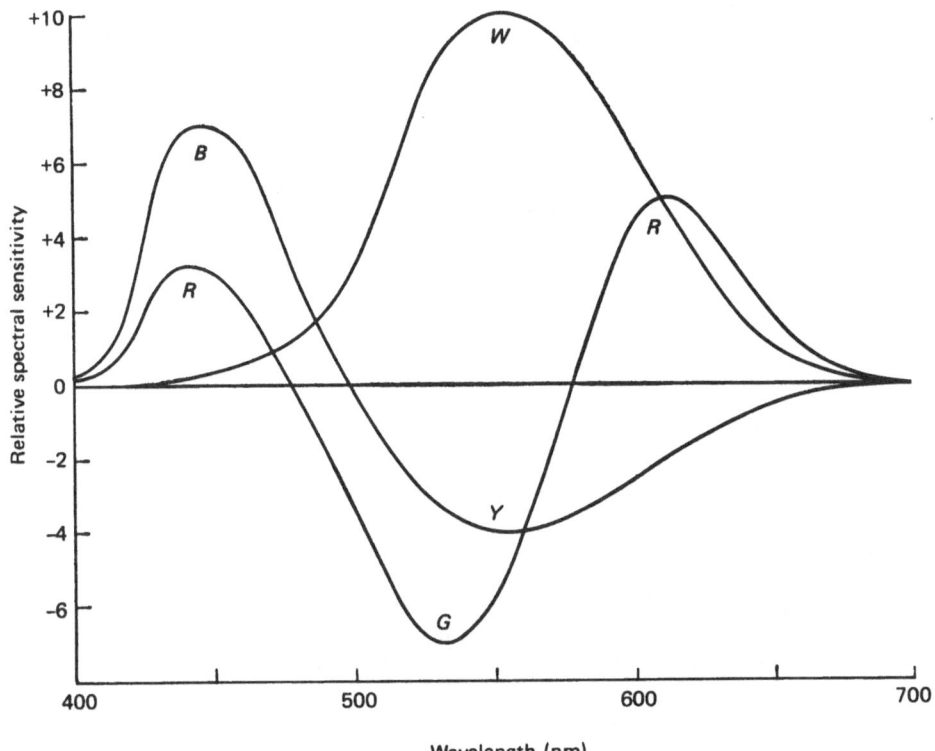

FIGURE 9.12 *The three photoreceptor absorption curves of the Hering opponent color theory, showing that both excitation and inhibition of spontaneous activity (unlike the solely excitatory processes of Figure 9.11) were thought to occur specifically in the three types of photoreceptor. The early Hering theory proposed that the R receptor was excited at both ends of the visual spectrum. The reader is cautioned to carefully note the differences between this set of hypothetical absorbtion curves and the superficially similar psychophysical data of Figure 9.10 (from Judd, 1951).*

excitatory and inhibitory processes holds at any given level of the nervous system, electrophysiological experiments must be carried out. It is the purpose of this section to specify the direct biological correlates of stimulus wavelength at each level of the ascending visual pathway.

A. The Photoreceptor

1. Rushton's Reflection Densitometry. One of the first direct optical measurements of the characteristics of cone pigments was reported by Rushton (1958), using a device that he had developed a few years earlier (Rushton, 1956). Rushton's device was essentially a very large automatic opthalmoscope as shown in Figure 9.13. The technique depends upon the fact that the pigments of the dark-adapted eye tend to absorb light, while a light-

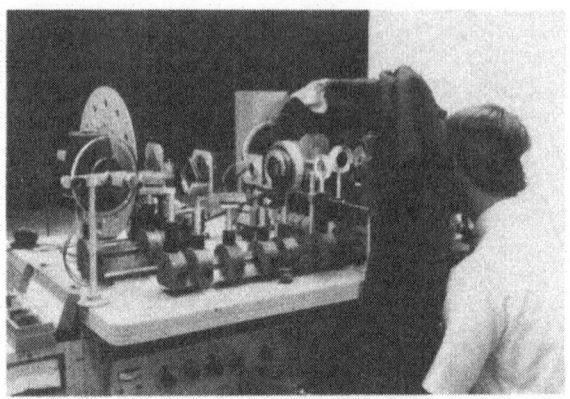

FIGURE 9.13 A photograph of Alpern's modification of the Rushton reflection densitometer, showing part of the optical chain, part of the electronics, and the subject in position (courtesy of Dr. Matthew Alpern, University of Michigan).

adapted eye reflects more of the incident light back from the rear of the eye —less light being absorbed by the bleached than by the unbleached pigment. The amount of light reflected back at the various wavelengths of the visual spectrum was determined first in the dark-adapted and then during the dark interval of a flickering adapting light. The difference between the two spectral absorption curves (the so-called difference spectrum), Rushton initially felt, directly reflected the absorption characteristics of the photoreceptor pigments.

Rushton's technique required several successive steps, which we should clarify by spelling them out in detail. First, an absorption spectrum was determined by measuring the reflected light from the dark-adapted eye. Then a second absorption curve was determined following bleaching with red light, for example. The second absorption curve was then subtracted from the first to give the difference spectrum. Then after all of the red-sensitive pigment had presumably been removed in this manner, a second bleaching was carried out, using a strong white light and a second difference spectrum calculated by subtracting a third absorption curve from the first. A typical pair of these two difference spectra is shown in Figure 9.14. The key datum is that the peak of the two difference curves has been shifted by the successive bleaches.

Rushton's early interpretation of these data was that the two difference curves predominantly reflected the absorption spectra of two different pigments, the first mainly that of a yellowish-orange-sensitive pigment with a peak absorption at about 590 nm, and the second that of a yellow-green-sensitive pigment with a peak absorption at about 540 nm. Pointing out that there was no practical way to measure the blue curve (if there indeed was one), Rushton (1958) concluded that he only had direct evidence of the absorption spectra of two of the cone pigments. In 1959, Weale used a similar technique and obtained similar data. However, sometime later, both Rushton (1964) and Ripps and Weale (1964) reinterpreted the meaning of these difference spectra and stated that they now felt that the retinal densitometry techniques do not reflect accurately the individual absorption

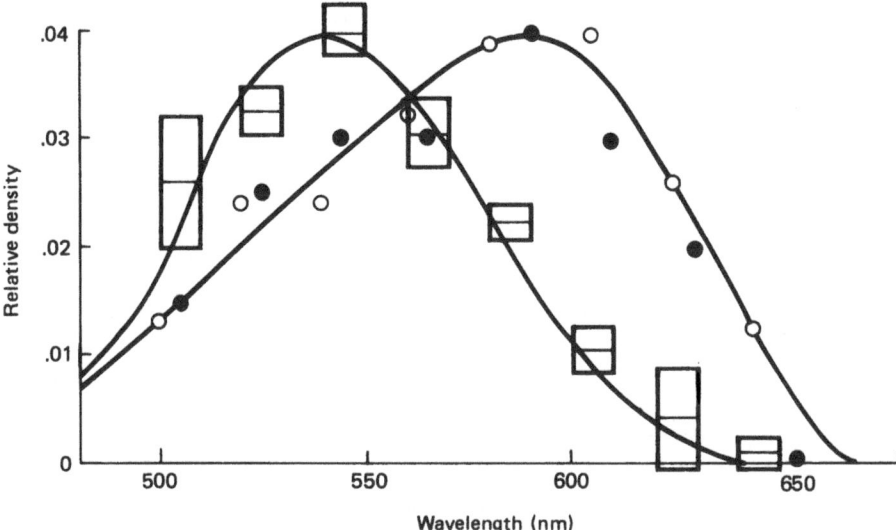

FIGURE 9.14 *Difference spectra originally believed to be of two of the normal cone pigments of the normal eye. These data are no longer believed to have that significance, but rather to be a more complicated mixture of cone response characteristics. Originally, Rushton believed that the right hand curve (tracing the course of points marked with O and •) reflected the absorbtion of a long wavelength sensitive pigment and the left hand curve (tracing the course of the rectangles) reflected the absorbtion of a medium wavelength sensitive pigment (from Rushton, 1958).*

spectra of any of the classes of the foveal cones when more than one pigment is present. In the special situation in which one of the two measurable pigments may be missing, it is probable, they believe, that valid estimates of the remaining system can be made, since any influence of the blue or short wavelength system seems to be undetectable with this technique. But, for mixtures of pigments, the results are now considered to be equivocal. Retinal densitometry is now used mainly as a means of tracing the temporal course of dark adaptation rather than as a means of specifying absorption spectra (Rushton, 1962, 1964).

Brown and Wald (1964) have also questioned the validity of the techniques of reflection densitometry as a means of specifying the spectral absorption curves of cone pigments.

2. Direct Microspectrophotometric Studies of Single Cones. In 1964 two remarkable papers, which will have the most important implications for all theories involving cone absorption spectra, were published. As noted, one of the main issues of controversy in color vision theories up to recent years has been the specification of the fundamental triad of primary colors, which were assumed to exist in the retina. All of this controversy, however, could be laid to rest if an extremely difficult technical *tour de force* could be executed, namely, the determination of the absorption spectra of individual cones in the human retina. This ideal experiment was actually carried out nearly simultaneously by two groups (Marks, Dobelle, and MacNichol, 1964, and Brown and Wald, 1964), using newly developed and nearly identical techniques of microspectrophotometric measurement.

Briefly, the procedure involves the passage of a tiny beam of light, demagnified by being passed through an inverted microscope, through a single cone. The light absorbed by the cone could be determined by comparing this tiny beam of light with another light beam that did not pass through any equivalent absorbing material. This arrangement is shown in Figure 9.15. A measurement of the difference in the energy of the two beams was made at many monochromatic wavelengths across the visual spectrum. It should be noted, however (and this point has been especially prominent in a criticism of these data by Sheppard, 1968), that only a very few cells had been sampled in this most difficult technical experiment. In fact, Brown and Wald's entire paper is based on one rod and only four cones from the extracted retina of a human cadaver, and Marks, Dobelle, and MacNichol report only the absorption curves of seven monkey cones and two human cones. Nevertheless, the agreement in their data is remarkable. Figure 9.16 shows the absorption difference spectra of the four cones measured by Brown and Wald. One peaks at 450 nm, two at 525 nm, and the fourth at 555 nm. Marks, Dobelle, and MacNichol's data, as replotted in Figure 9.17, show three groups peaking, they state, at 445 nm, 535 nm, and 570 nm, respectively.

Hopefully, if these data are substantiated and do not turn out to be sampling errors produced either accidentally or by virtue of the fact that cells with absorption spectra that fall into these particular categories are, for some reason, more likely to be sampled than others, then much of the classical controversy will be laid to rest. The major significance of this work lies in the fact that they directly and definitely specify the width and peak sensitivity of the absorption spectra of the primate color primaries. Of special interest to theories of quality coding is the fact that there are points on the spectrum at which all three curves overlap, and, thus, a stimulating light at certain wavelengths will stimulate all three receptor systems to some degree.

Unfortunately, although nearly a decade has passed since the original reports, there have been no replications or extensions of these findings reported in the literature. The presumption is that they do correctly reflect the grouping of three visual photopigments for primates, but rigorousness demands that at least a note of caution be mentioned at this point.

More extensive data for the cones of the goldfish have, however, been reported by Marks (1965). One hundred thirteen separate runs were made on single cones, using the same sort of microspectrophotometric measuring procedure described above. Figure 9.18 is a histogram, showing the peak sensitivities measured in this group of spectral response determinations. Clearly, in this case, there is also a clustering of the peaks into just three main groups centered at 455 nm, 530 nm, and 625 nm. These findings are quite comparable to the primate data, although the right group seems to peak at a longer wavelength in the goldfish than in the primate.

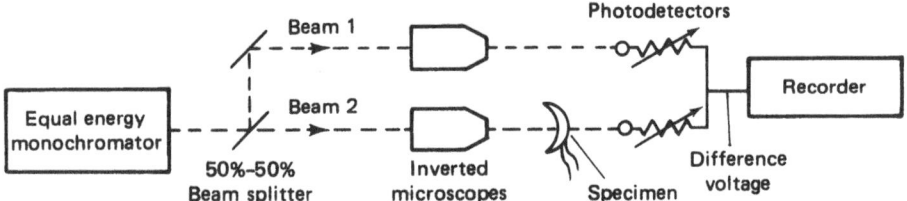

FIGURE 9.15 *Diagram of the components of a recording microspectrophotometer. The output beam of a constant energy monochromater, is split by a half silvered mirror. Both half beams are demagnified by inverted microscopes. Beam 1 then passes through the specimen, while Beam 2, the reference beam, does not. The differences in the balanced output of a pair of matched photodetectors is, then, a direct measure of the absorbance of the specimen as the wavelength of the illuminating light is scanned.*

3. Electroretinographic Studies. The electroretinogram, the long-lasting graded potential produced by the retina when it is stimulated with light, can also provide a means of indirectly estimating the absorption characteristics of visual cones. This technique has been applied both to human and infrahuman preparations in a number of different ways. Witkovsky (1968) and Burkhardt (1968), in a pair of articles published simultaneously, both examined the effects of chromatic adaptation on the electroretinogram of the carp and goldfish, respectively. While different components of the electroretinogram responded in somewhat different manners, all of their data were consistent with the notion that adaptation with different colored lights and measurement of the *b* wave of the ERG produced a very few residual response curves with different peak sensitivities. Both of the authors considered this to be indicative of the fact that the photoreceptors were of a small number of different types and that each type was filled with chemicals that had their peak absorption at relatively widely spaced points. Although, as we noted in our chapter on transduction, the spectral absorption curves of different animals will differ slightly because of the species-specific details of the opsin, it is interesting to compare the peak absorptions suggested by the data from these animals with those of the previous section on primates. Witkovsky concluded that the residual ERG action spectra following chromatic adaptation obtained from the carp reflected the effects of four pigments with absorptions peaking at 482 nm, 517 nm, and 660 nm, respectively. Burkhardt, however, working with the goldfish, was only able to specify the peak sensitivity of the blue and red receptor system that appeared to peak at 450 nm and 620 nm, respectively.

The electroretinogram has also been used with human subjects by Riggs, Johnson, and Schick (1966) in an ingenious manner. A stimulus pattern consisting of alternating bars of different color lights was presented to the observer. The intensities of the two lights were adjusted to produce equal electroretinographic responses. However, when the pattern was displaced, the chromatic change induced an electroretinographic response, which was presumably independent of the luminosity of the stimuli. The

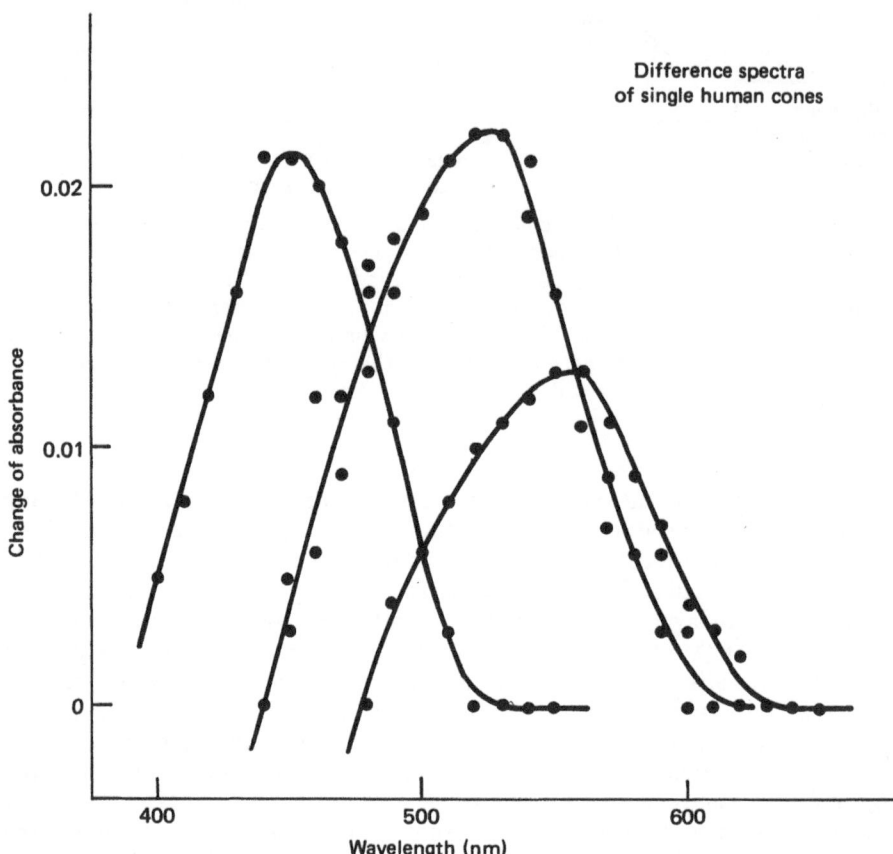

FIGURE 9.16 *The difference spectra, following bleaching with yellow light, of four human cones, measured by a direct microspectrophotometric procedure. One code peaks in the blue, two in the yellow-green, and one in the red. The color names "blue," "red," etc. are used here and elsewhere in our discussion of the biological data as a shorthand for the wavelength of the photic stimulus to which the receptor is most sensitive (from Brown and Wald, 1964).*

major factor determining the amplitude of this evoked response was the absolute difference in wavelength between the two colored lights. Riggs and his colleagues interpreted their data to be consistent with a trichromatic receptor system in the retina, but were scrupulously careful in noting that it was not possible to calculate specific spectral absorption curves on the basis of these data without making certain assumptions which, they felt, could not be justified on the basis of their results.

4. *Electrophysiological Recordings from Single Cones.* Another type of experiment, which can be used to determine the nature of the cone absorption spectra, is one in which the neural responses of individual photoreceptive elements are investigated. In this manner, the problem of analyzing the

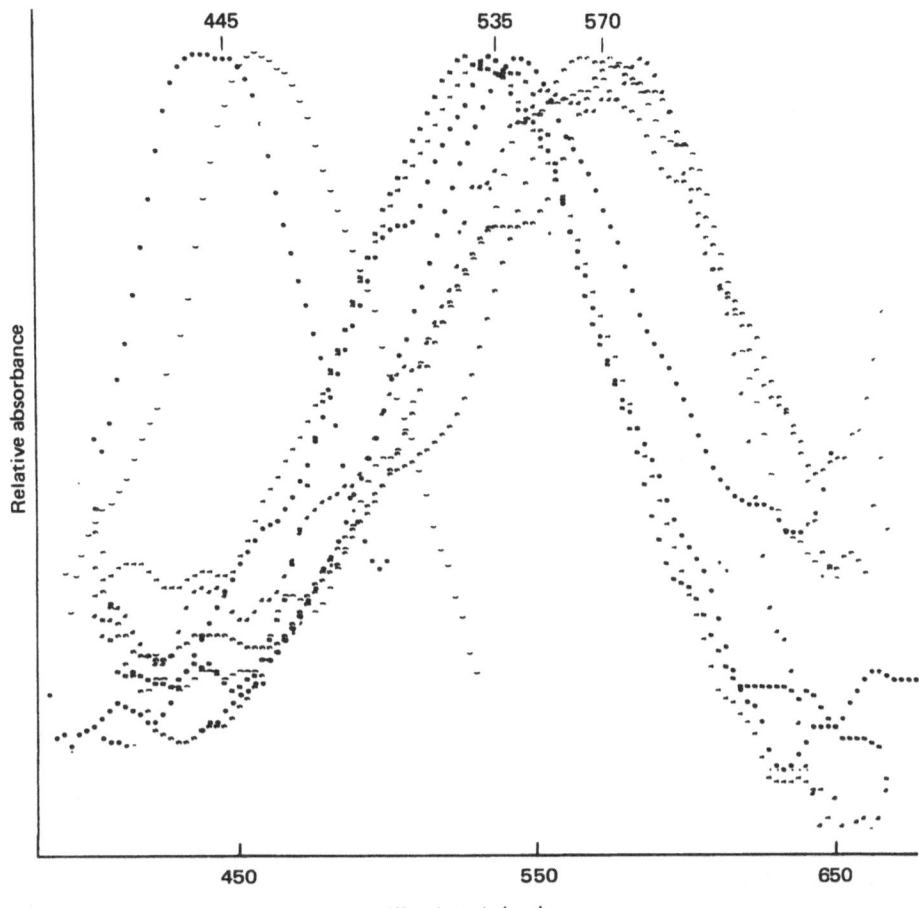

FIGURE 9.17 *Absorption spectra for 10 primate cones, showing the clustering of the responses into three different groups peaking in the blue, yellow-green, and red portions of the spectrum (from Marks, Dobelle, and MacNichol, 1964).*

complex integrated responses of a number of intermixed photoreceptor types with overlapping sensitivities is avoided. Because of the very small size of the vertebrate cone, such an experiment is technically extremely difficult, and its successful execution would be a *tour de force* of the highest order. Yet the task of inserting a microelectrode into a single cone has been accomplished on a number of different species. The first group to do so used the carp as their experimental animal (Oikawa, Ogawa, and Moto-kawa, 1959). However, we shall discuss a more recent study by Tomita, Kaneko, Murakami, and Pautler (1967), who also used the carp, but whose advances in technique allowed the accumulation of a much higher quality data base.

The success of a complex experiment, such as the one to be described here, often depends upon rather curious, and at first glance trivial, changes

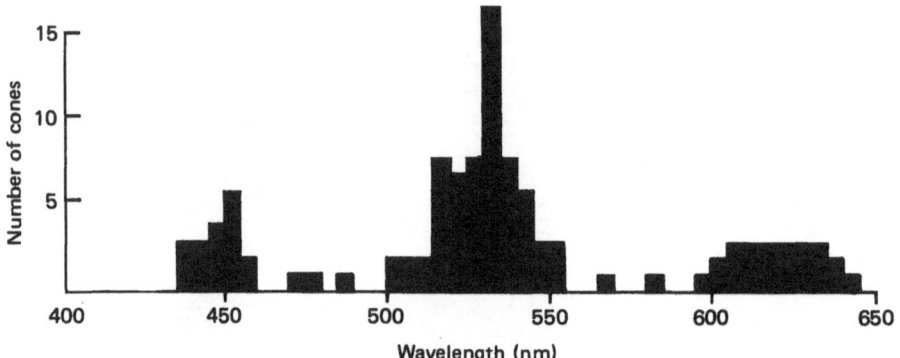

FIGURE 9.18 A histogram showing the peaks of the absorbance spectra of 113 goldfish cones, displaying the striking clustering into three different groups with sensitivities in the blue, yellow-green, and red portions of the spectrum (from Marks, 1965).

in procedure. Two important, though small, procedural developments were of special consequence in this study. Because the cone in the carp retina is so small, an ultramicroscopic capillary electrode was required to avoid massive destruction as the electrode penetrated the cell wall. Tomita and his group (Tomita, Murakami, Hashimoto, and Sasaki, 1961) had developed techniques for drawing out glass microelectrodes with points as fine as 0.1 μ. These electrodes, however, were still not sufficiently small to easily penetrate the cone cell membrane when they were simply advanced by a micromanipulator. The cell wall was sufficiently elastic so that the slowly moving microelectrode simply stretched the membrane under the low level of accelerative forces so generated. Tomita and his colleagues, therefore, invented a device that "jolted" the stage on which the retina was mounted as the electrode was advanced. The higher accelerations produced by this delicate jolting were sufficient to overcome the elasticity of the cell wall, and the electrode then penetrated into the interior of the cone. With this instrumentation, they were able to record a graded dc hyperpolarizing potential when the cone was stimulated by light. This potential was presumably the receptor potential itself and varied in amplitude depending upon the wavelength of the stimulating light. Incidentally, as noted in Chapter 4, it is now believed that all vertebrate visual receptor potentials are hyperpolarizations, suggesting that the effect of the breakdown products of the photochemical may be to reduce the membrane permeability rather than to increase it. This is confirmed by other experiments in which constant electrical currents are passed through the photoreceptor. Voltage measurements made during the period the stimulating light is on show a relatively large increase over those obtained during the dark period. A simple application of Ohm's laws dictates that this must be the result of increased membrane resistance, which is the same thing as decreased permeability. In invertebrates, most analogous receptor potentials appear

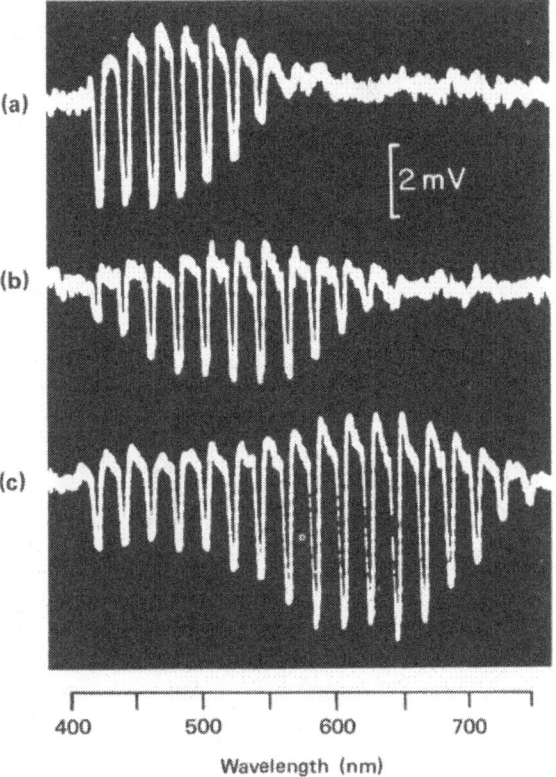

FIGURE 9.19 Graded potentials recorded from three different classes of carp cones exemplifying peak sensitivities in the blue, yellow-green, and red portions of the visual spectrum. The responses in this figure, it must be clearly noted, are not spikes, but are brief graded potentials produced by stimulating the cones with brief, though equal energy spectral pulses. Also note that the response to light is a hyperpolarization in all of these cases, downward being negative (from Tomita, Kaneko, Murakami, and Pautler, 1967).

to be depolarizing and probably result from increases in membrane permeability.

The exact site of entry of the microelectrode would, of course, be of some interest. The very small cross section of the outer segment of the cone makes it unlikely that Tomita's group had actually entered that part of the cell. Indeed, using an electrophoretic dye injection technique, Kaneko and Hashimoto (1967) subsequently showed that the electrode in these experiments was usually located in the inner segment of the carp's cone.

An automatic monochromator was used by Tomita and his colleagues to produce visual stimuli at wavelength intervals of 20 nm. The amplitude of the evoked receptor potential was recorded photographically for each wavelength interval from the face of a CRT, which had its x axis coupled to the wavelength control of the monochromator. The automaticity of the device was very important because even with these fine electrodes, a cone could be held active only for a few minutes. In 40 sec, an entire spectral response curve could be determined for an impaled cell ranging over the spectrum from 400 to 740 nm. A sample output of this scanning procedure is shown in Figure 9.19 for three cells typical of the population, which was more or less randomly sampled every time an electrode was advanced into

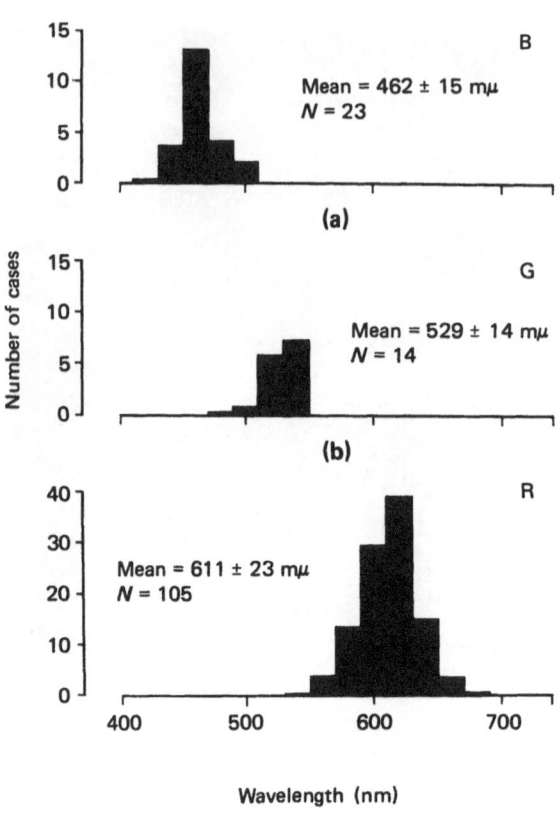

FIGURE 9.20 Histograms of the peak sensitivities of a larger sample of the three classes of cone responses shown in Figure 9.19. Once again it is clear that the cones in this animal have absorption spectra, which cluster into three widely spaced groups (from Tomita, Kaneko, Murakami, and Pautler, 1967).

the retina. The maximum amplitude of any of these negative-going receptor potentials is only 5 mV, yet the response curves are relatively smooth and noise free, a signal-to-noise ratio characteristic of the fine technique of this group.

Tomita and his colleagues were able to record the spectral response curves of 142 cells sufficiently well to include them in their analyses. The analyses are summarized in the histograms of Figure 9.20(a), (b), and (c). Three groups of response curves appear to emerge from this analysis. The spectral absorption curve does vary slightly from one cell to another in the retina of this fish, but whether this is true variation in the absorption characteristics or merely an artifact of these low-amplitude signals cannot be determined. Nevertheless, it is clear that there is a group of receptors whose peak sensitivity is in the short wavelengths at about 462 nm, a medium wavelength sensitive group with a peak sensitivity of 529 nm, and a long wavelength sensitive group with a peak sensitivity of 611 nm. Tomita and his colleagues also pooled all of their data for each group and plotted three average spectral absorption curves they believed to be representative of the total population. This is presented in Figure 9.21, and it can be seen that once again the familiar picture obtains—three relatively broadly tuned classes of receptors with peak sensitivities as indicated above. It should also be noticed that the long wavelength-sensitive pigment seems to have a

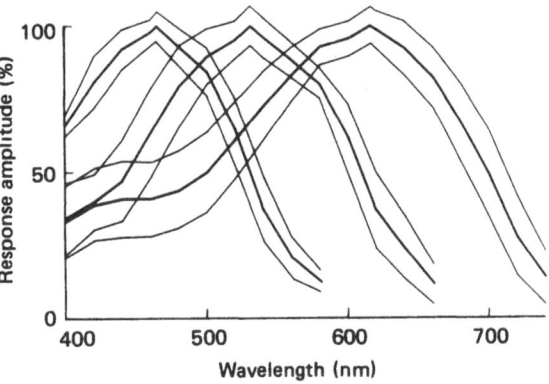

FIGURE 9.21 The average absorption spectra for the data of Figure 9.20. This figure further emphasizes the fact that the response curves are broadly tuned in relation to the full visual spectrum. Both mean values and variance limits are shown in this figure (from Tomita, Kaneko, Murakami, and Pautler, 1967).

sensitive tail, which extends well down into the shorter regions of the spectrum, and that this is fairly typical of most of the spectral functions we have discussed. The "red" pigment, therefore, is sensitive across almost the entire spectrum—a very broad band tuning indeed.

5. A Brief Summary of Retinal Color Coding. All of the data presented so far in this section support the conclusion that Young was essentially correct 170 years ago when he hypothesized three more or less broadly tuned receptors with peak sensitivities in the red, yellow-green, and blue portions of the spectrum. Collectively, these data put to rest a number of persistent controversies. With the exceptions of those practical applications of color mixture which may, for some procedural reason, require some other triad of primaries, there is no justification, theoretical or otherwise, for assuming any other triads of primaries than the ones identified by these studies. The narrowly spaced primaries of Hecht (1934) and Hurvich and Jameson (1957), though interesting, are simply nonphysiological and must be considered to be only mathematical fictions, which can exist only because of the fact that there is no psychophysically unique set in trichromatic color matching. Similarly, there is no evidence of any opponent process at the receptor level, all response functions being monophasic.

Acknowledging the fact that the data described above have been collected on several different species and that species differences do often lead to shifts in peak sensitivities, it still may be of some use to summarize the information contained in this section. This has been done in Table 9.2, which lists the peaks of the triad as determined in each of the physiological studies we have discussed in addition to the psychophysical studies (Stiles, 1949, 1959, Wald, 1964, 1966) which bear on this problem. In spite of the species differences and the differences in technique in each laboratory, the agreement among these measurements is quite high. There is little evidence of any fourth receptor in the yellow region, a fact that also puts to rest some notions of "primary yellow," or for that matter any sort of opponent process at the retinal level. But therein, of course, lies the rub, for as we ascend to the very next accessible level of neural coding—the bipolar layer of the retina—the picture changes in a surprising way.

TABLE 9.2. THE PEAK SPECTRAL SENSITIVITIES OF
TRICHROMATIC RETINAS DERIVED FROM SEVERAL SOURCES*

Study	Species	"B"	"G"	"R"
Brown and Wald, 1964	Man	450	525	555
Marks, Dobelle, and MacNichol, 1964	Man Monkey	445	535	570
Marks, 1965	Goldfish	455	530	625
Witkovsky, 1968	Carp	482	517	580, 660
Burkhardt, 1968	Goldfish	450		620
Tomita *et al.* (1967)	Carp	462	529	611
Stiles (Psychophysics) (1949, 1959)	Man	440	540	575
Wald (Psychophysics) (1964, 1966)	Man	430	540	575

* Note particularly that there are only two different groups of animals involved–primates
and teleost fish–and that two of the studies are psychophysical ones. This table clearly shows
that widely spaced visual primaries with peak sensitivities as indicated must now be accepted.
Trichomatic retinas have not, however, yet been demonstrated in other animals.

B. Color Coding Beyond the Photoreceptors

1. *The Retinal Horizontal and Bipolar Layers.* As thoroughly compelling as
the findings are that the photoreceptors are organized into a broadly tuned
trichromatic system, there is no *a priori* reason to believe either that the
coding schema remains the same or, for that matter, that it changes drastically as the signal ascends to higher portions of the visual pathway. The
basic premise of coding theory is that the representation scheme of patterns
of stimulus information may vary at different levels.

As if nature wanted to emphasize this point, we shall discover when
we consider the data for those cells that synapse with the receptors in the
outer plexiform layer—the bipolars and horizontal cells that they encode
color information in a completely different way than do the receptors. The
beginning of the story is actually based upon a misinterpretation of some
data that had originally been presented by Svaetician (1956) as representative of cone electropotentials. Later, MacNichol and Svaetician (1958) and
Svaetician and MacNichol (1958) modified this conclusion and stated that
the potentials they recorded in their experiments actually originated in the
inner nuclear layer.

The general procedure in these experiments was to insert a very fine
glass microelectrode into the retina of a fish. The potentials recorded, like
those recorded at the level of the photoreceptor, were purely graded signals

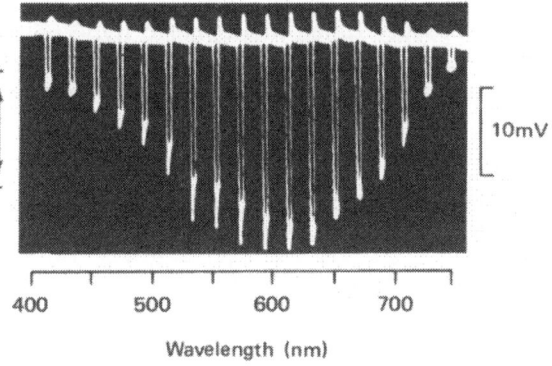

FIGURE 9.22 One type of graded potential obtained from the bipolar layer. In this example, the cell produces a hyperpolarization when stimulated with almost any wavelength light. This response, like that of the cone, is not a spike response, but only a series of brief graded potentials produced by equal energy stimulating pulses (from Tomita, 1965).

of varying amplitude with no evidence of spiking. The response functions recorded in their experiments, as the wavelength of the incident light was varied, were of two kinds. First, there were cells that had a very broad spectral sensitivity and responded solely by producing a graded hyperpolarization of varying amplitude. Figure 9.22 shows the response pattern of one of these cells. However, another major class of cells, which had a completely different pattern of response, was also recorded. With these cells, as the spectrum was scanned, the response of the slow potentials changed from a depolarizing to a hyperpolarizing response. Figure 9.23 shows the form of the response function produced by a cell that hyperpolarized in the blue region of the spectrum, but depolarized when the stimulating light was in the red end of the spectrum. Svaetician also originally reported the presence of cells that depolarized when the stimulating light was in the blue end of the spectrum, but hyperpolarized when the light was in the longer wavelengths, but in the later papers these findings could not be replicated. MacNichol and Svaetician (1958) associate the monophasic hyperpolarizing response with certain giant horizontal cells, while the opponent responses were assumed to be the product of bipolar cell activity.

However, the picture may be even more complicated than as described by Svaetician and his co-workers. Tomita (1965) has found that in addition

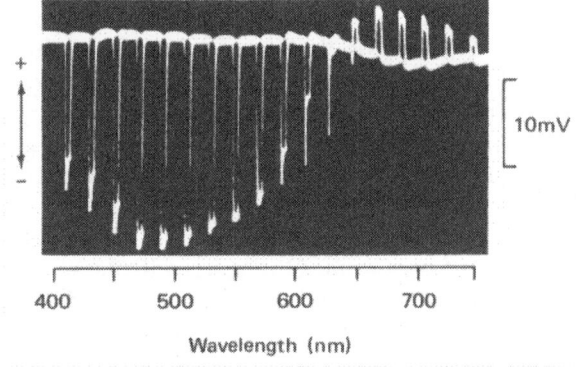

FIGURE 9.23 An opponent type of bipolar layer response. This response is also a graded potential and not a spike response. The cell hyperpolarizes in the blue-green end of the spectrum and depolarizes in the yellow-red end (from Tomita, 1965).

to the broadly tuned monophasic hyperpolarizing cells, and the cells that had adjacent spectral regions of hyperpolarization and depolarization, some cells (probably bipolars) in the inner nuclear layer responded with a triphasic response, which was hyperpolarizing at both ends of the spectrum, but depolarized in the middle range of spectral stimuli. The response of such a cell is shown in Figure 9.24.

The important general point that is made by the data is that the coding schema for colors has already begun to change at the second stage of neural processing. Considering the possible complexity of the interconnectives between the photoreceptors and the inner nuclear layer, this transformation can be understood, but it is still a surprising turn of events, for in one synaptic leap we are beginning to find elements of an opponent color system! Perhaps some of Hering's intuitions concerning color coding were not too farfetched, regardless of the fact that his theory of the photoreceptive process is so clearly wrong.

2. Amacrine Cells and the Ganglion Cells of the Optic Nerve. Third level neurons in the retina—the amacrine and ganglion cells—introduce a new factor into the coding scheme. Werblin and Dowling (1969) have shown in the mudpuppy, at least, that, unlike the receptors, these cells are able to propagate regenerative spike action potentials. Thus, the symbols available in the coding language are now different.

Although not very much is known of color coding in the amacrine cells, since the axons of the ganglion cells make up the optic nerve they are relatively accessible. Surprisingly, when one considers the relative ease with which ganglion cell potentials can be recorded (compared to bipolar responses, for example), there is a relatively contradictory set of data concerning color coding at this level. The first studies of their neural processing were carried out by Granit, who has summarized the main ideas of his work in an important book (Granit, 1955). Unfortunately, while the theoretical influence of Granit's book is still continuing, the details of his experimental work on ganglion cell color coding do not seem to have had the same persistence.

Let us consider one of Granit's papers in detail to understand the sort of findings he obtained and the techniques he used. Granit (1945) inserted glass insulated metal microelectrodes through the cornea into the retina of a cat. The signals that were recorded in this manner were trains of spike activity. The relative spectral sensitivity was measured by scanning with an equal energy spectrum after selective adaptation with colored lights. The number of responses that occurred in a fixed period of time was used as the response measure, but were normalized so that the strongest responses were indicated at 100 percent.

In this 1945 paper, Granit reported finding two different general classes of receptors. One group displayed relatively narrow (about 50 nm wide at the half bandwidth level with moderate stimulus intensities) spectral sensitivity curves, with center wavelengths at about 460, 540, and 600 nm. Figure 9.25 shows a set typical of this first class. In line with his previous work, he referred to those cells as the chromatic modulators and associ-

FIGURE 9.24 Another kind of bipolar layer graded response. In this case, the cell is not simply opponent, but is actually triphasic in response form. This particular cell hyperpolarizes in the short wavelengths, depolarizes in a middle band of stimuli, and then hyperpolarizes once again for even longer stimulus wavelengths (from Tomita, 1965).

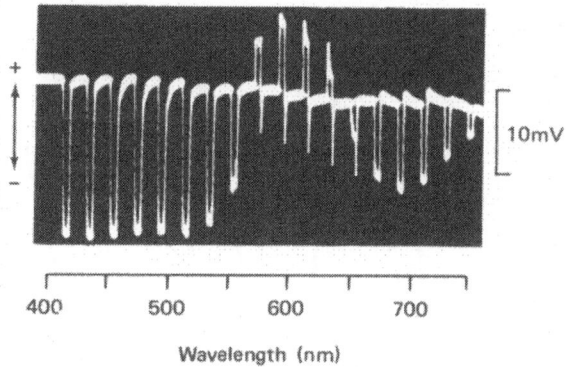

Wavelength (nm)

ated them specifically with the color receptors of the retina, although it seems almost certain now that a normal cat is really a dichromat and has only two kinds of cones. The second class of ganglion cell fiber observed in the cat's eye was characterized by a very broad spectral range—almost 125 nm wide at the half bandwidth level in some cases. Two types of these broadly tuned cells were observed. One had a peak sensitivity near that of the scotopic luminosity curve, and it was, therefore, referred to as a scotopic dominator, while the other had a peak near that of the photopic luminosity curve and was referred to as the photopic dominator. In all, the five different types of cells, three "modulators" and two "dominators," provided the basis for Granit's "modulator-dominator" theory of neural coding. It must be clearly noted that this theory assumes a trichromatic basis for color coding at the level of the ganglion cells. Granit is quite specific about this point (see pages 134–135 of Granit, 1955). Thus, modulator-dominator theory is just another version of the now-familiar Young-Helmholtz theory, but expressed in neurophysiological terms at the ganglion cell level.

However, the results of another important study of ganglion cell responses carried out by Wagner, MacNichol, and Wolbarsht (1960) on goldfish retinas led these investigators to conclude that the neural coding mechanisms in the ganglion cells were opponent rather than trichromatic in nature. In this case, however, the term "opponent" has a different meaning. In the more peripheral levels of the retina, opponent mechanisms were reflected as decreases or increases in the level of polarization of a cell membrane and were thus graded potentials. In the ganglion cell, we are now talking about rates of spike firing, and the opponent mechanism is reflected by a decrease or increase away from the spontaneous spiking frequency. The amplitude of the specific neural response involved—the spike—of course, remains constant.

Wagner and his colleagues used microelectrodes made of a platinum and iridium alloy to record ganglion cell potentials from the excised retina of goldfish. Their data indicate a much more complicated pattern of action than the one suggested by Granit. For example, in addition to the differential opponent spike rate response, the color of the incident light also

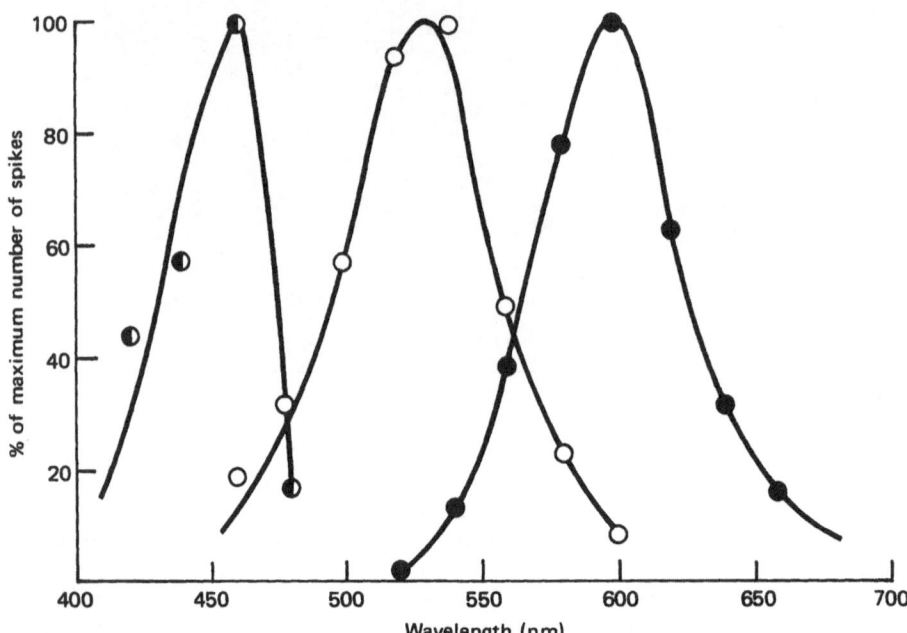

FIGURE 9.25 *Three spectral response curves for ganglion cells of the class that Granit referred to as modulators. This sort of finding was the basis of his assertion that there was a trichromatic system at the ganglion cell level of the retina. This assertion is not now believed to be correct (from Granit, 1945).*

strongly affected the temporal "on" and "off" responses of the cells. Some cells were stimulated to respond with a burst of activity at the beginning of the stimulus when the stimulus was of a short wavelength, while at longer wavelengths the response produced was a purely "off" response. Other cells behaved in just the opposite fashion. The spontaneous activity of some cells was inhibited by a stimulus. Some cells fired in a sustained manner rather than in an "on-off" fashion. To further complicate the picture, some cells changed their pattern of response as the intensity of the stimulating light varied.

Figure 9.26 shows the pattern of response of a typical opponent cell that produced "on" responses for wavelengths about 500 nm, and "off" responses for wavelengths greater than 600 nm, and combined "on-off" responses in the middle regions of the wavelength spectrum. The two separate "on" and "off" curves were interpreted by Wagner and his colleagues as being representative of opponent color mechanisms, but in this case the main coding mechanism appeared to be the relative amount of "on" and "off" activity rather than the opposite polarity of response observed in the bipolar cells. Motokawa, Yamashita, and Ogawa (1960), in a study aimed at the general problem of receptive fields of the carp's ganglion cell, report data that essentially support the Wagner, MacNichol, and Wolbarsht findings.

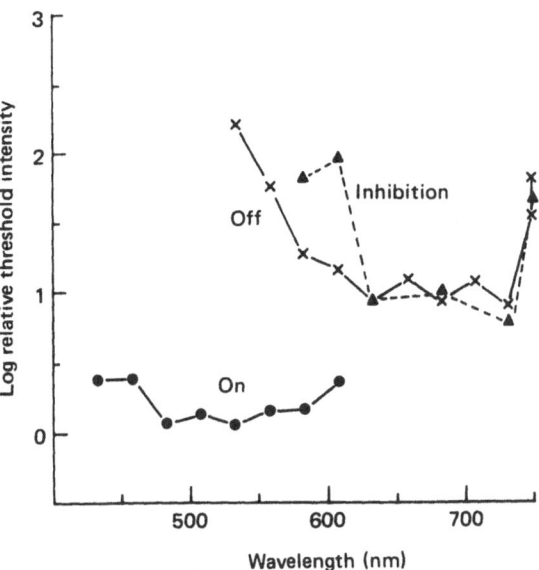

FIGURE 9.26 Another form of ganglion cell spectral sensitivity, in which the "on" and "off" spike responses of the same cell have quite distinct spectral sensitivities. This is another unusual form of opponent process. The vertical coordinate indicates the intensity of the stimulus required to produce a criterion response (from Wagner, MacNichol, and Wolbarsht, 1960).

Thus, the data that have been obtained by Granit (see p. 503), on the one hand, and by Wagner, and by Motokawa and their respective colleagues, on the other, are quite contradictory. Whether this is a species difference (which is unlikely considering the variety of species Granit used) or is due to some other procedural differences cannot be determined at this time, and future experiments will have to definitively unravel the apparent contradiction. Considering the coding mechanisms in prior and successive levels, it appears that Granit's work is misleading in some way, but of this we cannot be certain, for in addition to the temporal complexities we have just mentioned, some new work suggests there are also some chromatic-spatial interactions involved in the receptive field organization of these cells that further complicate the subject of ganglion cell color coding.

Daw (1968) and Gouras (1968) have both been interested in the receptive field structure of the color-sensitive ganglion cells of the goldfish and monkey, respectively. Both experimenters find that each animal displays a center-surround antagonistic receptive field arrangement similar to that we have already discussed for monochromatic stimuli in Chapter 9. But in this case not only did the temporal and spatial dimensions interact, but the chromatic dimensions of the stimulus also became involved in a very intricate way. Perhaps the complexity of the interaction can best be emphasized by simply quoting one of Daw's summary statements, which holds, in general if not in detail, also for Gouras' findings in the monkey.

> Most cells (49%, Type O) also gave a peripheral response with an "on" response to green light, and an "off" response to red light in the periphery, as well as an "on" response to red light and an "off" response to green light in the centre (or vice versa).
>
> (DAW, 1968, p. 567.)

This is an extreme example of a case in which one neural code—the spike frequency pattern—is overlappingly sensitive to many aspects (space, time, and quality in this case) of the stimulus and probably contributes to the definition of equally many dimensions of the perceived experience.

The main point of these findings from the ganglion cell is to emphasize the variety of functions contributing to the response of this third-order cell. In addition to the ones we have already measured, the overall spatial and temporal pattern of the stimulus is certainly also involved. For example, the spatial distribution of the stimulus can also produce differential effects. One reason that Granit's findings may have diverged so much from these other studies is that he often used diffuse light stimuli. Many of these effects occur only with more localized stimuli. On the other hand, Daw also reports that his effects are maximized when the spots are not very tiny, but of some intermediate size.

Another point made by Gouras is also important to note. One of the two types of ganglion cells observed by him seemed to be sensitive to the output of two types of cones in a way that is not too dissimilar to the opponent mechanisms we have so far discussed. The other type of ganglion cell was, however, more like a simple trichromatic mechanism, although it, too, could be both inhibited and excited, depending upon the portion of the receptive field in which a particular color stimulus fell. Thus, even at the ganglion level, there appears to be some redundancy in the coding as well as the overlapping we have just described. Clearly, we have here a most complicated example of overlapping and redundant coding, of which the whole story has not as yet been told.

3. The Lateral Geniculate Body. The next stage of neural processing for which data are available is the thalamus. The ganglion cell axons, which make up the optic nerve and optic tract, ascend without any further synaptic interaction until they arrive at the thalamic lateral geniculate bodies, and, therefore, little integration or recoding of any consequence can occur between the retina and this central level. Most of our knowledge of chromatic coding in the lateral geniculate body is based on the work of DeValois and his colleagues (DeValois, Smith, Kitai, and Karoly, 1958; DeValois, 1960; DeValois, Jacobs, and Jones, 1963; DeValois, 1965; DeValois, Abramov and Jacobs, 1966; DeValois and Jacobs, 1968). DeValois, Abramov, and Jacobs' paper (1966) is the best summary source, and it is upon this paper that we shall concentrate our attention.

The general technique used by DeValois and his colleagues was to drive KCl-filled glass microelectrodes into the various layers of the monkey's lateral geniculate body and thus more or less randomly sample the pattern of activity of single cells during periods of stimulation with spectral colors. Because of the relative size of the cells and the electrode and of the response magnitude, they felt that all of their recordings were probably extracellular. The potentials recorded in their experiments were not graded potentials, but bursts of spike activity similar to those recorded in the ganglion cell axons of the optic nerve.

DeValois had earlier shown that the activity induced in the various layers of a cat's lateral geniculate differed with regard to their time course rather than representing the chromaticity of the stimulus. [A separate representation of red, green, and blue responses from each eye in each of the six layers had been hypothesized by Le Gros Clark (1949) to explain the multilayered anatomical organization of this thalamic center. But this idea was definitively dispatched by these new findings.] Some layers contained cells that predominately produced "off" responses, some "on" responses, and some both "on" and "off" responses, but all color information was represented in all six layers by one or another of these coding mechanisms.

All of the cells that were encountered displayed moderate amounts of spontaneous activity, usually varying between 5 and 10 spikes/sec, and as we shall see, this spontaneous activity was absolutely critical in characterizing the response pattern of each cell. After a cell was located, brief flash stimulation with 12 different wavelengths of light was used to determine the relative response of the cell as a function of the chromaticity of the stimulus.

Over the course of the experiment, DeValois and his co-workers were able to study 147 cells that displayed some sort of chromatic response function. These cells divided into two groups. One group produced a response function which was such that in one part of the spectrum the steady firing was increased by the stimulus, while in another part of the spectrum the activity was decreased. These cells were termed spectrally opponent cells. One example of such a cell's response is given in Figure 9.27 as a function of stimulus wavelength. On the other hand, a second group of cells, which either uniformly increased or uniformly decreased its activities as the stimulus flashes scanned across the spectrum, was also found. These cells were termed nonopponent excitors or nonopponent inhibitors, respectively.

The opponent cells were further classifiable into four different groups, depending upon the spectral locus of the excitatory and inhibitory region. Two long wavelength excitatory types exhibited peaks in the red and yellow regions, while two short wavelength excitators exhibited peak increases in their activity either in a green or blue region.

Typical spectral sensitivity curves for the six different types of cell are shown in Figure 9.28(a) through (f). DeValois, Abramov, and Jacobs conclude by suggesting that the spectrally opponent cells are the ones primarily responsible for the representation of color, whereas the overall brightness information is represented by both the inhibitory and excitatory nonopponent cells. Once again, at this level it is clear that simple notions of trichromaticity do not well describe the behavior of the sample cells.

The data obtained in these experiments emphasize a number of other important facts. First, whatever is the spectral sensitivity and the nature of the coding of the individual neurons that represent chromaticity throughout the ascending visual pathways, there is virtually no evidence of any very narrow or narrowly spaced spectral sensitivity curves. Rather, it seems always to be the case that relatively broad and broadly spaced response curves are found. DeValois' work also suggests one other important point, namely, that the relative amount of activity among the three or four systems is probably more important than the absolute amount of neural activity in a single system in the representation of chromatic information.

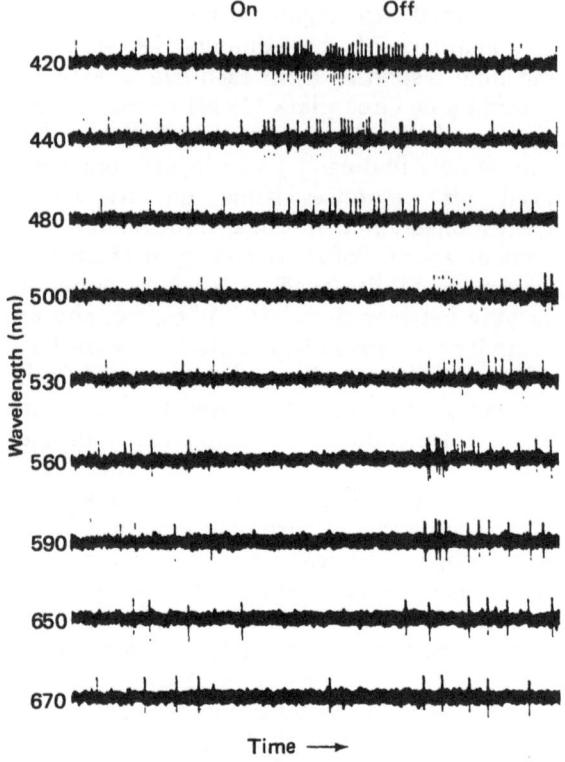

FIGURE 9.27 A sample of the type of opponent response observed in a lateral geniculate neuron as a function of the frequency of the stimulating light. In the short wavelength end of the spectrum, this cell produced a substantial "on" response. In the long wavelength end, it produced a substantial "off" response. This is another form of opponent coding (from DeValois, 1965).

A significant caveat, which might be worthwhile to mention concerning this and related work that deal with the response of cells with varying levels of spontaneous activity, is that there always remains the possibility of a bias concerning the sample of cells from which the experimenter records. We have already seen how the level of spontaneous activity is associated with the response type of a given cell. Since there would be some tendency to miss cells that do not have any appreciable spontaneous activity, this might be reflected in a somewhat distorted picture of what is going on at any particular neural level. The apparent predominance of the opponent mechanisms may be more a result of this sampling bias than the true biology of the situation.

Wiesel and Hubel (1966) have also studied the responses of color-sensitive cells at the level of the lateral geniculate body of the thalamus. They, however, were concerned with another aspect of the problem. They noted that the antagonistic center-surround receptive field arrangement explored by Kuffler and others and the color mechanisms explored by De-Valois and his colleagues both were examples of opponent mechanisms. In the one case, the opposing stimuli fell on different spatial locations, while in the other, the opponent stimuli lay in different portions of the visual spectrum. The question they asked concerned the behavior of single cells in this situation. Are individual geniculate cells capable of responding to both kinds of opponent mechanisms or are the spatial and chromatic codes conveyed separately through separate systems? It turned out, as they pursued their experiments, that most cells differentially sensitive to color were also differentially sensitive to some aspect of the spatial pattern and vice versa. Hubel and Wiesel observed four different types of cells in the various layers of the lateral geniculate body. Type I included antagonistic center-surround arrangements with the center being maximally sensitive to one color and the surround being maximally sensitive to another. Type II cells showed no center-surround ararngement, but did show opponent color mechanisms similar to those described by DeValois over a limited spatially homogenous receptive field. Type III cells had the same spectral sensitivity in both the center and surround of an antagonistically organized field, while Type IV had a central excitatory field surrounded by a large inhibitory field in which the peak spectral sensitivity was always shifted more or less to the longer wavelengths with regard to that most vigorously exciting central field.

Thus, Hubel and Wiesel conclude that most cells were affected more or less both by the spatial and chromatic dimensions of the stimulus. This is clearly a situation in which the neural coding mechanisms is overlapping, just as intensity and color interact in other situations. It is an effective warning to us to be sure that, whatever our coding schema turn out to be for a given dimension, we always make it quite clear that the statement "all other things being equal" is conspicuously appended either explicitly or implicitly.

4. Single Cell Responses in the Visual Cortex. In spite of the enormous complexity of the cellular response patterns of the visual cortex to spatio-temporal patterns (see, for example, in Chapter 8) the spatio-temporal complexity observed by Hubel and Wiesel and by Spinelli, it is still possible to find evidence of differential spectral sensitivity among single cortical cells. Motokawa, Taira, and Okuda (1962), for example, were able to insert tungsten microelectrodes through holes in the skull of monkeys directly into the visual cortex, so that extracellular responses could be recorded from single cells. Stimulus lights of 15 different wavelengths were intensity modulated with neutral density filters until all had equal constituent energy. Each was then flashed in succession for ½ sec with 8-sec interflash intervals. In this manner, the spectral response function of these cells at different wavelengths could be determined. The cells, which were surveyed, typically showed the on and off behavior patterns found at so many other levels of the visual pathway.

As it should be expected, there seemed to be very many different factors influencing the behavior of these cortical cells. The general arousal state of the animal influenced the cellular response substantially, and it was necessary to continuously monitor the EEG to be sure that the preexperimental surgical anesthesia effects were completely overcome. During the experiment, the monkeys were immobilized with Flaxedil—a curarelike substance—and rigidly fixed in a holding apparatus.

The results were quite surprising. In our discussion of the coding of color in the ascending visual pathway, with the exception of Granit's some-

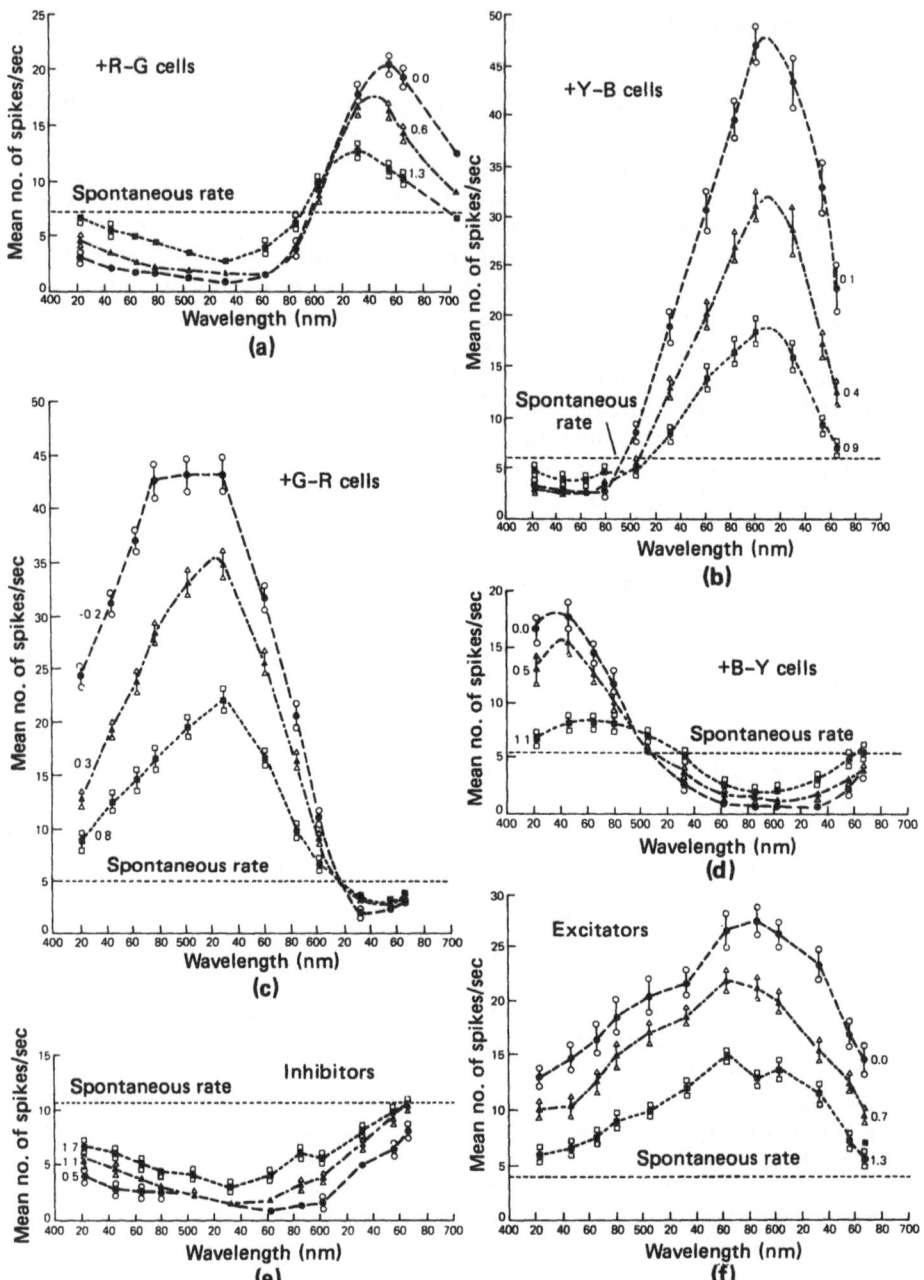

FIGURE 9.28 *The various types of spectral response curves observed in the lateral geniculate body. (a) A cell which was inhibited in the short and excited in the long wavelengths. The crossover points defines this as a +red-green opponent cell. (b) A cell which was inhibited in the short and excited in the long wavelengths. The crossover point defines this as a +yellow-blue opponent cell. (c) A cell which was excited in the short and inhibited in the long wavelengths. The crossover point defines this as a +green-yellow opponent cell. (d) A cell which was excited in the short and inhibited in the long wavelengths. The crossover point defines this as a +blue-yellow opponent cell. (e) A cell which is inhibited over the entire visual spectrum. This is defined as nonopponent inhibitory cell. (f) A cell which is excited over the entire visual spectrum.*

what atypical findings and Gouras' second type of ganglion cell, there was little evidence of simple monophasic trichromatic representation from the very earliest synaptic contact in the retina. Opponent type operations of one sort or another seemed to be the main coding mechanism all the way up through the lateral geniculate body. However, although Motokawa and his colleagues found several different kinds of response patterns, they found some cells, at least, that were at least partially trichromatic in their coding scheme. Figure 9.29 is a plot of their data for a particular group of 22 cells for which they were able to successfully track the entire response spectrum using an "on" response as the criterion. The data have been pooled for both cortical cells and cells that Motokawa and his colleagues felt were probably extensions of the optic radiations, but the overall pattern is clear. The familiar picture of three broadly tuned receptor groups with peak sensitivities at 460 nm, 530 nm, and 620 nm[1] is found once again. Thus, information originally encoded in terms of trichromatic mechanisms and subsequently re-encoded in terms of opponent mechanisms has re-emerged at the cortical level once again in the language of a trichromatic code.

Some of the cells, however, exhibited a sort of behavior, which Motokawa, Taira, and Okuda classified as opponent type responses. These cortical cells seemed to have different behavior patterns for the "on" portion of their responses and for the "off" portion. The sensitivity of the "on" responses for some cells peaked in a very narrow range at the long wavelength end of the spectrum. Surprisingly, the "off" responses of these same cells displayed a peak of evoked activity at the short wavelength end of the spectrum. Both the "on" and "off" portion of these opponent processes, therefore, were excitatory in nature. In this case, however, they were distinguished in terms of whether the short or long wavelength ends of the spectrum maximally excited the "on" or "off" portions of the response. Figure 9.30 shows this type of response pattern for a typical cell with a peak "on" activity centered at about 620 nm and a peak "off" activity centered at about 480 nm.

In addition to these cells that showed a single peak of sensitivity for either the "on" response or the "off" response, some cells, which displayed double peaks of sensitivity in both the "on" and "off" responses, were also observed by Motokawa and his colleagues. Figure 9.31 displays this kind of response pattern.

Andersen, Buchmann, and Lennox-Buchthal (1962) have also explored the behavior of single cells in the monkey cortex, using a flash technique in which the visual stimuli were only 8 msec long. In this case, there would be no way to separately compare the "on" and "off" effects. In general, their

---

[1] This, of course, does not agree with the spectral sensitivity of the monkey's red cone, which, on limited evidence, appears to peak at 570 nm.

This is defined as a nonopponent excitatory cell. The horizontal dotted lines in each case define the spontaneous level of activity, and the small numbers indicate the log attenuation of the stimulus with respect to the maximum stimulation level. Each curve in these figures is, thus, for a different stimulus intensity. The color names are defined by what human observers report. We do not know what this animal sees (all figures are from DeValois, Abramov, and Jacobs, 1966).

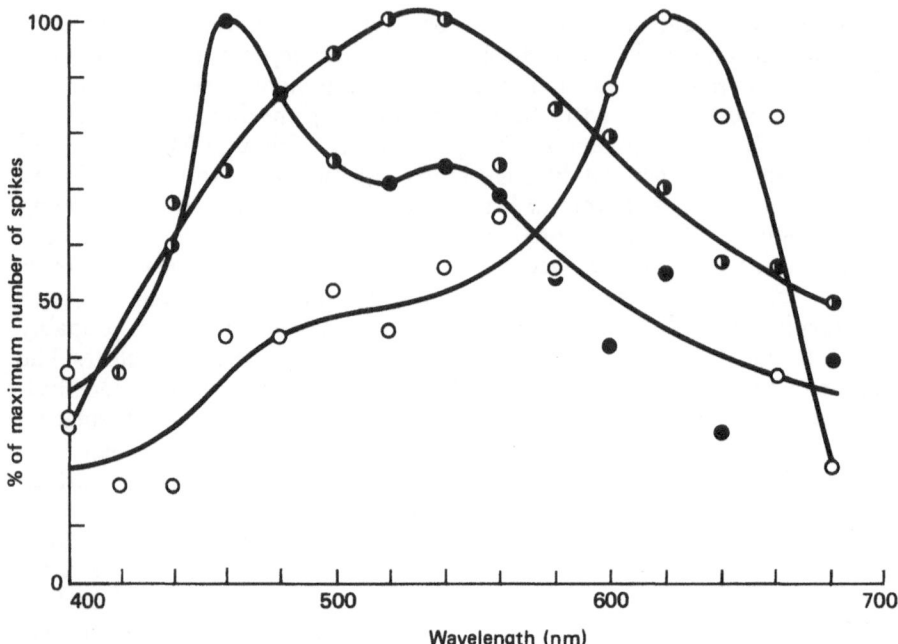

FIGURE 9.29 In the primate cerebrum, some evidence of trichromatic coding is seen once again. The figure shows the spectral sensitivities of some trichromatic cell types in the monkey's visual cortex (open and half-filled circles) and the optic radiation (filled circles). All responses in this case were from cells that gave strong "off" responses (from Motokawa, Taira, and Okuda, 1962).

findings can be characterized as showing no evidence of either trichromatic or opponent codes of any kind. Each cell seems to respond to a characteristic band of spectral wavelengths, but there was no evidence of any clustering into three or more groups. Perhaps more interesting is their finding that the specific sensitivities of the individual cells were very labile—a cell with a narrow response band might change suddenly to become responsive to white light and all monochromatic frequencies. This shift, which was not reversible, seemed to be associated with the type of anesthesia used in this experiment—a clear warning of the possible pollution of what otherwise might seem to be a relatively straightforward experiment by ostensibly insignificant technical details.

Finally, we may call attention to Hubel and Wiesel's (1968) work on the monkey striate cortex. They found that cortical cells with any kind of color sensitivity were relatively rare, and even the few from which they could record seemed to be associated with all possible variants of the different kinds of temporal-spatial sensitivities (see Table 8.1) that were present in the monkey's brain. (Higher-order complex cells were not observed in this animal.) As they put it,

> . . . a satisfactory study [of cortical color coding] will probably mean recording from thousands, rather than hundreds of cortical cells.
>
> (HUBEL and WIESEL, 1968, p. 225.)

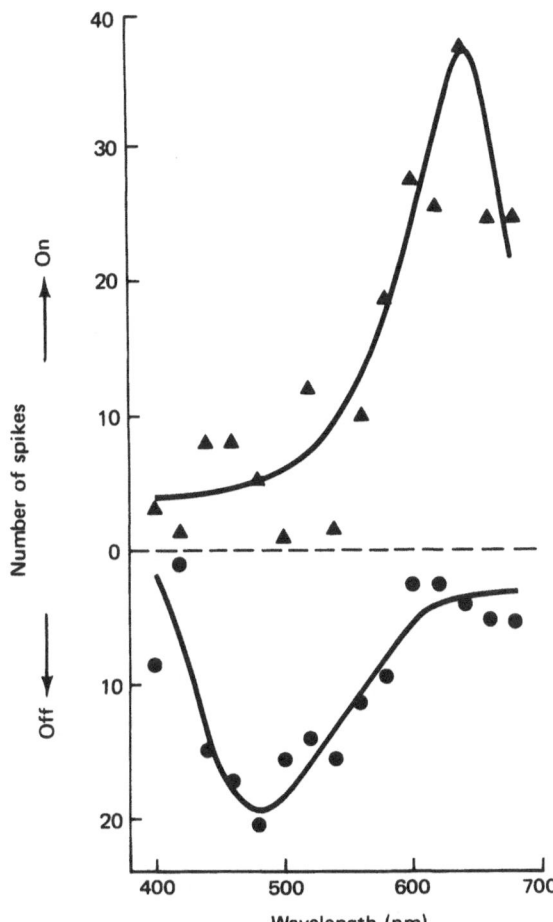

FIGURE 9.30 An opponent type process in a cortical unit in the monkey. This cell produces excitatory "on" responses and "off" responses, but in different regions of the spectrum. But as we saw in Figure 9.29, the "on" and "off" responses themselves might preserve some trichromatic codes (from Motokawa, Taira, and Okuda, 1962).

It is clear that this sort of data is only chipping at the peak of a horrendously complex system of cortical color coding and that much further work will have to be done to extend and rationalize these few observations. But what is clear is that the possible kinds of mechanisms for the encoding of color at the cortical level are several and diverse as well as being intermingled with mechanisms for the representation of time, space, and intensity.

V. A CONTEMPORARY MODEL

As one examines the history of color theories, it seems that the only real biological controversy that existed between the trichromatic theory and the opponent color theory concerned the nature of the photoreceptive process itself. That controversy is clearly resolved at this point in the history of the problem. The receptor processes are trichromatic and it is entirely probable that three different chemicals reside in each of three different kinds of cone. Though we have no idea what the nature of the anatomical or bio-

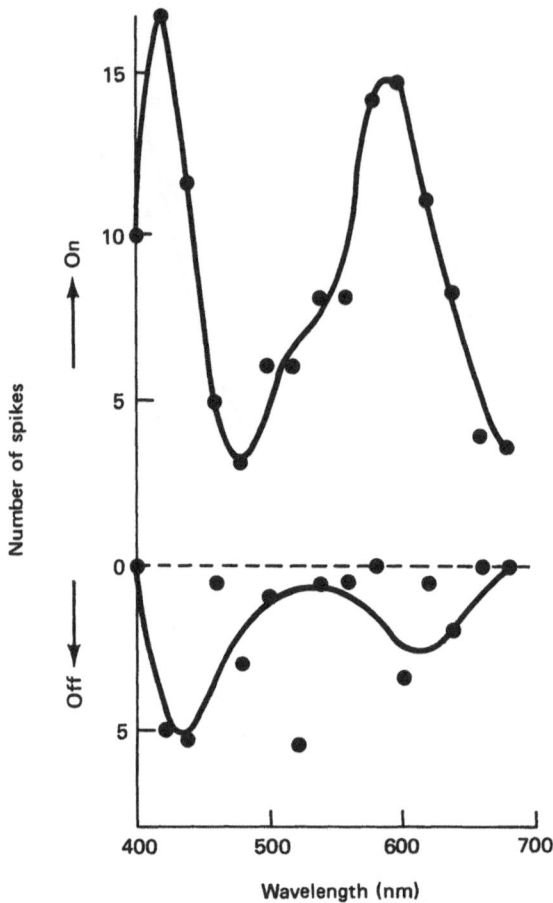

FIGURE 9.31 A curious cortical cell response, which was triphasic in its opponent mechanism. Both the "on" and "off" responses were excitatory at both ends of the spectrum, but to a lesser degree in the middle (from Motokawa, Taira, and Okuda, 1962).

chemical difference among the three cones is that allows each to acquire or manufacture a different type of photochemical with a characteristic absorption curve, it is quite clear that this is exactly what they do. Furthermore, the difference in the absorption spectra of the three pigments is specifically attributable to the difference in three different kinds of opsins, the large macromolecular moeity, a single form of retinal₁ presumably, according to Wald's theory, being common to all three.

The data concerning retinal photopigment absorption also resolve another one of the major issues that distinguishes the various trichromatic mathematico-descriptive theories from one another. The nature of the triad of trichromatic fundamentals is now established beyond any reasonable controversy. The three photochemicals have absorption spectra that are about 100 to 150 nm wide and peak at 450 nm, 530 nm, and either 575 nm for primates or 620 nm for the fish, respectively. Any further attempt to use primaries with significantly different characteristics is inappropriate and can only give rise to what is essentially a mathematical fiction based on the psychophysical fact that any triad can be used for color matching as well as neglect of the biological data.

The success of a trichromatic theory in describing the nature of the absorption pigments and in putting to rest that specific part of the Hering theory that postulated opponent photochemical properties does not, however, mean that all notions of opponent mechanisms in the visual system must also be discarded. It is quite clear that trichromatic coding mechanisms are only infrequently found once one is past the photoreceptor layer. From the bipolar cell layer onward, apparently the neurophysiological data do support the idea that a single cell can operate to encode color information in a manner that comes closer to what we call opponent mechanisms than it does to the trichromatic ideas.[2] However, the re-emergence of trichromatic mechanisms possibly in the optic nerve and in the cortex should also be a warning that information, whatever the language it is encoded in at any particular level, is essentially preserved as one ascends the visual pathway. Trichromatic recoding by subsequent mechanisms is not only possible, but has been observed in at least a few instances.

The major premise, which we are compelled to accept, once again, is the notion of equivalent but different encodings of the same information at different levels in the ascending pathways. The rapprochement of the trichromatic theory and opponent color theory is based on the fact that mechanisms associated with one or the other of the two views, can exist sequentially at different levels of the nervous system without any inherent contradiction.

Theories of color based on different neural coding schemes at different levels are generally called *state* or *zone* theories and have been present in the literature, though relatively unnoticed, for the past 70 years. Most of these zone theories, unlike the classical theories of Young-Helmholtz or of Hering, are patently neurophysiological in their conceptualization. In this regard, they go quite far beyond the matter of the absorption spectra of the retinal receptors. Over the years, the names of Von Kries, Schrodinger, Adams, Müller and Judd have been associated with the zone, state, or in the nomenclature of this book, *level theory*. Perhaps the most fully worked out zone theory is actually that of Hurvich and Jameson, whose championing of the opponent aspects is somewhat better known. Although their aim was to provide support for an opponent color theory, their papers clearly affirm the notion that the code may differ at each level. Their work is of special interest because they, more specifically than any of the others, speculate about the nature of the transformations that might account for the re-encoding of the output from a trichromatic retina to a central opponent mechanism.

The Hurvich and Jameson theory (1957) assumes a particular trichromatic set of photoreceptors in the retina and subsequent opponent color mechanisms. However, it is primarily a theory based on psychophysical

---

[2] The words "color," "red," "green," and "blue" are used here and earlier in this chapter in a way that may distress or confuse some readers. They are meant to be used by the author as shorthand terms for long, medium, and short wavelength photic stimuli as defined by the subjective experiences that would be produced by these wavelengths if observed by a normal human subject. We are not suggesting that there is any color sensation in any of the neurophysiological preparations being discussed. A similar statement must be made concerning the use of such words as sweet, salty, fragrant and high or low pitch in later chapters.

findings and, as such, is by itself incapable of confirming anything about the details of the central opponent processes. As we have seen, there are several different ways in which opponent processes may be coded. Furthermore, the major specific photochemical assumption of their original theory, that of narrowly spaced pigment absorption curves, has been rejected and replaced with a more modern set (Jameson and Hurvich, 1968). Much to their credit, Hurvich and Jameson (1957), anticipating future developments in neurophysiology, specifically noted that some plausible method for converting from a trichromatic coding in the retina to a central opponent mechanism must be hypothesized if their model was to have any possible substance. In 1957 they were faced, in addition, with the equally plausible alternatives of assuming that the three photoreceptor substances were each isolated in separate cones or that combinations of any two photoabsorptive pigments could exist in a single cone. In the light of the evidence which has been forthcoming since then, it is feasible to ignore the latter alternative and consider only the case in which a single pigment is present in each cone.

Figure 9.32 (adapted from Hurvich and Jameson, 1957) shows a hypothetical set of connections, which might account for the conversion of trichromatically coded retinal information to a central opponent color system in one synaptic jump. The three circles represent the three types of cones. In the original drawing, Hurvich and Jameson labeled these circles α, β, γ because the primaries in their hypothetical system were all assumed to be in the yellow region of the spectrum. However, based on the directly measured absorption spectra of the three pigments, it is not inappropriate for us to return to the older nomenclature—R, G, and B—indicating long wavelength, medium wavelength, and short wavelength sensitive substances, respectively.

The three circles representing the photoreceptors are connected by single stage communication links to the three opponent cells represented by the attached pairs of rectangles. Each of the three types of retinal receptor has three outputs, two of which may be excitatory or inhibitory as required, while the third is solely excitatory. Two of the outputs go to opponent type "neural units." These units are cell or cell combinations which, while not specifically identified by Hurvich and Jameson, can now be assumed to be either second-order neurons in the inner nuclear layer or combinations of these second-order retinal units. The important fact is that whatever these neural units are, they must, in some way, respond differentially as a function of the relative balance between the inputs from the receptor cells. Hurvich and Jameson believe that the two opponent neural units indicated in Figure 9.32 are specifically involved in the chromatic encoding, while the third cell or cell system is associated with the overall luminosity, a function of the cumulative output of the three cells. This third mechanism was originally considered by Hering to be also an opponent system, but in the light of the data then current, Hurvich and Jameson considered it to be a nonopponent overall brightness system.

A necessary premise for the Hurvich and Jameson re-encoding idea is that the effect of the output of any of the three photoreceptors may be either inhibitory or excitatory on the two hypothetical chromatic opponent

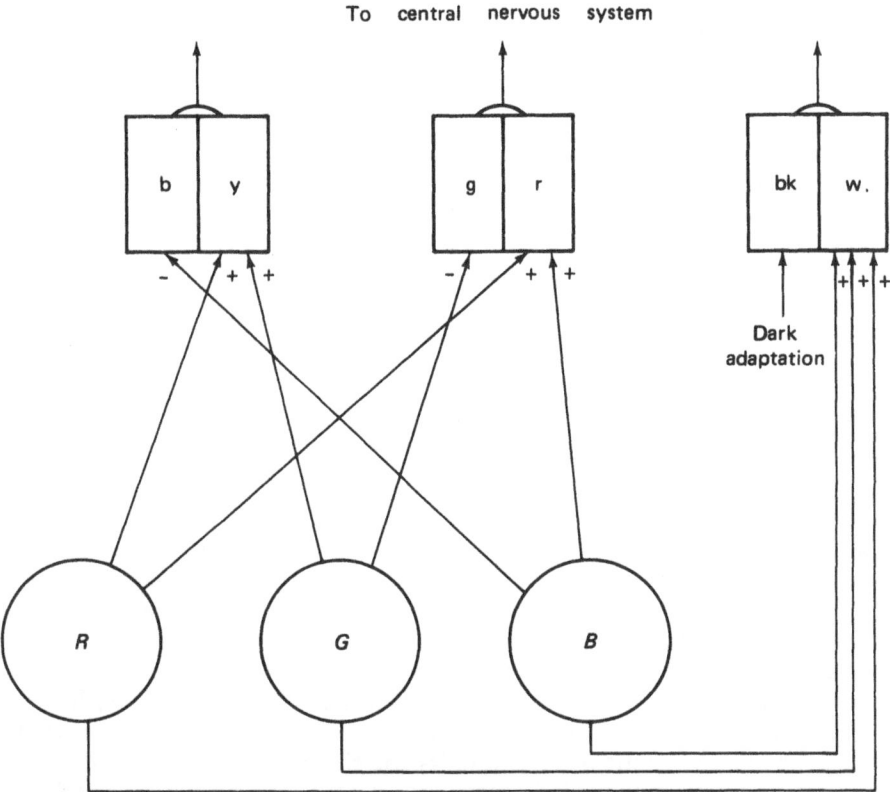

FIGURE 9.32 A schematic sketch of a plausible neural mechanism, which could convert a trichromatic (R, G, and B) photoreceptor coding scheme to a more central opponent mechanism (b-y, g-r, and bk-w) (adapted and modified from Hurvich and Jameson, 1957).

neural units. A red receptor, for example, as indicated in Figure 9.32, tends to excite both the blue-yellow and the green-red opponent units. The output of the green receptor, on the other hand, tends to excite the blue-yellow opponent unit, but inhibit the green-red opponent unit. The blue receptor, finally, has outputs that tend to excite the green-red unit, but inhibit the blue-yellow unit. All three units tend to contribute to the excitation of the black-white unit. (Incidentally, this schema is slightly different than the original Hurvich and Jameson model, but in what is believed to be a simplifying and clarifying manner.)

How, then, are colors encoded by the opponent system? Table 9.3 illustrates at least one coding scheme, which might be used to represent differences in both hue and saturation. If a light from the red end of the spectrum is used as a stimulus, then the blue-yellow and the green-red opponent units both increase in the amplitude of their activity or in some other way selectively respond in a positive sense. This is indicated by a + in both columns in the table. If the red light is a very saturated red, then the

TABLE 9.3 A POSSIBLE CODING CHART FOR AN
OPPONENT COLOR CODING SYSTEM (SEE TEXT FOR FULL DETAILS)

	b/y	g/r	bk/wh
Unsaturated Red	+ +	+ +	+ +
Saturated Red	+	+ +	+
Unsaturated Green	+ +	− −	+ +
Saturated Green	+	− −	+
Unsaturated Blue	− −	+ +	+ +
Saturated Blue	− −	+	+

total amount of activity will be limited mainly to the output of the red
receptor (++), and the activity of the black-white and the blue-yellow units
will be relatively low (+). On the other hand, if the light is relatively unsaturated and contains a relatively large amount of other colors, this state
can be reflected by large amounts of activity (++) in each of the chromatic
opponent units and in the output of the black-white receptor. Thus, for this
red light, hue and saturation are encoded by a relative amount of activity
among the two chromatic opponent units and the black-white receptor.

Similarly, an unsaturated green light would lead to increased activity
in the black-white and blue-yellow systems (++), as well as a substantial
decrease in the relative amount of activity (− −) in the green-red system.
A very pure green, however, would lead to only a slight increase (+) in
the black-white and blue-yellow cell outputs, but still produce the same
(− −) decrement in the green-red system. In the same way, a stimulus light
from the blue end of the spectrum would result in a substantial decrease
(− −) in the amount of activity in the blue-yellow opponent unit, but a
greater or lesser amount of activity in the opponent green-red and nonopponent black-white units, depending upon whether or not the light is
saturated.

The enormous strength of this sort of coding scheme is that a zone
theory allows us to consider a system that is at once both trichromatic and,
at different levels of the ascending pathway, opponent in operation. Another important advantage of this hypothetical system is that it once again
directs our thinking toward a system in which the *relative* amounts of activity in the several subunits are critical to the specification of hue rather
than the absolute amount of activity in any system. Thus, the same red,
with any given degree of saturation, can occur at many different levels of
brightness. Although there are some changes of hue with brightness level
(the Bezold-Brucke effect), this idea is in general agreement with the overall stability of hue at various brightness levels. The discrepancies, which
do exist, are probably due to the fact that the nonopponent black-white

system is probably considerably more complicated than the one postulated in this obviously oversimplified model.

In Hurvich and Jameson's (1957) discussion, they were able to show that a wide variety of other visual phenomena could be explained in a relatively straightforward manner by their zone model. If we ignore the very obvious discrepancy of the spectral absorption curves of the triad of primaries, their model did a relatively good job in handling such diverse phenomena as wavelength discrimination, chromatic adaptation, and much of the color blindness data. With regard to this latter problem, the notion of different coding mechanisms at different levels of the nervous system is particularly valuable in helping to understand how some color blindness may be due to shifts or absences in photoreceptor absorption spectra, while others may be due to neural processes at more central levels. Hurvich and Jameson felt, for example, that protanomaly and deuteranomaly were probably due to shifts in the absorption spectra of the receptor photo-pigments toward shorter wavelengths and longer wavelengths, respectively. On the other hand, deficiencies in some more central green-red or yellow-blue opponent neural systems, they feel, are more closely linked to the dichromatic protanopia, deuteranopia, and tritanopia.

In sum, then, color coding throughout the visual pathway seems to be characterized by several kinds of recoding at different levels. At the most peripheral level, a trichromatic system based on three different kinds of photopigment underlies the initial transduction. However, at the very first synapse, this trichromatic mechanism seems to be re-encoded into opponent type systems, which are maintained in one form or another with few exceptions all the way to the cortex. It should be noted that the specific nature of the opponent processes, that is, the particular code employed, varies in ways that make the opponent processes differ as much among themselves as they do from the trichromatic mechanism. Opponent processes in the inner nuclear layer, at least in part, seem to be reflected in the opposite amplitudes and directions of polarization of graded potentials. In the lateral geniculate body, on the other hand, the opponent mechanism seems to be encoded by an increase or diminution in the rate of spontaneous spike action potential activity. Finally, there is some evidence in the cortex that the opponent mechanisms are encoded by a different peak spectral sensitivity for the "on" and "off" responses of single cells in addition to the suggestion that trichromatic patterns of response re-emerge at this level.

The overall impression that one acquires from the neurophysiology of chromatic responses is that there are probably a large number of different neural codes for visual quality operating at different levels (and even occasionally at the same level) of the visual pathway. There is, in this sense, no single code for quality in the visual system, but a number of different manners of representing stimulus wavelength information—information that remains, regardless of the neural language, more or less constant, until it activates that state of the nervous system at which it becomes equivalent to the experience of color.

Another theme that permeates all of the data we have discussed is the interplay of color-coded information and temporal and intensive information. The "on-off" system is obviously evolved to encode temporal discontinuities in the visual stimulus; yet in our discussion we often see instances in which the "on-off," "on," or "off" activity is also modulated by the spectral characteristics of the stimulus. Rates of firing of a given neuron are also affected by both the color and the intensity of the stimulus. In the ascending visual pathways, it is clear, therefore, that a single cell does not operate uniquely as a color encoder or as a time encoder or, for that matter, as a spatial or intensity encoder either. Any cell anywhere in the visual pathway that is sensitive to light would probably show some modulation of its activity when any of these stimulus dimensions are varied. The specific meaning of the different attributes of a visual stimulus, therefore, must in some way be functionally rated to a balance and comparison of the relative amounts of activity in a large number of different places. This is a sort of mechanism that is quite different from the labeled-line hypothesis, which asserts that the activation of a single key neuron is uniquely associated with some single attribute of the stimulus. Thus, in some broader sense, the entire visual system, and not only the quality code, must operate as a sort of opponent system, and Table 9.3 might well be expandable into some much more elaborate comparison scheme to represent the encoding of the total dimensionality of the visual stimulus.

CHAPTER 10: THE NEURAL CODING OF SENSORY QUALITY—AUDITION

I. THE KEY PSYCHOPHYSICAL DATA

A. Frequency Analysis and Pitch Discrimination

If the eye can be best characterized by the data of color synthesis or mixture, the ear is best described as an analyzer. The fact basic to audition is that the auditory system is capable of separating to some degree a complex mixture of different sounds into its components. The ability, for example, to hear a particular instrument in a performing orchestra or a particular voice in the noisy hubbub of a cocktail party makes our analysis of the phenomena of auditory pitch perception fundamentally different from those of visual hue perception.

Although this ability to analyze complex tones is present to a first approximation in human psychophysical processes, it should be understood that it is not as comprehensive a capability as many would have us believe. Ward (1970) has been particularly vigorous in his rejection of the generality of this "quarter-truth" (of frequency analysis) and has noted that vibratos are not frequency analyzed, nor are pulses, nor are many of the musical sounds encountered in our everyday life. Nevertheless, the idea of the general ability to analyze some signals is so ingrained in the scientific literature of audition and is a possible explanation of a sufficiently large number of situations to make it an important factor in any discussion of the basic theory of auditory coding.

If one looks at the pressure pattern of a complex acoustic waveform, it is clear that the capability of the auditory system to analyze sounds might, in some way, be analogous to the Fourier analysis process we discussed in

Chapter 2. Indeed, shortly after Fourier presented his mathematical theory as a means of analyzing and specifying the characteristics of mechanical oscillations, Ohm postulated a set of auditory laws that was based on the idea of the frequency analysis. Ohm's assertion, however, was not simply a statement that complex acoustic stimuli *could* be analyzed into a unique set of sinusoidal components, a notion already implicit in Fourier's work and the nature of the physical acoustic stimuli, but rather that the auditory system *did* exactly that analysis, and that the results were observable in the behavior of the organism.

The ability, or perhaps better, the partial ability, to analyze an acoustic stimulus into separate components is closely intermingled with the issue of the specific psychophysical effect of different acoustic frequencies. To a first approximation, different frequencies of stimulation give rise to different experiences of *pitch*—the term analogous to hue in the visual sense and representing the quality dimension for this modality. However, just as the color of a light may vary in attributes other than simple hue (it may, for example, vary in saturation as well), the single dimension of pitch (such as that produced by a pure stimulus frequency) does not completely describe the qualitative dimensions of a more complex tone. All musical instruments, for example, produce not single pure tones, but, rather, a complex mixture of the fundamental note and the overtones produced by the mechanics of the instrument. The quality of this mixture of tones, a concept which is separate from the pitch of the individual components, is known as the *timbre* of the instrument.

Other temporal properties of the tonal pattern beyond the frequency of the stimulating tone can also contribute to the quality of the sensation. Repeated oscillation of the temporal intensity pattern (amplitude modulation) varies a quality of the sensation known as *tremulo*. Oscillation of the frequency pattern (frequency modulation) produces an experience of *vibrato*. These temporal properties of the stimulus, however, are more comparable to those that produce flicker in vision or vibration in somatosensation than to color or touch and will not be further considered here.

The major qualitative dimension in audition is pitch, and just as it is difficult to describe what it is that we mean by a red or a green, it is also difficult to describe what is meant by a high or low pitch. The best manner of definition is an operational one. High pitches are associated with high-frequency stimulation and low pitches with low-frequency stimulation. Thresholds and subjective magnitudes also vary with frequency, however; the greatest sensitivity occurring between 1000 and 3000 Hz.

It should be also noted in passing, that the pitch of a pure tone does change to some degree as the intensity of the signal varies. Generally, the alteration in pitch with intensity shifts is greater at either end of the auditory frequency spectrum than in the middle region around 1000 Hz, where the threshold is the lowest. The effect has, over the years, been studied by numerous investigators and is considered to be important in some theories of auditory encoding, but at best it is a second-order effect, the perturbing effects of which can best be considered after our theories of auditory encoding have been developed to the point that the first-order effects have been satisfactorily accounted for. We shall, therefore, not deal with the issue further in the present discussion.

The discrimination of frequency differences is a related and exceedingly important matter, which we have already introduced when we discussed spatial interactions. This was done because of the well-known fact that much in the way of frequency discrimination is accounted for by the preneural spatial mechanics of the fluid-filled cochlea. Frequency discrimination was assumed to be, at least in some regards, closely analogous to visual spatial interactions. As a reminder only at this point, we should also note that frequency discrimination as it is often measured, with a warbling technique in which two alternatively presented tones are adjusted for equality of pitch, is very fine—of the order of 1 to 4 Hz within the range from 50 to 3000 Hz as was shown in Figure 7.6. This is a remarkably fine sensitivity, corresponding to $\frac{1}{10}$ of 1 percent of the frequency over much of this region. This ability to discriminate between nearby frequencies is one of the basic capabilities that must be explained by any theory of auditory encoding. In light of the broadly tuned nature of the peripheral auditory receptive mechanism, this has proved to be one of the most challenging points of contention among the competing theories.

Just as in vision, the apparent disagreement between the fine psychophysical frequency discrimination and the broadly tuned mechanical and neural mechanisms in audition has often been resolved by attributing successive sharpening mechanisms to the various levels of neural processing. (See, for example, von Békésy's 1967 book on sensory inhibition.) We have already detailed some of the objections to such an approach. It should also be noted that there is no *a priori* reason from the point of view of coding theory why the psychophysical discriminations should necessarily be isomorphic (to the extent that each is equally finely tuned) to the responses at any level of the nervous system. An equally good argument might be made for the representation of psychophysical fine tuning by discriminations of the differences between overlapping broad neural distributions (in the vein of signal detection theory) without resorting to any spatial isomorphism. This is a topic we shall deal with further in the later parts of this chapter and in the final summary of Chapter 11.

B. The Pitch of Combined Stimulus Frequencies

If one continuously increases the output frequency of a single sine wave acoustic stimulus, there is a corresponding continuous and monotonic increase in the pitch of the sound. Thus, to a first approximation at least, pitch is directly related to the energy of the particular frequency component of the stimulating tone. However, there are a large number of other auditory phenomena, most of which are associated with the perception of tones produced by combining acoustic frequencies, which seem to show that under many conditions, pitches are perceived that may be totally unrelated to the energy spectrum of the stimulus.

Before we discuss the details of these phenomena, it would be well to note that there are two possible general approaches toward an explanation of such a fact. First, it may be that frequency and pitch are simply not as directly related as suggested by the simple monofrequency experiment. On the other hand, it may be that this association does hold, but that in some manner distortions produced by nonlinear mechanical and neural auditory processes introduce the signal frequencies that are missing in the stimulus pattern itself. An analysis of this issue, therefore, is of the greatest significance in establishing the strengths and weaknesses of several of the alternative theories of auditory coding.

1. *Beats and Difference Tones.* When two frequencies of physical oscillation occur simultaneously in some medium, there is a waxing and waning of the amplitude of the combined oscillation at a frequency equal to the frequency difference between the two. Figure 10.1 shows the effect of adding two sinusoids on the amplitude of oscillation of the combined acoustic wave. The waxing and waning of the intensity of the combined wave is a purely physical phenomenon and is perfectly predicted simply by the linear addition of the two signals. In an auditory environment, if two sound waves are so mixed, an observer will report that he hears the waxing and waning or *beating,* as it is usually known, of intensity (if the difference in the two frequencies is quite small) in addition to the two individual components. As the frequency difference between the two sound waves increases, the intensity of beating passes through stages that have been variously reported as vibratos and burrs until at a specific frequency difference (which is determined by the frequencies of the individual components), a new continuous smooth tone is heard. This new tone corresponds in pitch to a sensation induced by a single oscillation equal to the difference between the two real sound waves. At this stage, the percept is no longer one of varying intensity, but of a pure and continuous additional tone. The important and disquieting fact about this phenomenon is that if a perfect frequency analyzing system examined the signal, then it would be shown that *there was no energy of any kind at the difference frequency.* Thus, it seems that the association between stimulus frequency (and the power of the signal at that frequency), on the one hand, and pitch, on the other, breaks down. The auditory system seems to be in some way responding not to the energy content at a specific frequency, but to the envelope of the composite wave—an envelope that has exactly zero energy content. It is only in a nonlinear system, which can introduce distortions, that frequencies corresponding to the envelope frequency with nonzero power become physically present.

The question then arises: are the beat frequency energies actually introduced by some nonlinear distortion in the auditory system, thus salvaging the notion that a given frequency signal is the main correlate of the auditory pitch? Or alternatively, is the auditory system in some way sensitive to the periodicity of the signal, even though the energy content of the periodicity be zero? As we shall see, this is the crux of much of the controversy among the various theories of auditory pitch perception.

In addition to the particular difference pitch, the beating we have described here (which is functionally related to the difference between two interacting frequencies), there are also many other kinds of summation and

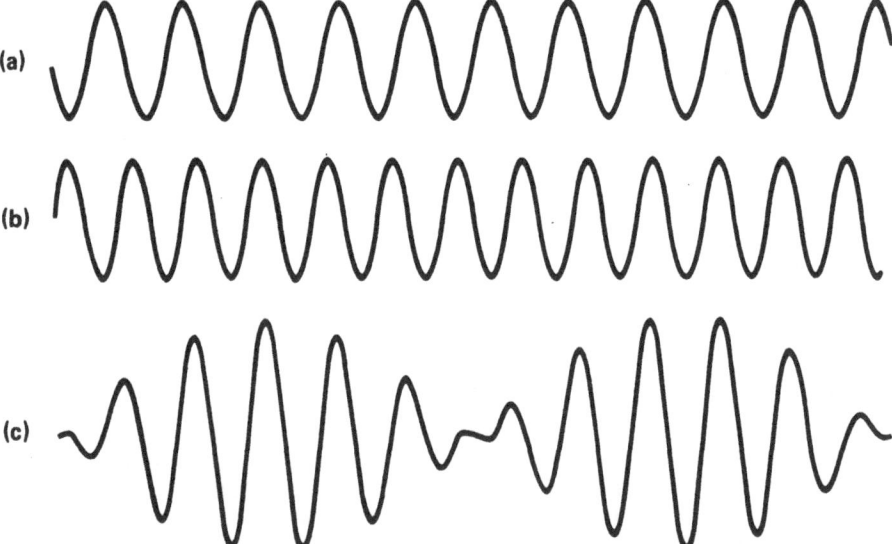

FIGURE 10.1 *When two oscillations of nearly identical frequency [(a) and (b)] are combined, the sum is a beat frequency equal to the frequency difference between the two.*

difference combination pitches. Summation or difference pitches, corresponding to frequencies equal to integral multiples of the sum of two stimuli can also be heard in many other situations. We shall discuss some of the other major combination pitches in the following sections.

2. The Seebeck Siren. Seebeck (1841) many years ago performed some experiments with a pneumatic siren that are closely related to this question of combination tones. His sirens (whistles might be a better term) were made from rotating disks containing perforations, which alternatively closed and opened a source of compressed air. In this manner, he was able to produce patterns of acoustic pulses that were composed of known mixed frequency components long before electronic equipment was developed. Seebeck used Fourier's mathematical analysis techniques to show that combinations of two high frequencies produced physical stimuli with very little energy at frequencies corresponding to pitches that were very strongly heard.

For example, if a frequency pattern such as that shown in Figure 10.2(a) was presented, a smooth high-frequency tone was heard. However, if every second puff of air was displaced very slightly as shown in Figure 10.2(b), then a tone one octave lower [equivalent to the experience produced by a stimulus pattern like that in Figure 10.2(c)] was heard. However, upon Fourier analysis of the stimulus pattern of Figure 10.2(b), it could be shown that there was virtually no energy present at the frequency represented by Figure 10.2(c). Thus, once again there appeared to be a perceived

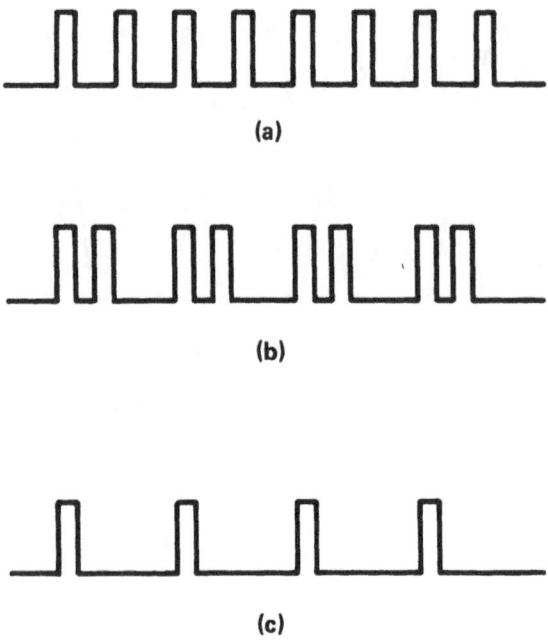

(a)

(b)

(c)

FIGURE 10.2 A simple sketch illustrating the Seebeck siren effect. An equal interval series of pulsed compressed air blasts (a) sounds like a pure frequency. If every other blast is slightly displaced in phase as is (b), a second tone is heard one octave below the original signal. It has a tone equivalent to that produced by the pattern in (c). However, there is no physical energy at the frequency of (c), and the problem is thus raised of how a place coded system could possibly respond with the pitch of (c) to the stimulus frequency pattern of (b).

pitch associated with a virtually zero energy stimulus component. The Seebeck experiments, like the beat phenomenon, therefore, represent an apparent deviation from the basic assumption of association of a given pitch with the energy content of a given frequency component that is implicit in Ohm's acoustic law.

3. The Missing Fundamental or the Residue. If several waves with frequencies of, for example, 500, 600, 700, and 800 Hz are mixed together, the combination produces an additional tonal experience comparable to the effect produced by a 100-Hz tone. Fletcher had originally reported this phenomenon in 1935 and had named it the missing fundamental. However, as Licklider (1951a) points out, it is not at all clear whether this is the correct term, for clearly both the difference tone and the common fundamental of all of these component frequencies are both equal to 100 Hz. The question thus arises: which of these two possible options—the common fundamental or the common difference—is responsible for the perception of the 100-Hz tone? Schouten (1940) repeated Fletcher's experiments with stimulus frequencies equal to 300, 500, 700, and 900 Hz and found that the perceived tone was still equivalent to that produced by a 100-Hz tone. Thus, the notion of a "missing fundamental" is the correct terminology, and this phenomenon is not a difference tone in the true sense of the word.

Schouten (1938, 1940) has been among the most active investigators in pursuing the question of the missing fundamental over the years. He has coined the term "the residue" to describe the residual tonal experience of a frequency fundamental whose physical energy content is zero in the stimulus, and which can exist even though supposedly canceled by a tone of equal frequency but opposite polarity. Schouten, therefore, concluded that even if the tone had been introduced by nonlinear distortion in the ear, this cancellation procedure was not able to remove its effect. This finding further suggests that the tonal experience is not linked to the energy of the stimulus frequency.

4. Tones in Random Noise. Huggins and Licklider (1951) were able to demonstrate that even random noise, which presumably has energy distributed at all frequencies, could take on specific tonal qualities under certain conditions. The experimental conditions they used involved a frequency dependent phase shifting mechanism. A 360-deg phase shift, a delay of one full cycle, was introduced for the high-frequency components of a noise signal. For low-frequency components, no phase shift was introduced, but at some narrow intermediate range the phase shift gradually changed from 0 to 360 deg. The original signal was amplified and fed into one side of the pair of earphones, while the signal with this specific pattern of phase shifts was fed into the other ear. In this situation, Huggins and Licklider report that a very faint tone is heard at about the center frequency band at which the phase shifter shifts over from no low-frequency shift to the high-frequency phase shift.

The Huggins and Licklider induced tone phenomenon occurs only below a crossover frequency of 1000 Hz and is best between 400 and 800 Hz. Fascinatingly, this same interesting phenomenon has been used by Licklider (1962) and von Békésy (1963a) to support the opposing frequency and place theories of hearing, respectively.

Miller and Taylor (1948) have also shown that if a white noise signal is interrupted at about 200 or 300 Hz, observers would also report a tonal quality at about the frequency of the interruption. The interesting and significant part of all of these data is that the spectrum of white noise is continuous, with energy at all frequencies with or without the interruptions. Yet in some manner, the interruptions and phase shifts apparently are introducing some new characteristic information, which could be deciphered as tonal experiences in much the same manner as zero energy beats, or missing fundamentals are heard.

In sum, there are a number of phenomena of combination tones, which seem to suggest that the simple notion of a unique correlation of stimulus frequency energy and pitch experience does not hold. The data suggest that there might be some way in which the purely temporal characteristics or periodicity of the stimulus, independent of the Fourier energy components, can produce the experience of tone.

As we have noted, there is also another possible explanation, namely, that the energy at the perceived frequency is introduced by nonlinear distortions of the input signal. Although the answer to this question is primarily one that will have to be answered by empirical mechanical and neurophysiological inquiries, Small (1970) has summarized a considerable amount of psychophysical evidence, which suggests that the arguments for the introduction of energy by nonlinear distortions cannot be supported as an explanation of pitch of combination signals.

Briefly, his reasons, as paraphrased by the author, include:

1. Subjects are able to detect combination pitches at very low sound pressure levels, which presumably would be within the range of linearity of the mechanical parts of the auditory mechanism (Thurlow and Small, 1955).

2. If a signal is added to a mixed signal with opposite phase, but intensity equal to the combination pitch, it would be expected that the combination pitch, if a real physical entity with nonzero energy content, would be canceled. In fact, Schouten's experiments show that the difference tone is not canceled. Thus, Small feels that the residue is probably not due to the presence of real energy (Schouten, 1938).

3. If a second signal is introduced with a frequency quite close to a combination pitch with zero energy such as a beat tone or a residue, it might be expected that there would be beating between the two tones. In fact, in this situation there is no perceived beating, again suggesting that no real energy has been introduced (Schouten, 1938).

4. If a second tone is introduced which would otherwise mask the combination pitch, it does not, in fact, do so. The presumption, therefore, is that the normal lateral interaction mechanisms do not come into play, because the cochlear places so stimulated are not adjacent. It is suggested, therefore, that the information about the combination pitch is carried by neurons other than the usual ones associated with that frequency (Licklider, 1954, and Small and Campbell, 1961).

5. A stimulus with a frequency corresponding to that which would produce a combination pitch can be used to selectively fatigue the region of the cochlea that would be expected to be associated with the combination pitch. In this case, however, the combination pitch is still heard, and its continued presence suggests, once again, that the information associated with the induced combination pitch is not carried by that region of the cochlea normal for that frequency. The generation of the combination pitch, Small therefore concludes, is not due to the presence of energy at that difference frequency, but dependent purely on the periodicity of the signal (Small and Yelen, 1962).

However, as we shall see later when we consider the physiological data, there is accumulating evidence that combination frequencies are actually observable in the cochlear microphonic and the auditory nervous response. The arguments cited by Small and these physiological findings, therefore, are apparently incompatible and cannot be reconciled at this particular stage in the history of the problem.

C. Masking and the Notion of Critical Bands

In the previous chapter when we discussed spatial interactions, we considered much of the data concerning masking of one tone by another. There is no need to repeat that discussion at this point; however, there is a set of phenomena which are closely related to the notion of masking to which we shall now attend. These findings deal with the concept of critical bands or bandwidths within which certain auditory phenomena remain essentially constant. It is difficult, because of the many different ways in which the notion of critical bands has been used throughout the auditory literature, to precisely define their meaning and significance other than operationally. The best way to introduce the notion, therefore, is to describe an experiment in which the critical bands are measured.

The classic determination of critical bandwidth has usually been carried out using a masking technique as summarized by Scharf (1970). Fletcher (1940), for example, used three monofrequency stimuli in his studies of the critical bandwidth, two of which were used to mask a third, the frequency of which was halfway between the two masking tones. Zwicker's (1956) more modern study of the problem substituted for the masked monotone a very narrow band of noise with its center frequency halfway between the two monotone maskers, but the findings of the experiments are, for all practical purposes, identical. The frequencies of the two masking tones initially are set very close to the center frequency of the noise, but in successive stages are moved further and further apart, one masking tone increasing in frequency, while the other decreases in frequency. As the frequency separation of the two masking tones increases, there is at first little change in the threshold of either the noise or the monotone, but at a given separation, the masking effect suddenly begins to decrease, indicating that the interaction is no longer as strong. The separation of the two tones at that point of sudden change is defined as the critical bandwidth for that particular center frequency.

Critical bands can be measured with a number of other nonmasking techniques. For example, complex sounds made up of several frequencies do not vary in intensity as the constituent frequencies vary over the critical bandwith. However, once the mixed tones begin to fall outside the critical bandwidth, the loudness of the combination begins to increase. Furthermore, thresholds of complex signals are not affected by signals outside the critical bandwidth. Much of these data have been summarized in Scharf's chart, which is reproduced in Figure 10.3. The critical band is seen to be relatively constant in its width from about 100 Hz up to about 500 Hz, after which it increases up to a maximum width of about 2000 Hz when measured at 10,000 Hz.

In general, the critical band data have been used as support for a place theory of auditory frequency coding. Critical bands are assumed to be explained by spatial interactions comparable to those explaining, for example, frequency discrimination (see Figure 7.6). Obviously, a critical band cannot be simply identified with the differential frequency measure, for it is 20 to 50 times as wide, but this ratio remains relatively constant as one scans the auditory frequency spectrum, and some less direct relationship may exist.

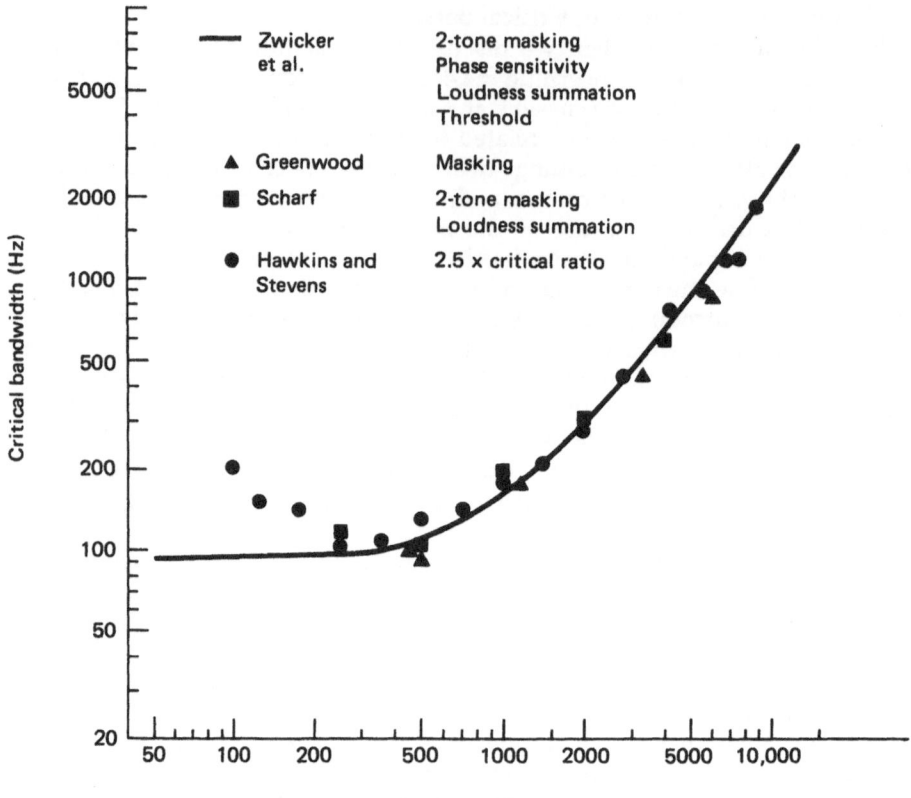

FIGURE 10.3 *A summary of the data prepared by Scharf from several experiments on the critical bandwidth. The source of the data is indicated in the legend on the figure (from Scharf, 1970, from data by Greenwood, 1961; Hawkins and Stevens, 1950, and Zwicker as well as from Scharf's own data).*

These, then, represent a brief sampling of some of the psychophysical phenomena of importance, which must be explained by any theory of auditory pitch. Obviously, the sampling is incomplete and cannot begin to do justice to all of the work done by so many psychophysicists in the last 50 or even 100 years. However, we are fortunate to have had an extraordinarily good book become available only recently. Tobias (1970) has edited a volume entitled *Foundations of Modern Auditory Theory*, in which a large number of the leaders in the field have presented a set of what is undoubtedly one of the most readable and authoritative statements on these problems to have appeared in many years. The reader who would like more complete details of these and related materials is directed to this very important treatise and especially to the work of Small (1970) and Scharf (1970) for more detailed discussion of the present material.

II. THE COMPETITIVE THEORIES

No discussion of contemporary auditory pitch theory can be responsibly carried out without extensive acknowledgment of the remarkable analysis of the problem by Wever (1949) in his book *Theory of Hearing*. Wever's book—scholarly, critical, and erudite—effectively summarizes both the history and the interrelationships of the various theories of pitch perception that have evolved over the past century. Most of the discussion in the following section will be, therefore, based on his analysis.

Pitch theory has in general, over the years, been characterized by a controversy over the anatomic level at which the tonal analysis (implied by Ohm's acoustic law) is carried out. Analysis is thought to be peripheral (cochlear) in some theories, but central in other descriptions. Peripheral analysis theories usually assume a loss of temporal fidelity early in the pathway. The central analysis theories necessarily required that a reproduction of the original temporal pattern of the acoustic signal be carried in some manner to the central nervous system, where a frequency analysis can presumably be carried out. On the basis of these premises, the two main general classes of auditory pitch theory have come to be called the place theories (all of which assume peripheral spatial analysis in the cochlea) and the frequency or periodicity theories (all of which assume central analysis after transmission of signals with high temporal fidelity to the central nervous system).

In the following portion of this section, we shall consider the place and frequency theories separately and trace the historical development of each. We shall distinguish among the varieties of each theory, noting the key differences among each.

A. Place Theories

Although all place theories agree, in principle, that the main mechanism for auditory pitch encoding is a peripheral analysis of stimulus frequencies in the cochlea, they do not all agree how this spatial analysis comes about. Place theories began to emerge almost as soon as some of the earliest notions of the cochlear anatomy were uncovered. Characteristically, each theory was quite closely tied to some physical theory that was then of contemporary interest. Whatever the dominant current technology, someone, it seems, was always able to rephrase the auditory coding problem in terms of an analytical mechanism based on that technology. Organ pipes, harps, elastic tubes, hydraulic waves, and so on, all became models of the acoustic place analyzing mechanism.

Table 10.1 adapts and extends a part of a table Wever prepared to describe the various place auditory theories. The emphasis in this table is on the specific mechanism that has been used to account for cochlear place localization. Two major classes of place theories can be used to encompass the entire variety of historical theories: those dependent upon resonant properties of the cochlear tissues and those dependent mainly upon the dynamics of waves in the cochlea. We shall now consider the details that distinguish between the resonance and wave versions of auditory place theory.

TABLE 10.1 AUDITORY PLACE THEORIES
(ADAPTED FROM WEVER, 1949)

	I. Resonance Place Theories		
	Date	Theorist	Critical feature
Dependent on resonance of tuned elements	a. 1605 — Bauhin		Differentially tuned air-filled cavities of various shapes and sizes
	b. 1672 — Willis		Two air-filled cavities, differentially tuned
	c. 1683 — Duverney		Differentially tuned elements of bony lamina
	d. 1707 — Valsalva		Differentially tuned elements of organ of Corti
	e. 1760 — Cotugno		Differentially tuned elements of organ of Corti
	f. 1867 — Helmholtz		Differentially tuned arches of Corti
	g. 1870 — Helmholtz, as influenced by Henson and Hasse		Differentially tuned transverse fibers of basilar membranes
Dependent on membrane resonance	h. 1867 — Hasse		Membrane resonance properties of tectorial membrane
	i. 1898 — Ewald		Standing waves on the basilar membrane
	II. Wave Theories of Place		
Independent of cochlear mechanics	a. 1894 — Hurst		Traveling bulge produced by interaction of original and reflecting wave
	b. 1900 — Ter Kuile		Traveling bulge produced by curtailed monodirectional waves
Dependent on basilar membrane mechanics	c. 1928 — von Békésy		Positions of maximum amplitude of a traveling wave as a function of basilar membrane properties
	d. 1946 — Zwislocki		Position of maximum amplitude of a traveling wave as a function of basilar membrane properties
Dependent on tube mechanics of the cochlea	e. 1931 — Ranke		Pulsations in elastic tubes
	f. 1937 — Reboule		Pulsations in elastic tubes

1. Resonance Place Theories. The notion of resonance is a simple one. Each physical object has a natural frequency of vibration and will tend to vibrate at that frequency more easily than at any other. Thus, energy can be transferred from a medium to a tuned object with maximum efficiency at its resonant frequency. In many instances, this transfer of energy can occur with no serious consequences. A violin string will tend to hum along at its resonant frequency when stroked or even when it is simply present in a noisy environment. A strong tone can also, however, cause a finely tuned object to destroy itself if the energy absorbed at the tuned frequency is much greater than the limits of physical strain of the object. In a trivial case, a crystal goblet can break after absorbing energy at its resonant frequency. With more serious consequences, bridges—particularly suspension bridges—unless carefully detuned with appropriate damping devices, can be sent into such violent oscillations that they can collapse. Perhaps one of the most striking examples of this was the Tacoma Narrows Bridge disaster in Washington, which collapsed in 1940 shortly after it was built. The bridge—a suspension type—hung in a windy valley, and the blowing of the wind, like the bowing of a violin string, was sufficient to make the bridge violently oscillate, and finally collapse. Similarly, stimulation with energies of mixed spectral distribution is often capable of exciting a set of tuned physical resonators to individually vibrate at amplitudes proportional to the power of each of their individual resonant frequencies.

When notions of tuned resonators were formalized in the seventeenth century, it almost immediately became obvious to some of the early students of audition that the resonance phenomena might possibly provide an explanation for some of the mysteries surrounding pitch perception in the human auditory system. Bauhin (1605) was the first to suggest that the inner ear was composed of a collection of air-filled cavities (analogous to organ pipes) of various sizes and shapes, each of which resonantly vibrated in tune with a particular frequency of airborne oscillation. Seventy years later Willis, astutely noting the absence of such a hypothetical system of cavities, suggested a modification of this hypothesis. The main change in his suggestion was that the relative amount of oscillation of only two particularly tuned resonant cavities was the key differentiating process. Unfortunately, his theory, like Bauhin's, had a serious defect. The necessary cavities simply did not exist.

The first really modern resonance place theory of audition was offered by DuVerney in 1683. His idea was based on the then newly discovered fact that the cochlea had a bony shelf—the osseus lamina —extending completely along its length. This bony lamina was discovered to vary in width, decreasing with distance from the oval window. Since long strings were known to resonate at lower frequencies than short strings, he assumed (incorrectly as it turned out) that the resonators in that cochlea were arranged so that low tones were localized near the oval window. High tones were thought to be localized at the extreme apical end of the cochlea.

In the eighteenth century, Valsalva and Cotugno added a most important notion. They both agreed that the resonating structure was not the bony lamina, but was in some way associated with the soft tissues, which were becoming ever more frequently observed as microscopic and dissection technique became increasingly efficient. Cotugno specifically assumed that the soft tissues of the organ of Corti were arranged in strands like the strings of a musical instrument and that the resonant vibrations of these strings were directly associated with specific tonal sensations.

Among other important points of Cotugno's theory was the fact that he, for the first time, properly assigned the basal portion of the cochlea to high tones and the extreme apical end to low tones. Although we now know this to be, in fact, true, his idea was based on an incorrect assumption. Cotugno, still assuming that a stringlike resonator mechanism was operative and knowing that the basilar membrane is wider at the apex than at the base, fortuitously made the right decision. As we shall see, however, it is clear that the width of the basilar membrane has nothing to do with place localization, and thus, while Cotugno was right about the basilar membrane locus of low and high tones, he was completely wrong in the reasons he used to support his argument.

The most famous of all of the resonant place theories was that presented by Helmholtz in two versions in 1857 and 1870, respectively. Wever's discussion of the details of the Helmholtz theory and of the manner in which it was presented is a classic example of the supremacy of style over content, for Wever makes it quite clear that the Helmholtz theory was little more than a rehashing of Cotugno's ideas of resonant strands in the organ of Corti. In the first version of the theory, Helmholtz, much impressed by the discovery of the arches of Corti, assumed that these microstructures were the resonant elements. However, shortly thereafter, Hensen (1863) showed that these units did not vary sufficiently in size to serve this role. Helmholtz, in the 1870 version of his theory, therefore, found it necessary to assume that transverse bands of the basilar membrane, operating independently of each other, were the tuned resonators. Unfortunately for his theory, subsequent studies showed even this modification to provide an inadequate basis of resonant discrimination for simple physical reasons. This can be elucidated by considering the tuning formula for a resonant string, which is given by the following equation:

$$f = \frac{1}{2L} \sqrt{\frac{T}{M}} \tag{10.1}$$

where f is the resonant frequency of the vibrating string; L is its length; T is the tension on the string; and M is its mass. This means that the tuned frequency of a vibrating string can be increased either by decreasing its length or its mass, or increasing its tension. There is little reason to assume that there is much in the way of a mass difference as one scans various portions of the basilar membrane, and even then, it was realized that there is little variation in the tension across the basilar membrane from one end to another. Thus, the major portion of the frequency difference must be attributable to string length. Unfortunately, the width of the basilar membrane varies only from about 0.1 to 0.5 mm; thus, string length could only vary by about 5 times. Considering that the auditory frequency range varies over a ratio of almost 1000 to 1, it is clear that simple vibrating string resonance is not adequate to account for the full range of tonal experiences.

The notion of resonantly tuned portions of the basilar membrane as the primary analysis mechanism, therefore, did not seem to be acceptable. Subsequent workers turned to the possibility that the properties of a continuous elastic membrane, rather than a vibrating string, might be invoked to account for the localization differences of the auditory spectrum. In 1867, Hasse called attention to the fact that the tectorial membrane was possibly resonant, but perhaps the most interesting resonant membrane theory was Ewald's 1898 extension of the notions inherent in the vibration of a cymbal or of what had been more generally called the Chladni plate. Metal disks, when struck, vibrate in elaborate patterns of standing waves. These waves can be made visible by dusting sand on the plate. The patterns will differ for plates of different size, mass, or thickness and for plates that are damped at different points on their surface. Ewald noted that since the vibratory pattern of the plates also varied as a function of the driving frequency, that auditory place localization might be accounted for in terms of this sort of membrane or platelike resonance of the basilar membrane. Unfortunately, most of the considerations that lead to the rejection of the tuned basilar membrane "string" also lead to the rejection of this hypothesis, even though the mathematical description of a two-dimensional vibrating plate is not so simple and the reasons for rejecting this idea not so apparent.

In sum, then, resonant place thories demand too much variance of the physical parameters of the delicate tissues of the basilar membrane to adequately explain auditory place localization. The mechanical properties of the tissue simply are not appropriate to permit the generation of highly localized place coding on the same basis that the operation of a harp string or a Chladni plate may be explained. The historical development of the resonance place theory, however, was very important, for there was a convergence on a very important premise on the part of all versions—namely, that it is the location along the basilar membrane that is the key correlate of stimulus frequency and, thus ultimately, pitch.

2. Wave Place Theories. If the physics of the cochlea made it impossible to accept any resonant place theory, was there any way in which localization of component frequencies could be accomplished on some other mechanical basis? In the years following Helmholtz's presentations, this question was repeatedly asked and a number of answers proposed by many investigators. The general theme, which ties all of their alternative answers together, is one that assumes that the behavior of the fluids in the inner ear, the medium through which waves are propagated, is critical. In other fluid dynamic situations, it could be shown that different wave patterns are produced by different driving frequencies. Thus, the wave or hydrodynamic properties of the fluids and the cavities of the inner ear offer a possible mechanism for establishing place representation, even though more primitive ideas of local resonance have had to be discarded. All of the theories we shall discuss in this section hypothesized mechanisms for the production of different wave patterns by virtue of the dynamics of fluid-filled tubes. But all theories are not the same in one or another aspect. The difference in wave pattern has been attributed by some to the elastic properties of the basilar membrane and by some to the tubelike characteristics of the entire cochlear cavity. Other theorists have suggested, however, that the wave patterns can be explained without any reference to the mechanical properties of the cochlea, but rather by simply assuming certain temporal relationships of time-varying sinusoidal signals in any medium.

Shortly after the difficulties with the Helmholtz resonance theories were noted, Hurst (1894) and Ter Kuile (1900a and b) suggested their versions of traveling wave theories. Both of their theories assumed a traveling bulge whose dynamics were independent of any of the mechanical features of the cochlea, but depended only upon the time course of the acoustic wave. Hurst suggested that when a wave of compression occurred in the air, it initiated a traveling wave moving from the oval window up the basilar membrane toward the heliocotrema. This wave was reflected from the apical end of the cochlea and, on its return, collided with one of the next cycles of the stimulus compression wave. The collision of the initial and reflected waves resulted in a bulge, which moved on the basilar membrane with its location at any given time dependent on the frequency of the stimulating wave. In fact, of course, the theory would not involve only a single bulge, but an intricate pattern of traveling bulges, depending upon the complexity of the incoming signal.

Ter Kuile's idea was very similar, but it did not even involve the collision of an outgoing and reflected wave—merely the fact that the distance between a wave of compression and a wave of rarefication for a given sound frequency was dependent upon its frequency. Thus, a wave or bulge, once started, would be inhibited mechanically by its own opposite phase at times that would correspond to places on the basilar membrane. The attractiveness of these theories is that they do not require any major differential mechanical properties of the cochlea beyond uniform elasticity.

Ranke (1931) and Reboul (1937) have also suggested place theories that depend only on the elastic properties of the tubelike cochlea. Their theories grew out of the hydrodynamic models, which were developed in the twentieth century to describe such phenomena as pulsations in veins and arteries. Unfortunately, the cochlea is a cavity in bone, a relatively inelastic material and displays few of the properties of a vein. For this reason, their hypotheses have never had a very great deal of popularity in modern theory.

The nonresonant place theories that are most prominent now are wave theories in which localization is dependent mainly upon the combined physics of the basilar membrane and the cochlear fluids. Specifically, von Békésy has proposed that limited mechanical elasticity and rigidity of the basilar membrane is sufficient to account for the formation of traveling waves whose amplitudes vary as they pass down the cochlea. The point of maximum amplitude has been shown by von Békésy to vary as a function of the frequency of the stimulating frequency in a way that explains many auditory phenomena. Because so much of von Békésy's theory is intimately involved in direct measurements, we shall consider his ideas in detail in the next section on the biological data. As a brief prelude, it is perhaps appropriate to say that his ideas have the greatest possible popularity today.

This, then, is the general history and a categorization of place theories, both of the resonance and wave types. We shall now turn to the other major category of auditory theories, in which the analysis is considered to be primarily central and which assume little, if any, analysis in the periphery.

B. Pure Frequency, Periodicity, or Telephone Theories

It is interesting to note that the group of theories that we shall now discuss arose primarily as reaction to the deficiencies of place theory in explaining all aspects of auditory pitch perception. The initial dates of the early presentations of the frequency theories fall in the second half of the nineteenth century—about the same time as the technology of telephonic communication was emerging and about the time that the pulsative nervous activity with varying interpulse frequency had first been observed. There was, for all practical purposes (according to Wever's history), no historic antecedent of frequency theories as there had been of the place theories. The reasons for this are clearly understandable in the context of the history of the problem. The anatomical discoveries of the preceding two centuries had repeatedly shown that the cochlea was a spatially extended organ, and the musical technology of the seventeenth, eighteenth, and nineteenth centuries was filled with instances of stringed instruments and resonant tubes. When the criticisms of the resonance theories began to be appreciated, however, some of the early workers apparently decided to bypass the issue of analysis. Many of the early frequency theorists simply ignored the problem of peripheral analysis or at least deferred it by assuming that information about the frequency pattern was transmitted relatively intact to the central nervous system.

Hopefully, it is obvious at this point in our discussion that there is no reason why frequency reproduction would not be a perfectly feasible means of pitch encoding. Coding theory makes no *a priori* requirement that pitch or any other quality be ultimately encoded by some spatial localization dimension. Various states of periodic neural activity are possible coding schema for acoustic frequencies, even if the frequencies of neural representation have shifted several octaves from the frequencies of the acoustic stimulation. This is a valid notion as long as the transforming relations are in some way interpretable by the central nervous system.

The use of the word *periodicity* as an alternative for the word *frequency* emphasizes that there is, in fact, something fundamental about the repetitive interval pattern as a candidate coding dimension for pitch that goes beyond average interval. Because of the fact that no recoding is assumed in the frequency theories beyond reproduction of the temporal

TABLE 10.2 AUDITORY FREQUENCY THEORIES
(ADAPTED FROM WEVER, 1949)

	Date	Theorist	Critical Feature
1	1865	Rinne	A critique of place theory
2	1885	Voltolini	All hair cells are capable of encoding all frequencies like a telephone
3	1886	Rutherford	Direct neural time representation up to 15,000 Hz; Complex tone decoded centrally
4	1892	Ayers	Field of grain—the hair cells are freely floating
5	1895	Bonnier	Basilar membrane is the responding tissue
6	1908	Hardesty	Tectorial membrane is the responding tissue

pattern, there is probably no psychophysical means to definitively prove that a frequency theory is true in the same way that a place theory may fall or be sustained on the basis of the detectability of envelope frequencies with no energy content. Frequency theories, therefore, are particularly dependent upon the direct neurophysiological evidence for support or disconfirmation.

Von Békésy (1963a) also notes another important point. Classic frequency theories, influenced by the then emerging technology of the telephone, had two separate and independent postulates. First, the general idea that the frequency pattern of the acoustic stimulus was preserved in the neural signal was axiomatic. The second postulate, modeled on the diaphragm in the mouthpiece of the telephone, asserted that all portions of the basilar membrane oscillated in unison and that all portions, therefore, have the capability of encoding all frequencies of acoustic stimulation. Direct observations, mostly carried out by von Békésy himself, refute this second postulate, but do not necessarily force us to reject the first one, and it is that notion rather than the second that shall be the major theme of the brief history of frequency theories that follows. Once again, our guide in this discussion must necessarily be Wever's (1949) extraordinarily well-written and comprehensive book.

Table 10.2 adapted from Wever (1949) lists the more significant of the pure frequency theories that have been proposed over the years. Most frequency theories differ only in certain minor anatomical and functional assumptions. Rutherford, the best known of the frequency theorists, ex-

TABLE 10.3 COMBINED AUDITORY PLACE AND FREQUENCY
THEORIES (ADAPTED FROM WEVER, 1949)

	Date	Theorist	Critical feature
1	1896	Meyer	Nonlinear elasticity of basilar membrane
2	1918	Wrightson	Summation of input signals
3	1930	Fletcher	Duplex theory
4	1949	Wever	Volley theory

pressed the common key idea when he postulated nerve action potential
frequencies of up to 14,000 Hz. Ayers, Bonnier, and Hardesty, three of
the less well-known frequency theorists, differed from one another mainly
in emphasizing the role of the hairs, the basilar membrane, and the tectorial membrane, respectively, as the sensitive medium, but all agreed
that the nervous activity essentially reproduced the temporal pattern of
the stimulus and that this pattern was transmitted to the central nervous
system, where it was analyzed by undefined mechanisms. It is, in fact,
this basic premise concerning the temporal properties of individual neurons
in the frequency theories, an axiom on which all of the theorists agreed,
upon which all of them collectively fall. Early in the twentieth century
with the development of the new electronic measuring techniques, it was
clearly and definitively established that the transmitted spiking rate of individual neurons never exceeded 1000 Hz and that direct reproduction of
any frequency greater than that *by a single neuron* was, therefore, impossible.

C. Combined Place and Frequency Theories
The individual difficulties with some of the early place theories and the
early frequency theories led some workers to the notion that a combined
place and frequency theory might be better able to serve as a model of
auditory pitch encoding. Wever (1949) also relates the history of these
combined theories. We have summarized his discussion in Table 10.3.
     Wrightson and Keith (1918), for example, had proposed a theory,
which was based essentially on the wave mechanics of a traveling bulge,
but which assumed that acoustic frequencies were represented at specific
frequency dependent places on the cochlea by nerve impulse firing rates.
The spatial distribution of frequency dependent information was not,
however, in his theory a result of any mechanical analytical process, for
according to Wrightson, the fluids of the inner ear were all incompressi-
ble, and all locations were capable of responding equally to each input

frequency. The spatial localization was thought to be due, rather, to a superimposition at any point of the activity produced by a given input frequency with the activity produced by any other frequency. Thus, complex incident waves produced patterns of neuronal activity that were rapid at some critical places and less rapid at others. Place localization in Wrightson's theory was, therefore, irregular in that there was no regular sequence of cochlear locations associated with the auditory spectrum. The specific locations of maximum activity, however, were the key correlates of input frequency. Unfortunately, his theory assumed not only that there was a one-for-one correspondence between stimulus and neural frequencies, but even worse, that each cycle of the stimulus produced four nerve action potentials. Thus, the problem posed by the inability of the neuronal firing rate to keep up with the stimulus frequencies was multiplied rather than simplified and the incompatibility with the neural data accentuated.

Meyer (1896) also used a hydraulic wave model to describe how different places on the cochlea responded to different frequencies of acoustic stimulation. Meyer was also particularly interested in showing how these different places of activation interacted mechanically on the surface of the basilar membrane to produce combination tones. Nevertheless, his theory also specifically states that there is a one-to-one correspondence between the neural response frequencies and stimulus and is thus, in major part, a frequency theory and is, therefore, subject to the same difficulties as all of the rest.

Perhaps the first of the truly modern combined theories of auditory quality was that proposed by Fletcher (1930). Fletcher was among the first, if not the first, to explicitly suggest that there is both frequency and place coding in the cochlea for different ranges of the stimulus frequencies. He stated, primarily on the basis of physical analogies and masking data, that high tones were more likely to be represented by place localization. Fletcher's conception of the mechanism for a place localization was resonance in a manner very similar to the original Helmholtz harp string, but slightly different in formulation. The main difference was that the length of the resonant elements was supposed to occur in the tuning equation as a square rather than in the linear form of Equation (10.1). The reasoning for this is somewhat obscure, but to quote Fletcher directly:

> Most authors who have tried to make a simple analysis of this problem have assumed that the frequency of resonance is inversely proportional to the length, w, of the cross fibers, but this analysis makes it inversely proportional to w^2. This is because it was assumed that the effective mass due to the vibrating liquid, which is associated with a small portion of the basilar membrane, decreases as w decreased. In other words, the effective vibrating volume is just sufficiently wide to cover the basilar membrane.
>
> (FLETCHER, 1930, p. 319.)

The main advantage of a system dependent upon the square of the length of the harp string, according to Fletcher, was that it allowed one to take

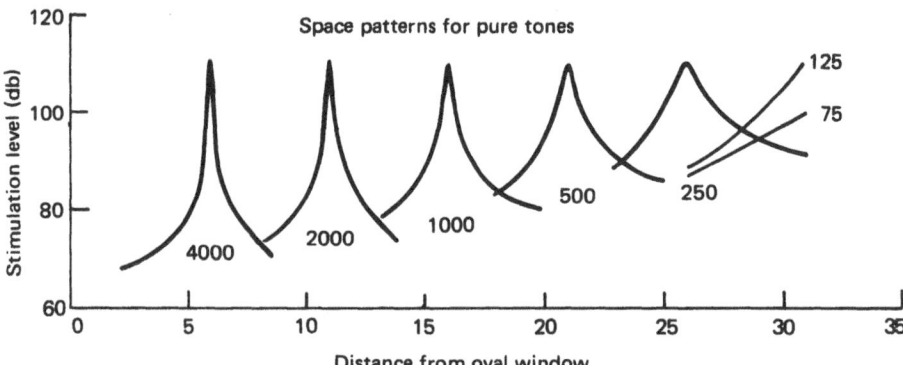

FIGURE 10.4 *The narrow (and now known to be incorrect) frequency turning curves of mechanical displacement along the basilar membrane according to Fletcher, 1930.*

advantage of the known 5 to 1 variation in the width of the basilar membrane to give a variation in tuning sufficient (in conjunction with an assumed 10 to 1 variation in basilar membrane tension from the basal end to the apex) to give a differential range of resonant oscillation varying from 86 to 16,000 Hz. Fletcher's theory assumed very narrow bands of activities produced by these resonant mechanisms as shown in Figure 10.4, although his theory did also allow a considerable broadening of this area of activity as the intensity of the stimulus was increased. He also assumed a sort of primitive phase locking in which the nerve impulse frequency followed the input signal oscillations, but only up to some maximum frequency. It is explicit in Fletcher's writing that this frequency following was also to be considered a code for low-frequency sound signals, and his theory, therefore, represents a historical precedent in the formulation of a duplexity theory of pitch encoding.

The most significant attempt to salvage some sort of temporal coding for stimulus frequency is the combined place and frequency theory known as the volley theory, which was presented by Wever himself in his 1949 book. Wever's ideas had a number of features that have been persistent in modern thinking, but also several that are difficult to maintain in the light of recent evidence. Briefly, Wever's theory was that both *resonance place* and *frequency* types of coding were to be found in auditory mechanisms. He, like Fletcher, supported the very important notion that the frequency theories were best able to handle some of the low-frequency signals, while place principles seemed best able to account for higher-frequency discriminations. This is an idea that has become the backbone of modern theories, as we shall see later in this chapter. On the other hand, to extend the range of application of the frequency principle, Wever suggested an idea, which he called the volley principle.

The basic idea of the volley principle is shown in Figure 10.5. This hypothetical synchronization of nervous activity in parallel fibers is spe-

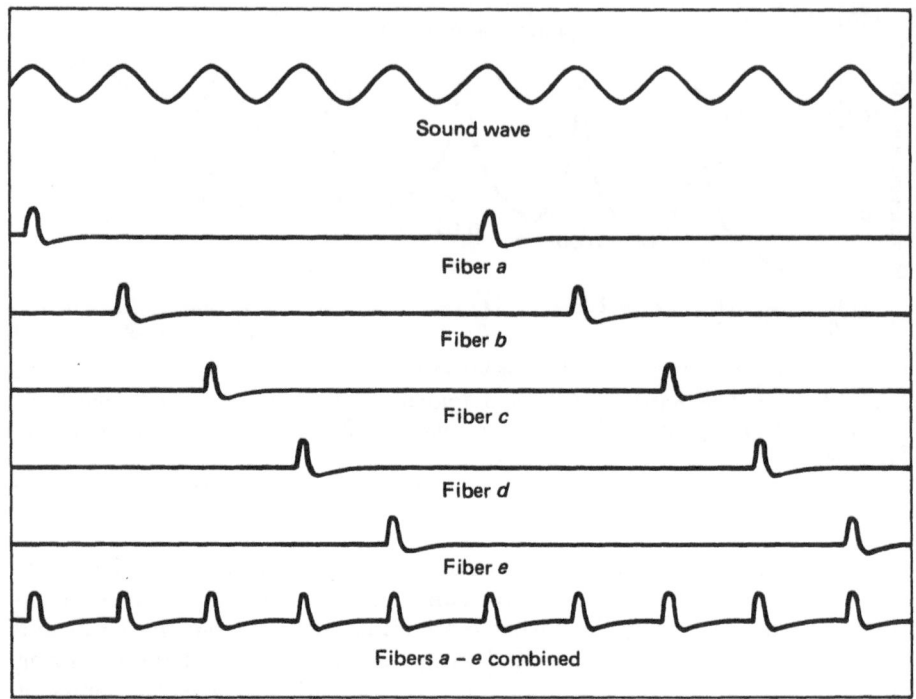

FIGURE 10.5 A diagram demonstrating the basic premise of the volley theory. The motion is that a group of nerves, none of which is individually capable of firing at the frequency of a sound stimulus, can collectively convey the necessary frequency information (from Wever, 1949).

cifically invoked to deal with the problem of how the limited frequency response range of a single auditory neuron could possible represent the very high frequencies at the middle and upper portion of the range of acoustic perception. Wever suggested that if one neuron could not do the job, perhaps several working together might be able to do so. Thus, in this figure, we see how a group of five neurons, each capable of firing only once every millisecond, collectively might be able to fire at a 5-kHz rate. Originally some critics thought that this level of synchronization was simply asking too much of the nervous system, but recent work (Rose, Brugge, Anderson, and Hind, 1967) suggests that these early critics were too modest in their estimate of the synchronization capabilities of the acoustic nerve and that, in fact, such volleying may actually be occurring. It now seems as if the major issue is to determine the range in which volleying can work and the upper limits of this type of frequency encoding, rather than to determine if it does work at all.

This, then, concludes our brief survey of the classic theories of auditory quality coding. The theories, historically, can be seen to be characterized by either the place or the frequency representation of different acoustic frequencies, and most recently by a trend which seems to rationalize the two approaches. At this point, it is necessary to turn our attention from theory to neurophysiological data, for in the past two decades a particularly high quality of experimental evidence, which is directly relevant to the neurophysiological postulates of the classic theories of audition, has been accumulating.

III. THE BIOLOGICAL DATA

Classical auditory theories differ somewhat from classic theories of visual quality in that they are, in general, much more specific about the neurophysiological mechanisms of nervous transmission. Specific assumptions have been made in almost all instances concerning the details, not only of the receptor mechanisms, but also of the patterns of neural encoding of the messages ascending toward the central nervous system. The net result of this orientation is that many features of the auditory theories are directly subject to empirical testing. We shall follow the same sequence used in the discussion of the visual modality, namely, to look at the encoding processes at various stages of the ascending auditory pathway. In this way, it is hoped that we shall be able to resolve some of the controversial issues raised by the psychophysical data and either reject or confirm some of the specific neural postulates of each type of theory. In the following section, we shall first examine what is known of the mechanical action of the cochlea in order to evaluate the various notions of cochlear function and coding and then the neural response patterns. We shall then consider the various coding schema used at higher levels of the pathway in order to evaluate what spatial and temporal parameters seem to be called into action at these levels to represent auditory quality.

A. The Cochlea

1. The Wave Mechanics of the Cochlea as Elucidated by Direct Visual Observation. Although it is quite certain that models and theories and indirect, but suggestive, findings are important in the development of our understanding of the various mechanisms of the auditory system, it is also quite clear that direct observations of the mechanical action of the cochlea would be of the greatest importance in selecting among hypothetical alternatives. It is also quite certain that the scientist almost single-handedly responsible for the development of the direct observation methods and the elucidation of the actual physical response in the cochlea is Georg von Békésy, who in 1961 received the Nobel Prize, primarily for his contributions in this area. Although others have contributed to this field in recent years, von Békésy's papers on this topic, which began in 1928, are still the best contemporary general statements on the mechanical and hydrodynamic aspects of cochlea function. Fortunately for the interested student, all of von Békésy's papers up to 1960 have been collected and translated and have been published as a single volume (von Békésy, 1960).

In the early 1920's, von Békésy had turned his attention to the problem of the cochlear localization of sounds. His interest in this problem and the publication of his theories and findings continued for the next three decades. The primary anatomical technique he used involved the decalcification of a portion of the temporal bone removed from a fresh cadaver. A dental-type grinding tool was then used to remove a small portion of the bony wall, exposing the apical end of the basilar membrane. Because of the entrance angle in his early studies, only about one-third of the basilar membrane was usually brought into direct view by the technique. Tiny carbon or alumina particles suspended in a saline solution were then flushed into the cochlea and allowed to deposit themselves on the basilar membrane. These deposited particles made clearly visible these otherwise nearly transparent tissues. The action of the basilar membrane could then be directly observed with a microscope as a function of the frequency or amplitude of the stimulating tone produced by either an earphone or a tuning fork.

One of von Békésy's first observations with this preparation was that there were no standing wave patterns as had been suggested by Ewald. There were, instead, patterns of traveling waves initiated, which moved from the oval window toward the heliocotrema at the apical end of the cochlea. By using stroboscopic illumination, von Békésy was able to observe these traveling waves in what was effectively slow motion and observe their velocity direction and amplitude as the stimulus characteristics varied. Another early observation was that there were observable displacements at the apical third of the cochlea only when lower-frequency stimuli were used. Frequencies higher than 300 or 400 Hz apparently were not capable of producing deformations anywhere within the region of the basilar membrane that von Békésy could see. Thus, the notion that the apical end is the region of localization of the low-frequency tones was supported and at least tentative support given for the suggestion that high-frequency tones might be localized near the oval window.

Another early and exceedingly important observation in this germinal study was that the traveling wave did not have the same amplitude throughout its visible course. Rather, there appeared to be a gradual increase in the amplitude of the wave of distortion on the basilar membrane as it came into view, and then a decrease as it moved past some point of maximum amplitude. Figure 10.6 shows the amplitude of the wave of distortion at two different positions of the wave produced by a 200-Hz signal as it moves along the basilar membrane. Note particularly the outer dashed line, which is the envelope of the maximum amplitude of the wave. This particular frequency peaks at a distance of 28 mm from the stapes. Other frequencies were seen to peak at other locations.

The substance of this very important contribution by von Békésy is that *the maximum amplitude of the traveling wave occurs at a different locus as a function of the frequency of the acoustic stimulus*. In later years, he was able to extend his direct observations of the cochlear vibrations by cutting out other small portions of the bony wall in different preparations and thus determine the point of maximum vibration up to about 1600 Hz. Figure 7.7 presented the results of this series of experiments. These data indicate the point on the cochlea at which the maximum amplitude of

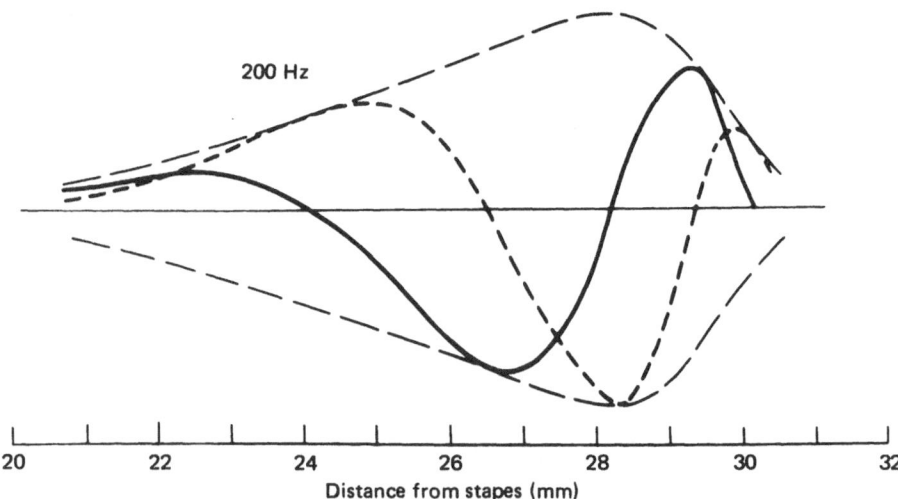

FIGURE 10.6 A drawing showing the observed amplitude and position of a traveling wave produced by a 200-Hz signal at two different instants as indicated by the solid and inner dashed lines respectively. The outer dashed line indicates the envelope of maximum amplitudes for all positions. The maximum amplitude of this outer envelope occurs at different locations for the different frequencies (from von Békésy, 1947).

vibration occurred for a given set of test frequencies. Figure 10.7 is a more detailed presentation of the overall amplitude pattern as a function of cochlear locus of the traveling wave for seven different frequencies. In this modified way, then, exceedingly compelling support is given to notions of place encoding of all stimulus frequencies above 50 Hz.

Another important finding from these direct observations of cochlear vibrations was von Békésy's demonstration that the pattern, wherever maximized and for whatever frequency, is extremely broad. There was never any sharply defined region activated by even the purest monofrequency. This is a critical observation, because it stands in sharp contrast to the fine frequency discriminative ability displayed in psychophysical tests. Furthermore, it also contrasts with many of the earlier theories of cochlear localization that proposed sharp tuning due to resonance.

At first glance, the psychophysical and neurophysiological sets of data seem almost antagonistic, for von Békésy reports that stimuli differing in frequency by as much as 20 to 40 Hz did not exhibit noticeably different patterns of basilar membrane response. Yet subjects can discriminate signals that differ by as little as 2 or 3 Hz in psychophysical experiments. Over the years this discrepancy has led a number of workers, including von Békésy, to speculate about mechanisms that sharpen the response of the system to allow for better discrimination. Usually these discussions revolve around the possibility of neural interaction of a spatial sort like those found in the visual system that we have already discussed in Chapter 7. Von Békésy (1967) has published an entire volume dealing

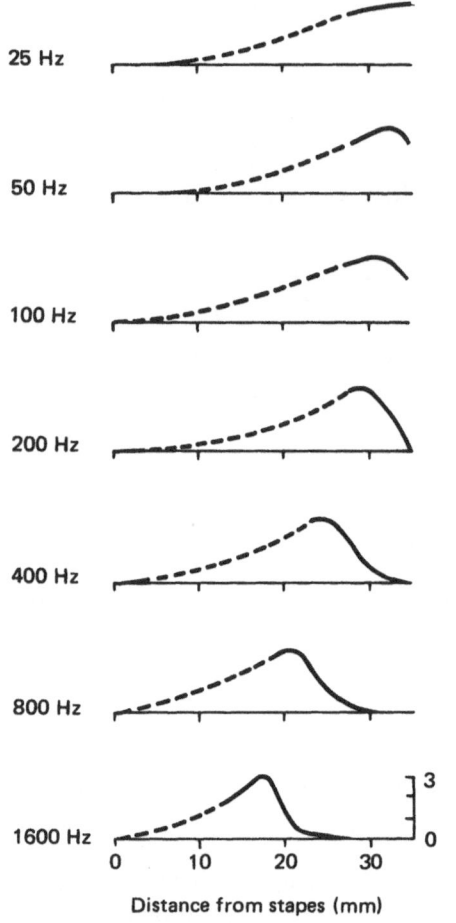

25 Hz

50 Hz

100 Hz

200 Hz

Relative amplitude

400 Hz

FIGURE 10.7 A set of seven amplitude envelopes similar to the one shown in Figure 10.6, showing the difference in the localization of the maximum as a function of the stimulus frequency. Note that the peak amplitudes produced by the higher frequencies tend to be located more toward the oval window and those produced by the lower frequencies near the heliocotrema (from von Békésy, 1949b).

800 Hz

1600 Hz

0   10   20   30

Distance from stapes (mm)

with the problem of neural interaction and its general relevance to many different perceptual phenomena. But the reader is also reminded of the absence of evidence supporting central sharpening. Tonndorf (1970), however, points out that there is some reason to believe that there may be some sharpening in the mechanical system itself, which would explain why even first-order neurons (see below) appear to have narrower tuning curves than does the cochlea mechanical apparatus.

It should be noted, at least in passing, that von Békésy's experiments have been criticized for a number of different reasons. In a separate section of his 1960 book, he has considered these issues and replied to them. First, some critics had noted that the amplitude of the stimuli he used had been very high and suggested that perhaps the responses at these stimulus amplitudes gave a distorted picture of what was actually going on. Von Békésy's rebuttal centered around the fact that over the range of stimulus intensities that produced any observable response, the amplitude of the response was linear. He felt that it was, therefore, highly unlikely that at lower intensities, the stimulus would become nonlinear and thus, in any fundamental way, be different from that observed at his experimental levels.

A second criticism was that there might be some change in the elasticity of the basilar membrane after the death of the experimental subject. Von Békésy noted that there was a 100 to 1 difference in the stiffness of the basilar membrane from one end of the cochlea to the other and that, therefore, any small postmortem change in this critical property could have little effect on the general outcome. Finally, the criticism was made that an opening in the cochlear wall might change the tube properties of the cochlea. However, von Békésy was able to show that this was not the case—only the amplitude of the response seemed to be affected by the hole and not the shape of the response.

In discussing these comments, von Békésy also reported another important discovery. The specific physical parameter of the basilar membrane, which is responsible for the production of traveling waves and the specific shape of these waves, is the stiffness of the basilar membrane. It is upon this mechanical property that place localization on the cochlea is dependent, and it is the wave action on the more or less stiff sheet of the basilar membrane that must take the place of tuned resonance in any modern place theory of auditory quality coding. We shall discuss this point further later in this chapter.

Other workers have recently extended von Békésy's direct observation technique to related problems. Among the foremost of these scientists to apply the technique has been Tonndorf (1962), who cosidered the problem of the auditory analysis of mixed acoustic frequencies. He introduced a complex wave consisting of a combination of a 50- and a 100-Hz tone after first stimulating the cochlea with the two tones separately. Figure 10.8 (a) shows the displacement pattern along the basilar membrane for the two tones individually. Each has a maximum amplitude in approximately the locus observed by von Békésy. When a mixture of the two tones was introduced into the ear, however, the resulting displacement function showed a bimodal "humping" consistent with a theory of simple Fourier analysis into component frequencies by the mechanical action of the cochlea. This is shown in Figure 10.8 (b). Thus, there appears to be a physical correlate of Ohm's acoustic law visually observable in the shape of traveling waves on the basilar membrane.

2. The Wave Mechanics of the Cochlea as Elucidated with the Mossbauer Effect—A Promising Technique. When a radioactive source moves about in space, there is a shift in the frequency of any radiation emitted by that source. This Doppler shift of frequency can be used as a remarkably sensitive means of recording very small velocities. The sensitivity is such that velocities as small as a few feet a year, for example, can be measured with appropriate gamma ray detection and measuring equipment. The shift in the gamma radiation frequency as a function of the velocity of the source is known as the "Mössbauer effect" and has been applied, because of its exquisite sensitivity, to the measurement of the motion of the basilar

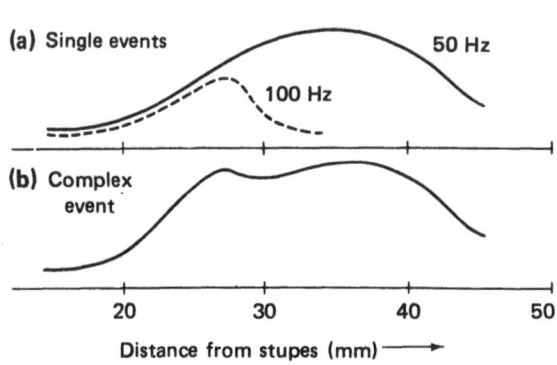

(a) Single events   50 Hz

100 Hz

(b) Complex
    event

20   30   40   50

Distance from stupes (mm) ⟶

FIGURE 10.8 Envelopes of traveling waves. (A) shows the envelopes for a 50- and a 100-Hz tone, respectively, while (B) shows the envelope of the combined stimulus. This form of response is considered to be evidence for acoustic frequency analysis at the level of the basilar membrane, since two peaks corresponding to the components of the combined wave appear in the latter's amplitude envelope (from Tonndorf, 1962).

membrane. Johnstone and Boyle (1967) seem to have been the first to apply the technique in a preliminary study, but a much more complete experiment resulting in a much more comprehensive set of data has been reported by Rhode (1971).

The general technique described by Rhode involves the surgical opening of the cochlear cavity and the placement of a small cobalt-57 radioactive source on the basilar membrane not far from the round window. The site of the observation in this case was, therefore, quite different from that used by von Békésy, most of whose observations were made near the apical end of the cochlea. All of the measurements made by Rhode on about 20 squirrel monkeys unfortunately were recorded from almost exactly the same single point on the basilar membrane. The velocity of the movement at this point was directly measured with the Mössbauer apparatus and, from this basic measure, the amplitude and phase distortions of the motion calculated.

The fact that the measurements were made at only one place on the basilar membrane (in addition to comparison measurements on the malleus of the middle ear) restricts the general importance of Rhode's application of the Mössbauer technique to the problem under discussion. The data obtained are clearly limited to the tuning of that single point; it remains for some future investigator to perform the tedious and difficult task of sampling the spatial distribution of the cochlear response at a very large number of positions to give the full and complete story of cochlear localization. However, it is clear that some of the more important features of the von Békésy theory of traveling wave localization are confirmed in Rhode's experiment.

Rhode determined the amplitude of the response to frequencies varying from 1 to 10 kHz for both the malleus and the basilar membrane, and then calculated the ratio of the amplitudes to give a more accurate description of the tuning of the basilar membrane. The ossicular chain, of course, has its own fundamental mechanical properties, and it is the transfer of energy between ossicles and the basilar membrane that criti-

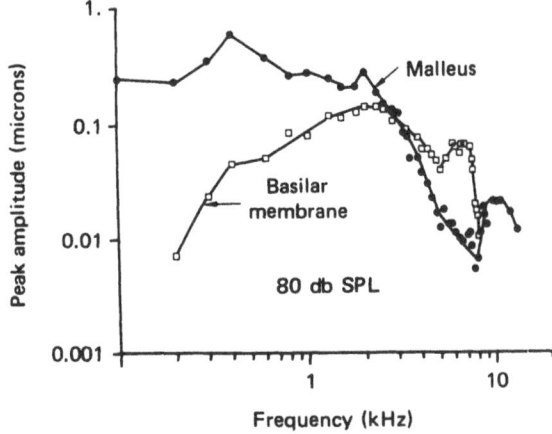

FIGURE 10.9 Amplitude of vibration as a function of stimulus frequency measured with the Mössbauer effect both at the malleus and at a single point on the basilar membrane near the oval window (from Rhode, 1971).

cally defines the response pattern of the basilar membrane, not the relation between the amplitude of oscillation of the basilar membrane and the external acoustic stimulus; that latter relation being confounded by the dynamics of the ossicles. Figure 10.9, for example, shows the absolute amplitude measurements for both the malleus and the basilar membrane. When stimuli of varying frequency are presented, clearly the response function of both was broadly tuned and quite unlike the sort of curve one would expect from either the known psychophysical or neurophysiological data. When the response functions of amplitude of the basilar membrane response are divided by that for the amplitude of the response of the malleus, however, a transfer ratio, which more clearly depicts the specific differential sensitivity of the basilar membrane, is obtained. Figure 10.10 is an example of such a ratio tuning curve. This curve clearly reflects the peaking of the tuning curve at about 8 kHz. Thus, this portion of the cochlea seems to be a region that is primarily associated with the place representation of 8-kHz tone, a finding which once again is consistent with the notion that high tones are spatially localized at the basal end of the cochlea.

An additional important observation contained in the graphs shown in Figure 10.10 is that the ratio curves do not perfectly overlap for the three different sound pressure levels used. This is an important observation, for these nonconstant ratios suggest that there is, indeed, a nonlinearity of the transfer function of the basilar membrane. This is extremely important, for it points to the anatomic level at which some of the combination tones might be introduced into the auditory message, namely, the initial mechanical cochlear analysis.

Another interesting point noted by Rhode is that the threshold for auditory signals has an amplitude that is only a small fraction of an angstrom unit, thus confirming indirect calculations made many years earlier. Clearly, the Mössbauer technique is going to be extremely important in helping to definitely resolve the problems of cochlear mechanics.

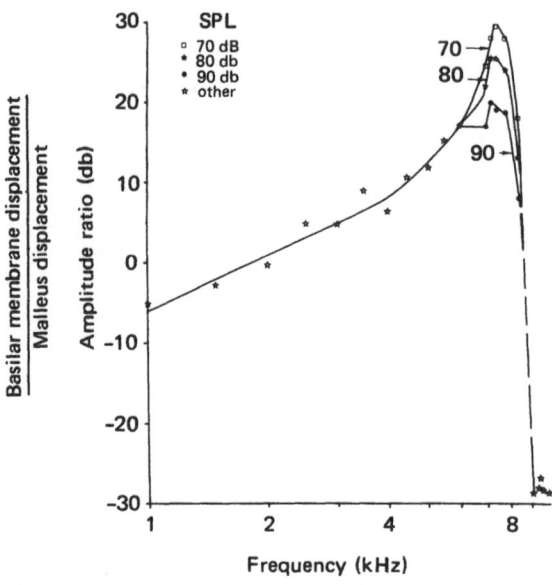

FIGURE 10.10 A set of curves calculated as a ratio of the two curves shown in Figure 10.9 for three different stimulus amplitudes. The curve in this graph is much closer in form to the conventional tuning curve with which we are more familiar. This location near the oval window is seen to have a peak sensitivity to stimuli with frequencies close to 8kHz. The discrepancy in the three curves near their peaks indicates that the basilar membrane is acting in that region as a nonlinear mechanism (from Rhode, 1971).

3. *Induced "Lesions" of the Cochlea—Reversible and Irreversible.* Another method for approaching the problem of cochlear localization is to disable a portion of the cochlea and determine what, if any, deficiencies appear in a subject's audiogram. There are several possible ways to selectively deactivate a portion of the cochlea. One is to take advantage of the fact that there is a transient period of selective diminished responsiveness following exposure to moderately intense acoustic stimuli, and to make before and after audiographic measurements with human subjects. Measures might be made of either the temporary threshold shifts (TTS) or of the temporary loudness shift (TLS) following loud acoustic stimulation. An alternative technique is to selectively and permanently damage portions of the cochlea with antibiotics, mechanical devices, or very intense sounds, and then compare psychophysically obtained audiographic data with postmortem inspection of the damage. This sort of experimental manipulation, of course, can only be applied to infrahuman subjects, although occasionally human clinical and postmortem data have been available. First, let us consider the preadaptation technique with moderately loud sounds.

The classical and probably still the definitive paper using the preadaptation technique with human subjects is the work of Davis, Morgan, Hawkins, Galambos, and Smith (1950). Following stimulation with single stimulus frequencies, they measured complete audiograms. In these postadaptation records, they did not find specific losses at sharply defined tonal bands. Their findings showed, rather, a generalized hearing loss for all tones with higher frequencies than the adapting frequency. Figure 10.11 depicts this pattern of acoustic loss for several adaptation frequencies. Furthermore, and quite surprisingly, the maximum hearing loss did not occur at the adapting frequency itself but, rather, usually at a fre-

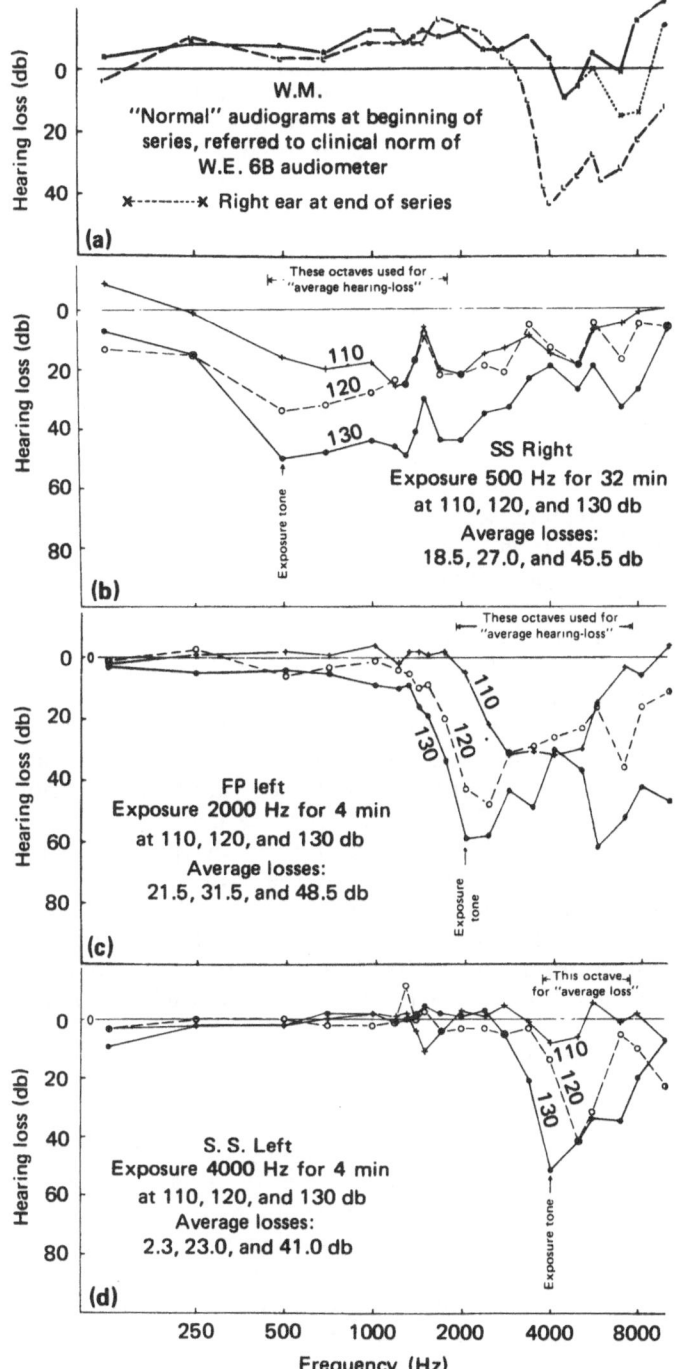

FIGURE 10.11 *Hearing losses that are produced by sustained exposure to pure tones. (a) Shows the normal audiogram before and after the test series. (b), (c), and (d) show the effects of stimulation with 500-, 2000-, and 4000-Hz stimulation at the levels and for the durations indicated. Low-frequency stimuli tend to impair hearing all across the spectrum. High-frequency stimuli tend only to impair higher-frequency hearing (from Davis, Morgan, Hawkins, Galambos, and Smith, 1950).*

quency half an octave higher. It may be hypothesized that these effects are correlated with the direction of movement of the traveling curve, which moves from the high tone encoding region at the basal end of the cochlea to the low tone encoding region at the apical end. Presumably, a very intense sound frequency would deactivate all more basal portions of the basilar membrane, in addition to the portion at which it produces its peak amplitude of deformation.

A similar finding obtains when selective cochlear destruction is carried out with drugs, which act selectively on the cochlea. Stebbins, Miller, Johnsson, and Hawkins (1969) used the antibiotics kanamycin and neomycin, which are known to produce specific destruction of the hair cells, to achieve selective cochlear destruction. The destructive action of these drugs begins at the basal end of the cochlea and gradually, with continued administration over a period of months, works its way progressively toward the apex. Stebbins and his colleagues first measured the normal audiograms of five rhesus monkeys with some ingenious animal psychophysical procedures (see Stebbins, 1970), and then administered drug doses for periods varying from one to six months. After a given period of time, during which progressive cochlear degeneration occurred, the animal was retested and then immediately sacrificed and microscopic examinations made of the then existing cochlear structure. Missing axons in the cochlear nerve, degeneration of hair cells, and even massive destruction of the organ of Corti were observed by Stebbins and his colleagues after one-to-six-month periods of antibiotic administration. Associated with this neural deterioration were deficiencies in the audiogram. These deficiencies were characterized by sharp cutoffs of the high-frequency components, but little loss in the low-frequency regions. The amount of high-frequency hearing loss increased with the passage of time until there was a broad range of tonal deafness after about six months of antibiotic administration. Figure 10.12 shows the general trend of increasing hearing loss as a function of frequency for increasing drug administration periods.

Associated with these relatively sharply cutoff hearing losses were equivalent sharp cutoffs of the limits of hair-cell destruction as determined in the postmortem. Figure 10.13 shows the anatomic destruction as measured by the number of hair cells remaining at various positions along the basilar membrane after various periods of drug administration. Obviously, the one animal to whom neomycin had been administered for a short time had been far more grossly affected by that treatment than had those animals who had received kanamycin, a less toxic antibiotic.

The general results of this experiment, therefore, are consistent with those of the adaptation experiments described above. Small lesions at the basal end of the cochlea seem to be associated with the loss of only very-high-frequency tonal coding. As the lesion increases in size, including more and more of the basal end of the basilar membrane, there is a gradual increase in the amount of loss of lower-frequencies hearing loss with ever lower frequencies dropping out in sequence.

Another way of experimentally producing controlled lesions along portions of the basilar membrane is "simply" to insert a probe and

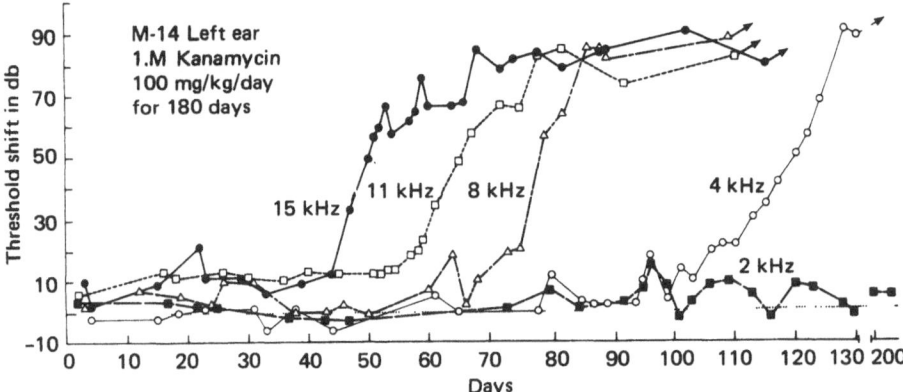

FIGURE 10.12 *Hearing losses as a function of duration of antibiotic treatment for four different frequencies. Obviously, high-frequency sensitivities are lost earlier than low-frequency ones, and this loss is correlated with destruction of the basal end of the organ of Corti in the earlier stages of drug administration (from Stebbins, Miller, Johnsson, and Hawkins, 1969).*

mechanically destroy these delicate tissues. This sort of experiment is, in reality, quite technically difficult to execute, but in some instances it can be done. For example, auditory effects of mechanical destruction of portions of the cochlea have been reported by Gross (1952) and Schuknecht and Neff (1952). Each of these experiments involved the loss of increasing amounts of the cochlea in a series of guinea pigs starting at the apex, the most surgically accessible region. Both found that increasing the area of destruction increased the bandwidth of low-frequency tones that were no longer perceived, and involved more and more high-frequency tones according to behavioral tests.

Guinea pigs are not people, however, and human data are always of prime interest. Unfortunately, it is not ethically possible to surgically manipulate the living human cochlea just for the purposes of an experiment of this sort. Therefore, what data are available have always depended upon accidental cochlear injuries, as measured with audiograms taken during life and subsequent postmortem examination of the tissue loss. Bredberg (1968) has recently published a monograph, in which a series of such studies was carried out. He discovered that, in general, degeneration at the basal end of the cochlea was associated with severe hearing loss for speech sounds, while degeneration at the apical end only modestly affected speech perception. This is probably due to the special importance of middle and high frequencies to speech perception and also supports the notion of high-frequency localization at the basal end of the cochlea.

A final type of selective deactivation experiment exaggerates the temporary hearing loss produced by a moderately intense adaptation tone. In this case, the ear is flooded with very-high-intensity sound waves of a single frequency for an extended period of time, and the experimenter then

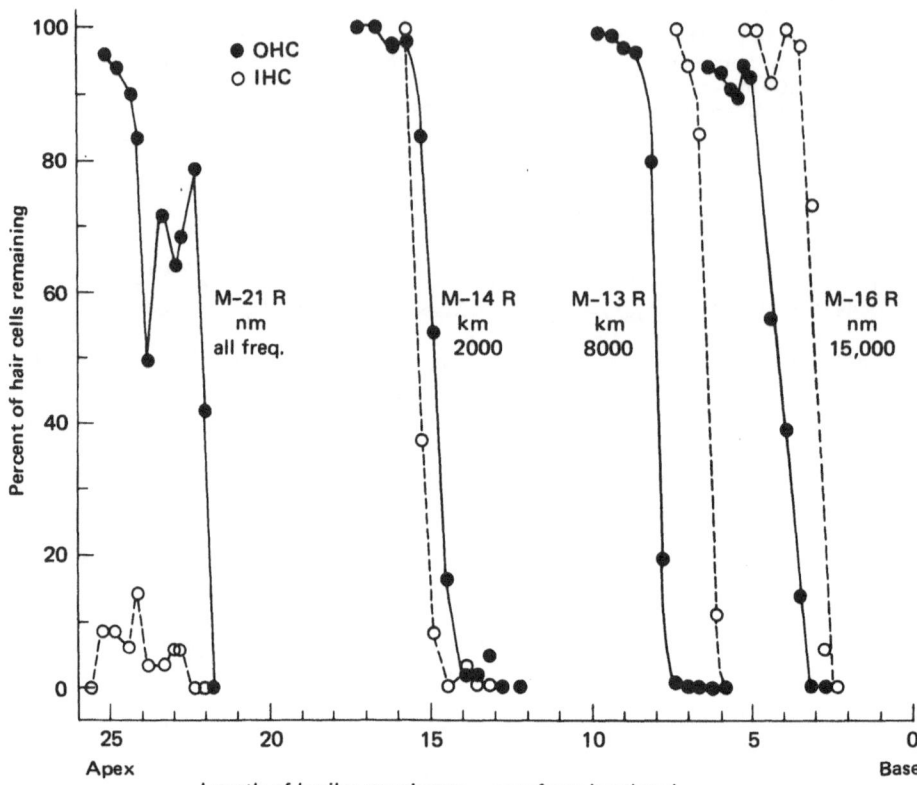

FIGURE 10.13 Curves showing the degree of damage to the inner (IHC) and outer (OHC) hair cells as a function of the type of antibiotic and the duration of the period over which it is administered. Monkeys 16, 13, and 14 were given kanamycin sulfate for 5, 28, and 180 days, respectively, resulting in increasing amounts of damage. Monkey 21 received neomycin sulfate for only 15 days, but in this brief time had much more severe damage to the organ of Corti than that caused by even longer periods of administration of kanamycin sulfate. This was particularly true for the inner hair cells, which were almost totally destroyed in this brief time (from Stebbins, Miller, Johnsson, and Hawkins, 1969).

examines the anatomical destruction produced by the various frequencies. This sort of experiment was initially performed by Smith (1947), who found that low-frequency tones produced broad bands of cochlear destruction near the apex, while high-frequency tones produced narrower bands of destruction closer to the oval window. Unfortunately, for the simplicity of the story we want to tell, when the cochlear microphonic correlates of such destruction were measured (Smith and Wever, 1949), the effect of any destruction stimulus frequency was found to be very widely spread across the auditory spectrum. But as we know, the microphonic is picked up simultaneously from widely spaced portions of the cochlea. Low tones, however, did produce a generally greater deficit than did

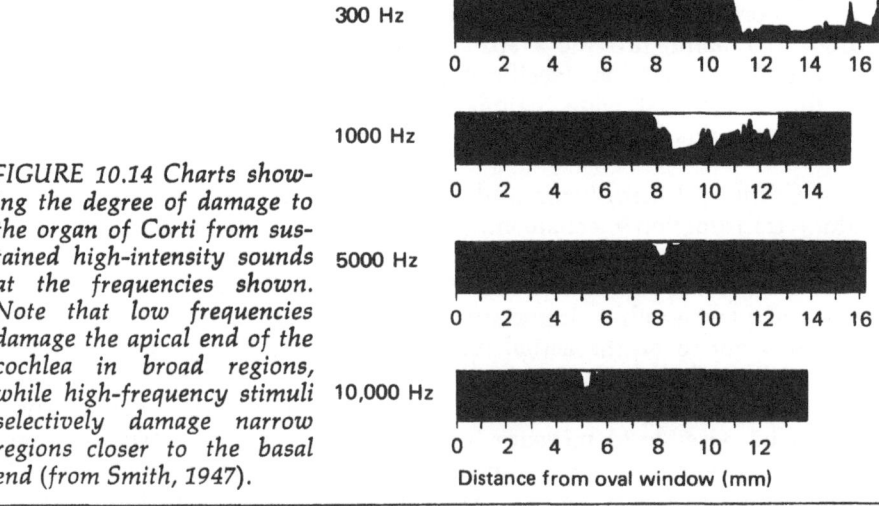

FIGURE 10.14 Charts showing the degree of damage to the organ of Corti from sustained high-intensity sounds at the frequencies shown. Note that low frequencies damage the apical end of the cochlea in broad regions, while high-frequency stimuli selectively damage narrow regions closer to the basal end (from Smith, 1947).

high-frequency tones. Figures 10.14 and 10.15 show that range of anatomical destruction and the sort of impairment of the cochlear microphonic produced by various stimuli.

All of these data are characterized by a single theme: low tones appear to be represented by activity predominantly broadly localized at the apical end of the cochlea, while high-frequency tones seem to activate

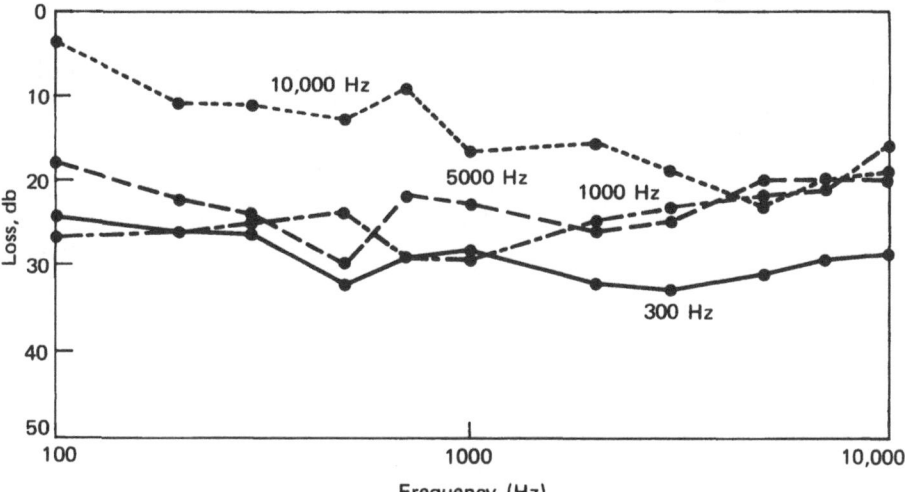

FIGURE 10.15 The effect of sustained high-intensity tones on the production of the cochlear microphonic. Though there is no solely local decrease in the sensitivity, low tones do produce a greater impairment than do the high tones, a fact which is in agreement with the wider spread of low-frequency responses and the widely dispersed source of the microphonic (from Smith and Wever, 1949).

narrower portions of the cochlea near the basal portion. The data do not, on the other hand, provide a strong argument for a unique localization of specific frequencies at specific places. Rather, all of it generally supports the notion that wide regions of cochlear activity are produced by even pure stimulus frequencies.

4. *The Cochlear Microphonic and Localization.* In our discussion of the auditory transduction mechanism, we have already introduced the cochlear microphonic as a possible candidate for the role of the receptor potential. Over the years, a number of investigators have suggested that it might also play another important experimental role, even if ultimately it is shown not to be the actual receptor potential. The general idea was that a small, but not microscopic, electrode, if placed on the basilar membrane, might pick up potentials only from that immediate region. Thus, it should be possible to measure tuning curves and other response functions of local points by using the cochlear microphonic as an indicator (a useful sign even if it is not a code). Such data would contribute greatly to our knowledge of the localization of acoustic frequencies on the basilar membrane. One of the first studies that interpreted the cochlear microphonic in this way was reported by Tasaki, Davis, and Legouix (1952). They used a differential electrode configuration to show that electrodes placed in the first basal turn of the cochlea picked up microphonics associated with all frequencies, while at the third turn only low frequencies produced recordable responses. But there is some controversy surrounding this approach. For example, Dallos, Schoeny, and Cheatham (1971) have shown that microphonics recorded in the cochlea contain all frequencies at all electrode positions.

The current view is that the cochlear microphonic response recorded with a gross electrode is not the restricted output of a very small region of the cochlea, but rather is the cumulative response of a rather broad region. In fact, Dallos and his co-workers believe that some portions of the cochlear potentials that are picked up at one end of the cochlea may actually come from the other end. They have, however, suggested a means of discriminating local from distant cochlear microphonics, based upon a differential recording system in which two electrodes are placed in the scala vestibuli and scala tympanni, respectively. Since it had been definitively established that the cochlear microphonic is generated in the basilar membrane, recordings from the two electrodes on either side of the membrane should be 180 deg out of phase. Only those signals that have a perfect 180-deg phase difference can be assumed to be associated with local activity, while signals with other degrees of phase shift would be considered to be generated at some distant locus. Figure 10.16 (a), (b), and (c) shows the phase angle response data as a function of frequency for electrodes positioned at various positions (one at each of the first three turns) of a guinea pig's cochlea All three of the response curves show some evoked microphonic potentials across the entire stimulus spectrum utilized. Not all responses, however, have the 180-deg phase angle characteristic of locally generated signals. These curves may be interpreted as indicating that all frequencies includ-

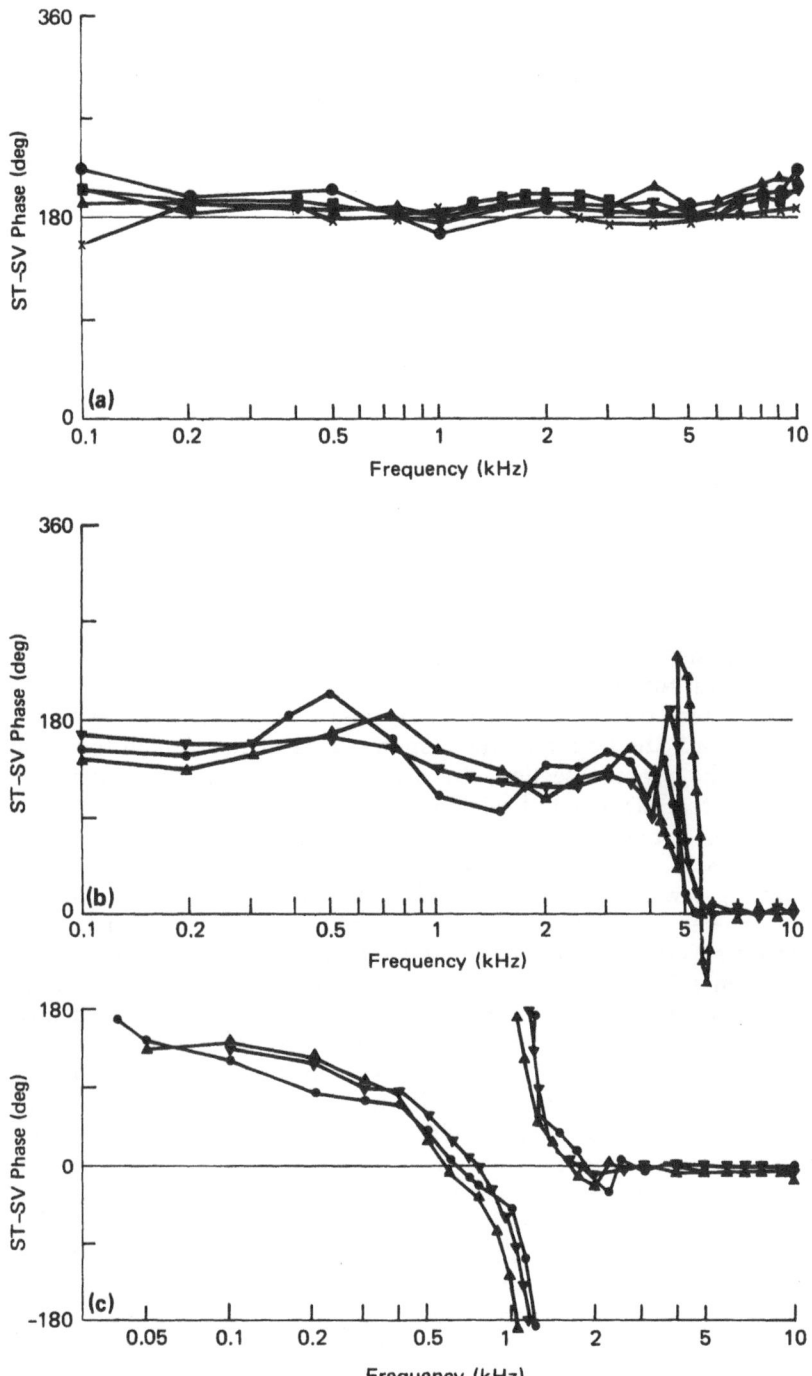

FIGURE 10.16 Phase angle measurements of the cochlear microphonic between the scala tympani (ST) and the scala vestibuli (SV) as a function of stimulus frequency. (a) As recorded in the first turn of the cochlea of five guinea pigs. (b) As recorded in the second turn of the cochlea of three guinea pigs. (c) As recorded in the third turn of the cochlea of three guinea pigs. See text for full details (from Dallos, Schoeny, and Cheatham, 1971).

ing the very highest used (19 kHz) produce cochlear microphonics in the first turn. In the second turn, only microphonic potentials up to about 3000 Hz are produced locally, while at the third turn only very-low-frequency tones produce local cochlear microphonics. These data, therefore, also speak to the same point made in several different ways in this section—namely, in general the cochlear responses produced by low tones are localized at the apical portion of the cochlea, while the responses produced by high tones are localized mainly at the basal end and central region of the cochlea.

In sum, then, some form of cochlear spatial localization of stimulus frequencies appears in the findings obtained with almost all of the different experimental methods we have discussed. Implicit in all these findings, therefore, is a very strong support of place theory at the cochlear level for the frequencies above 40 or 50 Hz. Below this limit, however, it seems that direct observations and indirect electrical measures all fail to show any differential localization.

B. The Response Area at Various Levels of the Ascending Auditory Pathway

In our previous discussion of spatial interactions, it was necessary to briefly introduce the notion of the response area of neurons in the auditory system. In the present section, we shall complete our discussion of this important set of data, emphasizing their current role in the support of place theories of auditory quality coding. The notion of response area was introduced by Galambos and Davis (1943), and their work has engendered a continuing series of follow-up studies. Galambos and Davis were interested in the response patterns of single auditory nerve fibers and explored the combined effect of stimulus intensity and frequency on the evoked spike response frequency. Glass microelectrodes, filled with KCl, were inserted through a surgically prepared opening in the skull of a cat into the auditory nerve so that potentials were recorded from single cells. Their initial observations suggested that each probed cell had a characteristic tuning curve such that its threshold was lowest at one particular frequency, but that frequencies on either side of their best frequency were also able to excite the nerve if their intensities were high enough. As the frequency difference between a stimulating frequency and the best frequency increased, the amplitude of the stimulating frequency had to be progressively higher to elicit a neural response. The function representing the response area thus defined is V-shaped on a graph, in which frequency is plotted along the horizontal coordinate, and the necessary stimulus amplitude for a criterion response is plotted along the vertical coordinate.

Figure 7.14 showed the general pattern of response as observed by Galambos and Davis for four auditory nerve neurons. This figure, now considered to be a classic, displays many of the important features that have been substantiated by more recent studies. One of the most significant of the features of this response curve is that it is not symmetrically V-shaped. The high-frequency cutoff region is steeper than the low-frequency cutoff. Furthermore, the width of the tuning curve is quite large. At the top of each of the curves, the width may be anywhere from 1500 to 3000 Hz, and this basic width increases as one goes from cells with low center frequencies to cells with higher center frequencies. This absolute increase in width with increase in frequency is often not appreciated, because these curves are always plotted on logarithmic horizontal axes, which obscure the increase in absolute bandwidth. On the other hand, it is also important to consider that the absolute width of the tuning curve may be less important than the ratio of the bandwith to the central frequency. Kiang (1965) has suggested the use of the traditional engineering "Q" ratio to define the sharpness of the tuning curve:

$$Q = \frac{\text{center frequency}}{\text{width of response area 10 db above threshold}} \qquad (10.2)$$

and has plotted the Q's for a large number of auditory nerve fibers. This plot is reproduced in Figure 10.17 and shows that the relative sharpness of tuning, at least as measured with the Q index, gradually increases with center frequency above 2 kHz, a conclusion that is the complete opposite of that drawn from the absolute width data. Nevertheless, whichever view of the trend in width one accepts, the general conclusion that must be drawn from these data is that neurons of the auditory nerve do not exhibit anywhere near the same degree of narrow responsiveness at normal listening levels that is reflected in psychophysical tests of frequency discrimination.

Over the years, a large number of workers have investigated the response curves of auditory neurons at other levels of the ascending pathways. Galambos (1952) himself and Gross and Thurlow (1951) have worked at the level of the medial geniculate body; Tasaki and Davis (1955) and Rose, Galambos, and Hughes (1959) at the level of the cochlear nucelus; and Hind (1960) and others at the level of the cortex. Moushegian, Rupert, and Galambos (1962) were the first to show that there were inhibitory areas within the excitatory response areas at some levels, in addition to the adjacent inhibitory response area originally shown by Galambos (1944) and further developed by Greenwood and Maruyama (1965). (See Chapter 7 for a complete discussion of this material.)

Because small differences in the details of procedure often make the results from different labs incomparable, Katsuki (1961) made a very important contribution to the problem when he studied the response areas at all of these levels within the confines of a single laboratory, with a single technique, and on a single species. Figure 10.18 reproduces his figure, showing the response curves recorded from the auditory nerve, the inferior colliculus, the trapezoid body, and the medial geniculate levels, respectively. We have already discussed in Chapter 7 the importance of this finding in raising a question of the existence of central sharpening.

Another distinction among cells at the various levels is also included in these data, to which our attention has been called by Simmons (1970). He points out that, at all levels, investigators have found both moderately wide response areas, like the ones we have been discussing, and also,

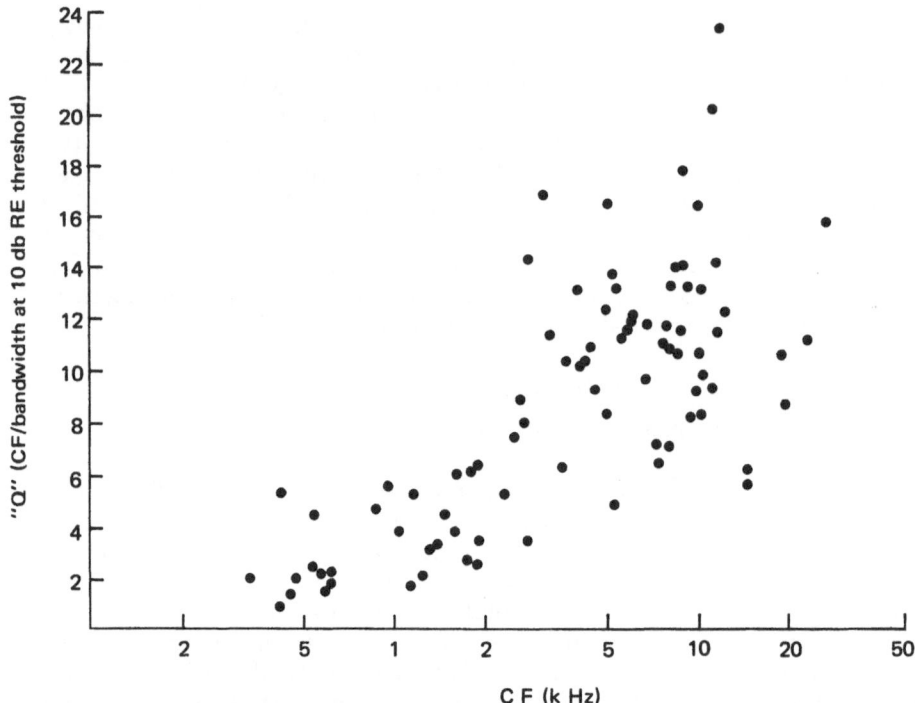

FIGURE 10.17 The sharpness of tuning curves as a function of frequency as measured with the Q metric. Sharpness in the space of this unit tends to increase as the center frequency increases, but there is little change in Q for cells with center frequencies below 2 kHz (from Kiang, 1965).

usually, a smaller population of cells that seem to have very broad response areas, some even extending to over 10,000 Hz. The analogy of these very broad response area cells to the nonopponent broad band cells in the visual system is striking. Both may be capable of encoding the overall levels of stimulus intensity independent of the component frequencies of the stimulus.

Because each of the auditory neurons seem to be associated with a restricted band of frequencies, and each cell is also presumed to represent the activity of a relatively narrow region of the basilar membrane (its tonal receptive "field"), these data generally are also thought to provide strong support for place theories of pitch representation and peripheral acoustic analysis.

C. Tonotopy—The Spatial Localization of Frequency Dependent Responses at Various Levels of the Auditory Pathways

Another traditional set of data, which has often been invoked to support the notion of place coding in the auditory system beyond the cochlea, is known by the generic name of tonotopic organization. Tonotopy deals with the spatial organization and localization of cells with different best

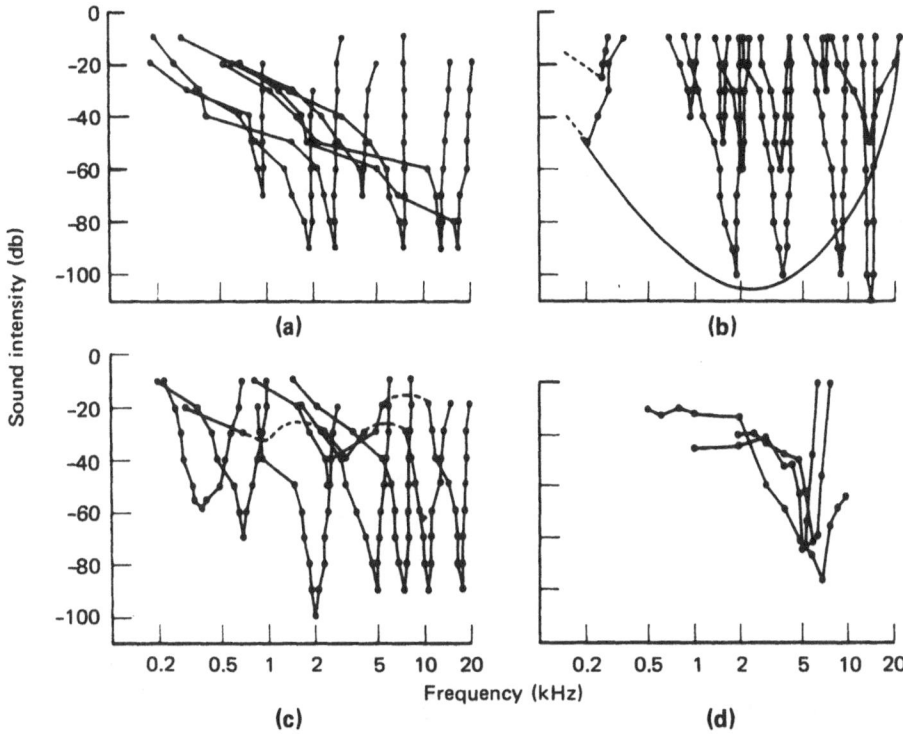

FIGURE 10.18 *Response areas of auditory system neurons recorded at four different levels of the ascending pathway.* (a) *At the level of the cochlear nerve.* (b) *At the level of the inferior colliculus.* (c) *At the level of the trapezoid body.* (d) *At the level of the geniculates. Note that the response areas are of almost constant width as one ascends the pathway (from Katsuki, 1961).*

frequencies at various levels of the ascending auditory pathway. The general procedure to produce a tonotopic map has been to locate a large number of cells that display optimum frequency behavior and to determine their spatial interrelationships.

Kiang (1965) has reported briefly on the spatial localization of cells in the auditory nerve of a cat with best frequencies varying from 400 to 30,000 kHz. Figure 10.19 displays his results for four different electrode penetrations, in which best frequencies were successively determined for a substantial number of these cells. Clearly, the best frequencies are not randomly scattered about in the acoustic nerve, but as we might have expected from he orderly way in which the neurons emerge from the basilar membrane to form the auditory nerve, there is a relatively well-ordered arrangement. The auditory nerve is apparently arranged in a spiral pattern. Cells whose center frequencies are high may be found first in a penetration and then, progressively, cells with medium and low best frequencies; or this order may be reversed. Such an arrangement would be explained by a spiral arrangement of the neurons in which the high-

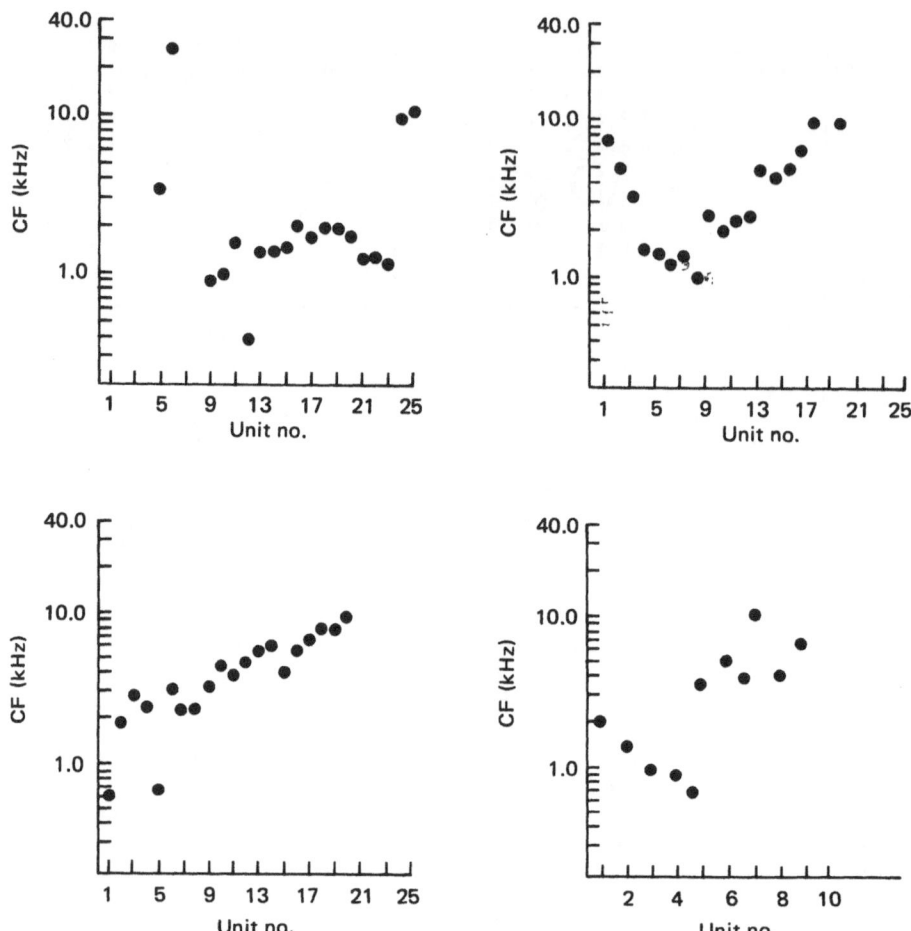

FIGURE 10.19 *Four electrode penetrations in the auditory nerve, showing the sequence of tonotopic organization at this peripheral level. These data are suggestive of a spiral organization in a regular frequency order. Cf-center or best frequency (from Kiang, 1965).*

frequency cells were on the outside at some points, while at other points low-frequency cells were on the outside.

Goldberg and Brown (1968) have also been able to demonstrate a similar kind of spatial or tonotopic organization in the medial superior olivary nucleus of the auditory pathway of a dog. Figure 10.20 shows the nature of the spatial arrangement of units with best frequencies within the range of 500 to 11,800 Hz. Low frequencies were found to be represented in the dorsal portion of this nucleus, while high frequencies were mostly found in the ventral portion. These investigators concluded that there is a more or less continuous gradation of the intermediate frequencies as one passes along the body of this nucleus from the dorsal to the ventral position.

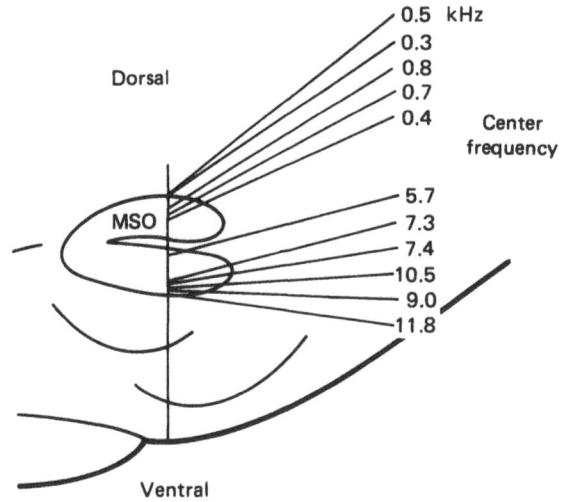

FIGURE 10.20 An electrode penetration showing the tonotopic organization of the superior olive of the dog. The dorsal lobe is seen, in general, to have cells with lower best frequencies than the ventral lobe (from Goldberg and Brown, 1968).

Similar measurements have been made for cat's midbrain by Aitkin, Anderson, and Brugge (1970). Glass-insulated platinum-iridium electrodes were inserted into the dorsal, central, and ventral nuclei of the lateral lemniscus, as well as in the central nucleus of the inferior colliculus. All electrode penetrations successively sampled a very regular system of tonotopically organized cells. Best frequencies were usually found to regularly increase during the experiment if the insertion was made from the dorsal side of the midbrain. Therefore, Aitkin and his colleagues concluded that low frequencies were localized dorsally and high frequencies ventrally throughout this entire system of midbrain nuclei. Cells were found with best frequencies, which varied from about 200 Hz to about 22,000 Hz.

The tonotopic organization of the cortex has been studied both with compound potentials (Tunturi, 1952) and with single cell preparations (Hind, 1960). Tunturi (1952), using gross electrodes to record compound evoked potentials in the cortex of the dog, found an exceedingly interesting pattern of organization in which various loci were excited differentially not only by different stimulus frequencies, but also by various stimulus intensities. Thus, the activation of a particular point in a topically organized two-dimension grid defined both acoustic stimulus frequency and intensity. Figure 10.21 shows this most extraordinary example of two-dimensional place encoding.

Hind (1960), on the other hand, using indium-filled glass microelectrodes, was able to look at the distribution not of groups of cells but of single cells. His experiments, however, were not as comprehensive and only sampled a single line of cells across the first auditory area of the cat's brain. Figure 10.22 shows that the best frequencies of these cells decreased from about 40,000 Hz to about 500 Hz as the electrode was successively positioned more and more posteriorly. It should also be noted

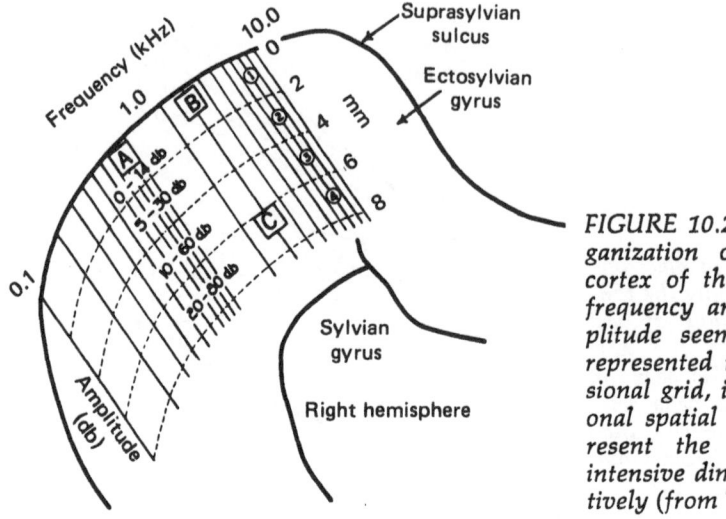

FIGURE 10.21 Tonotopic organization of the auditory cortex of the dog. Stimulus frequency and stimulus amplitude seem to be jointly represented in a two-dimensional grid, in which orthogonal spatial coordinates represent the qualitative and intensive dimensions, respectively (from Tunturi, 1952).

that these regions were bilaterally activated. Either ear seemed to produce the same pattern of responsiveness at each cortical locus.

Thus, at all levels of the ascending pathways, there appears to be some degree of well-ordered topographic representation of the tonal spectrum. Most noticeably absent from all of these data, however, are cells whose best frequencies are very low—below 100 or 200 Hz.

D. Phase Locking at Various Levels of the Auditory Pathways

As impressive as the evidence is that there is place representation throughout the auditory system, there is still a great lacuna which, up to now, has gone almost completely undiscussed. This lacuna concerns our knowledge of what is happening at very low frequencies. The direct physiological observations made by von Békésy (1960) at the apex of the cochlea, it should be recalled, did not show any distinguishing spatial pattern for any tones below 50 Hz. Similarly, even the most comprehensive studies of the response area (as perhaps best exemplified by the work of Kiang, 1965) of auditory nerve fibers never show cells with center frequencies less than 200 Hz. How, then, could one possibly account for the representation of very-low-frequency sounds and the ability to discriminate stimulus frequency differences of a couple of hertz in a 30- or 40-Hz signal with only a place-encoded system?

The answer to this question may lie in the findings of a series of studies that have been concerned with the relationship between the phase of the stimulus wave and the time at which spikes are generated in both the auditory nerve and higher levels of the nervous system. This mechanism, which operates mainly at low frequencies, may provide a means for the preservation of the temporal information of the stimulus, specifically as a temporal pattern, in the ascent throughout the auditory pathway. It, thus, suggests a possible use of periodicity as a code for pitch within this lower-frequency range. Such a coding mechanism would represent

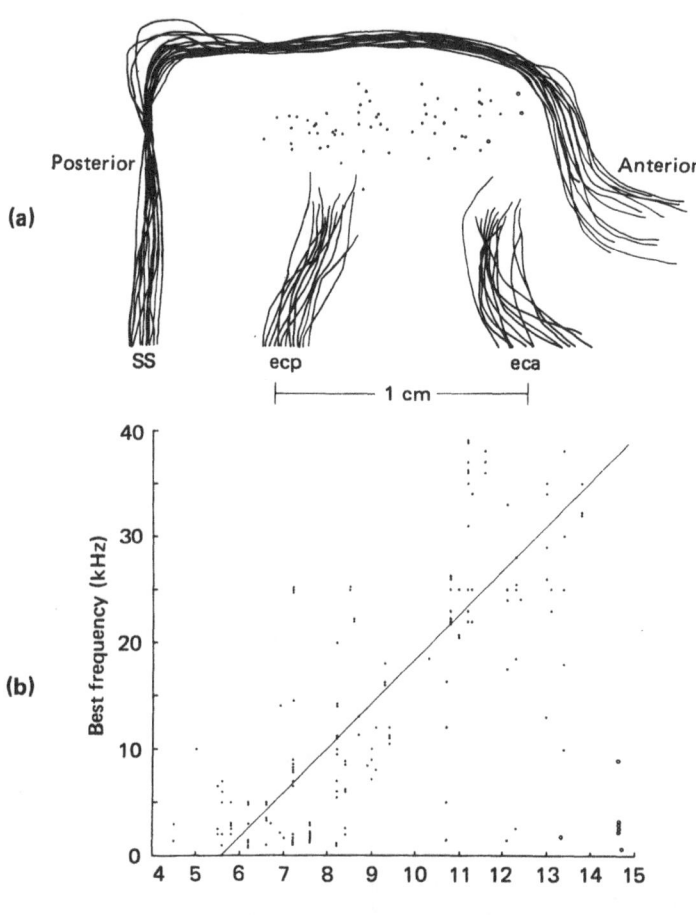

FIGURE 10.22 *A tonotopic map of the cat's auditory cortex. (a) Shows the points at which recordings were made from single cells. (b) Shows the relationship between best frequency and cortical locus (from Hind, 1960).*

an additional coding scheme for the representation of low tone information and would provide a means of filling the gap in which no neurophysiological place mechanism has been shown to operate.

The temporal pattern reproduction mechanism, which seems to fill the need for some means of representing low-frequency temporal pattern, has been called *phase locking*. The basic notion is that at low frequencies, a neuron is capable of always firing at the same point or phase of the acoustic oscillation. Figure 10.23[1] represents this sort of action for a

---

[1] Though this figure looks very much like Figure 10.5, which represented volleying, it should be kept clearly in mind that the two are very different. Volleying is the cumulative action of many neurons. Phase locking occurs within a single neuron.

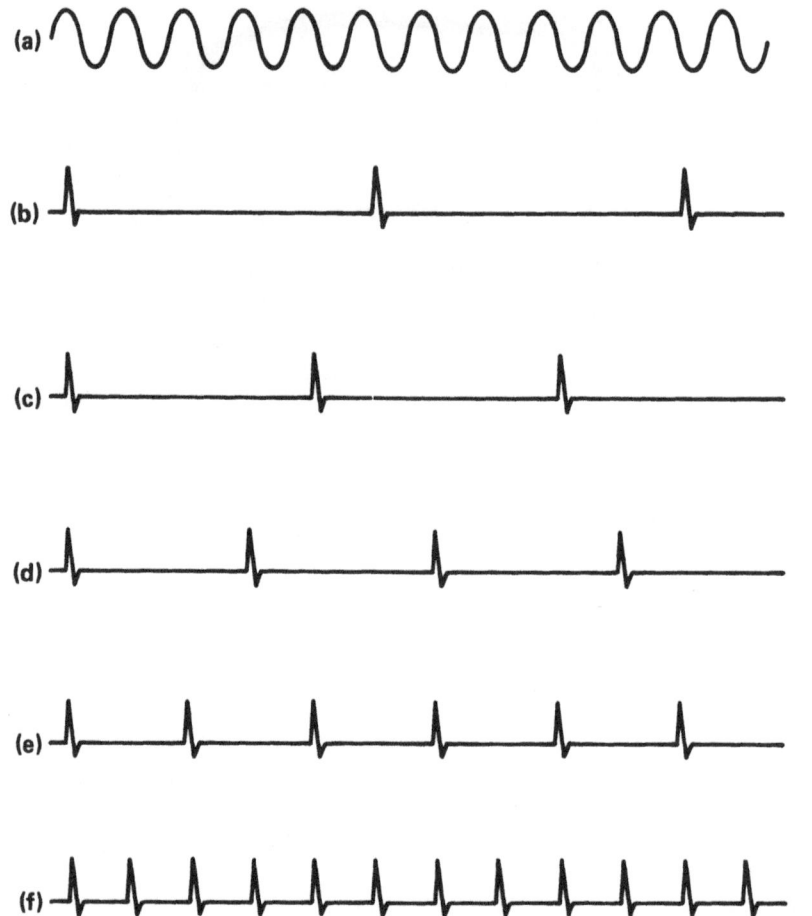

FIGURE 10.23 Drawing showing the basic characteristics of phase locking. In the separate parts of this figure, a phase locked signal is seen that always fires at the same phase of the stimulus sine wave, but that may fire every fifth, fourth, third, second, or first wave up to the physiological limit of the cell. In this figure, unlike Figure 10.5, all responses are in the same cell.

hypothetical cell, which is responding at every fifth wave for low stimulus intensities, but then increases its spiking to every fourth, every third, every second and, ultimately, to every wave of the stimulus as the intensity increases. The important point in the present context is that each spike occurs at the same place on the stimulus waveform. Phase locking was first described by Galambos and Davis (1943) in the cochlear nucleus, but has been shown to exist even at the level of the auditory nerve. The concept has been developed most fully by Tasaki (1954) and most recently by Rose and his colleagues at the University of Wisconsin.

One of the main issues with which our discussion must deal is the usable upper frequency limits of this phase locked activity. Direct physiological observation sets an upper limit on the ability of the auditory system to transmit frequency patterns directly, even if it does not tell us exactly for what region the periodicity is a useful and true code. The upper limits of phase locking so measured are surprisingly high. Tasaki reports phase locking for stimulus frequencies up to 2000 Hz, and Rose, Brugge, Anderson, and Hind (1967) report phase locking up to 5000 Hz. Of course, in these latter situations, precise phase locking might occur only every tenth stimulus wave; it is not being asserted that neurons fire at these rates. Thus, the frequency region over which his mechanism might work is quite a bit larger than simply the 20- to 50- or 200-Hz region over which place encoding seems not to operate. However, whether or not it is so used is another and independent question.

The full significance of this type of experiment can be appreciated best by considering the work of Rose, Brugge, Anderson, and Hind (1967) in more detail. These investigators used a squirrel monkey as their experimental animal and inserted glass micropipette electrodes into the auditory nerve. Responses were acquired and plotted in the form of interval histograms by an on-line digital computer. Figure 10.24 shows a typical output of this computer display for a range of stimulus frequencies varying from 412 to 1600 Hz. Clearly, the intervals between successive responses are either at or in integral multiples of the interwave duration —a mode of response which is characteristic of phase locking up to the highest frequency stimulus used. We must reiterate, however, that this result does not mean that the observed cell is necessarily firing at a rate equivalent to the stimulus frequency. Most of the time the cell does not fire on each successive stimulus wave, but only at integral multiples of the fundamental stimulus frequency. The important point is, no matter how many waves are skipped, a response is much more likely to occur at a particular phase of the stimulus wave than at any other point. The more intense the stimulus, the more likely the neuron is to fire every cycle of the stimulus.

These findings suggest that Wever's notion of volleying just may have a physiological basis after all. The synchronization requirements of his theory, which seemed so excessive initially, actually turn out to be met by a real physiological candidate code. Whether phase locking is capable of being decoded by some periodicity or interval detector at higher levels of the nervous system remains problematical, however.

As one proceeds further up the auditory pathway, however, the extreme range of phase locking found in the periphery is not maintained. Aitkin, Anderson, and Brugge (1970), for example, report that such synchronized responses can be found only up to stimulus frequencies of about 1000 Hz at the level of the lateral lemniscus.

By the time the signal has reached the level of the cortex, however, a completely different picture obtains. Brugge, Dubrovsky, Aitkin, and Anderson (1969) have shown that not only is there no phase locking at this level, but there is, in fact, *no* repetitive responses of the cortical cells of auditory areas 1 and 2 to maintained acoustic stimuli. Most cortical

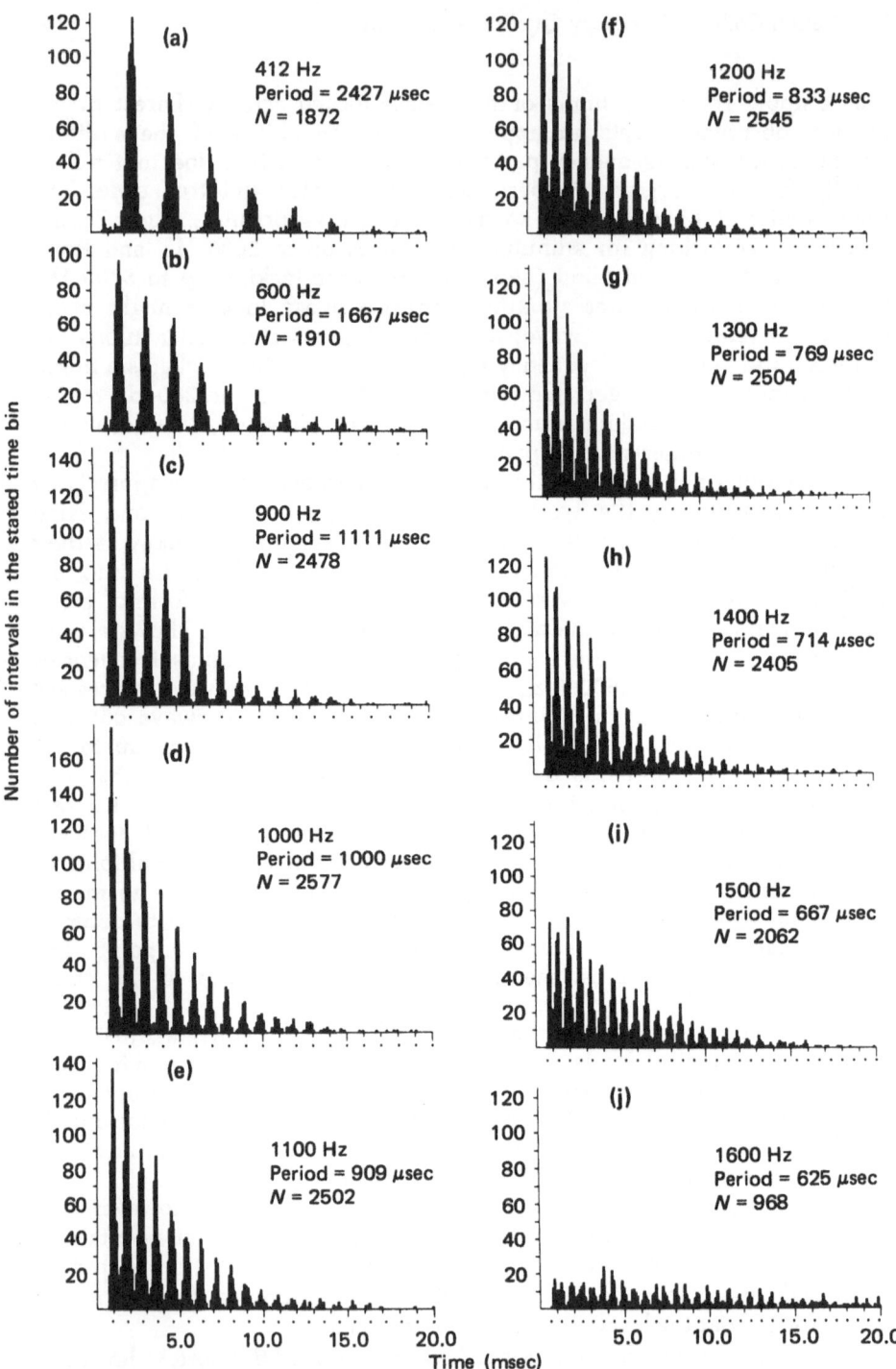

FIGURE 10.24 Phase locking in a real preparation. These figures show phase locked responses from 412- to 1600-Hz stimulus frequencies. Though the responses clearly tend to fire at a particular phase, these interval histograms clearly show that considerable amounts of skipping may occur at all frequencies (from Rose, Brugge, Anderson, and Hind, 1967).

cells, quite to the contrary, seem to respond with but a single spike or a very short burst to pure tonal stimuli of any duration. Goldstein, Hall, and Butterfield (1968) showed a more diversified pattern of responses (on, off, and continuous firing) in the cat's auditory cortex, but their findings also display no evidence of phase locking at this level.

The implication of these findings from the level of the auditory cortex is obvious. It means that either the frequency information conveyed by the phase locked periodic stimulus has been extracted and re-encoded into some new dimension at some lower level of the auditory pathway or it has, quite to the contrary, been lost. In spite of the exquisite fidelity of the frequency pattern maintained up to the level of the brain stem, phase locking is not even available to be considered as a candidate code at the cortex.

In sum, frequency codes do seem to be available at lower centers in the form of phase locked signals. This is so even if the firing frequencies of individual cells do not come close to reproducing the stimulus frequencies as would be required by a classical telephone theory. The capacity for volleying, as suggested by Wever, seems to exist, however, because of the high degree of synchronization displayed by phase locked signals, and may represent the basis of a sort of frequency code for sounds in the low-frequency range. However, phase locking does not occur centrally.

E. Neurophysiological Data Pertaining to the Problem of Combined Stimuli

The problem of the neurophysiological basis of coding of combination tones, such as the missing fundamental, Schouten's residue, beats, or summation tones, is of fundamental importance because these phenomena, more than any other body of data, contradict the basic ideas of place coding that are supported by so many other findings. The problem has been subject to some neurophysiological research in recent years and can be subdivided into two questions. First, do frequency energies corresponding to the combination tones appear in any neurophysiological record from any level? Second, if such energy is present at a given level, what is the locus of the nonlinear distortion, which is responsible for its introduction?

Let us first consider the simpler question of whether or not combination tones are present in neurophysiological recordings at any level. One way to approach this problem with regard to cochlear responses is to also use the cochlear microphonic as an indicator of the action of the basilar membrane. Sweetman and Dallos (1969) have reported the results of just such an experiment and have found that the basilar membrane does not appear to have associated with it any traveling wave action at the frequencies of combination tones. However, if the cochlear microphonic is looked at in another way, simply with regard to whether or not this electropotential itself exhibits the combination tone, then Dallos (1969) has shown the presence of electropotential power corresponding to the combination frequencies.

The next stage at which we can look for some evidence of neural energy at the combination frequencies is the auditory nerve. Kiang (1965) has shown that the cat's auditory nerve fibers fire in bursts at the frequency of the beat tone when a 1532-Hz tone and a 1527-Hz tone are

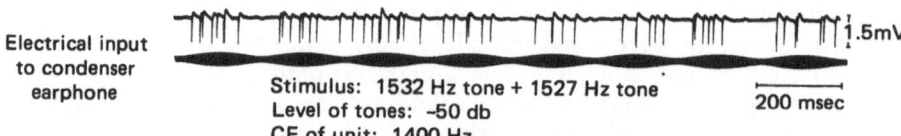

FIGURE 10.25 Neural detection of acoustic stimulus beats. This figure shows a stimulus (lower trace) made up of 1532- and 1527-Hz stimuli along with the 5-Hz beat frequency produced by their interaction. Although there is no energy at the beat frequency, there is an associated tendency to cluster neural responses at the point of maximum amplitude of the beat (from Kiang, 1965).

mixed. Figure 10.25 shows the response of a single cell from his experiments, in which the periodic firing of the nerve response at the frequency of the beating stimuli can be clearly seen.

Since the distortion does not appear in the mechanical action of the basilar membrane, but difference tones are observed in the cochlear microphonic and the acoustic nerve response, it might be that the distortion is perhaps introduced in the transduction process by some nonlinear action of the hair cells. However, it is known (see Chapter 4) that the cochlear microphonics are surprisingly linear over wide ranges of their dynamic range. The suggestion, therefore, is that the distortion occurs at the locus at which the cochlear microphonic is converted into the synaptic graded action potentials or perhaps even where the mechanisms responsible for the conversion of the postsynoptic potential into spike action potentials operate in the dendrites of the cochlear nerve neuron. Clearly, the data at this time are inconsistent, and much is yet to be done to resolve this dilemma.

Another alternative suggestion, which could also resolve this apparent inconsistency, is that the cochlear microphonic is not, in fact, an important part of the sensory communication process and, indeed, should not be considered as the receptor potential. But once again we ask questions for which no comprehensive answers are currently available.

Lest the complexity or controversy that surrounds this issue be underestimated, the reader is referred to Sweetman and Dallos' (1969) paper for a complete discussion of the arguments that have been put forth by a number of investigators concerning the mechanical or neural locus of the nonlinear mechanism for the introduction of combination tone energy. Perhaps all that can be said now is that this is one of the very controversial issues in auditory theory, and that there is insufficient evidence on either side of the question to completely resolve it at this time.

This, then, concludes our review of the biological data that are believed to be relevant to the problem of auditory quality coding. We shall now present a more or less contemporary view of a possible auditory quality coding system that incorporates these findings.

IV. A CONTEMPORARY MODEL
The last two decades, in which we have seen a flowering of neurophysiological findings, have changed the nature of auditory theorizing equally

as drastically as the changes that have occurred in visual quality theory. In addition, surprising support has been forthcoming for some of the older notions of auditory quality coding that had previously been based mainly on physiological intuition and indirect inferences from the psychophysical data. It seems safe to conclude now that both place and frequency mechanisms are probably operating to encode auditory quality, and thus contemporary auditory models must, like the current visual theory, be a compromise of past ideas rather than an absolute rejection of one or more competing prior theories. In the visual system, the compromise between the trichromatic and the opponent color theory was based upon the conversion of trichromatic processes into opponent processes, and vice versa, as one passed from one level to another in the visual pathway. In the auditory system, however, the compromise seems to be based on a completely different common meeting ground, namely, that the frequency and place principles seem to operate in parallel in different regions of the auditory spectrum.

Before we discuss the details of a contemporary theory of neural quality coding, we must consider another closely related issue concerning the mechanical action of the basilar membrane which has been discussed by von Békésy (1956). The question he asked is: are the various theories, particularly with regard to cochlear mechanical function, really as different one from the other as they may at first seem?

To answer this question, von Békésy first classified the four main theoretical approaches in terms of the specific nature of basilar membrane motion predicted by each. The resonance place theories are characterized by oscillatory motion at highly localized regions—the tuned resonators are assumed to be laterally independent of one another. The telephone or frequency theories, on the other hand, were characterized by their authors as having simultaneous and in-phase action that extended over substantially all of the basilar membrane. Traveling wave theories stood in some intermediate position, because traveling wave motion extends over wide portions of the basilar membrane for most frequencies even if all of the points were not doing the same thing at the same time. Rather, a wave of action varying in amplitude and moving from the basal end to the apical end of the cochlea is postulated by traveling wave theorists. The standing wave theories, on the other hand, also had widely distributed patterns of cochlear action, but these patterns were assumed to be static and not to move when stimulus conditions were constant. Figure 10.26 displays the differences among the various theories with regard to membrane response as shown in one of von Békésy's drawings.

Von Békésy pointed out that all four of these modes of action could be made to occur in any membrane, if only two of its mechanical properties—the stiffness and the coupling between adjacent parts—could be varied. If the stiffness of a membrane is relatively high and the coupling between adjacent points relatively low, then the action typical of local resonators occurs. If the stiffness is kept high but coupling between adjacent points is increased, then the whole membrane tends to vibrate as a whole, and the response pattern associated with the frequency theory occurs. On the other hand, if the membrane stiffness is decreased and the

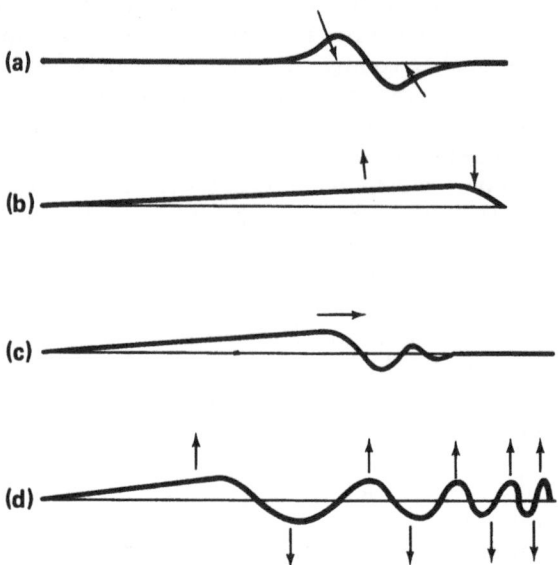

FIGURE 10.26 Drawing of four different patterns of basilar membrane action
that are predicted by four different theories of auditory pitch encoding. The
resonance theory (a) predicts a local vibration at a particular place. The telephone
or pure frequency theory (b) predicts a total synchronous involvement of the
entire basilar membrane. The traveling wave theory (c) predicts a moving wave
with a peak amplitude at a particular place, and the standing wave theory (d)
predicts stationary patterns of up-and-down oscillation across the entire basilar
membrane. Von Békésy has pointed out that any of these four patterns can be
produced in the same tissue if one has control over the stiffness and coupling
of the tissue. The key problem in basilar membrane mechanics, therefore is to
determine these physical properties. Measurement and direct observation now
provide firm support for the traveling wave theory (from von Békésy, 1956).

coupling between the adjacent parts is relatively low, then the mechanical
properties of the membrane are such that traveling waves occur. But if
the coupling between the adjacent parts of the membrane is increased
while the stiffness is kept low, then oscillations can actually reach the end
of the membrane and be reflected to result in standing waves.

On the basis of these ideas, von Békésy suggested that the problem
of which theory of cochlear mechanical action truly held could be resolved
simply by measuring the physical properties of the basilar membrane.
He actually made a number of different sorts of observations over the
years to answer this question. In one instance, he pressed a small probe
directly against the basilar membrane and observed the distortion pattern
so produced microscopically. These observations of the elastic properties
of the basilar membrane as well as the direct observations of its dynamics,
he feels, all support a traveling wave place theory of basilar membrane
mechanical action with low stiffness and low coupling. The other biological data we have already considered also confirm the general nature of the
traveling wave hypothesis for signals with frequencies greater than 50

Hz, and this particular form of the place coding hypothesis must now be considered as a major building block of all modern theories of auditory quality.

All of the biological data that we considered, however, indicate the same curious absence of any place encoding mechanism for frequencies lower than 50 to 100 Hz. For signals below this limit, therefore, there is little possibility that a traveling wave mediated cochlear place theory could possibly explain pitch and pitch discrimination. There are, on the other hand, large amounts of data that show that at the lower levels of the auditory system, there is excellent temporal reproduction of low-frequency tones up to 1000 Hz. Even though this frequency pattern information does not seem to be preserved at higher levels of the pathway, and true stimulus frequency reproduction of any kind certainly does not seem to occur at that level of the cortex, it is possible that the lower-frequency range may be represented by some sort of periodicity or volley type of code in the peripheral nervous system.

It is not possible to precisely define the exact range of each of the two modes of encoding (place for high stimulus frequencies and temporal pattern for low stimulus frequencies). Most probably the low frequencies are represented increasingly less well by the purely temporal code for signals over 100 Hz. On the other hand, place candidate codes seem not even to be available for frequencies below 50 to 100 Hz. Thus, it is likely that there is an intermediate region in which both codes may be simultaneously active. This region may be very broad, for phase locking as we have seen extends up as high as 5000 Hz, and place as low as 50 Hz.

The notion that higher frequencies are mainly encoded by place representations and lower frequencies by frequency reproduction is known as the duplexity theory of auditory quality. Clearly, both Fletcher's duplexity theory and Wever's resonance-volley theory are examples of duplex hypotheses, and both of their models include many of the features of both the classic place and frequency theories. Unfortunately, both Wever and Fletcher originally chose to associate their models with resonant analytical mechanisms, whose proposed role we now feel certain is truly played by the hydrodynamic traveling wave action described by von Békésy.

The basic elements of the most widely accepted contemporary model of auditory pitch encoding may now be thought of as including:

1. Fletcher's introduction of the duplexity idea with low tones being encoded by a frequency code and high tones by a place code.
2. Von Békésy's introduction of the notion of the traveling wave as the key mediator of cochlear spatial analysis for higher frequencies. While action is widespread, maximum amplitude occurs at places specific to stimulus frequency.
3. Wever's intuitive leap in suggesting the volley principle as a means of extending the range of application of the frequency code.
4. The notion of an intermediate region, probably between 50 and 1000 Hz, within which dual place and frequency representation holds.

Auditory theory historically has provided a fertile ground for the intermingling of new ideas from the engineering and biological sciences. A
major example of the fusion of such ideas is illustrated by the work of
J. C. R. Licklider (1951a, 1959), who has suggested that neural correlational
mechanisms analogous to the time series analyses developed by Wiener
(1949) and Lee (1960) play an important role in the perception of both
combination tones and binaural stimulus spatial localization. Licklider's
(1951a) original statement of his ideas proposed a two-part or duplexity
theory, which assumed a von Békésy-like spatial analysis, followed up by
an autocorrelational mechanism, which was able to extract the information
inherent in the envelope of combination tones. Licklider based his ideas
on the fact that there were two kinds of pitch (as evidenced by the two
musical names for pitch—tone height and tone chroma), but this is probably an unnecessary complication; there is plenty to explain if we simply
consider that there are both low and high tones and that both nonzero
energy tones and zero energy combination tones must be encoded.

It was implicit in Licklider's suggestion that spatial analysis is used
for most frequencies. But the major thrust of his attention was directed
at the autocorrelational mechanism for the extraction of combination
tone information. He assumed that there was some neural structure that
introduced systematic delays into the signals emanating from each
cochlear locus. These selectively delayed signals were then integrated
(converged) in a manner such that a neural analogue of the autocorrelational transform was produced. Autocorrelation (see Uttal, 1968, pp.
182–188) has the property of processing the information in a time series
in such a way that periodic information is extracted, regardless of the
energy content of the particular frequency. Thus, even zero energy signals
would appear in the autocorrelogram. Such a mechanism would be most
helpful in explaining the perception of zero energy combination tones if it
is ultimately shown that nonlinear distortions are not, in fact, responsible
for the introduction of real physical energy at the combination frequencies.

Licklider's most recent statement (1959) expands this highly speculative notion of a duplex system including an autocorrelator into a triplex
theory. The added component in his new statement is a neural net
capable of cross-correlating the signals to the two ears to determine spatial localization, but this is a problem that is not germane to the pitch perception issue discussed here.

The major implication of Licklider's work in the context of our present discussion is that it proposes a third mechanism for pitch encoding.
In addition to frequency and place representation, his theory suggests that
low-frequency information can be conveyed along place coded channels
which are, under normal conditions, associated with high-frequency information representation. Licklider assumes that the autocorrelator can
extract from the high-frequency channels information that can be interpreted as low pitches.

In conclusion, it appears that both the early place and frequency
theorists were each partially right. While the notion of simple resonance
and sharp localization of frequencies across the cochlea can no longer be

accepted in the light of modern biological data, it is clear that the concept of moving patterns of activity with different loci of maximum amplitude for different frequencies must be one of the cornerstones on which any modern model must be built. On the other hand, there is no physiological evidence of any differential place localization for the very lowest frequencies below 50 or 100 Hz. But phase locking of exquisite fidelity has been shown for lower frequencies, thus unencumbering us from the supposed limits on the response frequencies of individual nerves. The data on the neural representation of combination tones are equivocal, and no firm conclusions can be drawn at this time; however, it does at least appear that there are hypothetical mechanisms that could produce the responses associated with these complex stimuli, even though there is zero energy associated with their power spectrum.

Another important point that permeates the literature on auditory pitch representation is the fact that the response patterns are all very broadly tuned. The patterns of displacement of the basilar membrane, as shown by a number of different kinds of experiments, extend over wide regions of that tissue, and no sharp localization is ever evident. We have already spoken of the possibility that neural sharpening and even mechanical sharpening may improve this to some extent, but even at the highest levels of the auditory system, there is no evidence that the tuning is sharpened anywhere near the degree that is suggested by the psychophysical data. Clearly, the key variable for the representation of pitch is not so much the particular place as it is the relative amount of activity of a number of different places. This notion of broadly tuned receptors with overlapping fields of activation is closely analogous to the ideas that underlie modern models of visual quality, a point which will emerge again in the next chapter and which we shall discuss in general terms at its end.

CHAPTER 11: THE NEURAL CODING OF SENSORY QUALITY—THE OTHER SENSES AND A SUMMARY

In this chapter, we turn our attention to the "other" senses—somatosensation, gustation, and olfaction. All three of these topics suffer from a handicap, which has long inhibited the conceptualization and formalization of their respective theories of quality—namely, there is no single dimension of the stimulus that can be varied to systematically scan the range of microqualities assumed to be included within each of these macromodalities. For that matter, it is not clear whether there is, indeed, as much of an analogy between taste and vision, for example, as there is between sweetness and vision. It is entirely possible that the "other" senses are, in fact, conglomerates of a number of sensitivities, which are individually more like vision and audition than the collective terms (like taste) themselves. Previous attempts to cluster all of the tastes into a single sense may be merely an expression of the general similarities in locus and function rather than any more fundamental link among them. Be that as it may, there is a substantial difference in the way these three senses are dealt with in comparison to vision and audition. The questions asked are framed in a much more discrete form—stimuli are members of certain classes, which do not vary in microquality and, thus, do not vary continuously into one another. Such questions as qualitative difference thresholds are not routinely examined, nor is it exactly clear what the result would mean if they were. Rather, questions of specificity and nonspecificity of the receptors to the discrete classes of stimuli are more often encountered in our discussion.

In the following chapter, we shall discuss the material in much the same way that we have done previously. We shall first consider the key psychophysical data, then the competitive theories and the biological data, and finally attempt a synthesis of a contemporary theory. Often, as we shall see, it will be the case with this material that the specification of the research question is tantamount to the statement of the theory. Furthermore, as we shall also see, theory in these "other" senses often takes the form of possible receptor transductive mechanisms rather than more central coding mechanisms. We have already (in Chapter 4) discussed some of the material that is thus of relevance to the problems of quality representation considered in this chapter. The reader may want to review that material at this point.

I. SOMATOSENSATION

A. The Key Psychophysical Data

It is somewhat surprising to realize that there is virtually no direct experimentation relating to somatosensory quality discrimination. As one scans the somatosensory literature of the past few years, one appreciates the absence of experiments that might provide a psychophysical base for neural theories of somesthetic quality discrimination. Most of the effort in the cutaneous and body senses seemingly has been directed at their temporal, spatial, or intensive attributes.

The main reason for this paucity of information on somatosensory quality coding is, as we have noted, that there is no unique dimension of variation along which the complex percepts of the bodily senses can continuously and concomitantly vary. There is no somatosensory spectrum of stimuli in the same way there is a visual or auditory one. It seems almost as if we were dealing with not one, but a grab-bag of individual senses or modalities, each of which is more closely allied with vision or hearing than is the collective we call somatosensation. Even then, it is hard to appreciate what might be meant by the quality of, for example, different cold, different hot, or different touch experiences. Itch, touch, and tickle simply do not vary among or within themselves in the same way that hues or pitches do.

The result of this shortage of experimental data on somatosensory quality is that often the hoariest observations or almost casual anecdotal evidence are invoked to explain various theories of somatosensory quality. It is almost as if the somatosensory experiences were qualitatively "punctate" (we are either touched to a particular spatial, temporal, or intensive extent or we are not touched), just as the various cutaneous receptors have classically been considered to have been localized in a spatially punctate manner throughout the skin. Pain and proprioception, two noncutaneous somatosensory sensations, also seem to be this same "single quality" sort of experience, and it is hard to find words to describe different microqualities within these somatosensory experiences. For these reasons, the classic question in somatosensory quality coding has always been: what are the neural mechanisms that allow us to discriminate one of the many somatosensory experiences from another (for example, on what basis do we discriminate touch from cold)? We usually do not ask in somatosensory research how we discriminate different microqualities of the same sensory modality (different kinds of touch, for example) from one another.

Clearly, if the basic problem is formulated in this manner, then the classification of the different somatosensory modalities takes on an especially important role. Over the years, many authors have attempted to develop such classification schemes, but a particularly interesting one has recently been put forth by Sinclair (1967). We reproduce his taxonomy of the somatosenses in Table 11.1. Most of the sensory experiences listed in Sinclair's taxonomy are relatively straightforward, and nothing would be gained by any further attempt to define them more specifically. A few of the terms, however, should be elaborated upon.

Paraesthesia is the sensation of pins and needles that can be produced by any one of a number of abnormal conditions. Sinclair classifies paraesthesia in both the contact and pain groups, because certain aspects of its occurrence are painful, while others are not. In some instances, it seems more like a complex touch experience. *Dysaesthesia* refers to an abnormal condition in which a painful experience is produced by what would under normal conditions be a touch stimulus. *Causalgia* is also a pathological condition characterized by a well-localized burning pain. *Protopathic pain* is the general category for diffuse and general pain and is a term that arises out of the duplex theory of somatosensation propounded by Head (1920). *Kinaesthesia* is the sense of position of various parts of the body.

TABLE 11.1 SINCLAIR'S TAXONOMY OF THE
SOMATOSENSATIONS (FROM SINCLAIR, 1967)

Contact Group

Touch, pressure, vibration, tickle, tactile paraesthesiae

Pain Group

Superficial "pricking," deep "aching," discomfort, itch, painful paraesthesiae, dysaesthesiae, causalgia, and "protopathic" pain

Thermal Group

Cold, warm

Sensory Blends

Cold pain, wetness, smoothness, heat, etc.

Position

Sense of position in space, kinaesthesia

With the exception of kinaesthesia, there is some question whether these other "senses," which are generally considered to be painful pathologic conditions, really deserve to be treated as separate entities. All of them are more or less like the burning or pricking pains described elsewhere in this schema and may only truly represent unusual ways of pain induction rather than separate modalities. This is but one example of the sort of semantic difficulty encountered in somatosensory quality theory.

Thus, we see that while a historical set of "modalities" has been gradually agreed upon over the years, there is little in the way of hard data on somatosensory quality discrimination. The only real psychophysical milestone in that glacial development has been the report by Blix (1884) that the modalities of touch, warmth, and cold were apparently organized in a punctate manner. Yet even this simple and persistent "fact" has been challenged (Kibler and Nathan, 1960) and may not be acceptable as a general basis of somatosensory theorizing.

Since the late nineteenth century, there has been almost nothing of significance to report with regard to the psychophysics of somatosensory quality. In the important *Handbook of Experimental Psychology*, Jenkins (1951) has virtually nothing further to say about somatosensory quality, *per se*, nor does psychophysical data that would add to our knowledge of somatosensory quality appear in the two most recent volumes on somesthesis: a Ciba Symposium volume entitled *Touch, Heat and Pain* (de Reuck and Knight, 1966) and the very important volume on *The Skin Senses* (Kenshalo, 1968). All recent work seems to have been concentrated on the temporal, intensive, or spatial attributes of this group of modalities.

B. The Competitive Theories

The main controversy in somatosensory quality coding has always been between those who champion a specificity approach and those who believe that more complicated neural action patterns are necessary to define the cutaneous and proprioceptive microqualities of Table 11.1. The general thesis of the specificity theorists is that the various mechanical and thermal stimuli are analyzed by relatively narrowly tuned (that is, sensitive to only one kind of stimulus) responsiveness of the encapsulated and free nerve endings in such a way that different places are activated by different stimuli. The further assumption of specificity theorists is that the output of each of these units is subsequently associated with the different experiences. The pattern theorist, on the other hand, assumes that somatosensory mechano- and thermoreceptors are all broadly tuned and that each responds to some degree to a broad spectrum of the cutaneous and proprioceptive stimuli. However, since each receptor is tuned slightly differently from its neighbors, the pattern of activation of a group of receptors is different depending upon the stimulus. The relative amount of activity in each of the family of involved receptors is assumed to be the key code. Now let us consider these points of view in detail.

1. Von Frey's Specificity Theory. The classic formularization of the specificity theory was that enunciated by von Frey (1895). His original theory was based on Blix's (1884) observations of the punctate localization of the sensory experiences and contemporary anatomical observations, which showed that a variety of cutaneous receptor types could be microscopically identified in the skin. Clearly, von Frey was also considerably influenced by Müller's "law" of the specific energy of nerves, which assumed an equivalent specificity in the function of the sensory nerve fibers leading away from the receptors. What could have been more reasonable in light of this knowledge than the assignment of the perceptual experience of punctate localization to the anatomically punctate end organs? Specifically, von Frey assumed that there were four cutaneous senses—touch, warmth, cold, and pain. As indicated by Table 11.1, we now believe that this classification is incomplete, for von Frey's original four categories omit many of the other important cutaneous experiences. There has, from time to time, been some argument that the other experiences such as itch, tickle, or pressure are derived experiences created from combinations of these four basic senses, but no empirical support for such an idea has been really compelling. Von Frey specifically assigned a single receptor type (as defined by the anatomic investigations) to each of these four supposed basic senses. Free nerve endings were assumed to subserve pain; Meissner corpuscles, touch; Ruffini cylinders, warmth; and Krause end bulbs, cold.

A more recent corollary of the von Frey receptor specificity theory has been the association of specific nerve fiber diameters with specific cutaneous modalities. Touch was assumed to be mediated by the largest fibers and pain by the smallest. Warmth and cold messages were presumed to be handled by intermediate sized fibers. This set of ideas was based in part on the sequential dropout of the various senses when the blood supply of the arm was cut off by a sphygmomanometer cuff inflated above the systolic pressure. Larger nerve fibers were thought to be disabled first, and it was also believed that touch sensitivity disappeared first. The order of sensory dropout, however, has been shown by Sinclair and Hinshaw (1950) to depend upon a very large number of factors and that the order of dropout can, under some conditions, even be reversed. Furthermore, some drugs, which selectively affect pain, seem to desensitize nerve fibers nonspecifically with regard to size. Generally, Sinclair (1967) concludes that the idea of associating axonal diameter with specific experience is not tenable at the present time.

In Chapters 3 and 4, when we discussed receptor anatomy and transduction, it became rather clear that some of the anatomical assumptions implicit in von Frey's formalization were inaccurate. First, it was noted that there is virtually no authenticated correlation between the receptor types and the sensory spots. Second, Loewenstein and his colleagues have clearly shown that the encapsulation of at least the Pacinian corpuscle (and it is the encapsulation that contributes most to the uniqueness of the anatomy of the corpuscular end organs) could be almost totally stripped off without changing the overall function of the end organ (even though it did affect the shape of the generator potential).

Another argument against the specificity theory has always been that the cornea displays a wide range of sensory experiences, but contains only free nerve endings. Yet free nerve endings, in traditional specificity theory, are the receptors that were associated specifically only with pain. Another criticism raised occasionally has been that there really are almost too many different types of receptors. While initial categorizations led the early microscopist to suggest only a few modal types, more recent microscopy has suggested that there is really a continuum of anatomical types ranging from free nerve endings to the most elaborately structured encapsulations even within a single animal.

If these basic premises, seemingly almost necessary prerequisites for the von Frey theory, do not receive modern support, must we necessarily reject the von Frey theory entirely? Melzack and Wall (1962) have considered this question and have made an analysis of von Frey's contributions that is worthy of the greatest attention. It was their judgment that von Frey's theory is not, in fact, a single conceptual structure, but is really a mixture of three different notions, each of which is capable of being looked at and dealt with separately from the other two in the light of modern data. Melzack and Wall consider the three separate and independent assumptions of the von Frey theory to be:

1. The physiological assumption:
   Skin receptors are differentiated to respond selectively to different mechanical stimuli.
2. The anatomical assumption:
   A single receptor lies beneath each cutaneous sensory spot.
3. The psychological assumption:
   Each dimension of somesthetic experience is associated on a one-for-one basis with a specific dimension of neural experience.

The first assumption, as Melzack and Wall note, pertains almost exclusively to the physical tuning of the receptors and a definition of the adequate stimulus for each receptor type. The question here is a conceptually simple one; namely, are some forms of energy capable of activating one or another cutaneous receptor more easily than any of the other forms? But the simplicity of the question is not matched by an equal ease in the conceptualization of definitive experiments. A formidable obstacle to a simple experimental answer to this question is that almost all of the cutaneous senses, no matter of what type, are not only responsive to mechanical stimuli but also, as chemical systems, are sensitive to changes in the temperature of their environment. Therefore, it is not always clear exactly what the spectrum of energies is that one should be comparing to determine the fineness of tuning. Yet according to Melzack and Wall, if there is anything to be salvaged from von Frey's theory, its essence is within the scope of this first assumption.

Melzack and Wall most promptly dispose of the second of the three assumptions, which concerns the relation between the sensory spot and the individual receptor, citing the lack of correlative evidence that has already been summarized in Table 3.3.

The third assumption of the von Frey theory, on the other hand, is rejected by Melzack and Wall on more or less indirect grounds. First, they feel that von Frey's assumption of a one-to-one correspondence between a single dimension of sensation and a single dimension of the nerve patterns just does not hold as a general premise of neural coding. Their criticism is at least partially founded on psychophysical grounds. The variation of brightness with the wavelength of a visual stimulus or pitch with the intensity of an auditory stimulus suggests that the one-for-one relationship does not hold. Furthermore, they also raise the question of whether the four basic cutaneous senses von Frey has chosen are any more likely candidates for the role than any other set.

This latter point brings us to the next main point of view concerning the neural coding of somatosensory quality pattern theory. Melzack and Wall, in rejecting the von Frey psychological assumption, champion in its place a theory, which proposes that it is the overall spatio-temporal pattern of nerve impulses that determine the quality of the sensation.

2. Pattern Theory. What has come to be called cutaneous pattern theory was originally developed as an alternative to the specificity theory of von Frey. The main impetus to pattern theory was derived from the electro-physiological findings of the 1930s, 40s and 50s. From the very first days of these exciting neurophysiological explorations, it became clear that the responses of neurons were not related, in any simple manner, to stimulus type. Nafe (1929) was probably the first to more or less explicitly reject the labeled line hypothesis implicit in von Frey's theory and to introduce the notion of the "spatio-temporal pattern of nerve impulses" as a possibly more important means of coding somatosensory quality. The most energetic championing of these pattern ideas in recent years can be found in the writing of Weddell and his group. Weddell (1955) reviewed the literature on the subject (including what is probably the best bibliography of the work of his own group) and summarized all of the evidence with the following sentence:

> It is clear from an analysis of this literature on somesthesis (culled from widely differing fields of experimental work) that sensory experience is now being considered in terms of a spatio-temporal pattern of nervous activity rather than a series of discrete connections within a limited number of modes.
>
> (WEDDELL, 1955, p. 132)

The key premises of the pattern theories were:

1. The receptors are not highly specific, but are broadly tuned to respond, albeit differentially, to a wide variety of physical stimuli.
2. In so responding, these receptors generate a pattern of activity that defines, by virtue of the relative amount of activity in the various neurons, a given sensory experience.

The original formulators of the pattern theories rejected completely the notion of specificity in the receptors and, instead, believed that all mechanical distortions produced equivalent neural responses if the physical energies were the same. This statement is probably no longer acceptable to even the most ardent supporters of contemporary pattern theory. Rather, in its place has emerged the notion that receptors respond to broad ranges of stimuli but with differing sensitivities. Thus, it is now considered to be the relative amount of activity, rather than the absolute amount that is critical in defining sensory quality in the somatosensory system, as well as in the auditory and visual ones.

The most up-to-date statement of pattern theory is also presented in Melzack and Wall's (1962) paper. The general goal of that paper was to provide a rapprochement between the theories of receptor specificity and that aspect of the pattern theory that assumed completely nonspecific receptors. Melzack and Wall concluded that one would have to accept the fact that receptors respond to finitely wide "ranges" of stimuli and that, beyond the receptor levels, spatio-temporal pattern representation must predominate. It is clear, therefore, that their statement, in spite of the fact that they wish to accept some form of limited specificity and decry the lack of precision of the classic pattern theories, is itself certainly a statement of a pattern theory. One of their main contributions was to explicitly state some of the axioms that such a modern pattern theory must have. Because of their succinctness in the statement of these axioms, we quote them here in their entirety:

1. *Skin receptors have specialized physiological properties for the transduction of particular kinds and ranges of stimuli into patterns of nerve impulses rather than modality-specific information.*
2. *Certain aspects of temporal and spatial patterns of impulses produced by stimulation of the skin may be filtered out presynaptically by the properties of terminal arborizations.*
3. *Central cells can detect some characteristics of stimuli from the impulse patterns arriving from the skin by their properties of threshold, temporal summation and adaptation.*
4. *Central cells can detect some characteristics of stimuli from the impulse patterns arriving from the skin by their property of spatial summation.*
5. *Central cells can detect some characteristics of stimuli from the impulse patterns arriving from the skin as a result of the special connexions of afferent systems.*
6. *More than one nerve impulse from a single afferent fiber, or more than one fiber carrying single nerve impulses, is essential for central cells to detect the characteristics of a sensory stimulus.*
7. *The somesthetic system is a unitary, integrated system comprised of specialized component parts.*
8. *Every discriminably different somesthetic perception is produced by a unique pattern of nerve impulses.*
   (MELZACK and WALL, 1962, pp. 353–354.)

Clearly, Melzack and Wall's contribution and emphasis are aimed at a general statement of the integrative capability of central nervous cells; there is very little detail to distinguish their "theory" from the pattern theory enunciated by Weddel or Nafe other than the less than infinitely wide tuning of the receptors. But this is a general deficiency of "pattern" theories, or for that matter of all statements that use the word *pattern* to describe manifold variables. Melzack and Wall's great contribution was to establish a precise frame of reference and to define the form a theory must take, even if they do not specify the details of the elements of that framework. Pattern theories of the sort proposed by Nafe, Weddell, or Melzack and Wall are all precursors of a more general sensory-coding theory, but do little more than emphasize the multidimensionality of sensory quality codes and reject the notion of specific labeled lines as the single code for sensory quality.

Nevertheless, by considering these alternative points of view, we hopefully have acquired some perspective of the critical questions that must be asked to fill in the details of the ultimate theory. One question is a transductive one: are the receptors broadly or narrowly tuned? The answer to even this superficially simple question will be difficult to acquire for the reasons we have mentioned. Another important question refers to the coding scheme of the transmitted messages. What specific dimensions of the neural response are actually conveying the information associated with stimulus quality at each of the levels of neural coding in the ascending somatosensory pathways? We shall explore the biological data that are relevant to each of these questions in the next section.

C. The Biological Data

1. Are Somatosensory Receptors Specific or Multimodal? In spite of the apparent disagreement between the proponents of the specificity and pattern theories, there is now emerging a sort of consensus with regard to the issue of the neurophysiology of receptor specificity. Perhaps the best way to illustrate this is to quote directly from three of the most modern statements of somatosensory coding theory. First, let us see what Rose and Mountcastle (1959), writing in the very important *Handbook of Physiology,* have to say. It should be noted that these authors generally support a modified specificity theory.

> *Whatever opinions one may hold about the way tactile stimuli arouse sensations it is fundamental to recognize that there are some receptors which are specifically sensitive to such stimuli. Conclusive evidence in this respect is provided by studies of discharges, usually of single units, when mechanoreceptors are activated by natural stimuli. In many of these studies [Adrian, Cattell, and Hoagland, 1931; Adrian and Umrath, 1929; Adrian and Zotterman, 1926; Andrew, 1954a, b; Andrew and Dodt, 1953; Boyd and Roberts 1953; Cattell and Hoagland, 1931; Fitzgerald, 1940; Gernandt and Zotterman, 1946; Hensel and Zotterman, 1951; Hogg, 1935; Loewenstein, 1956; Ness, 1954] the existence of a specific receptor is inferred from the behavior of the neural discharge; in some [Alvarez-Buyella*

and De Arellano, 1953; Gray and Malcolm, 1950; Gray and Matthews, 1951a, b; Gray and Sato, 1953], the receptors themselves were iden- tified.

(ROSE and MOUNTCASTLE, 1959, p. 391.)

And also:

> The problem of sensitivity of mechanoreceptors to other than tactile stimuli has attracted but casual interest of most observers, chiefly because it is known that thermal and painful stimuli charac- teristically cause discharges in the smaller spectrum of fibers. Never- theless, it was observed by Adrian & Umrath [1929] that thermal stimuli did not excite the mechanoreceptors they studied, and Hogg [1935] stated that thermal and chemical stimuli are less effective in the frog in activating large fibers than small ones and that the reverse is true for tactile stimuli. Hensel & Zotterman [1951] recently pre- sented interesting data on the response of some mechanoreceptors to cold. In the tongue of the cat they found mechanoreceptors not sensitive to strong thermal stimuli as well as thermoreceptors un- responsive to tactile excitation. In addition to these receptors they also found a group of fibers which responded both to pressure and to cooling. The response to cold differed in important aspects from the response of a typical thermoreceptor for the response occurred only to very low temperatures and rapid cooling (while thermorecep- tors respond with a sensitivity to about a tenth of a degree below 40°C) and it adapted to extinction within a few seconds (while a typical response to cooling persists for as long as the stimulus is applied). How to interpret such a response to cooling is an open question. It is conceivable that it represents a secondary effect due, for example, to a displacement of a mechanoreceptor through vaso- constriction, although this interpretation is considered as rather unlikely by the authors.

(ROSE and MOUNTCASTLE, 1959, p. 392.)

Melzack and Wall (1962), considering exactly this same question of recep- tor specificity, state:

> There is now considerable evidence to show that many skin re- ceptors respond to at least two classes of environmental energy. This is particularly striking in the reports of a large number of peripheral fibers whose receptors are sensitive to both pressure and tempera- ture (Hensel and Zotterman, 1951; Hensel et al., 1960; Hunt and McIntyre, 1960a, b; Lele and Weddell, 1959; Wall, 1960). Even recep- tor-fiber units that respond to hair movement may also respond to temperature change if it is sufficiently intense (Hunt and McIntyre, 1960a). In addition, the physiological properties of Pacinian corpuscles are affected by skin temperature (Loewenstein, 1959), so that it is likely that the transducer activities of virtually all mechanoreceptors are modified by warming or cooling the skin.

This does not mean, however, that every receptor responds to the full range of all environmental stimuli. First, receptors vary in their threshold to pressure stimulation. The thresholds of receptor-fiber units to pressure were found by Wall (1960) to vary from low to high threshold in a continuous distribution, with no signs of any particular subdivisions in the curve. Second, receptor-fiber units that respond to cooling or warming of the skin (including those that also respond to mechanical stimulation) show peak sensitivity within only narrow ranges of temperature change. These response maxima are distributed over a wide range (see Hensel and Zotterman, 1951; Hunt and McIntyre, 1960a, b) and the data of the available studies suggest that they form a continuous distribution.

(MELZACK and WALL, 1962, pp. 342–43.)

This is a position which is generally in accord with that of Sinclair (1967), who says:

The adequate stimulus for a given end organ is nowadays defined [Ruch, 1961] as the form of energy to which the receptor is most sensitive, and can be determined by monitoring the discharge from the end organ during exposure to various kinds of stimulation. By this means it can be shown that certain end organs are aroused by one kind of energy much more readily than by others. Such findings include the Pacinian corpuscle, which responds preferentially to deformation [Loewenstein, 1961b], and the facial pits of rattlesnakes, which respond preferentially to infrared radiation (Bullock and Diecke, 1956). Others are less selective, and may be readily activated by two or more forms of stimulation.

The evidence for this last statement is derived from experiments in which recordings are taken from what are presumed to be "single fibres" [p. 23]. It is of course possible that different kinds of receptor may be borne on one and the same fiber. However, it is more likely that all the receptors connected to a single fiber are of the same general kind. If this is so, the discovery of impulses in this fiber in response to two or more forms of stimulus must mean that the particular kind of receptor which it bears is sensitive to two or more forms of energy.

Weddell and Miller (1962) give examples, taken from the literature, of endings with apparently multiple sensitivities. Many of these examples concern endings which respond to thermal stimulation as well as to another form of energy, and a special difficulty arises in such cases, since change in temperature can alter charge transfer through mechanically excited receptor membranes and so cause variations in the frequency of impulses recorded, though temperature may not in itself excite the end organ (Ishiko and Loewenstein, 1961). Thus, the responses to mechanical stimulation of Pacinian corpuscles and of the "touch corpuscles" of Pinkus can be considerably influenced by temperature (Inman and Peruzzi, 1961;

> *Werner and Mountcastle, 1965), but in neither case can the cor-*
> *puscles be classed as thermoreceptors.*
>
> (*SINCLAIR, 1967, pp. 49–50.*)

One might ask at this point: is there any inherent contradiction among any of these three statements? The answer is probably no; there is not. Rose and Mountcastle's championing of specificity theory is thoroughly qualified in the summary statement of their chapter to include some pattern notions, and clearly the idea of secondary effects of temperature, for example, opens the door to nonspecific influences. And neither Sinclair, on the one hand, nor Melzack and Wall, on the other, demand that all stimulus energies be equally effective (as measured in some comparable energy scale) in eliciting neural activity. They simply point out that there are cells activated by more stimuli than solely touch or temperature. Probably when pressed, all of these authors would reject the extreme specificity implicit in von Frey's theory, as well as the complete nonspecificity suggested by the early pattern theories of Weddell.

Very little research on the problem of touch specificity has been reported in the 1960s. Among the few important findings were the discovery and description of the anatomy and physiology of a new receptor unit by Iggo and Muir (1969). These workers found the clustered structure of Merkel cells, which was shown in Figure 3.37. Though Iggo and Muir were highly committed to the notion that specificity was still a perfectly defensible position, even their description of the new touch corpuscle included the fact that temperature, as well as mechanical forces, could affect the output of the unit. Interestingly, the activity of the Iggo corpuscle, as this end organ is usually known, increased as the skin temperature was reduced. This result clearly indicates that the output of the unit was capable of being modulated by more than simply mechanical stimuli. From another point of view, evidence of nonspecificity was also evident in their observation that the corpuscle's response was dependent not only upon the amplitude, but also upon the velocity of a stimulating displacement.

The problem of warmth and cold reception is particularly complicated because of the fact that any chemical system varies in its rate of reaction as the temperature of its environment shifts. Thus, a "specific" heat receptor could arise as a direct result of the thermal conditions on the metabolic resting processes of the cell. It is not even completely convincing when cells are shown to operate in the opposite direction—lowered temperatures producing higher response rates—because of the possibility of reduced inhibitory interactions from other cells, which may have their activity decreased by cooling.

There is a rather substantial body of information on the thermal sensitivities of single cutaneous neurons that, for the most part, is rather contradictory. Hensel (1968), in a discussion of some of his recent work on thermal receptors, notes that there are many different types of cells responsive to cold and warmth in different manners. Some are apparently not specifically sensitive to the absolute level of cold, but do respond to cooling. Some operate in the opposite manner and are sensitive to warming, but not to absolute temperature levels. Some of the warm and cold cells are also responsive to mechanical stimulation, while others are not.

Table 11.2, which has been compiled by Murray (1966), lists a wide range of neurons, which increase their rate of firing in response to temperature reductions. This list includes encapsulated and free cutaneous receptors as well as central neurons and also tabulates the source of the data.

After considering that a very varied group of receptors would be required to initiate all of these observed thermal effects, Murray concluded that the thermal sensitivity is more probably a general responsiveness of any nerve membrane. The diversity of thermal effects is a strong argument against any specificity theory that asserts that each receptor responds solely to a single type of stimulus.

In sum, it appears that the preponderance of data does not support the notion that somatosensory receptors are highly specific or narrowly tuned. Even the receptor structures, which are described by the most committed proponents of specificity theory as being relatively specific, often display some sort of sensitivity to at least thermal stimuli and often to other stimulus parameters.

From all of this, we must conclude that neither the strict specificity of the von Frey school nor the complete nonspecificity of the early pattern theories comes close to adequately describing the true state of affairs to be found in somatosensory quality coding. In fact, while many somatosensory receptors seem to respond to several different kinds of energy and to several of the parameters of mechanical energy, each seems to have a lowest threshold to some single stimulus class. This is a sort of broad tuning, displaying a "best" threshold that is analogous to the response areas of the auditory system or the peak spectral response of a visual cell. Unfortunately, the discontinuous nature of the stimulus continuum in the somatosensory system makes it difficult to quantify this notion in a way that would make the analogy less than a superficial one.

2. Can a Single Somatosensory Fiber Carry Multiple Sensations? Because the problem of quality coding in somatosensation is so vaguely defined, data that show specific neurological correlations with human psychophysical data are of particular importance. Many authors have worked with electrical stimuli in somatosensation as an alternative to the natural stimuli because of the ease with which the stimulus parameters can be controlled. A considerable amount of progress has been made in studying temporal and spatial discrimination using these stimuli. However, it is always the case that there is virtually no quality variation with variation in the characteristics of an electrical stimulus other than a sudden onset of pain as some critical intensive threshold is passed or as there is a change in the current pathway. A small crack in the skin, for example, will lead to a painful prick at a stimulus intensity that is hardly felt when the skin is intact. The reason for the difference is that the current in the former case is channeled entirely through a small region, while in the latter case it is distributed over a wide

TABLE 11.2   A TABLE OF NEURAL STRUCTURES THAT INCREASE THEIR RATE OF FIRING AS A RESULT OF BEING COOLED (FROM MURRAY, 1966)

Preparation	Sensitivity (impulses/sec/°C)	Reference
Mammalian tongue and skin	-30, -55	Hensel and Boman, 1960; Hensel, Iggo, and Witt, 1960; Iriuchijima and Zotterman, 1960
Ampullae of Lorenzini	-90, -40	Hensel, 1955; Sand, 1938
Crustacean leg motor nerves	-40	Dorai Raj and Murray, 1962
Mammalian skin mechanoreceptors	-30	Witt and Hensel, 1959
Lateral line organs of *Xenopus*	-4	Murray, 1956
Stretch receptors, crustacean	-1·5	Florey, 1956
Stretch receptors, fish	-0·3	Sand, 1938
Various invertebrate central neurones	-1	Kerkut and Taylor, 1956

area. Variations in current density, therefore, are associated in this case with a change in perceived quality.

More typically though, low intensity electric stimuli produce a sort of perceptual thump (Uttal, 1959, 1960), which is constant from one stimulus pattern to another. Never in the experience of most who have worked with this stimulus was there any suggestion of a synthetic wetness, warmth, cold, or tickle, regardless of the place or frequency of electrical stimulation.

The absence of a wide range of qualitative effects with electrical stimulation suggests that a major factor in the coding of quality in the somatosensory system is, as was suggested by the pattern theorists, the spatiotemporal patterning of the nervous response. More specifically, it suggests that unsynchronized signals with variable timing and variable relative amounts of activity are critical in defining the quality of the sensation. The electrical stimulus, however, probably acts directly on axons rather than through the mediation of the receptors, and thus tends to hypersynchronize the nerve action potentials. Such a highly unphysiological stimulus as an electrical pulse may, therefore, essentially wipe out all of the critical timing and phase information, which is normally necessary to signal the different somatosensory qualities.

If it is the case that the relative phasing and temporal relations of a number of neural units are required for the specification of the quality of a cutaneous sensation, then a new question arises. Can any qualitative information be conveyed along a single neuron? Surprisingly, this question has been asked using a most unusual preparation—the human. Hensel and Boman (1960) performed a somewhat unusual experiment involving experimental surgery on human subjects. A small twig of the radial nerve in the forearm was exposed during a brief operation while the subject was under general anaesthesia. Following the surgery, the subject was awakened, and relatively conventional neurophysiological recording electrodes (glass tubes filled with KCl-soaked cotton wick) were applied to measure nerve impulses from nerve fibers dissected free from the exposed nerve twigs. The novel and important part of the experiment, however, was that the subject was able to describe the sensations produced by normal mechanical and thermal stimuli that were applied to his skin. The skin was then explored to determine what kind of stimuli were effective and what the shape of the receptive field was for each examined neuron.

A major finding of Hensel and Boman's work concerned the problem of specificity. It turned out that both highly specific and multimodal fibers were observed in their experiments. The specific fibers were usually sensitive only to touch stimuli applied to their receptive areas, but there was also a unique case of a cell that responded only to cooling. All of the multimodal cells examined in this highly unusual preparation were sensitive to both touch and cooling. Furthermore, in all of the multimodal cells, which constituted over 70 percent of the sample of radial nerve fibers, the activity of the cell increased as the skin was suddenly cooled, but was inhibited if the skin was warmed. Figure 11.1 plots the response rate of one of these cells to both kinds of stimuli. Note particularly the difference in the time course to each type of stimulus.

In the context of the present discussion, another very important finding was that a touch sensation could not only be induced by the activity of a single fiber, but even more amazingly, a conscious tactile experience could be produced when only a single spike was evoked in that single neuron. On the other hand, Hensel and Boman found that the experience associated with the cooling of the skin was not evoked until a relatively long stream of signals was elicited. The fact that the thermal fibers were often spontaneously active suggests that some statistical trend would be required for a thermal change to be detectable, and, thus, the requirement for the long response train makes good sense. On the other hand, if we recall the very rapid adaptation (a single nerve action potential at the onset of even a continuing mechanical stimulus as was the case in the Pacinian corpuscle), then the importance of a single spike to a touch experience also becomes clear.

3. An Example of Macrotemporal Quality Coding in the Spinal Cord. If we look at Figure 11.1, it is clear that the time course of the responses elicited by touch and thermal stimuli is quite different. This may be due to the physics of the stimuli or to some property of the receptor, but in any event there is inherent in this differential response pattern another candidate neural code—the macrotemporal pattern of activity of a single fiber. Wall and Cronly-Dillon (1960) have studied the response of single second-order cells in the spinal cord of the cat and have shown that there are many individual spinal cells that seem to respond to different kinds of stimuli with different temporal response patterns. Such multimodal cells may reflect one of two possible anatomical arrangements. They may respond to multimodal stimuli, because they are receiving inputs from nonspecific receptors responsive to several different kinds of stimuli. On the other hand, they may also be acting as centers of convergence for inputs from several different kinds of specific receptor cells, each of which is capable of responding only to a single kind of stimulus. Nevertheless, for these cells at this coding

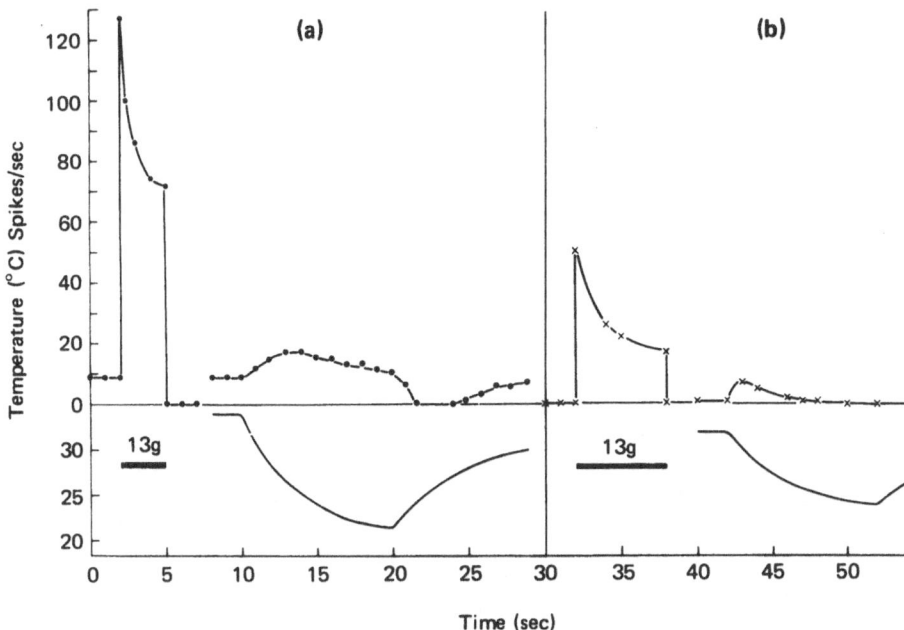

FIGURE 11.1 *The response curves of two human peripheral somatosensory neurons (a and b) graphed by plotting the spike impulse frequency as a function of the type and magnitude of both a 13 gram mechanical and a thermal stimulus. Note the difference in waveform between the firing pattern produced by cooling and that produced by a mechanical stimulus (from Hensel and Boman, 1960).*

level, at least, the notion of labeled lines is—as we shall see—demonstrably inapplicable, for they convey multimodal information.

By suggesting that the macrotemporal pattern of the spike action potentials is a candidate code for quality, Wall and Cronly-Dillon raise the possibility that a single cell should be capable of carrying multimodal quality information. To determine whether or not this was actually the case, they surgically exposed the spinal cord and determined the response pattern to a variety of natural stimuli.

If the stimulus was a sustained light pressure, they found that the response pattern of a single spinal neuron was a brief burst of activity when the stimulus was first applied. The intensity of the stimulus was apparently represented by the duration of this burst, but was not related to its frequency. The same cell could also be activated by heating the skin, but in this case the macrotemporal response pattern was a sustained increase in the spontaneous activity, the frequency of which was associated with the magnitude of the temperature change. For thermal stimuli, the response of the cell did not tend to diminish over time, but was sustained for as long as the stimulus was present. If the stimulus was a (presumably) painful one (the attribution of pain being based on avoidance responses on the part of the cat) produced by attaching a small clamp to the skin, the response pattern was a highly irregular high-frequency pattern with interspike interval spacing approaching a random distribution. This burst of activity was usually followed by a period of response depression below spontaneous levels when the clamp was removed. On the other hand, if Cowhage, a powerful itching substance, was applied to the cat's skin, a rapid and regular series of bursts of high-frequency activity was produced.

Wall and Cronly-Dillon also applied vibratory stimuli to the cat's skin and observed phase locking at the frequency of the stimulus (or at multiples of it depending upon the stimulus intensity) very similar to the phase locking phenomenon we have previously discussed in the auditory nerve.

Figure 11.2 summarizes the varied response patterns of a single cell to the various stimulus types used by Wall and Cronly-Dillon in their experiments. If these findings can be generalized, it seems that somatosensory signals, rather than being solely encoded by specific receptors and parallel labeled lines, are at least in part encoded by macrotemporal patterns in a single neuron. It is also possible, however, that for some reason associated with the details of this technique, Wall and Cronly-Dillon may have been sampling a rather peculiar set of neurons, which conveyed information that had converged from a number of distinct receptor classes, but were not typical of the transmission neuron at the pathway.

Indeed, other experiments at higher levels of the nervous system suggest that it is more usual to find highly specific somatosensory cells than large numbers of multimodal ones. For example, if we consider the level of the cortex, the general picture that emerges is one of individual cell specificity, even though most of the cutaneous modalities seem to project to the same primary somatosensory area. Individual cells have been shown by Mountcastle (1957) and by Morse, Adkins, and Towe (1965) to respond most often to only a single type of natural stimulus. Morse and his colleagues found that while most cortical cells were activated by touch and a few to touch and hair bending or pressure, only a few cells in his sample displayed the same multimodal sort of representation observed in the spinal cord by Wall and Cronly-Dillon.

D. A Contemporary Model

With such a sparse background of psychophysical data, such obscure definitions of the somatosensory qualities, and such vigorous controversy over specificity versus broadly tuned receptors, it is difficult to give a simple and coherent statement of a contemporary model of somatosensory quality coding. It seems clear that with regard to receptors, there is little evidence for any specificity fine enough so that only a single form of physical energy would be capable of stimulating a given receptor. On the other hand, there is ample evidence that the tuning is not so broad that all stimuli can act as equally effective agents in eliciting activity. There appears to be evidence for encoding, which is both modality specific and multimodal at all levels of the ascending somatosensory pathways, and thus some sort of pattern theory seems to be required to play the role in somatosensation that relative response rates obviously play in audition and vision. But this new pattern theory is at least tempered by the fact that peripheral receptors do exhibit a

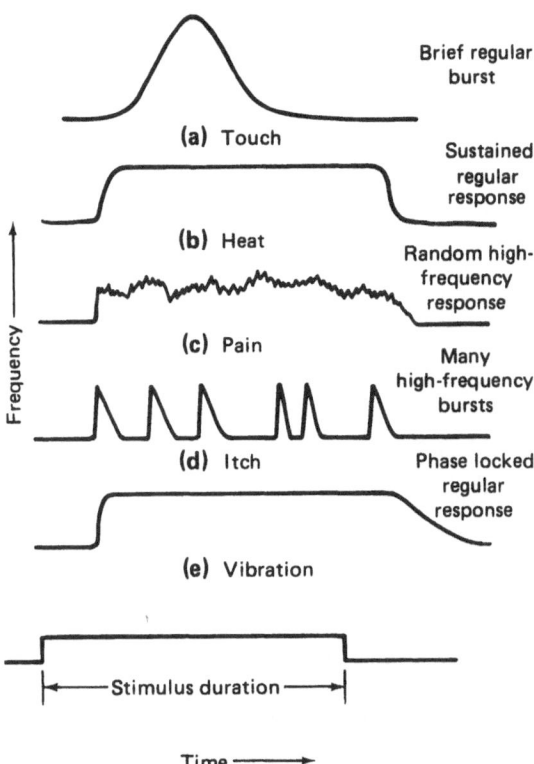

FIGURE 11.2 A set of drawings showing the spike action potential frequency pattern as observed in spinal neurons of the cat as a function of the quality of the applied stimulus (this figure is adapted from the discussion in Wall and Cronly-Dillon, 1960).

moderate degree of specificity. Clearly, what must be rejected is the pure specificity—labeled line premise of the von Frey school and the completely nonspecific tuning championed by the early pattern theorists. The conceptual compromise in this case is one in which the data seem to be forcing theory to converge toward an intermediate position, but, in sum, both classic theories must be rejected.

Is there any possibility that some feature other than receptor morphology might be the critical factor in defining the limited degree of specificity that is observed? Loewenstein and Rathkamp's (1958) work was most important in showing the ineffectiveness of the exterior capsule in defining the specificity of the Pacinian corpuscle. Presumably, this fact can be generalized to all other encapsulated endings. However, it is also possible that the nature of capsules, coupled with their location in the skin, may in some indirect way account for a modest form of specificity. It might be postulated, for example, that receptors close to skin ridges are more likely to be influenced by delicate touch stimuli. More deeply embedded cells, on the other hand, may in some way be selectively stimulated by thermal or pressure-evoking stimuli. But all of this is still in the realm of speculation and cannot be considered a comprehensive statement of somatosensory quality coding.

II. GUSTATION

A. The Key Psychophysical Data

As was the case with the somatosensory modalities, there is no single dimension of variation of any physical stimulus that is capable of sequentially producing the full range of gustatory sensations. Rather, gustation seems to be also characterizable as a group of separate but interacting senses rather than a continuum along some single qualitative dimension. There is nothing in our taste experiences that corresponds to the continuous gradation in hue or pitch in vision or audition as the respective stimuli vary. Furthermore, there is very little in our language that reflects any ability on the part of humans to distinguish among different kinds of sweetnesses or sours. Gustatory experiences more often seem to be characterized as conglomerates of more or less independent sensations rather than as fused or unitary perceptions.

For these reasons, over the years of research in this area, there has been little psychophysical experimentation that is specifically directed at such problems as taste discrimination, absolute taste identification, or, until very recently, much related to the synthesis of complex tastes from basic ones. Rather, the qualitative dimension in gustation has been more or less ignored at the psychophysical level, and most attention directed at the intensive effects of different chemicals that are assumed to produce a certain predefined sensory quality.

It is not certain, of course, whether our language reflects the details of our biology sufficiently well to draw any inference from the fact that classically we have defined four gustatory primaries. Yet history and anecdote have consistently restated the hypothesis that there are four, and only four, primary tastes—sweet, sour, bitter, and salty. To describe what is meant by each of these would be difficult if it were not for the fact that a particular archetypical chemical has come to be associated with each of these tastes. Sweetness is defined as the experience produced when solutions of sucrose are placed on the tongue. Quinine, in dilute enough solutions to be at all palatable, produces what is by common agreement referred to as a bitter experience, and dilute concentrations of acids like hydrochloric produce a sour sensation. The salty experience produced by NaCl, for example, is also well enough known. The host of other gustatory sensations, the classical view holds, is produced by mixtures of these four fundamentals.

The result of this ill-defined system of gustatory experience is to introduce an element of semantic confusion into the vocabulary used in psychophysical and neurophysiological experiments, which may explain some of the apparent disagreement between psychophysical and neurophysiological data we shall encounter later in our discussion. The words *salty, sweet, sour,* and *bitter* are psychological terms describing four primitive taste sensations reported by human observers. On the other hand, there are four prototypical chemicals or "basic taste stimuli," which are known to produce these sensations in man. They are the four we have just mentioned: sodium chloride, sucrose, hydrochloric acid, and quinine compounds, respectively. It is not certain that it is appropriate to call sodium chloride a salty stimulus in an animal experiment, however. Several authors have suggested that the nomenclature should be somewhat more guarded than the somewhat loose use of the term "salty" when used in animal studies. The words *basic taste stimuli* are now conventionally used to refer to the four chemicals, and the term *primary* or basic tastes to refer to the sensations reported in human experiments. Confusion of the two sets of words leads to considerable difficulty in understanding the relation between the two domains.

A major problem remains, however. Are these really the only four fundamental tastes, or are there more hidden away in the history of our vocabularies? So many investigators assume that these are the "fundamentals" that most modern literature seems to simply accept this idea as a given axiom. As we shall see later, however, there is little physiological support for such a notion, and shifting criteria of discriminability could alter the number of chemicals that are accepted as fundamentals.

The empirical question thus arises: is it possible to stimulate all other taste experiences by mixing various ratios of four archetypical basic taste stimuli? This is a difficult experiment to do in a clear-cut fashion, primarily because it is difficult to find a verbal response repertoire that adequately describes the resulting tastes. The reasons for this paucity of classificatory terms are multiple. First, the words may simply not be there. It is interesting how often we refer in our daily language to compound terms like bitter-sweet, sweet-and-sour, or metallic, all of which suggest that it is very difficult to find simple terms to describe taste experiences in the same way we note the differences between red, green, and blue. Furthermore, the taste of many food substances is determined by many factors other than the chemical composition of the substance. The term "flavor" is a sensory term, which probably contains quite a few more stimulus dimensions than simply the four basic tastes. Smell and the mechanical texture of the food have much to do with its flavor. Temperature is also known to affect the taste of substances to a considerable degree. In practical experience, we do not not usually taste nice neat aqueous solutions of the four taste stimuli, but complex, lumpy, temperature-varying chemicals of widely different textures.

In spite of these difficulties in defining and quantifying the gustatory response repertoire, a few attempts have been made to synthesize taste experiences. One of the first attempts to determine if tastes could be synthesized from the four basic taste stimuli was reported by Skramlik (1921). His approach was not to attempt to synthesize natural tastes, but rather to see if a variety of artificial tastes manufactured from a mixture of inorganic salt solutions could be matched by the four basic chemicals mentioned above. His results indicated that it was possible to reproduce any of the tastes of the unknown salt solutions by mixing appropriate proportions of the four standard substances.

Other attempts to confirm or deny the existence of four basic gustatory sensations have usually involved some aspect of the fact that the various areas of the tongue do not respond equally well to all four of the basic stimuli. Figure 11.3 shows a top view of the tongue and the areas that have been classically associated with the specific gustatory sensations. It must be emphasized that these areas are not rigidly demarcated or unique. It seems as if the pattern of arrangement is more in terms of overlapping spatial dis-

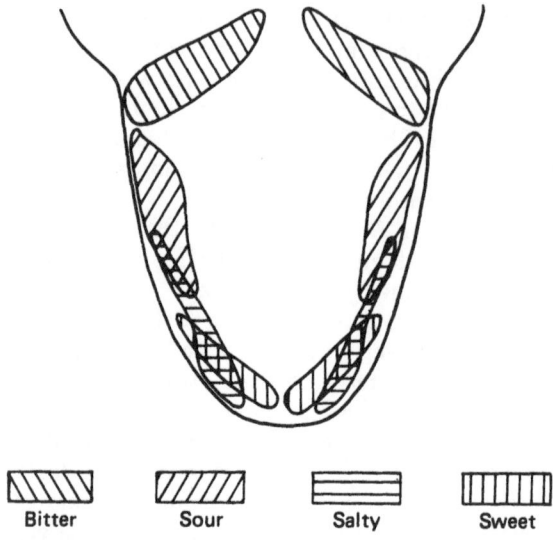

FIGURE 11.3 *A drawing of the tongue, showing the areas that seem to have maximum sensitivity to the indicated substances. But remember that the sensitivity for any stimuli is not zero any place (see Figure 11.4).*

tributions than in terms of precisely defined taste areas. The classic data defining these areas are that of Hänig (1901) and are shown in Figure 11.4, where the sensitivity of various parts of the tongue is plotted in terms of some vaguely defined threshold measure. This figure shows better than Figure 11.3 that the more or less general sensitivity to salty substances is maximum near the front and along the side of the tongue; sour substances are most easily transduced along the side near the center of the tongue; sweet substances near the tip (explaining perhaps why we lick an ice cream with the tip of our tongue); and bitter substances near the back of the tongue. But at no place on the tongue is the sensitivity to any one basic taste stimulus zero. All areas are, to some extent, sensitive to all substances.

The use of electrical stimuli as a nonadequate means of evoking gustatory experiences with varying quality in human subjects is a technique that has been used for many years. Some of the early experimenters working with Voltaic cells noted the tastes of the generated dc currents. Most recently, von Békésy (1964c) has improved upon the technique by using pulsed electrical stimuli, an improvement which prevents almost all of the electrolytic disassociation of salivary substances. Since electrolytically decomposed substances have their own tastes, this had been a major contaminent of early electric taste experiments.

In von Békésy's experiment, pulse trains that lasted for a few seconds and that varied in frequency from about 10 to 200 Hz were used. The results of his study are complicated, but are very important, since they represent virtually the only modern data on gustatory quality. First of all, von Békésy found that there was a very strong effect of electrode size. If the electrode was large (about 70 mm²), then variations of stimulus frequency allowed as many as three different types of gustatory experiences to be evoked when the current intensity was near threshold. If the electrode was medium sized (about 3 mm²), then at most two basic tastes could be evoked

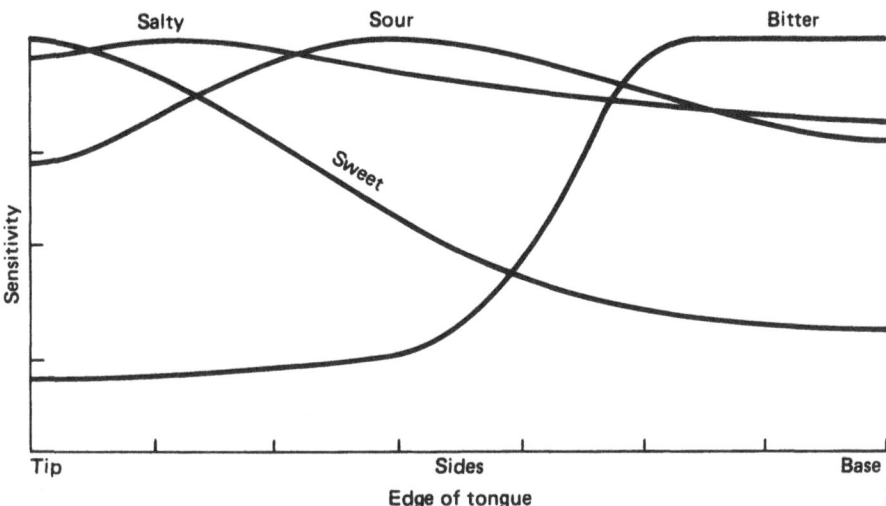

FIGURE 11.4 Distribution of gustatory sensitivities on the tongue varies from the tip to the base of the tongue but, once again, note that it is nowhere zero for any of the four basic tastes (figure from Boring, 1942, after Hänig, 1901).

at different stimulus frequencies. If the electrode was small (about 0.3 mm^2), then only one quality could be evoked no matter what the frequency of stimulation. A small electrode, therefore, was used in subsequent experiments to study the localization of quality. Von Békésy more or less randomly sampled various papillae scattered across the tongue and generally found that subjects reported that each produced only one of the four basic tastes when stimulated electrically.

In addition to finding only four different classes of subjective response, von Békésy also noted that there was a characteristic optimum frequency of electrical stimulation to activate each of the four different receptor types. This tuning phenomenon, analogous to the auditory one, suggested that salty and sour receptors are most responsive at about 40 Hz, and sweet and bitter receptors are most easily stimulated when the stimulus frequency is about 70 or 80 Hz. These response areas for the gustatory receptors are shown in Figure 11.5. The meaning and origin of this functional difference is obscure, to say the least.

The major difficulty with von Békésy's study is that the same results would be obtained if the subjects had only four taste names to use even if there was, in fact, a greater variety of sensations. There is no *a priori* way to tell whether or not the receptor mechanism or the vocabulary is the critical determining feature in this situation. Certainly, some of the sensations so produced were quite different from those obtained with natural chemical stimuli. One subject, for example, reported that the sweetness produced by low intensity electrical stimuli was "angelic"—a choice of words suggesting that it was quite a novel sort of experience. Von Békésy's explanation of this was that while natural stimuli are not pure, but have "overtones" produced by their partial stimulation of the other four recep-

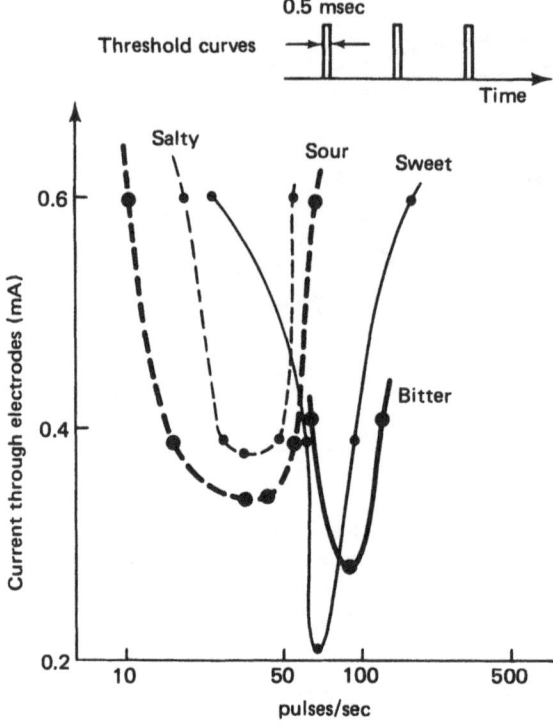

FIGURE 11.5 Pulse electrical stimulation of taste papillae produces response curves analogous to those found in the auditory system. These curves indicate the electrical current necessary at various frequencies to produce the four basic taste sensations. Salty and sour can be seen to have lower best frequencies than sweet and bitter but sweet and bitter require lower energies per pulse (from von Békésy, 1964c).

tor types, the electrical sweetness is uncontaminated by the other three basic tastes.

Von Békésy concluded from this research that the gustatory receptors are highly specific. In doing so, his point of view reflects what has been the classic view, that of specificity, and updates the older work of Allen and Weinberg (1925), who drew almost the same conclusions with electrical stimuli many years ago. Allen and Weinberg's work has been criticized on a number of grounds that may also be applicable to von Békésy's electro-stimulation experiments. The reader is referred to Amerine, Pangborn, and Roessler (1965, p. 42) for a critical discussion of this matter.

Von Békésy (1966), however, has gone on to use adequate chemical stimulation in a way that overcomes many of these criticisms and that adds, he believes, further support to his hypothesis that papillae are individually sensitive to only one of the four basic taste stimuli. His technique was remarkably direct. He simply stimulated individual papillae by dropping a small drop of the test solution on them. To do so, however, required an ingenious technical development—vacuum erection of individual papillae. One of the initial observations reported in this study by von Békésy was the fact that individual papillae were generally not effectively stimulated by a drop of the solution on their exposed ends. Rather, responses were elicited with much lower concentrations when the fluid was placed on their side. The side of a papilla, however, is not exposed under normal conditions,

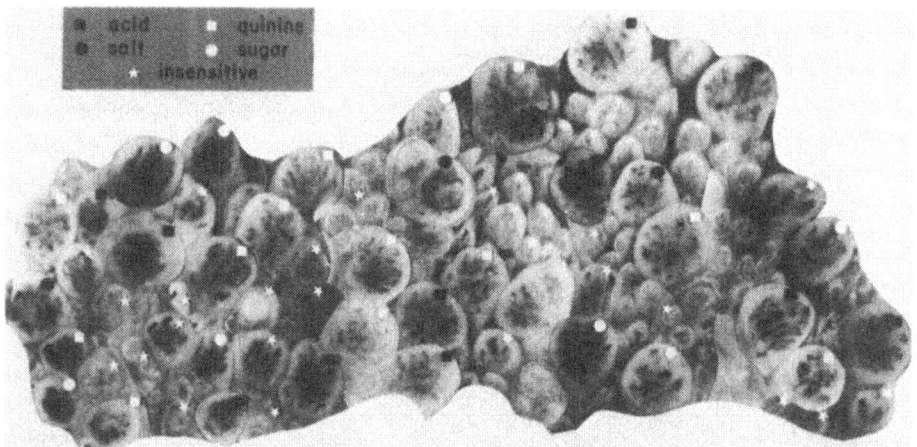

FIGURE 11.6 *Photograph showing the papillae distributed on the tip of the tongue. Von Békésy believes that each one is specific to a single taste substance and has so identified each one. Whether or not this is true, it is certainly evident that all of the basic tastes are represented to some degree even at the tip of the tongue (from von Békésy, 1966).*

and thus the erection technique was required. To erect a papilla with a vacuum, a small suction tube was placed on the tip of the papilla and lifted. Once lifted out from among its neighbors, a papilla would typically remain erect for several minutes, and solutions could be quite conveniently placed anywhere on its surface. The general result of this procedure, according to von Békésy, was that each papilla (with some curious exceptions) also responded to only one of the four basic taste stimuli.

Figure 11.6 (from von Békésy, 1966) shows a group of papillae marked with their specific sensitivities. This figure is taken from the tip of the tongue, but obviously all four basic tastes are represented even in this region. It is also interesting to note that there are also a large number of totally insensitive papillae. On the two subjects with whom von Békésy worked, there was a high degree of correlation between the results obtained with electrical and chemical stimulation, a finding that helped to strengthen his notion of papillar specificity to only one of the four taste stimuli.

Other experimental evidence that has been used to support the specificity hypothesis that there are four, and only four, gustatory primary receptor modalities revolves around the actions of a group of curious substances, which are capable of modifying or blocking one or more of the taste qualities. Perhaps the most interesting of these substances, is the taste-modifying berry known as the miracle fruit. Daniell (1852) was the first to describe the surprising effects of this southwest African berry. After chewing on a miracle fruit, even sour substances taste sweet. In the lands in which this berry is indigenous, it is frequently eaten in conjunction with foods that are naturally sour to make them more palatable.

Bartoshuk, Dateo, Vandenbelt, Buttrick, and Long (1969) have performed one of the few controlled psychophysical experiments utilizing the miracle fruit and have found that the effect could be most properly described as a sweetness generator rather than a converter of sourness to sweetness, as it is usually reputed to be. Miracle fruit adds sweetness to produce a sweet-and-sour taste, but does not diminish the sourness of the food. Apparently, the critical substance in the fruit is a specific enhancer of the action of sweet receptors and not an inhibitor of the action of sour receptors. Two groups of investigators (Henning, Brouwer, van der Wel, and Francke, 1969; and Kurihara, Kurihara, and Beidler, 1969) have extracted the active agent from the miracle fruit and have found it to be a rather large organic molecule with a molecular weight of about 42,000. The action of the fruit was shown by both groups not to be due to any chemical modification of the sour food itself, for the addition of the sweetness does not occur no matter how long the juice of the miracle fruit and the food were mixed together. The action is definitely exerted on the receptors of the tongue, for after putting miracle fruit in the mouth, all sour foods taste sweet to some degree. Henning and his colleagues have named the active substance of miracle fruit *miraculin*.

Another natural plant product, gymnemic acid, has exactly the opposite effect. It has been known for almost a century that the leaf of a plant, which grew wild in India, had the capability to suppress sweetness. Originally, it was also thought to suppress bitter tastes, but it is now known that it does not actively affect bitterness. Bartoshuk and his group (1969), for example, definitively showed that the substance was quite specific in its suppression of sweetness, but was incapable of diminishing the taste response to either sour, salty, or bitter substances.

Both gymnemic acid and miraculin, thus, appear to have a very specific action on the sweet receptor systems and little action on any of the other three basic tastes. The action of another flavor modifier, monosodium glutamate, is much more complex. Generally, this substance is said by some to enhance the natural flavors of many different kinds of food, but not to have any taste of its own. Others believe it to be able to suppress unpleasant tastes. However, Amerine, Pangborn, and Roessler (1965) state that the substance in its pure form does have a characteristic flavor—a sweet and salty combination as well as a peculiar tactile sensation in the mouth. Clearly, the action of monosodium glutamate is not yet well know enough to be definitively defined. It is known (Schaumburg, Byck, Gerstl, and Maskman, 1969) that it does produce a disease known as the "Chinese restaurant syndrome" if it is eaten in unduly large quantities. The skin becomes flushed and itchy, and there are accompanying headaches. Undoubtedly, it is a very potent biochemical, and some assert that it is so by virtue of its ability to increase Na^+ permeability. There have been some claims that it causes more or less permanent damage to the vertebrate brain.

These taste modifiers have also been useful in spelling out some discrepancies in the analogies drawn between electrical and chemical stimulation by von Békésy. It is not at all certain, for example, that the two modes of stimulation operate in exactly the same way. Bujas and Pfaffmann (1971) have shown that the sweetness produced with electrical stimulation is not blocked by the application of potassium gymnate (a derivative of gymnemic acid) in the same way as that produced with a chemical stimulus. They attribute this to the fact that electrical stimuli are probably activating neuronal axons directly and therefore bypassing the receptor mechanism, while the chemical effect is produced by activation of the usual receptor sites on the papillae.

In sum, the psychophysical evidence continually seems to evoke the use of the four basic taste words. Yet, as we have noted, it is moot whether this must be interpreted as a reflection of the underlying biological mechanisms or of the evolved language of gustatory experience. But it is clear that whatever the reasons, almost all psychophysical experiments seem to result in their authors drawing the conclusion of specificity. The next step in our analysis will be to determine whether or not there is any physiological evidence that supports this usual psychophysical conclusion. As we shall see, neurophysiological data support just the opposite view.

B. The Competitive Theories

There are no major schools of disagreement or very precisely defined theories of gustatory quality coding beyond the receptor other than a more or less general disagreement between specifists and pattern theorists. Rather, there are a couple of questions that seem to be appreciated by all as having not yet been answered. One of these questions concerns the nature of the specific or quasi-specific action at the receptor that accounts for taste differentiation. This is really a matter of transduction dynamics, and we have discussed most of the relevant issues in Chapter 4. The other major issue is one to which we have already repeatedly referred. It is essentially the same issue as was raised in the somatosensory system: are the receptors finely tuned to narrow ranges of stimuli or are they relatively nonspecific in their response repertoire? To answer this and related questions, we must now turn to the neurophysiological data.

C. The Neurophysiological Data

1. Gustatory Receptor Potentials. Kimura and Beidler (1961) have recorded what is apparently a receptor potential from both the rat and hamster. KCl-filled glass microelectrodes were inserted into single cells of a taste papilla, and the signals recorded were fed to a dc coupled amplifier. The taste stimuli applied to the papillae were drops of NaCl, sucrose, quinine hydrochloride, and hydrochloric acid. The resulting potentials recorded from one sample cell were shown in Figure 6.32. This particular cell was found to respond to all four of the stimulus substances with a receptor potential that, while it varied in amplitude for the different sapid substances, was identical in rise time and shape for all four. Of the population of cells that Kimura and Beidler sampled, some displayed responsiveness to at least two, some to three, and many to all four of the basic taste chemicals. Kimura and Beidler at that time (1961) believed that this multiple sensitivity was due to a multiplicity of receptor types on each of the receptor cells, but of course rather broadly tuned individual chemoreceptive sites are an alternative hypothesis, which could equally well explain this nonspecificity.

A more recent analysis of the ionic origin of gustatory receptor potentials has been presented by Ozeki (1970). It is Ozeki's conclusion that there is some fundamental difference in the membrane processes that are activated by NaCl and quinine hydrochloride, respectively. To arrive at this conclusion, Ozeki inserted KCl-filled glass microelectrodes into gustatory receptor cells and recorded the electrotonic potentials produced by a series of applied constant current electrical test pulses superimposed on the receptor potential. The brief (100 msec) electrotonic potentials were purely passive electrical responses and merely reflected the momentary resistance of the membrane. His findings suggested that the action of NaCl on the membrane was to reduce the overall resistance of the membrane and thus reduce the electrotonic potentials. This is shown in Figure 11.7(a) by the reduction in the size of the brief electrotonic potentials produced by the test pulses during the period of the receptor potential compared to the unstimulated periods.

On the other hand, the response to quinine hydrochloride was quite different. Figure 11.7(b) shows that the membrane resistance actually increased when the cell was stimulated, for in this case the electrotonic responses to the test current pulses were enlarged during the period of the receptor potential. Ozeki concluded on the basis of a voltage clamp type of experiment that this increase in membrane resistance during stimulation with quinine hydrochloride was due to a specific decrease in the membrane permeability to K^+. However, the same sort of clamping experiment suggested to him that the decreased resistance reported during stimulation with NaCl was due to a specific increase in the permeability of the membrane to Na^+. Thus, the membrane action, which is the origin of the receptor potential produced by NaCl, seems to differ from that underlying the origin of the receptor potential produced by quinine hydrochloride. Whether similar differences occur with the other basic taste stimuli is still moot, but this sort of differential effect fits in fairly well with the specific ionic binding site hypothesis of the primary gustatory sensory action we discussed in Chapter 4. It also supports the notion of multiple receptor mechanisms on a single cell and, thus, nonspecificity.

2. *First-Order Fibers.* The nervous fibers primarily responsible for conducting taste information are cabled in two major nerve trunks—the chorda tympani and the glossopharyngeal nerve. These nerves are made up, in part, of fibers that synapse at the base of the taste receptor cells in the tongue, but other nongustatory fibers are also present. Because of their course from the tongue, these two nerves have been readily accessible to experimental neurophysiological inquiries for many years. There does appear to be some distinctiveness between the information conveyed by each of the two nerves, for the chorda tympani generally is not as responsive to sucrose and quinine as it is to sodium chloride and hydrochloric acid (Pfaffmann, 1970). On the other hand, the integrated response of the glossopharyngeal nerve seems to be more sensitive to sucrose and quinine than to the other two basic taste stimuli. The reason for this difference in "tuning" is probably due to the spatial distribution of the receptor sites serviced by each nerve. The glossopharyngeal nerve serves the base and side of the tongue, where

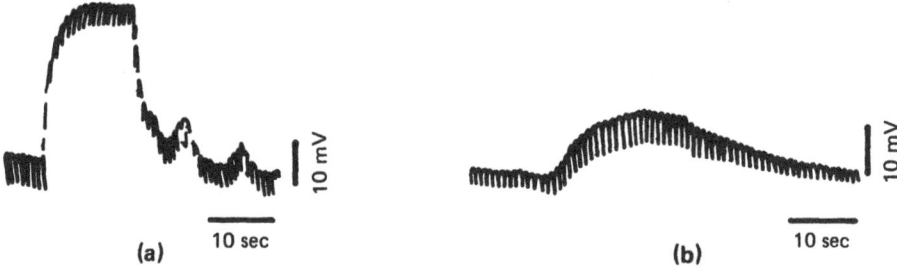

FIGURE 11.7 *Two receptor responses from a rat's gustatory receptor cell. The continuous curve is the receptor potential, while the small downward-going spikes are the potentials produced by a series of applied test stimuli. These spikes are, therefore, nothing more than the electrotonic potential produced by the action of the test current, and their amplitude is purely a function of the membrane resistance in accord with Ohm's law. (a) The response of the cell to NaCl. (b) The response of the cell to quinine hydrochloride. The small spikes decrease in size in (a) but increase in (b), indicating that the depolarizing membrane receptor potential in (a) is due to a decrease in membrane resistance, but in (b) it is more likely due to an increase in membrane resistance (from Ozeki, 1970).*

sweet and bitter receptors are more densely located. The chorda tympani, on the other hand, serves the tip and sides of the tongue. These differences are not absolute, but are only relative, and some sensitivity to all four basic taste stimuli exists in both nerves.

Studies of the taste sensitivity of individual chorda tympani nerve fibers have been almost routinely carried out for many years, providing continuing support for the observations originally made by Pfaffmann (1941). In general, multiple sensitivity of individual nerve fibers to all four taste stimuli is usually observed. Almost all of the fibers studied are sensitive to more than one of the four taste stimuli but, as with the Kimura and Beidler findings, to a variable degree for each individual cell. Thus, a given fiber might respond strongly to NaCl and less strongly to quinine, while a neighboring fiber might respond to the same pair of chemicals, but in the reverse order of sensitivity.

Cohen, Hagiwara, and Zotterman (1955) found a somewhat unusual pattern of responsiveness when they recorded from the cat's chorda tympani. The cat seems to have a type of fiber that is especially sensitive to distilled water. There were also fibers that were sensitive to acid alone or to quinine alone, but both the distilled-water-sensitive fiber and a similar salt-sensitive fiber usually responded to two or more of the four stimuli.

Pfaffmann (1955) composed a graph, which has currently taken on the status of a classic display of gustatory sensitivity. His notion was to show the respective sensitivities to the four basic taste stimuli (and in addition KCl) for a random sample of different neurons. This graph is reproduced in Figure 11.8 and shows what appears to be a quasi-random distribution of the sensitivities to five test chemicals. Whether or not this distribution was truly random has been debated vigorously in recent years, with Frank and Pfaffmann (1969) reporting perfectly random distribution of the sensi-

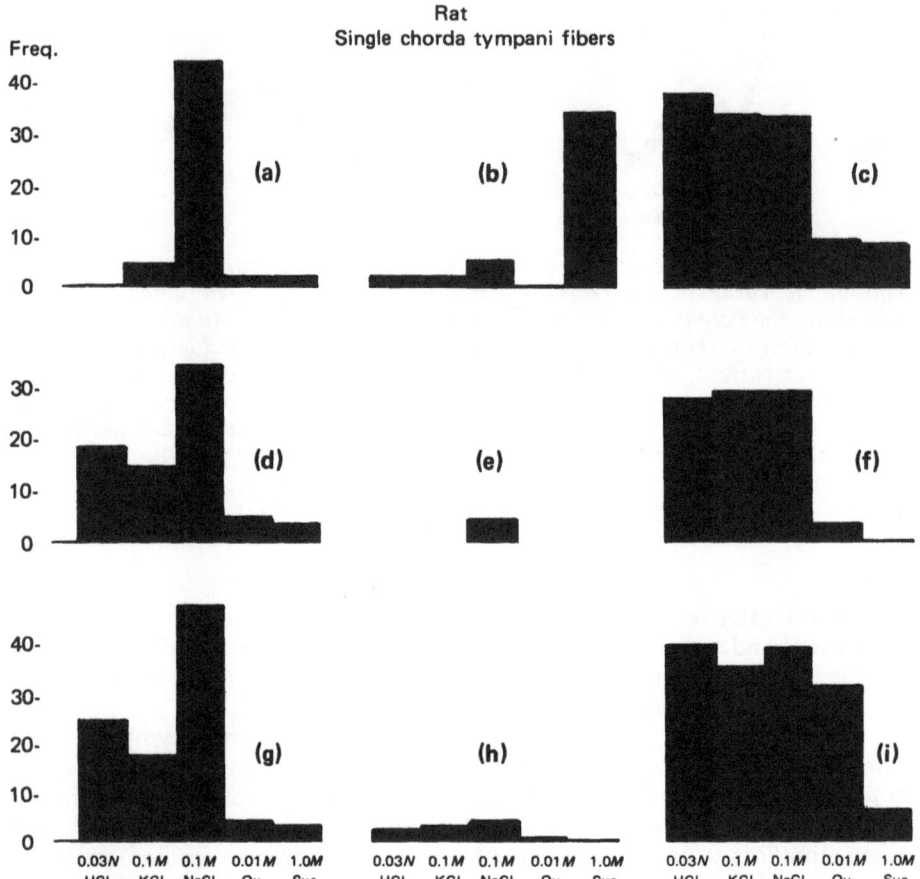

FIGURE 11.8 *A plot of the taste sensitivity histograms of nine chorda tympani responses in the rat to a set of five taste stimuli. Note that all of the cells respond to a greater or lesser degree to all stimuli (adapted from Pfaffmann, 1955).*

tivities to the various stimuli. Ogawa, Sato, and Yamashita (1968) report, however, that a statistical analysis of some similar data displays some correlations between pairs of the chemicals in some animals. Sato, Yamashita, and Ogawa (1969), for example, have found that in the rat there is a correlation between the responsiveness of a cell to quinine and to hydrochloric acid as well as a mutual correlation between these two substances and cooling. This triple association is a type of multimodality that had not been considered by the earlier investigators. Figure 11.9 shows the correlation patterns observed by Sato and his colleagues in both the rat and the hamster, presented in an unusual and interesting graphical manner.

The main import of these data is to suggest that while peripheral fibers seem not to be sensitive to a single chemical as had been postulated

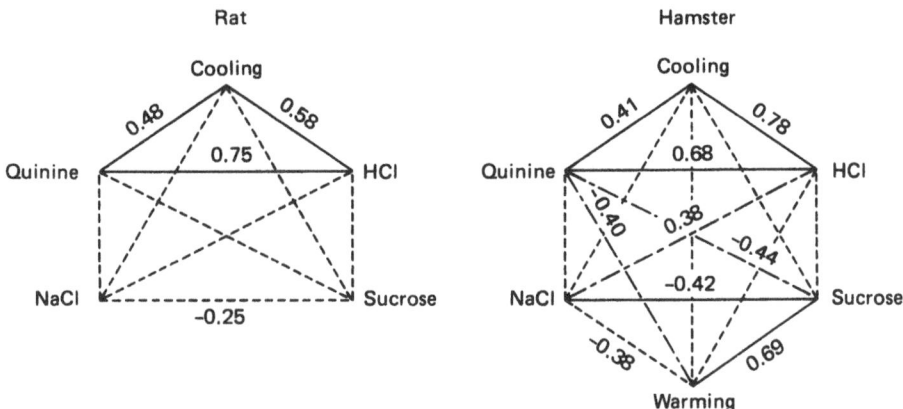

FIGURE 11.9 Correlation stars showing the relation among gustatory responses to four taste stimuli and two thermal stimuli (heating and cooling) for chorda tympani neurons in the rat and hamster, respectively (from Sato, Yamashita, and Ogawa, 1969).

by the classic specificity theories and seemingly substantiated by the psychophysical studies, they do seem to have sensitivities, in at least some animals, that are clustered or correlated. This is a statement of a very weak form of specificity, however, and it still must be concluded that the general picture that emerges from neurophysiological experiments still seems to speak for a relatively nonspecific pattern of gustatory neural action. Figure 11.10 from Sato, Yamashita, and Ogawa (1969) updates Pfaffmann's bar graphs for 28 chorda tympani cells in the hamster. It also indicates the relation among cooling, spontaneous activities, and the chemical sensitivities and is reflective of the sort of data that are the basis of the sort of correlagrams shown in Figure 11.9.

Frank and Pfaffmann (1969) have also studied the responses of the glossopharyngeal nerve to taste stimuli and find the same sort of nonspecificity of response that was observed in the chorda tympani. Cells, which responded to one, two, three, or even four of the basic taste chemicals, were found.

3. *Higher Centers.* An important contribution to the understanding of quality coding in any modality would be to have a single laboratory compare the neurophysiological response pattern at sequentially higher levels of the ascending pathway of a single species. The advantages of such an approach would accrue because of the standardization of stimulation and recording techniques without the "little" technical differences, which so often make the findings from separate laboratories completely incompatible. Fortunately, there is just such a report comparing chorda tympani and medullary responses by Doetsch, Ganchrow, Nelson, and Erickson (1969; see also Doetsch and Erickson, 1970). Their study is all the more remarkable because it probably is the first time that gustatory responses have been recorded

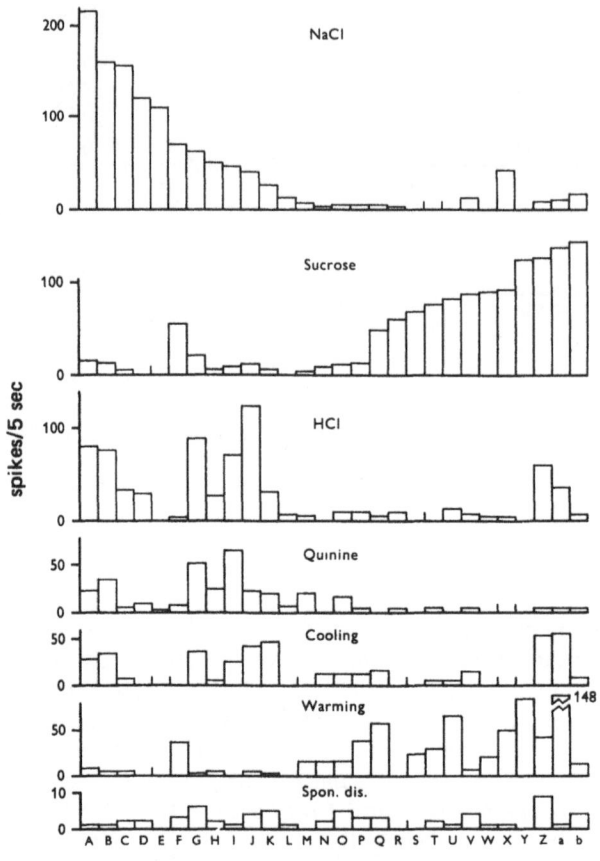

Chorda tympani fibers

FIGURE 11.10 Histogram showing the relative responsiveness of 28 hamster chorda tympani neurons to four taste stimuli and warming and cooling, as well as the spontaneous level of activity. Data like this provide the data base for the correlation stars of Figure 11.9 (from Ogawa, Sato, and Yamashita, 1968).

from the medulla. For a systematic interlevel comparison to be reported in a paper that also introduces a major new technique is a highly unusual, though thoroughly commendable, development.

The responses recorded at the chorda tympani simply confirmed the results we have already described in the previous section. The responses recorded from the medulla with KCl- or NaCl-filled glass micropipettes (which intracellularly detected the responses of single units) showed the same general pattern of nonspecific activity, but with a few notable differences. The general similarity was evidenced in the fact that all medullary cells exhibited the same multiple sensitivities to two or more of the taste stimuli as recorded in the peripheral nerves and, thus, can be said to be also broadly tuned. On the other hand, an unexpected difference between the two levels occurred in the temporal dynamics of the response. Surprisingly, Doetsch and his colleagues found that cells in the medulla fired at a rate five times *greater* than those in the chorda tympani. In some way a frequency multiplication had been produced as the signals crossed a single synaptic step. This finding is in sharp contrast to results from the visual and acoustic system which usually show a reduction in the maximum response frequency of which neurons are capable as one moves the recording electrode more centrally. In addition, another difference was that the initial burst of activity at the onset of a stimulus was relatively reduced at the medullary level, again a finding that differs from other systems in which turn-on transients are emphasized centrally.

Attempts by Doetsch and his colleagues to record responses from the thalamus and the cortex elicited by natural taste stimuli were generally unsuccessful in these experiments, although they were able to drive cortical cells and thalamic cells with electrical stimulation of the taste nerves.

Successful recordings at the level of the thalamus have, however, been reported by Frommer (1961). These thalamic taste areas are located in the general region that also subserves the tactile sensitivities of the tongue. Considering that the chorda tympani and the glossopharyngeal nerves both also convey tactile impulses from the tongue, this is an entirely expected finding. Frommer used insulated nichrome wires which were not sharpened, but simply cut off to produce a relatively large blunt end. These macroelectrodes were driven into the thalami of rats, which were kept under general anesthesia during the course of the experiment. Macroelectrodes of this sort detect the responses of a large number of single cells, which are pooled in the recording and show up in oscillographic records as a family of mixed amplitude spikes. Since these mixed records are so difficult to analyze directly, Frommer used an integrator to produce a running estimate of the total amount of neural activity evoked by the various taste stimuli. Figure 11.11 shows a typical record from an experiment in which a number of different stimuli have been applied to the tongue of the rat. The amplitude and time course of each response are of special interest in this record.

Because the records in Frommer's experiment are integrated measures of a population of cells, it is not possible to answer the question of single cell specificity directly for these thalamic responses. There is indirect evidence, however, that the coding mechanisms for taste stimuli are equally as broadly tuned here at the level of the thalamus as they are at the medullary and peripheral chorda tympani levels. This indirect evidence is that the relative *amplitude* of response to the basic taste stimuli does not seem to vary much between these levels. Frommer has compared his data with some data from these lower centers recorded by Halpern (1959) with a similar integrated output measure. He has summarized his comparison in a chart, which we reproduce here in Table 11.3.

It appears that there has been no successful attempt to record single cell responses from higher levels of the nervous system than the thalamus. The difficulty in defining a cortical area responsive to taste stimuli has been discussed by Oakley and Benjamin (1966). In general, they argue that it is not yet possible to find an area that is selectively sensitive to chemical

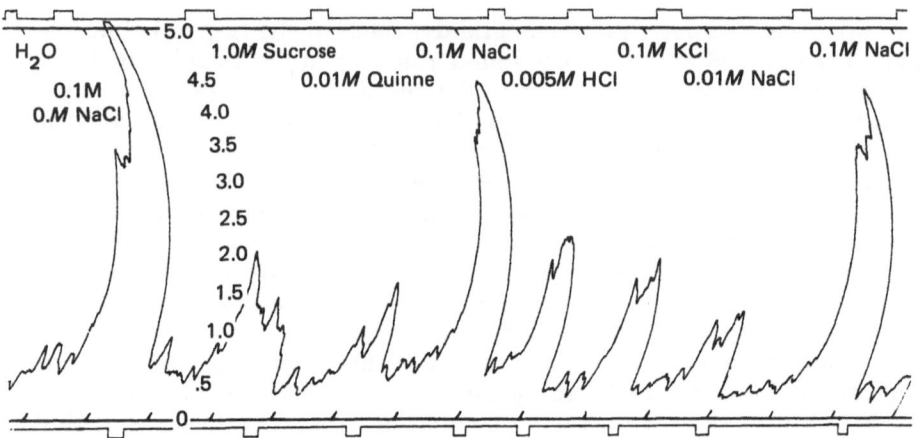

FIGURE 11.11 Output of an integrated recording from a gustatory thalamic relay as a function of a variety of taste stimuli of various concentrations. This chart runs in time from right to left (from Frommer, 1961).

stimuli, much less examine the response repertoires of the constituent neurons.

D. A Contemporary Model

As we have seen, the psychophysical data and the neurophysiological data for the gustatory modality generally do not agree with each other. For one reason or another, whenever a human subject is asked to make qualitative judgments, his responses tend to be classified into four words. These basic sensations—sweet, salty, sour, and bitter—recur throughout the psychophysical data, and stimulation with small electrodes or drops of fluid produces reports that support localized specificity. On the other hand, the neurophysiological data in gustation are perhaps more consistent than in any other sensory modality and yet in complete disagreement with the psychophysical data. Nonspecificity and multiple responsiveness to two or more of the four basic taste stimuli are regularly found at all levels of the ascending gustatory pathway.

The facts of the matter, therefore, are that in spite of the psychophysical evidence, the notion of specific labeled lines as the communication code for gustatory quality cannot be accepted. The restriction is simple enough. Before a neural dimension can possibly be nominated as a candidate code, it must be shown that it, in fact, exists. The subsequent question—are candidate codes true codes or merely electrophysiological signs of the stimulus quality?—can be approached only after the candidate codes are identified. In the case of gustatory coding, however, the basic requirement for candidacy is not met. There is no evidence in the physiological findings that a specific receptor labeled line mechanism is present. Therefore, an explanation of the psychophysical data must be sought elsewhere than in specificity theory.

TABLE 11.3 RESPONSE MAGNITUDE RELATIVE TO THAT PRODUCED
BY A STANDARDIZING 0.1M NaCl STIMULUS RECORDED AT THREE
LEVELS OF THE ASCENDING GUSTATORY PATHWAY (FROM
FROMMER, 1961, COMPILED FROM HIS OWN DATA AND
THAT OF HALPERN, 1959)

Chemical Stimulus	Relative Response Magnitude		
	Thalamus	Medulla	Chorda Tympani
0.1M NaCl	100	100	100
0.1M KCl	39.8	27.0	36.5
0.005M HCl	52.0	35.5	53.5
0.01M quinine HCl. . . .	21.8	22.8	15.5
1.0M sucrose.	33.8	30.0	44.0

The conclusion to which we are inevitably driven in this situation is
that gustatory quality coding is mediated by relative amounts of activity
generated in an associated group of broadly tuned neurons by receptors
that are equally broadly tuned. Broad tuning, in this case, means multiple
responsiveness to two or more of the basic taste stimuli. Certainly, we must
accept the fact that there are local differences on the tongue regarding
maximum sensitivities, but even these differences are spatially "broadly
tuned" with no unique localization at any locus.

The neurophysiological data, therefore, support a pattern theory of
gustatory quality of very much the same sort that we have already described for the somatosensory, auditory, and visual modalities. A quality is
apparently defined by the ratio of activity in a population of communication neurons. Workers in the field of gustation have coined a special term
for their data—"across-neuron patterning"; but this term refers to essentially the same idea expressed by the term "pattern theory." The key idea is
expressed by Pfaffmann's statement:

> . . . the same afferent fiber can convey different information depend-
> ing upon the amount of activity in another parallel fiber.
> (PFAFFMANN, 1959, p. 228.)

Thus, if two fibers are both sensitive to, say, NaCl and quinine, but one
responds more to quinine than to NaCl and the other responds more to
NaCl than to quinine, definitive information specifying saltiness and bitterness is conveyed by the relative rate of firing of the two fibers. Of course,
the situation is not this simple in the ebb and flow of all the solutions that
roll across the receptors of the tongue. In any real situation, there are not
just two fibers involved but many thousands. The principle, however, is just
the same—quality is defined by the relative amount of activity in a large
number of gustatory fibers.

III. OLFACTION
In any discussion of olfactory quality coding, there are also usually only two main issues of controversy. The first deals with the nature of the primary sensory action—the transductive mechanism—to which we have already directed major attention in Chapter 4. In the present section, we shall concern ourselves exclusively with the second issue—that of specificity versus broad tuning at the various levels of neural transmission. This question also often finds itself expressed in terms of whether or not there is a small family of fundamental or basic smells.

A. The Key Psychophysical Data
The basic psychophysical facts of olfactory quality coding are that the nose can detect the difference between a very large number of stimuli and that the human observer has a very large repertoire of verbal responses to describe this variety of experiences. Over the years, many different systems of odor names have been developed. We have already discussed one of them, Amoore's seven basic smells, in Chapter 4. But there is a sense of arbitrariness about this scheme, which even Amoore (1969) himself has recently come to acknowledge. In addition to the more or less classic classification systems, Amoore has added to this table a new list of 27 smell names, which have been distilled from a search for specific anosmias. An anosmia is a smell "blindness" and, curiously, smell blindness seems to be relatively specific. The characteristics of the usual anosmia is such that the observer is smell-blind to only a very specific chemical or group of chemicals. All other olfactory sensitivities appear to be relatively unaffected. Amoore ingeniously hit upon the idea of simply placing advertisements in various journals asking for communications from anyone who was unable to smell something his friends and associates could. From the many responses he received with this imaginative research technique, Amoore was able to sort out what he believed to be 27 specific anosmias—all others were related by virtue of the chemical similarities of the substances described by his correspondents. This new smell name schema and the older more classic systems have been summarized by Amoore and are reproduced in Table 11.4. Clearly, the historical trend has been toward more and more "basic" smells, and it is probably the case that this reflects a more realistic picture of the underlying biology than does the simple quadrichotomy of the basic taste experience or the sevenfold classification of the older smell theories. Unfortunately, the richness of the vocabulary in the olfactory domain does not reduce the complexities of the semantic problem to any significant degree. It is quite possible that even this enlarged response repertoire is not completely able to cope with the true range of discriminable sensations.

Modern psychophysical studies of olfactory quality, which are not actually studies along the intensive dimensions, are, as in gustation, few and far between. Perhaps one of the most interesting is a study reported by Amoore (1970) in his new book entitled *The Molecular Basis of Odor*. The general procedure called for subjects to rate the similarity between an unknown chemical and the seven standard chemical substances of the early Amoore theory (see our Chapter 4). The subject was given a rating scale for each of the seven basic substances. If a substance smelled completely dissimilar to one of the substances, it was to be rated 0; if extremely similar, it was to be rated 8. A set of rating scales used in this way gives a sevenfold numerical code defining the olfactory quality of an unknown, which hopefully could approximate the relative contribution of the seven basic smells to the sensation indicated by the unknown chemical. When the seven basic smell stimuli themselves were given as unknowns, the general result should be to produce a table in which all the entries along the diagonal are quite high and all others quite low. As we can see from Table 11.5, this is, in fact, what happens.

In addition to providing a validation measure, this sort of data also allows us to provide some sort of a similarity ordering of the seven basic smells on the basis of adjacent values of the rating scale. A seven-number characteristic, analogous to a power spectrum analysis of an acoustic stimulus can, in this manner, be attached to each and every unknown smell. The approach is complicated by the fact that the seven basic smells may not, in fact, be the true fundamentals and certainly do not represent points along a continuous single dimension. Rather, each basic smell is a discrete point on a multidimensional continuum of shape, size, and electrovalence. Nevertheless, there is considerable advantage to future studies in simply having a characteristic numerical descriptor, no matter how biased it may be, over the bare statement that a given chemical may smell a little fruity and a little pungent.

A similar technique of similarity judgments had been used by Wright and Michels (1964) to evaluate the similarity of a large group of organic odorants. Their work was originally carried out to evaluate the applicability of an infrared theory of olfactory primary sensory action, but generally showed no support for this thermal absorption hypothesis. However, their data have been analyzed by Døving (1970) in a most interesting way, which is helpful in arriving at an understanding of the reasons so many different smell-naming schemes might have evolved. Døving applied a hierarchal clustering technique, originally developed by Johnson (1967), to describe the Wright and Michels data. The results of this hierarchal clustering procedure are best depicted in a tree such as that shown in Figure 11.12. This figure is not only interesting in terms of the associations that are shown among the various chemicals, but because it also suggests that variable decision criteria may be the main reason that 3, 4, 7, or even 27 different basic smells are variously suggested by olfactory theorists. For example, if the decision for the establishment of odor classes was relatively loose, as indicated by the semicircular arc (a) drawn near the base of the tree in Figure 11.12, then only a very few basic smells would be suggested. Another class would be indicated wherever the arc cut a branch of the tree. However, if the criteria for clustering are very strict, as represented by the semicircular arcs (b) and (c) drawn near the tips of the branches of the tree, then the classification scheme would assume many discriminably different subgroups, as the arc in this case would cut many more branches. All of this is to say that whether one has many or a few basic smells (or, for that matter, basic tastes or basic touches) may depend more upon the decision criteria and the available vocabulary than upon the biology of the situation. In such a situation, consensual agreement would be very difficult to obtain.

TABLE 11.4 A TABLE COMPARING THE WIDE VARIETY OF CLASSICAL ODOR SYSTEMS WITH THOSE "BASIC SMELLS" OBTAINED IN A STUDY OF SPECIFIC ANOSMIAS (FROM AMOORE, 1969)

Line No.		Zwaardemaker 1895 30 (sub) Classes	Linnaeus 1756 7 Classes	Henning 1915 6 Classes	Crocker & Henderson 1927 4 Classes	Amoore 1952 7 Classes	Schutz 1964 9 Classes	Wright & Michels 1964 8 Classes
					General Odor Classifications			
1		Fruity						Hexyl-acetate
2		Waxy						
3		Ethereal				Ethereal	Etherish	
4		Camphor				Camphor		
5		Clove	Aromatic					
6		Cinnamon		Spicy				Spice
7		Aniseed						Benzo-thiazole
8		Minty				Minty		
9		Thyme						
10		Rosy						
11		Citrous		Fruity				Citral
12		Almond					Spicy	
13		Jasmine		Flowery		Floral		
14		Orange-blossom	Fragrant		Fragrant		Fragrant	
15		Lily						
16		Violet						
17		Vanilla					Sweet	
18		Amber						
19		Musky	Ambrosial			Musky		
20		Leek	Alliaceous					
21		Fishy						
22		Bromine						
23		Burnt		Burnt	Burnt		Burnt	Affective
24		Phenolic						
25	*	Caproic	Hircine		Caprylic			
26	–	Cat-urine						
27		Narcotic	Repulsive					
28		Bed-Bug						
29		Carrion	Nauseous					
30		Fecal						
31				Resinous				Resinous
32				Foul		Putrid	Sulfurous	Unpleasant
33					Acid			
34							Oily	
35	–						Rancid	
36							Metallic	
37								
38								
39								
40								
41								
42								
43								
44								
45								
46								
47								
48								
49								
50								
(Nonolfactory)						(Pungent)		(Trigeminal)

General Odor Classifications		Specific Anosmia Analyses			
Harper et al. 1968 44 Classes	Miscellaneous Additional	Reputed Specific Anosmias			
		27 Classes	Related Anosmias		
Fruity		λ-Undeca-Lactone			
Soapy					
Etherish; solvent		Ethylene-dichloride	Trichloro-ethylene	Benzene	Methyl cyclo-propyl ketone
Camphor; mothballs		1.8-Cineole	Naphthalene	p-Dichloro-benzene	Adamantane
Aromatic		Eugenol	Bonzyl alcohol	Anisole	
Spicy		Cinnam-aldehyde	Salicyl-aldehyde		
Minty		Menthone	Menthol	Tert-butyl carbinol	
		Thymol			
		Geraniol	Phenyl-ethanol		
Citrous		Geranial			
Almond		Hydrogen cyanide	Isobutyr-aldehyde		
Floral		Peme carbinol			
Fragrant					
		Ionone	Farnesol		
Vanilla; sweet		Vanillin	Benzyl salicylate	Anisic aldehyde	Cyclotene
Animal					
Musk		Macrocyclic musks (4)	Androstenol	Musk xylol	Versalide
Garlic		Allyl iso-thiocyanate	Phenyl iso-thiocyanate	Allicin	Propenyl-sulfenic acid
Ammonia; fishy		Hexylamine			
		Iodoform			
Burnt					
Carbolic					
Sweaty		Isobutyric acid	Phenylacetic acid	Caproic acid	
		Phenyl-isoyanide			
Sickly		Putrescine			
Fecal		Skatole	Indole		
Resionus; Paint					
Putrid-Sulfurous		Mercaptans (3)	Dimethyl disulfide	Thiophane	
Acid		Formic acid	Acetic acid		
Oily					
Rancid					
Metallic					
Meaty					
Moldy		2-Heptanone			
Grassy					
Bloody					
Cooked-vegetable		Methional			
	Sandal	Cedryl acetate			
	Watery				
	Urinous	Androsta-dienone			
(Pungent; & 5 others)					

TABLE 11.5 A RELATIONAL ANALYSIS OF THE SEVEN BASIC SMELL SUBSTANCES. HIGH SCORES INDICATE SIMILARITY AND LOW SCORES DISSIMILARITY (FROM AMOORE AND VENSTROM, 1966)

Odor	Eth.	Cam.	Mus.	Flo.	Min.	Pun.	Put.
Ethereal	6.3	1.2	0.6	1.1	1.1	0.4	0.1
Camphoraceous	1.0	6.2	1.2	1.3	2.1	0.2	0.1
Musky	0.5	0.5	5.9	1.9	1.2	0.3	0.0
Floral	0.7	1.3	1.8	6.3	1.7	0.1	0.0
Minty	0.6	1.7	0.6	2.4	6.7	0.2	0.0
Pungent	0.6	0.3	0.5	0.6	0.4	7.1	0.7
Putrid	0.3	0.2	0.3	0.1	0.1	1.5	7.0

B. The Competitive Theories

We have already described in Chapter 4 the various theories of olfactory transduction. These theories make up the major portion of theoretical controversy in this sensory field. Of the theories that are specifically concerned with the transmission code, there are only a few that are sufficiently rigorous in their development to merit discussion. The general attitude that seems to prevail among most workers in this field is that olfactory quality coding is mediated by patterned neural action similar to the "across-neuron" patterning we have already described for the gustatory system. The relative amounts of activity among a widely diverse system of receptors represent the critical information for the coding of quality from this point of view. O'Connell and Mozell (1969) phrase it this way in their recent statement of olfactory pattern theory:

> It is apparent that the absolute amount of activity in any receptor cannot by itself encode quality. . . . However, a coding system in which several cells have different response functions for the same odorant can encode quality independent of quantity.
>
> (O'CONNELL and MOZELL, 1969, pp. 60–61.)

As we shall see, most electrophysiological evidence supports this general notion. A somewhat different statement of a pattern theory has been presented by Hughes and Hendrix (1967). These investigators examined the specific frequency pattern of a compound bioelectric potential (similar to an EEG) recorded with stainless steel macroelectrodes from the olfactory bulb of a rabbit. Their recordings of the continuous fluctuating signals evoked with odorants were then power spectrum analyzed. Hughes and Hendrix discovered that there was a variation in the relative amplitude of various components of the frequency analyzed signals, depending upon the substance used as a stimulus. Generally, the higher the molecular weight of the odorant, the lower was the dominant frequency. Hughes and Hendrix have formalized this finding into a theory, which they refer to as the "frequency component hypothesis." In any evaluation of their theory, it must

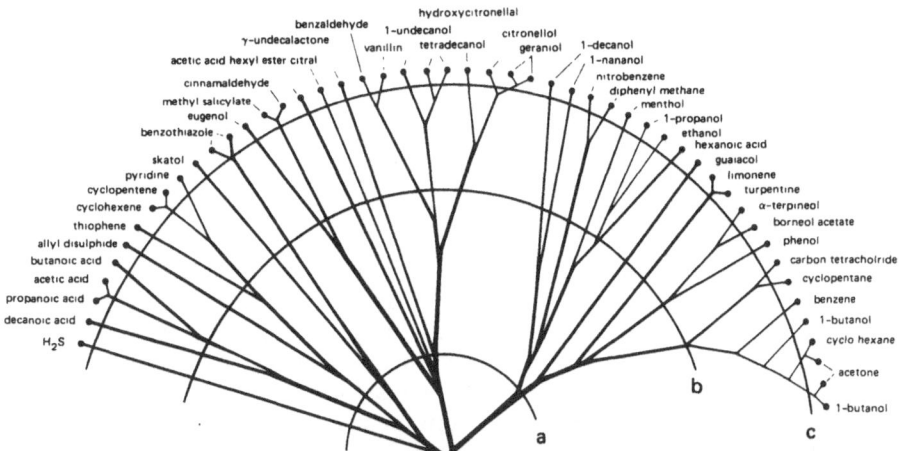

FIGURE 11.12 *An explanation of how decision criteria can affect the number of basic taste substances. If the tree shown in the figure (which is produced by a clustering technique) is divided at (a), representing relatively loose decision criteria for taste similarity judgments—smaller differences are ignored—then it is obvious that there are only seven "basic" smell stimulus classes. If however, the slice is made at (b), representing a more strict decision criteria for one's judgment of similarity, then there are, equally obviously, 26 "basic" smell stimuli. If the cut is made at (c), representing a very severe criterion before similarity is accepted, then there are equally obviously 39 "basic" smell stimuli (adapted from Døving, 1970, after data of Wright and Michels, 1964).*

be remembered that the signals they are recording are superimpositions of a very large number of individual cellular potentials. Since it is not known exactly what the relationship between these compound potentials and single cell potentials is, it is somewhat difficult to evaluate their significance in terms of a single cell oriented coding theory. In any event, it does not appear to differ from any other pattern theory of olfactory quality in its fundamental premises.

C. The Neurophysiological Data and a Contemporary Model

What are the neurophysiological findings that have provided such a consensus among olfactory theorists, all of whom seem clearly to be pattern theorists of one sort or another? If we recall that the anatomy of the olfactory system is very poorly understood beyond the olfactory bulb, it is obvious why the findings we shall now concern ourselves with are going to be limited in the number of levels that can be considered. Since we have already discussed differential effects on the generator potential, the reports we shall emphasize in this section will be limited almost exclusively to first-order responses in the nerve fibers of the filia olfactoria and to the responses of the second-order fibers in the olfactory bulb. Beyond that point, very little is known about the ultimate destinations of these second-order fibers or what sort of third-order fibers might be involved in central decoding.

However little is known of the anatomy, even less is known of the electro-physiology of these more central regions—not a single report could be found that discussed the neural responses of the olfactory system beyond the bulb.

First, let us consider the findings from the first-order fibers, which run from the olfactory receptors up through the cribiform bone into the olfactory bulb. Probably the most important of the few papers that have appeared describing results at this level is that of Gesteland, Lettvin, and Pitts (1965), who recorded from the primary neurons of the frog's olfactory system. These investigators found that the frog's olfactory neurons had a relatively lively amount of spontaneous activity and that the different chemicals used as stimulants in their experiments might either depress this activity or enhance it. Two chemicals that both produced an increase in activity in a single fiber in one location might both depress another fiber; or even, in a third fiber, one might enhance the spontaneous activity, while the other depressed it. In general, they were able to find no evidence of any highly selective specificity in any of their preparations.

O'Connell and Mozell (1969) have also studied neural responses in the filia olfactoria with a more highly purified set of odorants and report the same sort of nonspecificity observed by Gesteland and his colleagues. They do, however, note that the inhibitory action of some odorants was much less frequent and appeared in only one cell in their sample. This cell happened to have a very high rate of spontaneous activity, interestingly enough.

An argument against any highly specific receptor sites on the olfactory receptor cells has been made by Beidler (1965). He has recorded the action potentials from twigs of the trigeminal nerve. This nerve originates, in part, as free nerve endings in the olfactory epithelium. These free nerve endings have no specialized receptor structures, yet there is still the same sort of more or less generalized responsiveness to a large number of odorous stimuli that one finds in the neurons originating at the bases of the olfactory receptor cells. But there is also sufficient differentiation among the responses produced by the various stimuli to illustrate the same sort of quasi-specificity observed in the neurons of the filia olfactoria or of the second-order units of the olfactory bulb. The main impact of these data is that there is little reason to argue for highly specific receptor sites on the microvilli of the specialized olfactory receptor cells, if, indeed, the trigeminal nerve fibers show the same sort of response pattern without any specialized terminal structure other than free nerve endings.

Let us now consider second-order responses recorded from the olfactory bulb. Adrian (1953) was the first to report the existence of olfactory bulb cells that he believed were "tuned" to some specific odorant. On this basis, he suggested some sort of specificity among the second-order neurons of the olfactory system. Over the years, however, Adrian had been the principal remaining champion of olfactory specificity. In recent years, he has further suggested that there are regional differences in specificity to be found as one explores various areas of the olfactory mucosa (Adrian, 1956). Unfortunately, most modern work seems to support a less specific sort of coding.

One of the more important and novel recent single cell recording techniques has been developed by Moulton (1963), who used chronically implanted olfactory bulb electrodes and found that some chemicals tended to activate specific regions of the olfactory bud preferentially. A few years later (Moulton, 1967), he concluded that there was no electrophysiological evidence for differential coding in single cells other than perhaps a slightly lower threshold to some groups of chemicals in one or another cell. Moulton has, thus, also supported the notion that the key quality code is a spatiotemporal pattern of activity across the volume of the olfactory bulb.

Moulton (1965) believes that the following list includes the most likely possible codes for olfactory quality:

1. Broad regional differences in overall activity.
2. High sensitivity of a few individual sites.
3. Suppression of activity at a few individual sites.
4. Latency and rise and decay times.

All of these, it should be noted, are volume and compound neural codes rather than specific single cell mechanisms. It is probably most fair to say that the data are not yet conclusive. There appears to be some suggestion of some sort of spatial localization at both the mucosal and bulbar levels, but the technical difficulties in recording from the various levels of the olfactory system have made it impossible to give a firm foundation to any of the speculative ideas so far introduced. The main conclusion we can draw from experiments at the level of both the primary and secondary olfactory neurons is that here, too, there is no evidence of sharp specificity. At best, one could assume that there is a sort of relative specificity and that the key factor in quality coding is like all other quality dimensions—the relative amount of activity among a large number of neural units.

IV. AN INTERIM SUMMARY

As we look back over the material we have discussed in these last three chapters, it is clear that there are a number of important generalizations forced on us by the data. By far the most important is the conclusion that there is no finding from any sense modality that provides support for a highly specific, labeled line sort of quality coding mechanism. Almost all of the receptors sampled in the many experiments exhibit a sensitivity to a variety of effective physical stimuli. In the visual system, the half bandwidth of the cone spectral sensitivities are about 50 nm wide. In the peripheral portions of the auditory system, a high-frequency stimulus activates much of the basilar membrane. Individual chemoreceptors are affected quite generally by many different taste or odor-invoking chemicals, and even the individual and anatomically idiosyncratic mechanoreceptors of the skin often seem to be activated by many different forms of mechanical and thermal stimuli. Sharp specificity, when it does occur, is notable mostly because of its rarity.

Coupled with this broadly tuned operation of these neurons and receptors, however, is usually some sort of a peak sensitivity. Some chromatic stimuli, some acoustic stimuli, and some chemicals are capable of activating a given receptor more easily than other similar forms of stimulus energy. It must be emphasized that this peak in the sensitivity function is not equivalent to a highly specific response function. Most stimuli are dealt with in real life at suprathreshold levels, and, therefore, it seems relatively fair to say that many different stimuli are usually simultaneously activating a given receptor.

More than a century ago, a number of workers formalized the notion that whatever the nature of the stimulus, the excitation of a given sensory nerve could only give rise to a single form of experience. The formal statement has come down to us as *Müller's law of specific nerve energies*. Müller's law was originally stated as a law of macromodalities and of whole nerves. But a common extrapolation of the law of specific nerve energies holds that the excitation of a single nerve fiber would also give rise to a specific sensory microquality—a microquality being defined as a qualitatively discriminable experience within one of the major modalities. Red, for example, is a microquality of vision. This concept is intimately tied up with the idea of very specific receptors in both vision and somesthesis. When stimulated with stimuli different from the energy to which they were most sensitive, specific receptors, it was thought, would respond less strongly. However, it was thought that the excitation could only result in an experience indistinguishable from a lower intensity stimulus of the kind to which the receptor was most sensitive.

In recent years, there has been a gradual accumulation of evidence that suggests that while Müller and his contemporaries certainly were right in their formulation of the law of specific nerve energies in the context of the major modalities, the representation of the specific subqualities (or micromodalities) does not, in fact, follow this law. This point has been made specifically for the somatosensory system by Melzack and Wall (1962), but it seems to hold true as a general principle for all the senses. Erickson (1968) and Uttal (1969a) have both drawn attention to the general breakdown in Müller's law when it is applied to single fibers in all of the senses.

In other words, a single receptor cell cannot encode sufficient information to completely define a sensory quality. Rather, in each case it is necessary to postulate some sort of *comparative* process, which takes into account the *relative* characteristics of the activity from two or more different cells to define a microquality. Perkel and Bullock (1968) have recently pointed out that the *relative* phasing of the nerve action potential temporal sequence in two separate neurons may also be important. Relative activity need not be limited to comparisons in mean frequency or response amplitude alone.

If, therefore, comparisons are critical and we acknowledge the general fact that most receptors are broadly tuned to stimuli, then we must look at the law of specific energies of nerves in a somewhat different way than we have in the past. While we can appreciate that we shall never "hear" a light, it seems difficult to postulate absolute labeled line neural codes that can account for a specific sensory quality, without some basis for a *comparative* evaluation of the activities of several different neurons.

Thus, the specific-energies-of-nerves hypothesis does not appear to hold for any microquality or at the single cell level of discourse. Broadly tuned receptors do not permit such a mechanism, and there is increasingly ample evidence that relative amounts of activity in different neurons, or differences in time of arrival of two different signals, both of which are temporal comparisons of the activity in two different places, are available as neural codes.

The practical implications of such a change in our thinking are quite profound. At the very least (and even this minimal impact might be devastating to modern neurophysiology), we might be forewarned by Erickson's (1968) comment:

> If the Bell-Magendie-Mueller doctrine does not hold at the single neu-ron level, descriptions of the responsiveness of individual neurons will not show how the nervous system encodes stimuli.
>
> (ERICKSON, 1968, p. 456.)

Erickson has also considered many of the issues that we have discussed here. He distinguishes between narrowly tuned topographic representing neurons and broadly tuned nontopographic neurons in a way that differs from our general view that all receptor neurons are broadly tuned, but his paper is a lucid and important alternative discussion of these same important issues.

Coupled with the breakdown in the Müllerian law of specific nerve energies is the fact that there is a surprising lack of correspondence between many of the psychophysical data for sensory quality and the neurophysiological findings. Where specificity and precision of discrimination are terms that dominate any discussion of the perceptual domain, overlapping, broadly tuned, nonspecific patterns of neural response seem to be words that are more descriptive of the neurophysiological findings.

There are some major philosophical and technical issues that have to be considered with care concerning this lack of correspondence. We must first ask if it is really necessary that the psychophysical and neurophysiological data show isomorphism. Sharp psychophysical discrimination, from one point of view, need not be represented by equally sharp nonoverlapping bands of neural activity. It is entirely possible that some sort of statistical process could be acting, in which a "degree of confidence" of the difference between two different but overlapping distributions could mimic sharp discriminative abilities. The search for central neural mechanisms that "sharpen" the peripheral signal may, therefore, be somewhat futile from this point of view, and in general such sharpening does not seem to occur. Coding theory is perfectly flexible with regard to this issue, it should be noted, for broadly tuned overlapping distributions are acceptable coding mechanisms, even for highly discriminable phenomena at the molar level.

CHAPTER 12: EPILOGUE—EMERGING PRINCIPLES OF SENSORY CODING

And so we have completed our survey and discussion of the coding mechanisms, processes, and symbols that are of relevance to sensory theory. It certainly must have seemed to some readers that the parade of interesting experimental findings was never to end, in spite of the limited selection presented here. In fact, the list of experiments probably is never-ending in some practical sense, for as the author of any book such as this can certify, more or less relevant new papers are published at a rate with which no reviewer can keep pace.

As one surveys even the limited number of studies we have considered, there is a certain tendency to ignore a key fact, which we mentioned briefly at the outset—namely, that no single experiment is really of critical importance. Rather, it is the general perspective or global understanding gained from such a survey that is of historic consequence. Many different individual studies can make equivalent contributions to our theoretical models of the relationship between the mental and the physiological aspects of our world. The absence of any single study would hardly be noticed, so many others could serve the same role.

The purpose of this final chapter—the epilogue—is to sum up this book and to emphasize, by restatement, the general principles that transcend the individual findings. These are the conclusions and generalizations which, it is hoped, the reader will take away with him even though few should or could remember all of the details of each of the individual experiments. This summary material is in the form of a list of ideas, concepts, conclusions, and general principles and is presented quite dogmatically. Hopefully, sufficient argument and evidence have already been presented so that any further supporting discussion is unnecessary. In some instances, the items on the list represent facts which enjoy the consensual agreement of the psychobiological community. In other instances, they represent one side of what obviously is a vigorously debated controversy. In some cases, they represent the essence of some modern theory of general acceptance; in other cases, admittedly, they represent nothing more than the author's bias and personal perspective of what is necessary as a unifying premise. Through the entire list, however, it is hoped that there is a coherent and internally consistent perspective clearly apparent to the reader.

1. Neural activity is the sole basis and only significant concomitant of mental activity. Though the specific links between mind and brain may not yet have been found, this axiom must be basic to all of the conclusions and summations that follow. This premise is a modern statement of the classic monistic philosophy, which evolved from more primitive dualisms and asserts that mental activities are nothing more (nor less) than one function of the material nervous system.

2. With a very few exceptions, all physiological data are accepted as being accurate and true representations of the processes of the nervous system. Some data are biased by sampling errors; some may be misleading in terms of how they are interpreted; but there are very few studies that are demonstrably incorrect in terms of the quantitative aspects of the data.

3. Similarly, few psychophysical studies are incorrect in any factual sense. While some experiments in this domain may actually measure something other than they purport to, gross errors of fact are just as rare in psychophysics as in neurophysiology. It is particularly distressing, however, to have different psychophysical techniques give qualitatively different results even when both purport to be measuring identical biological phenomena. One or the other must be assumed to be misleading in such a case and preference should be given to the one suggesting finer discrimination.

4. The theoretical links that have been made between some neurophysiological and some behavioral findings, however, are not as definitive as some would suggest. We must never forget that when neurophysiological *data* are used to explain psychophysical *findings,* such data then become physiological *theories;* a point made most eloquently by Charles Harris.

5. The interpretations or theories we construct are based not only on the results we obtain from experiments, but also on the perspectives we currently hold. Similarly, the instrumental technology we use exerts a strong constraining influence on what results we obtain.

6. There is, at present, still no good general model of the relationship between neurophysiological data and mental phenomena, but the area of psychobiology that is most promising is the sensory one in which we compare afferent neural signal patterns and perceptual experience. This is so

because of the relative simplicity of the sensory pathways and the unique anchor that is provided by a sharply defined set of physical stimulus parameters.

7. There is a need for and the possibility of a general theory of sensory coding. Coding schema from each of the senses must be extracted and then synthesized into a common description of the neural representations of equivalent perceptual dimensions.

8. The essence of the sensory psychobiological problem is a comparison between the common dimensions of the perceptual experience and the dimension of the suggested or candidate neurophysiological responses. Comparisons of the relationship between the stimulus dimensions and the neural response (the domain of neurophysiology), on the one hand, and the stimulus dimensions and the perceptual responses (the domain of psychology), on the other, while interesting in their own right, do not speak directly to the psychobiological problem. Sensory psychobiology, as such, is the most researchable modern statement of the classic mind-brain problem.

9. A whole new set of logical and conceptual complexities is encountered when one attempts to solve the psychobiological problems that are not present in either the neurophysiological or the perceptual domains.

10. The sensory-coding aspect of the general psychobiological problem is multidimensional. Often it has been mistakenly asserted that the relationship between neural signal frequency and perceptual magnitude is *the* coding problem. In fact, we also have to consider the full range of spatial, temporal, and qualitative dimensions of the perceptual response, as well as the large number of candidate neural codes. An $\{m\} \times \{n\}$ correlation matrix must be completed for each level of the ascending pathway where $\{m\}$ is the set of common sensory dimensions and $\{n\}$ is the set of candidate neural codes.

11. In general, there is no *a priori* requirement for isomorphism between the dimensions of the neural signal and the perceptual response, or between different levels of the afferent pathway. Perceptual amplitude functions represented by spatial or temporal neural codes may easily be imagined. Spatial codes are often converted into temporal codes and vice versa. Furthermore, there is no need to assume that linear (or nonlinear) perceptual functions are represented by linear (or nonlinear) neural codes. All that is required is some sort of transformation relationship to allow any neural dimension of any form to represent any perceptual dimension of any other form.

12. Because the psychophysical experiment deals with the organism as a black box and examines only the input and output, little can come from psychophysical experiments, that can bear specifically on the problem of internal neural coding mechanisms. Two overtly similar perceptual processes may be represented by internal codes that are analogous in function, but different in their mechanisms and mode of operations. In only a few special cases does the molar behavior directly reflect the properties of internal single cells or cell classes.

13. The basic importance of the notion that different codes may operate at different levels of the ascending pathways cannot be over-

emphasized. Even within a single neuron, there may be several different manners in which the stimulus information pattern is represented. Within the entire ascending pathway of any sense, there are many. But none of these represents any more fundamental encoding of stimulus information than any other. They are all as equivalent as the representations of a concept in different languages by a line of human translators. History and technology have frequently led to the emphasis of one or another coding scheme, but this is an artifact of our strategies and perspectives and not a property of the biology of the sensory systems.

14. The great hope of a parsimonious theory of sensory coding capable of unifying the diverse theories proposed for each of the senses depends on the fact that identical codes may be used in the various senses at equivalent levels. If this turns out not to be the case, then the coding problem fractionates into a collection of individual tasks with little commonality. In fact, a comparison of the various dimensions for the various senses indicates that there are great commonalities. These commonalities are not always direct. It is sometimes difficult to establish exactly what are equivalent levels among senses, but once having done so, simplifying generalities often appear in great numbers.

15. There is a logical necessity for dealing with the physical stimulus as the initial reference and anchor point for all subsequent discussions. But it must be repeated that our dependence on the stimulus as a reference must not be allowed to confuse the true issue of psychobiology—namely, that the percept and the neurophysiological response bear a relation to each other in a way in which the stimulus is only indirectly involved. This view is a modern version of the classic dual aspect theory, one monistic philosophy proposed to explain the relationship between mind and body.

16. Transduction—the process of converting the physical energy of an external stimulus into a neurochemical event—is a multistage process. First, there is usually some nonneural modification acting on the physical stimulus that must be adequately considered to fully understand the transduction process. Second, for each sense organ there is some specific primary sensory action that must be identified. The primary sensory action is the final physical step prior to and responsible for the neurochemical energy release. Modern theory now states that the neurochemical transduction process itself must usually be defined in terms of some change in the properties of a receptor cell membrane in such a way that a graded nonpropagating intermediary signal is produced. This intermediary graded potential is known as a generator potential if the receptor cell has its own axon and if a propagated spike action potential is produced in that axon as a result of the presence of the generator potential. Otherwise, for those cells that do not have their own axons, it is known as a receptor potential. Receptor potentials lead to spikes in second-order neurons, but through the mediation of transynaptic activity, which is actually their main direct consequent. In some instances, we know a great deal about the primary sensory action but little about the actual production of the receptor potential (for example, in vision), while in other cases, our knowledge and lack of knowledge are reversed.

17. Most receptor cells display some sort of ciliated or elongated structure, which may be interpreted as the adaptive end product of evolutionary forces, which tend to increase receptor area without increasing volume and to extend the receptor membrane into regions in which they are likely to encounter the various physical stimuli.

18. Recent electronmicrographic and electrophysiological evidence has suggested that many receptors can be modulated in their sensitivity by efferent signals from the central nervous system. Specific postsynaptic sites have been observed on many receptor cells.

19. The afferent pathways of the various sense modalities are made up of only three or four neuronal links from the receptor to the most central portions of the nervous system. At the level of the cortex, though, extravagantly intricate interconnections occur. It is at this level that most of the really interesting information processing probably takes place. Unfortunately, we know virtually nothing about interactions at that central level and are just beginning to understand the full implications of spatial and temporal interactions at the more peripheral levels.

20. While the electrochemical properties of neurons are of considerable interest and help in understanding the underlying mechanisms of neuronal action, it should be remembered that the coding and information-processing properties of the nervous system are in a certain sense "technology independent." We might not be very much different animals if the same information processes were implemented with a totally different technology than the sodium-potassium-chlorine nerve membrane model, which is most widely accepted now.

21. The term *action potential* refers to a family of responses in which the electropotential of the membrane deviates from some resting level. The term no longer should be considered to include only the propagated regenerative spike action potential. Such a narrow definition ignores and downgrades the very important information-processing properties of graduated and nonpropagating signals. The spike is a highly useful and specialized action potential, but is only one of many different and equally important neural information codes. Many theories of coding pay far too much attention to the spike or give it some special meaning in the coding schema that cannot be justified in light of the multileveled schema now proposed.

22. The generally accepted explanation of nervous action potentials assumes a semipermeable neuronal plasma membrane. The exact structure of this proteinaceous and lipoidal structure is debated, but it is assumed that variations in the permeability of the membrane to sodium and potassium, in particular, are the key factors in all nervous action. This is known as the "membrane theory."

23. Though the emphasis in this book has been on the transmission of information patterns from the periphery to the central nervous system, we must also remember that these afferent signals can be modulated by efferent (centrifugal) signals in many ways. The introduction of this kind of feedback into the system extremely complicates any systems analysis, but cannot be ignored.

24. Information in the stimulus pattern is generally degraded as it passes up the afferent pathways. This is not to say that the reduction or

even addition of information is necessarily nonadaptive, but rather that the representations at higher and higher afferent levels differ ever more greatly from the original stimulus pattern.

25. The common sensory dimensions that have been suggested by psychophysicists and that must be explained in terms of neural equivalents are perceived quantity, perceived quality, a set of temporal discriminations, and a set of spatial discriminations.

26. The neural dimensions that have been suggested by neurophysiologists and that may be considered as candidate codes include place (the labeled line), the number of activated units, neural event amplitude, the shape of the response, the frequency of firing (as interpreted either with a counting or clocking process), macrofluctuations and microfluctuations in the frequency pattern, and temporal comparisons between two or more different places. In addition, we are just becoming aware of the possibility that higher-order statistical measures of spike trains, such as the standard deviation or even higher statistical moments, may be of significance and may possibly be candidate codes.

27. The process of definitively linking candidate codes and common sensory dimensions is complex and not always possible to do, but should be considered in terms of "Gedanken" experiments, even when they cannot be actually implemented.

28. There are a number of difficulties in electing an item from the list of candidate codes (members of which are on that list purely because of their demonstrated occurrence in a physiological experiment) to the list of true codes that exhibit identity functions with the common sensory dimensions. The mere existence of a neural dimension and its correlation with a perceptual one are not in themselves proofs that the neural dimension is equivalent or in any way identifiable with the covarying perceptual function. It must be determined that the candidate code is a true code rather than an irrelevant concomitant sign by testing its necessity and sufficiency. This generally has to be done in an experimental paradigm, which permits specific stimulus driving of the nervous signal rather than one that allows the pattern to be determined by the receptor's transduction functions. In sum, there is no *a priori* reason to expect that the mere existence of a candidate makes it a true code.

29. One must, furthermore, always be aware of potential dimension alternations at different levels and always be cognizant of the fact that a code at one level is no more fundamental than one at some other level. There is no *a priori* reason to expect isomorphism between codes and stimuli or between codes at different levels.

30. One must, furthermore, be aware of the possible confusion that can be introduced by overlapping or redundant codes. There is no *a priori* reason to expect a simple one for one coding scheme.

31. One must also be cognizant of species and interindividual differences as well as dynamic differences at different times in the same individual. There is no *a priori* reason to assume that all species and all individuals encode everything in the same way all of the time.

32. One must also be aware of the errors of perspective that can confuse the issue of coding. Sometimes our technology has directed, or rather

overdirected, our attention to only one of several important aspects of neural coding. The predominance of axonology before 1960 is one example of this misattention.

33. Similarly, we must always also be aware of the possible unrelatedness of two processes that may appear superficially to be similar, but that, in fact, are completely different at the level of their neural implementation. It is entirely possible that "ideas" may interact in a mutually inhibitory manner because of similar "meaning" in a way that is quite dissimilar to that occurring when geometrical contours interact, as one example.

34. The notion of thresholds has undergone an evolutionary development. We now tend to consider thresholds more in terms of statistical properties than as absolute lines of demarcation between the perceptible and the imperceptible. In fact, some would now argue that there is no threshold. The existence of measurable amounts of false positive responses in most experiments suggests that "below threshold" might be better phrased in terms of low probabilities of response than in terms of subthreshold imperceptibility. Signal detection theory provides a formal framework for this general new perspective in both psychophysics and neurophysiology.

35. The range of intensities of the stimulus to which most sensory systems can usefully respond is extremely wide. Since the neurological and psychophysical ranges (defined in terms of the ratio of the largest acceptable response to the smallest measurable one) are quite a bit smaller, response compression must play an important role throughout the nervous system. Two models, one based on a logarithmic law and one based on a power law, have been suggested. Neither fits all data, and each must be considered a useful approximation rather than a mathematical tool with fine predictive ability. Critical tests of the best fit of the two theories have been few and far between, and in some instances (for example, when power functions have low exponents), there is no way to discriminate between the two alternatives, nor between either and some other less simple descriptive relation.

36. In general, there appears to be little relation between the coefficients of the power functions that represent psychophysical magnitude functions and those that represent neurophysiological functions. Since differences in power function coefficients represent nonlinear relationships, there appears to be no way in which we can make these two domains isomorphic with these simple metrics. Psychophysical coefficients ranging up to 7.0 have been reported. Neurophysiological coefficients usually are less than 1.0 or go slightly over 1.0 only in certain peculiar situations. Clearly, there is much more measured with the psychophysical power functions than with the neurophysiological ones. Decision processes, experiential and semantic overtones all are mixed with the raw sensory magnitude in the psychophysical data.

37. However useful the power function is as a general metric of the course of an amplitude response dynamic, there is considerable evidence that suggests that it has no particular theoretical significance. Rather, its convenience rests in the fact that a wide range of different monotonic functions can be represented with this single metric—the exponent of a power function.

38. There is increasing evidence that some of the "complex" processing involved in what had classically been called perceptual experience is done in the most peripheral receptor tissues. As one example, most neurophysiological response compression appears to occur at the initial transductive level. Coefficients of approximating power functions are as low or lower than at all other levels. Near-linearity of information transmission beyond the receptor seems to be the rule in the quantity domain. Similarly, contour enhancement seems to be, in large part, a peripheral process.

39. Spatial convergence, a basic neurophysiological net property, leads to a reduction in spatial acuity and the development of such organizational structures as the receptive field.

40. Spatial and temporal divergence leads to a reduction in temporal acuity and the development of such organization structures as the psychological moment.

41. Lateral interaction is a fundamental organizational property of peripheral neural nets with profound implications. It accounts for the stabilization of the nervous system and specifically for certain perceptual phenomena like the Mach band contour enhancement. Contour enhancement, in general, may be thought of as a well-established psychophysical correlate of peripheral neurophysiological lateral interactions and occurs in one form or another in most of the senses.

42. Unfortunately, it has become almost something of a fad to apply lateral inhibitory interaction as a model for too diverse a family of perceptual phenomena. Psychophysical and neurophysiological evidence, as well as a comparison of the time scales involved, suggests that this may be a misdirection.

43. There is little evidence to suggest that lateral interactions comparable to those responsible for contour enhancement in the periphery also go on in the central nervous system.

44. There seems to be little to support any precise isomorphism of psychophysical data and neurophysiological findings at the single cell level in the spatial, temporal, or qualitative domains after one has passed beyond the problem of contour enhancement. Fine spatial, temporal, and qualitative discriminations seem to occur even though the cellular neural responses are widely diffuse in time and space.

45. While the absolute energetics of the stimulus are important in defining their neurophysiological and perceptual effects, recent evidence suggests that the spatio-temporal pattern of the distributions of energies may, in fact, be more important. Constant high-energy levels do not always produce constant high levels of response, and small deviations in the time-space pattern may make even a very-low-energy stimulus extremely effective. The spatio-temporal patterns of stimuli play an important role in defining the responsiveness of neuronal units at all levels of the nervous system in many different animals. Feature extraction mechanisms have been demonstrated to be of elaborate and intricate organization, although the relevance of these to the psychophysical findings has not yet been adequately elucidated.

46. Much as we would like to segregate the temporal and spatial dimensions in separate experimental manipulations, there appears to be too

close a relationship to actually do so in most practical situations. Taking a temporal snapshot, in which space is held constant at a single locus is the classic paradigm of neurophysiology. But this approach leads to the loss of much of the significant spatial coding information. Similarly, a spatial snapshot, in which the temporal aspects are fixed at a specific moment, also usually obscures the key variables. The spatio-temporal pattern may be no more divisible in psychobiology than it is in quantum or astronomical physics.

47. Visual space appears to be mainly encoded by static spatial patterns. All visual localization in two or three dimensions depends upon spatial localizations or disparities on the retinas and at higher levels of the nervous system. By contrast, auditory spatial localization seems to be mediated in large part by dynamic dimensions. The phase angle of a dichotic acoustic stimulus, along with the intensity differences, seems to account for most aspects of auditory spatial localization.

48. The classic and fundamental law of quality coding has been, until recently, Müller's law of specific nerve energies. In general, it now appears that it is not applicable at the level of the single cell or of the microquality within the great modalities. While we shall never see a "sound," it is clear that whether a visual neuron is signaling information that will be decoded as red, green, or blue is not specifically defined by which neuron it happens to be.

49. The actions of receptors and more central neurons encoding color or pitch or any of the other sensory qualities seem, rather, to be characterized by very broadly tuned curves. While these curves generally peak in one or more places, they often have widths equivalent to major portions of the total bandwidth of the stimulus domain.

50. The general quality code observable throughout all of the senses is the relative amount of activity in different places. Absolute place codes or highly specific labeled line notions (à la Müller) are, thus, being replaced as the key code in quality coding by relative temporal comparisons. If the neural encoding loses the information about the delicate phasing differences between the responses at different places, then most psychophysical qualitative distinctiveness is also lost, and only a bland sensory experience remains.

51. Many persistent theoretical controversies have now been resolved by direct observations. The absorption characteristics of the three chromatic photoreceptors are no longer really an issue, nor is the nature of the wave pattern produced by an acoustic stimulus on the basilar membrane. Direct observation of internal response, rather than theoretical interpretation or observation of indirect effects, is always preferable, especially in these instances in which the theory is based mainly on input and output functions. Such "black box" observations usually possess large numbers of potential mechanistic explanations, all of which can produce the same sort of molar behavior. Arguing from analogy of molar response form is not tantamount to proof of homology of internal structure.

52. The general finding in sensory quality psychophysics is of very fine discriminations between nearly alike stimuli. Neurophysiological findings, however, generally indicate that all neuronal units at all anatomical

levels are very broadly tuned and are responsive to a wide range of stimuli. This lack of correspondence between the fine psychophysical quality discrimination and the broad tuning of the nervous components, along with the frequent lack of correspondence between the psychophysical and neurophysiological quantity and space-time data, represents a major difficulty for any sensory-coding theory that requires isomorphism.

53. And finally, as the concluding statement of this book: even given that we all would agree that neural activity is the basis of all behavior, it is clear that there still is no satisfying general explanation of the relationship between the structure of our brains and the process of our minds. Clearly, one-for-one coding models cannot work, and equally clearly, neither our current technology nor theory has yet provided us with a clear picture of the relationship between neurophysiology and psychophysics. We need metrics that are adequate to compare the activity of *populations* of neurons and mental processes. It seems almost certain it is to some form of psychobiological statistics, which has not yet been formulated, that we shall have to turn to more fully understand neural coding. Since the responses of single cells do not correspond adequately with perceptual phenomena, then obviously it must be some ensemble aspect of larger groups of neurons in which the identity functions will ultimately be found. We noted that where the nervous system generally displays broad tuning and a lack of specificity, psychophysical functions usually display fine discriminative abilities. The important implication of this statement is that there must be some sort of a statistical analysis being performed such that the "central tendency" of a broad distribution of multicellular activity is extracted and converted to perception or thought. We are badly in need of a new theoretical breakthrough, akin to the statistical theory of gases, which does not depend upon individual neuronal behavior, but upon some more statistical notion of pooled or ensemble behavior of groups of cells. These new statistical ideas, like a statistical theory of gases, must be relatively insensitive to individual neuron behavior, yet be precise predictors when the central tendencies of the total population are evaluated. New theory and new technology for the study and analysis of ensemble activity represent the current frontier in the science of sensory coding.

It is probably well that we end this book on this note of the unknown. It is one of the most stimulating aspects of the sensory sciences that we do not know all of the answers to all of the questions and that there is much yet to be learned. It is a wide open and fertile field of exploration for those researchers who are able to cast off old conventions and prejudices and view the full and exciting range of problems in this area from new perspectives. The future most certainly belongs to them.

If this book has raised some questions and reoriented a perspective or two for the few who will lead this exploration, it will have achieved its goals.

SUGGESTIONS FOR FURTHER READING

This textbook, like any other, presents a selected sampling of a very large body of information. The full range of our knowledge of the sensory sciences is, of course, much broader than any single volume could encompass. In the following list, I have gathered together a sample of some of the more important, interesting, amusing, informative, or curious books, which may be the next step in the reader's introduction to the field of the sensory sciences. Some of the books are, admittedly, not technical tomes. The wonderful drawings of Escher or the beautiful photographs of Dröscher are examples of sensory phenomena and structures rather than solid scientific explanations of them. Some of the other books are highly technical volumes, which present the views of experts in the field without very much concern for the novice's limited experience. Hopefully, though, this list will provide the basis of a varied and eclectic perspective for the reader who is interested in pursuing this material further, without forcing any particular view on him.

Of course, these are just the books. There is, in addition, a wide variety of periodical journals in the field that publish the findings of sensory research. The reader may get a pretty good idea of the most important ones by looking through the bibliography of this book. Keeping abreast of all of the enormous number of relevant papers is, of course, impossible, but browsing, though a random process, is amazingly efficient in keeping oneself up to date in at least a selected small portion of the field.

Allport, F. H. *Theories of perception and the concept of structure*. New York: Wiley, 1955.

Alpern, M.; Lawrence, M.; and Wolsk, D. *Sensory processes*. Belmont, Calif.: Brooks/Cole, 1967.

Amerine, M. A.; Pangborn, R. M.; and Roessler, E. B. *Principles of sensory evaluation of food*. New York: Academic Press, 1965.

Amoore, J. E. *Molecular basis of odor*. Springfield, Ill.: C. C. Thomas, 1970.

Békésy, G. von. *Experiments in hearing*. New York: McGraw-Hill, 1960.

———. *Sensory inhibition*. Princeton, N.J.: Princeton Univ. Press, 1967.

Bender, M. B. *Disorders in perception*. Springfield, Ill.: C. C. Thomas, 1952.

Buchthal, F., and Rosenfalck, A. Evoked action potentials and conduction velocity in human sensory nerves. *Brain Res.*, 1966, 3:1–122.

Buddenbrock, W. von. *The senses*. Ann Arbor: Univ. of Michigan Press, 1970.

Bullock, T. H., and Horridge, G. A. *Structure and function in the nervous systems of invertebrates*. Vols. 1 and 2. San Francisco: W. H. Greeman, 1965.

Burkhardt, D.; Schleidt, W.; and Altner, H. *Signals in the animal world*. New York: McGraw-Hill, 1967.

Case, J. *Sensory mechanisms*. New York: Macmillan, 1966.

Cherry, C. *On human communication*. Cambridge, and New York: M.I.T. Press, Wiley, 1957.

Cobb, W., and Morocutti, C., eds. The evoked potentials. *EEG Clin. Neurophysiol.*, 1967, Suppl. 26.

Cold Spring Harbor Symposia on Quantitative Biology, Vol. 30 (Sensory Receptors), 1965.

Cornsweet, T. N. *Visual perception*. New York: Academic Press, 1970.

Corso, J. F. *The experimental psychology of sensory behavior*. New York: Holt, Rinehart and Winston, 1967.

Davson, H., ed. *The eye*. Vol. 4. *Visual optics and the optical space sense*. New York: Academic Press, 1962.

De Reuck, A. V. S., and Knight, J., eds. *Hearing mechanisms in vertebrates*. Boston: Little, Brown, 1968.

———. *Touch, heat and pain*. Boston: Little, Brown, 1966.

Deutsch, F., ed. *On the mysterious leap from the mind to the body*. New York: International Universities Press, 1969.

Dodwell, P. C., ed. *Perceptual processing: Stimulus equivalence and pattern recognition*. New York: Appleton-Century-Crofts, 1971.

Dodwell, P. C. *Visual pattern recognition*. New York: Holt, Rinehart and Winston, 1970.

Dröscher, V. B. *The magic of the senses*. New York: E. P. Dutton, 1969.

Eccles, J. C. *The neurophysiological basis of mind*. Oxford: Clarendon Press, 1952.

———. *The physiology of nerve cells*. Baltimore: Johns Hopkins Press, 1957.

———. *The physiology of synapses*. New York: Academic Press, 1964.

———. *Brain and conscious experience*. New York: Springer-Verlag, 1966.

Escher, M. C. *The graphic work of M. C. Escher*. New York: Hawthorn Books, 1960.

Euler, C. von; Skoglund, S.; and Söderberg, U., eds. *Structure and function of inhibitory neuronal mechanisms*. Oxford: Pergamon, 1968.

Field, J., ed. *Handbook of physiology. Neurophysiology*. Vol. 1. Washington: American Physiological Society, 1959.

Forgus, R. H. *Perception*. New York: McGraw-Hill, 1966.

Geldard, F. A. *The human senses*. New York: Wiley, 1953.

Gersuni, G. V., ed. *Sensory processes at the neuronal and behavioral levels*. New York: Academic Press, 1971.

Gibson, J. J. *The senses considered as perceptual systems.* Boston: Houghton Mifflin, 1966.

Giese, A. C., ed. *Photophysiology.* Vol. 2. *Action of light on animals and micro-organisms; Photobiochemical mechanisms; Bioluminescence.* New York: Academic Press, 1964.

Graham, C. H. *Vision and visual perception.* New York: Wiley, 1965.

Granit, R. *Receptors and sensory perception.* New Haven: Yale Univ. Press, 1955.

Green, D. M., and Swets, J. A. *Signal detection theory and psychophysics.* New York: Wiley, 1966.

Gregory, R. L. *Eye and brain. The psychology of seeing.* New York: McGraw-Hill, 1969.

Gulick, W. L. *Hearing. Physiology and psychophysics.* New York: Oxford Univ. Press, 1971.

Haber, R. N., ed. *Contemporary theory and research in visual perception.* New York: Holt, Rinehart and Winston, 1968.

———. *Information-processing approaches to visual perception.* New York: Holt, Rinehart and Winston, 1969.

Harris, J. D., ed. *Forty germinal papers in human hearing.* Groton, Conn.: Journal of Auditory Research, 1969.

Hartridge, H. *Recent advances in the physiology of vision.* London: J. & A. Churchill, 1950.

Hayashi, T., ed. *Olfaction and taste II.* Proceedings of the Second International Symposium. Oxford: Pergamon, 1967.

Hebb, D. O. *The organization of behavior.* New York: Wiley, 1949.

Hurvich, L. M., and Jameson, D. *The perception of brightness and darkness.* Boston: Allyn & Bacon, 1966.

Julesz, B. *Foundations of cyclopean perception.* Chicago: Univ. of Chicago Press, 1971.

Kabrisky, M. *A proposed model for visual information processing in the human brain.* Urbana, Ill.: Univ. of Illinois Press, 1966.

Kare, M. R., and Halpern, B. P. *Physiological and behavioral aspects of taste.* Chicago: Univ. of Chicago Press, 1961.

Katz, B. *Nerve, muscle, and synapse.* New York: McGraw-Hill, 1966.

Kiang, N. Y.-S. *Discharge patterns of single fibers in the cat's auditory nerve.* Cambridge: M.I.T. Press, 1965.

Kling, J. W., and Riggs, L. A., eds. *Experimental psychology.* 3rd ed. New York: Holt, Rinehart and Winston, 1971.

Koch, S., ed. *Psychology: A study of a science.* Vol. 1. *Sensory, perceptual, and physiological formulations.* New York: McGraw-Hill, 1959.

———. *Psychology: A study of a science.* Vol. 4. *Biologically oriented fields: Their place in psychology and in biological science.* New York: McGraw-Hill, 1962.

Kolb, L. C. *The painful phantom.* Springfield, Ill.: C. C. Thomas, 1954.

Kolers, P. A., and Eden, M., eds. *Recognizing patterns. Studies in living and automatic systems.* Cambridge: M.I.T. Press, 1968.

Leibovic, K. N. *Information processing in the nervous system.* New York: Springer-Verlag, 1969.

Lipkin, B. S., and Rosenfeld, A. *Picture processing and psychopictorics.* New York: Academic Press, 1970.

Loewenstein, W. R., ed. *Handbook of sensory physiology.* Vol. 1. *Principles of receptor physiology.* New York: Springer-Verlag, 1971.

Lowenstein, O. *The senses.* Baltimore: Penguin Books, 1966.

MacKay, D. M. Evoked brain potentials as indicators of sensory information processing. *Neurosci. Res. Prog. Bull.,* 1969, 7: 181–276.

McCleary, R. A. *Genetic and experiential factors in perception.* Glenview, Ill.: Scott, Foresman, 1970.

McLennan, H. *Synaptic transmission.* 2nd ed. Philadelphia: Saunders, 1970.

Mandelbaum, M. *Philosophy, science and sense perception: Historical and critical studies.* Baltimore: Johns Hopkins Press, 1964.

Meek, G. A. *Practical electron microscopy for biologists.* London: Wiley-Interscience, 1971.

Mellon, D., Jr. *The physiology of sense organs.* San Francisco: W. H. Freeman, 1968.

Meyer, M. F. *How we hear.* Boston: C. T. Branford, 1950.

Milne, L. and M. *The senses of animals and men.* New York: Atheneum, 1962.

Minsky, M., and Papert, S. *Perceptrons. An introduction to computational geometry.* Cambridge: M.I.T. Press, 1969.

Montagu, A. *Touching: The human significance of the skin.* New York: Columbia Univ. Press, 1971.

Mueller, C. G. *Sensory psychology.* Englewood Cliffs, N.J.: Prentice-Hall, 1965.

Neff, W. D., ed. *Contributions to sensory physiology.* Vols. 1–5. New York: Academic Press, 1965–1971.

Neisser, U. *Cognitive psychology.* New York: Appleton-Century-Crofts, 1967.

Ogle, K. N. *Researches in binocular vision.* Philadelphia: Saunders, 1950.

Osgood, C. E. *Method and theory in experimental psychology.* New York: Oxford Univ. Press, 1953.

Perkel, D. H., and Bullock, T. H. Neural coding. *Neurosci. Res. Prog. Bull.,* 1968, 6: 221–348.

Pfaffmann, C., ed. *Olfaction and taste.* Proceedings of the Third International Symposium. New York: Rockefeller Univ. Press, 1969.

Piéron, H. *The sensations.* New Haven: Yale Univ. Press, 1952.

Plonsey, R., and Fleming, D. G. *Bioelectric phenomena.* New York: McGraw-Hill, 1969.

Polyak, S. L. *The retina.* Chicago: Univ. of Chicago Press, 1941.

———, ed. *The vertebrate visual system.* Chicago: Univ. of Chicago Press, 1957.

Porter, K. R., and Bonneville, M. A. *Fine structure of cells and tissues.* 3rd ed. Philadelphia: Lea & Febiger, 1968.

Quarton, G. C.; Melnechuk, R.; and Schmitt, F. O. *The neurosciences.* New York: Rockefeller Univ. Press, 1967.

Ratliff, F. *Mach bands: Quantitative studies on neural networks in the retina.* San Francisco: Holden-Day, 1965.

Reichardt, W., ed. *Processing of optical data by organisms and by machines.* New York: Academic Press, 1969.

Rhodin, J. A. G. *An atlas of ultrastructure.* Philadelphia: Saunders, 1968.

Rosenblith, W. A., ed. *Sensory communication.* Cambridge and New York: M.I.T. Press, Wiley, 1961.

Ruch, R. C., and Patton, H. D., eds. *Physiology and biophysics.* 19th ed. Philadelphia: Saunders, 1965.

Schmitt, F. O. *The neurosciences: Second study program.* New York: Rockefeller Univ. Press, 1970.

Sheppard, J. J., Jr. *Human color perception.* New York: American Elsevier, 1968.

Sinclair, D. *Cutaneous sensation.* London: Oxford Univ. Press, 1967.

Smith, K. U. *Delayed sensory feedback and behavior.* Philadelphia: Saunders, 1962.

Smith, K. U., and Smith, W. M. *Perception and motion.* Philadelphia: Saunders, 1962.

Southall, J. P. C. *Introduction to physiological optics.* London: Oxford Univ. Press, 1937.

Stebbins, W. C. *Animal psychophysics: The design and conduct of sensory experiments.* New York: Appleton-Century-Crofts, 1970.

Symposia of the Society for Experimental Biology. No. XVI. *Biological receptor mechanisms.* Cambridge: University Press, 1962.

Teevan, R. C., and Birney, R. C., eds. *Color vision.* Princeton, N.J.: Van Nostrand, 1961.

Thompson, R. F. *Foundations of physiological psychology.* New York: Harper & Row, 1967.

Tobias, J. V., ed. *Foundations of modern auditory theory.* 2 vols. New York: Academic Press, 1970–72.

Uhr, L., ed. *Pattern recognition.* New York: Wiley, 1966.

Uttal, W. R. *Real-time computers.* New York: Harper & Row, 1967.

Uttal, W. R., ed. *Sensory coding. Selected readings.* Boston: Little, Brown, 1972.

Warren, R. M., and Warren, R. P. *Helmholtz on perception: Its physiology and development.* New York: Wiley, 1968.

Wathen-Dunn, W., ed. *Models for the perception of speech and visual form.* Cambridge: M.I.T. Press, 1967.

Weintraub, D. J., and Walker, E. L. *Perception.* Belmont, Calif.: Brooks/Cole, 1966.

Wever, E. G. *Theory of hearing.* New York: Wiley, 1949.

Wiener, N. *Cybernetics.* New York: Wiley, 1948.

Wiersma, C. A. G., ed. *Invertebrate nervous systems.* Chicago: Univ. of Chicago Press, 1967.

Wolstenholme, G. E. W., and Knight, J. *Taste and smell in vertebrates.* London: J. & A. Churchill, 1970.

Wright, R. H. *The science of smell.* New York: Basic Books, 1964.

Wyburn, G. M.; Pickford, R. W.; and Hirst, R. J. *Human senses and perception.* Toronto: Univ. of Toronto Press, 1964.

Zotterman, Y., ed. *Olfaction and taste.* Proceedings of the First International Symposium. New York: Macmillan, 1963.

———. *Progress in brain research.* Vol. 23. *Sensory mechanisms.* New York: Elsevier, 1967.

Zusne, L. *Visual perception of form.* New York: Academic Press, 1970.

BIBLIOGRAPHY

Ades, H. W. and Engström, H. Form and innervation in the vestibular epithelia. In A. Graybiel, ed., *The role of the vestibular organs in the exploration of space*. U.S. Naval School of Medicine: NASA SP–77, 1965, pp. 23–41.

Adey, W. R. The sense of smell. In J. Field, ed., *Handbook of physiology. Neurophysiology*. Vol. 1. Washington: American Physiological Society, 1959, pp. 353–548.

Adrian, E. D. Sensory messages and sensation. *Acta Physiol. Scand.*, 1953, 29: 5–14.

———. The basis of sensation—some recent studies of olfaction. *Brit. Med. J.*, 1954, 1: 287–290.

———. Transmission of information from the olfactory organ. In Problems of the modern physiology of the nervous and muscle systems. *Acad. Sci. Georgian S.S.R.*, 1956, 13–19.

Adrian, E. D.; Cattell, McK.; and Hoagland, H. Sensory discharges in single cutaneous nerve fibres. *J. Physiol.*, 1931, 72: 377–391.

Adrian, E. D., and Umrath, K. The impulse discharge from the Pacinian corpuscle. *J. Physiol.*, 1929, 68: 139–154.

Adrian, E. D., and Zotterman, Y. The impulses produced by sensory nerve endings. Part 3. Impulses set up by touch and pressure. *J. Physiol.*, 1926, 61: 465–483.

Aitkin, L. M.; Anderson, D. J.; and Brugge, J. F. Tonotopic organization and discharge characteristics of single neurons in nuclei of the lateral lemniscus of the cat. *J. Neurophysiol.*, 1970, 33: 421–440.

Alexander, J. *Colloid chemistry.* 4th ed. New York: Van Nostrand, 1937.

Allen, F., and Weinberg, M. The gustatory sensory reflex. *Quart. J. Exp. Physiol.,* 1925, 15: 305–420.

Allison, A. C., and Warwick, R. T. T. Quantitative observations on the olfactory system of the rabbit. *Brain,* 1949, 72: 186–197.

Allport, D. A. Phenomenal simultaneity and the perceptual moment hypothesis. *Brit. J. Psychol.,* 1968, 59: 395–406.

Alpern, M. Metacontrast. *J. Opt. Soc. Amer.,* 1953, 43: 648–657.

————. Movements of the eyes. In H. Davson, ed., *The eye.* 2nd ed. Vol. 3. *Muscular mechanisms.* New York: Academic Press, 1969. Pp. 1–214.

Alpern, M.; Rushton, W. A. H.; and Torii, S. The size of rod signals. *J. Physiol.,* 1970, 206: 193–208.

Alvarez-Buylla, R., and De Arellano, R. Local responses in Pacinian corpuscles. *Am. J. Physiol.,* 1953, 172: 237–244.

Amerine, M. A.; Pangborn, R. M.; and Roessler, E. B. *Principles of sensory evaluation of food.* New York: Academic Press, 1965.

Amoore, J. E. The stereochemical specificities of human olfactory receptors. *Perfum. Essent. Oil Rec.,* 1952, 43: 321–323.

————. The stereochemical theory of olfaction, 2, elucidation of the stereochemical properties of the olfactory receptor sites. *Proc. Sci. Sect. Toilet Goods Assoc.,* 1962, 37 (Suppl.): 13–23.

————. Current status of the steric theory of odor. *Ann. N.Y. Acad. Sci.,* 1964, 116: 457–476.

————. Psychophysics of odor. *Cold Spr. Harb. Symp. Quant. Biol.,* 1965, 30: 623–636.

————. A plan to identify most of the primary odors. In C. Pfaffmann, ed., *Olfaction and taste.* Proceedings of the Third International Symposium. New York: Rockefeller Univ. Press, 1969. Pp. 158–171.

————. *Molecular basis of odor.* Springfield, Ill.: C. C. Thomas, 1970.

Amoore, J. E.; Johnston, J. W., Jr.; and Rubin, M. The stereochemical theory of odor. *Sci. Amer.,* 1964, 210(2): 42–49.

Amoore, J. E., and Venstrom, D. Sensory analysis of odor qualities in terms of the stereochemical theory. *J. Food Sci.,* 1966, 31: 118–128.

————. Correlations between stereochemical assessments and organoleptic analysis of odorous compounds. In T. Hayashi, ed., *Olfaction and taste II.* Proceedings of the Second International Symposium. Oxford: Pergamon, 1967. Pp. 3–17.

Andersen, V. O.; Buchmann, B.; and Lennox-Buchthal, M. A. Single cortical units with narrow spectral sensitivity in monkey (*Cercocebus torquatus atys*). *Vision Res.,* 1962, 2: 295–307.

Anderson, A. B., and Munson, W. A. Electrical excitation of nerves in the skin at audiofrequencies. *J. Acoust. Soc. Amer.,* 1951, 23: 155–159.

Andres, K. H. Anatomy and ultrastructure of the olfactory bulb in fish, amphibia, reptiles, birds and mammals. In G. E. W. Wolstenholme and J. Knight, eds., *Taste and smell in vertebrates.* London: J. & A. Churchill, 1970. Pp. 177–193.

Andrew, B. L. The sensory innervation of the medial ligament of the knee joint. *J. Physiol.,* 1954, 123: 241–250. (a)

————. Proprioception at the joint of the epiglottis of the rat. *J. Physiol.,* 1954, 126: 507–523. (b)

Andrew, B. L., and Dodt, E. Deployment of sensory nerve endings at knee joint of cat. *Acta Physiol. Scand.,* 1953, 28: 287–296.

Andrews, D. P. Perception of contours in the central fovea. *Nature,* 1965, 205: 1218–1220.

Arden, G. B. Complex receptive fields and responses to moving objects in cells of the rabbit's lateral geniculate body. *J. Physiol.*, 1963, 166: 468–488.

Arvanitaki, A.; Takeuchi, H.; and Chalazonitis, N. Specific unitary osmereceptor potentials and spiking patterns from giant nerve cells sensory coding in a neural *in vivo* model. In T. Hayashi, ed., *Olfaction and taste II*. Proceedings of the Second International Symposium. Oxford: Pergamon, 1967. Pp. 573–598.

Attneave, F., and Arnoult, M. D. The quantitative study of shape and pattern perception. *Psychol. Bull.*, 1956, 53: 452–471.

Averbach, E., and Coriell, A. Short term memory in vision. *Bell Syst. Tech. J.*, 1961, 40: 309–328.

Barlow, H. B. Optic nerve impulses and Weber's law. *Cold Spr. Harb. Symp. Quant. Biol.*, 1965, 30: 539–546.

Barlow, H. B.; Blakemore, C., and Pettigrew, J. D. The neural mechanism of binocular depth discrimination. *J. Physiol.*, 1967, 193: 327–342.

Barlow, H. B.; Fitzhugh, R.; and Kuffler, S. W. Change of organization in the receptive fields of the cat's retina during dark adaptation. *J. Physiol.*, 1957, 137: 338–354.

Barlow, H. B., and Hill, R. M. Selective sensitivity to direction of movement in ganglion cells of the rabbit retina. *Science*, 1963, 139; 412–414.

Barlow, H. B.; Hill, R. M.; and Levick, W. R. Retinal ganglion cells responding selectively to direction and speed of image in the rabbit. *J. Physiol.*, 1964, 173: 377–407.

Barlow, H. B., and Levick, W. R. The mechanism of directionally selective units in rabbits retina. *J. Physiol.*, 1965, 178: 477–504.

———. Three factors limiting the reliable detection of light by retinal ganglion cells of the cat. *J. Physiol.*, 1969, 200: 1–24.

Bartoshuk, L. M.; Dateo, G. P.; Vandenbelt, D. J.; Buttrick, R. L.; and Long, L., Jr. Effects of *Gymnema sylvestre* and *Synsepalum dulcificum* on taste in man. In C. Pfaffmann, ed., *Olfaction and taste III*. Proceedings of the Third International Symposium. New York: Rockefeller Univ. Press, 1969. Pp. 436–444.

Bauhin, C. *Theatrum anatomicum*. Francofurti at Moenum, 1605. Cited in E. G. Wever, *Theory of hearing*. New York: Wiley, 1949.

Baumgartner, G.; Brown, J. L.; and Schultz, A. Visual motion detection in the cat. *Science*, 1964, 146: 1070–1071.

Baylor, D. A., and Fuortes, M. G. F. Electrical responses of single cones in the retina of the turtle. *J. Physiol.*, 1970, 207: 77–92.

Beatty, J., and Uttal, W. R. The effects of grouping visual stimuli on the cortical evoked potential. *Percept. & Psychophys.*, 1968, 4: 214–216.

Beidler, L. M. Comparison of gustatory receptors, olfactory receptors, and free nerve endings. *Cold Spr. Harb. Symp. Quant. Biol.*, 1965, 30: 191–200.

———. Anion influences on taste receptor response. In T. Hayashi, ed., *Olfaction and taste II*. Proceedings of the Second International Symposium. Oxford: Pergamon, 1967. Pp. 509–534.

———. Innervation of rat fungiform papilla. In C. Pfaffmann, ed., *Olfaction and taste III*. Proceedings of the Third International Symposium. New York: Rockefeller Univ. Press, 1969, pp. 352–369.

Beidler, L. M.; Nejad, M. S.; Smallman, R. L.; and Tateda, H. Rat taste cell proliferation. *Fed. Proc.*, 1960, 19: 302.

Beidler, L. M., and Smallman, R. S. Renewal of cells within taste buds. *J. Cell Biol.*, 1965, 27: 263–272.

Békésy, G. von. The variation of phase along the basilar membrane with sinusoidal vibrations. *J. Acoust. Soc. Amer.*, 1947, 19: 452–460.

————. The vibration of the cochlear partition in anatomical preparations and in models of the inner ear. *J. Acoust. Soc. Amer.*, 1949, 21: 233–245. (a)

————. On the resonance curve and the decay period at various points on the cochlear partition. *J. Acoust. Soc. Amer.*, 1949, 21: 245–254 (b).

————. Microphonics produced by touching the cochlear partition with a vibrating electrode. *J. Acoust. Soc. Amer.*, 1951, 23: 29–35.

————. Current status of theories of hearing. *Science*, 1956, 123: 779–783.

————. Sensations on the skin similar to directional hearing, beats and harmonics of the ear. *J. Acoust. Soc. Amer.*, 1957, 29: 489–501.

————. Funneling in the nervous system and its role in loudness and sensation intensity in the skin. *J. Acoust. Soc. Amer.*, 1958, 30: 399–412.

————. *Experiments in hearing.* New York: McGraw-Hill, 1960.

————. Hearing theories and complex sounds. *J. Acoust. Soc. Amer.*, 1963, 35: 588–606. (a)

————. Interaction of paired sensory stimuli and conduction in peripheral nerves. *J. Appl. Physiol.*, 1963, 18: 1276–1284. (b)

————. Olfactory analogue to directional hearing. *J. Appl. Physiol.*, 1964, 19: 369–373. (a)

————. Rhythmical variations accompanying gustatory stimulation observed by means of localization phenomena. *J. Gen. Physiol.*, 1964, 47: 809–825. (b)

————. Sweetness produced electrically on the tongue and its relation to taste theories. *J. Appl. Physiol.*, 1964, 19: 1105–1113. (c)

————. Taste theories and the chemical stimulation of single papillae. *J. Appl. Physiol.*, 21: 1966, 1–9.

————. *Sensory inhibition.* Princeton, N.J.: Princeton Univ. Press, 1967.

Best, C. H., and Taylor, N. B. *The physiological basis of medical practice.* 8th ed. Baltimore: Williams & Wilkins, 1966.

Bezold, W. von. Ueber das Gesetz der Farbenmischung und die physiologischen Grundfarben. *Ann. Phys. u. Chem.*, 1873, 150:221–247.

Bishop, P. O., and Davis, R. Bilateral interaction in the lateral geniculate body. *Science*, 1953, 118:241–243.

Blakemore, C., and Campbell, F. W. On the existence of neurones in the human visual system selectively sensitive to the orientation and size of retinal images. *J. Physiol.*, 1969, 203: 237–260.

Blakemore, C., and Sutton, P. Size adaptation: A new aftereffect. *Science*, 1969, 166: 245–247.

Blix, M. Experimentelle Beiträge zur Lösung der Frage über die specifische Energie der Hautnerven. *Z. Biol.*, 1884, 20: 141–156.

Blum, H. F. *Time's arrow and evolution.* Princeton: Princeton Univ. Press, 1955.

Boeckh, J. Inhibition and excitation of single insect olfactory receptors, and their role as a primary sensory code. In T. Hayashi, ed., *Olfaction and taste II.* Proceedings of the Second International Symposium. Oxford: Pergamon, 1967. Pp. 721–736.

Borg, G.; Diamant, H.; Oakley, B.; Ström, L.; and Zotterman, Y. A comparative study of neural and psychophysical responses to gustatory stimuli. In T. Hayashi, ed., *Olfaction and taste II.* Proceedings of the Second International Symposium. Oxford: Pergamon, 1967. Pp. 253–264.

Borg, G.; Diamant, H.; Ström, L.; and Zotterman, Y. The relation between neural and perceptual intensity: A comparative study on the neural and psychophysical response to taste stimuli. *J. Physiol.*, 1967, 192: 13–20.

Boring, E. G. *Sensation and perception in the history of experimental psychology.* New York: Appleton-Century-Crofts, 1942.

Boudreau, J. C., and Tsuchitani, C. Binaural interaction in the cat superior olive S segment. *J. Neurophysiol.*, 1968, 31: 442–454.

Boyd, I. A., and Roberts, T. D. M. Proprioceptive discharges from stretch-receptors in knee-joint of cat. *J. Physiol.*, 1953, 122: 38–58.

Boynton, R. M., and Whitten, D. N. Visual adaptation in monkey cones: Recordings of late receptor potentials. *Science*, 1970, 170: 1423–1426.

Brazier, M. A. B. The historical development of neurophysiology. In J. Field, ed., *Handbook of physiology. Neurophysiology.* Vol. 1. Washington: American Physiological Society, 1959. Pp. 1–58.

Bredberg, G. Cellular pattern and nerve supply of the human organ of Corti. *Acta Oto-Laryng.*, 1968, Suppl. 236: 1–135.

Brindley, G. S.; Du Croz, J. J.; and Rushton, W. A. H. The flicker fusion frequency of the blue-sensitive mechanisms of color vision. *J. Physiol.*, 1966, 183: 497–500.

Brown, J. L. The structure of the visual system. In C. H. Graham, ed., *Vision and visual perception.* New York: Wiley, 1965. Pp. 39–59.

Brown, K. T., and Murakami, M. A new receptor potential of the monkey retina with no detectable latency. *Nature*, 1964, 201: 626–628.

Brown, P. K., and Wald, G. Visual pigments in single rods and cones of the human retina. *Science*, 1964, 144: 145–151.

Brugge, J. F.; Dubrovsky, N. A.; Aitkin, L. M.; and Anderson, D. J. Sensitivity of single neurons in auditory cortex of cat to binaural tonal stimulation; Effects of varying interaural time and intensity. *J. Neurophysiol.*, 1969, 32: 1005–1024.

Brugge, J. F.; Dubrovsky, N. A.; and Rose, J. E. Some discharge characteristics of single neurons in cats' auditory cortex. *Science*, 1964, 146: 433–434. (abstract)

Buchsbaum, W. H., and Mayzner, M. S. The effect of line length on sequential blanking. *Psychon. Sci.*, 1969, 15: 111–112.

Buchthal, F., and Rosenfalck, A. Evoked action potentials and conduction velocity in human sensory nerves. *Brain Res.*, 1966, 3(1):1–122.

Bujas, Z., and Pfaffmann, C. Potassium gynemate and the sweet and bitter taste provoked electrically. *Percept. & Psychophys.*, 1971, 10: 28–29.

Buller, A. J.; Nicholls, J. G.; and Ström, G. Spontaneous fluctuations of excitability in the muscle spindle of the frog. *J. Physiol.*, 1953, 122: 409–418.

Bullock, T. H. Neuron doctrine and electrophysiology. *Science*, 1959, 129: 997–1002.

———. On the anatomy of the giant neurons of the visceral ganglion of *Aplysia*. In E. Florey, ed., *Nervous inhibition.* New York: Pergamon, 1961. Pp. 233–240.

Bullock, T. H., and Diecke, F. P. J. Properties of an infra-red receptor. *J. Physiol.*, 1956, 134: 47–87.

Bullock, T. H., and Horridge, G. A. *Structure and function in the nervous systems of invertebrates.* Vol. II. San Francisco: W. H. Freeman, 1965.

Burkhardt, D. A. Cone action spectra: Evidence from the goldfish electroretinogram. *Vision Res.*, 1968, 8: 839–853.

Burns, B. D. *The mammalian cerebral cortex.* London: E. Arnold, 1958.

Campbell, F. W., and Green, D. G. Monocular versus binocular visual acuity. *Nature*, 1965, 208: 191–192.

Campbell, F. W., and Kulikowsky, J. J. Orientation of selectivity of the human visual system. *J. Physiol.*, 1966, 187: 437–445.

Capek, M. *Philosophical impact of contemporary physics.* New York: Van Nostrand, 1961.

Carterette, E. C.; Friedman, M. P.; and Lovell, J. D. Mach bands in hearing. *J. Acoust. Soc. Amer.*, 1969, 45: 986–998.

Cattell, McK., and Hoagland, H. Response of tactile receptors to intermittent stimulation. *J. Physiol.*, 1931, 72: 392–404.

Cauna, N. The effects of aging on the receptor organs of the human dermis. In *Advances in biology of skin—Vol. VI—Aging*. Proceedings of the symposium held at the University of Oregon Medical School, 1964. New York: Pergamon, 1965. Pp. 63–96.

———. Light and electron microscopal structure of sensory end-organs in human skin. In D. R. Kenshalo, ed., *The skin senses*. Springfield, Ill.: C. C. Thomas, 1968. Pp. 15–28.

Cohen, M. J.; Hagiwara, S.; and Zotterman, Y. The response spectrum of taste fibres in the cat: A single fibre analysis. *Acta Physiol. Scand.*, 1955, 33: 316–332.

Cole, R. E., and Diamond, A. L. Amount of surround and test-inducing separation in simultaneous brightness contrast. *Percept. & Psychophys.*, 1971, 9: 125–128.

Cone, R. A. Early receptor potential: Photoreversible charge displacement in rhodopsin. *Science*, 1967, 155: 1128–1131.

Cone, R. A., and Brown, P. K. Dependence of the early receptor potential on the orientation of rhodopsin. *Science*, 1967, 156: 536. (abstract)

Cone, R. A., and Cobbs, W. H., III. Rhodopsin cycle in the living eye of the rat. *Nature*, 1969, 221: 820–822.

Conger, A. C., and Wells, M. A. Radiation and aging effect on taste structure and function. *Radiation Res.*, 1969, 37: 31–49.

Coombs, C. H.; Dawes, R. M.; and Tversky, A. *Mathematical psychology: An elementary introduction*. Englewood Cliffs, N.J.: Prentice-Hall, 1970.

Cornsweet, T. N. *Visual perception*. New York: Academic Press, 1970.

Corso, J. F. *The experimental psychology of sensory behavior*. New York: Holt, Rinehart and Winston, 1967.

Cox, D. R., and Smith, W. L. On the superposition of renewal processes. *Biometrika*, 1954, 41: 91–99.

Crawford, B. H. Visual adaptation in relation to brief conditioning stimuli. *Proc. Royal Soc. Lond.*, 1947, Ser. B., 134: 283–302.

Dallos, P. Combination tone $2f_1-f_h$ in microphonic potentials. *J. Acoust. Soc. Amer.*, 1969, 46: 1437–1444.

Dallos, P.; Schoeny, Z. G.; and Cheatham, M. A. Cochlear summating potentials: Composition. *Science*, 1970, 170: 641–644.

———. On the limitations of cochlear-microphonic measurements. *J. Acoust. Soc. Amer.*, 1971, 49: 1144–1154.

Daniell, W. F. On the *Synsepalum dulcificum* De Cand.; or, miraculous berry of Western Africa. *Pharm. J.*, 1852, 11: 445–448.

Dastoli, F. R. On comparison of interactions of a "bitter-sensitive protein" from porcine tongues with human taste thresholds. *Nature*, 1969, 223: 524–525.

Dastoli, F. R.; Lopiekes, D. V.; and Price, S. A sweet-sensitive protein from bovine taste buds. Purification and partial characterization. *Biochemistry*, 1968, 7: 1160–1164.

Dastoli, F. R., and Price, S. Sweet-sensitive protein from bovine taste buds: Isolation and assay. *Science*, 1966, 154: 905–907.

Davidson, M. L. Perturbation approach to spatial brightness interaction in human vision. *J. Opt. Soc. Amer.*, 1968, 58: 1300–1309.

Davies, J. T. A theory of the quality of odours. *J. Theoret. Biol.*, 1965, 8: 1–7.

———. Recent developments in the "penetration and puncturing" theory of odour. In G. E. W. Wolstenholme & J. Knight, eds., *Taste and smell in vertebrates*. London: J. & A. Churchill, 1970. Pp. 265–291.

Davis, H. Some principles of sensory receptor action. *Physiol. Rev.*, 1961, 41: 391–416.

―――. A model for transducer action in the cochlea. *Cold Spr. Harb. Symp. on Quant. Biol.*, 1965, 30: 181–190.

Davis, H.; Morgan, C. T.; Hawkins, J. E., Jr.; Galambos, R.; and Smith, F. W. Temporary deafness following exposure to loud tones and noise. *Acta Oto-Laryng.*, 1950, Suppl. 88: 5–57.

Davis, H., and Silverman, S. R. *Hearing and deafness* (3rd ed.). New York: Holt, Rinehart and Winston, 1970.

Daw, N. W. Colour-coded ganglion cells in the goldfish retina: Extension of their receptive fields by means of new stimuli. *J. Physiol.*, 1968, 197: 567–592.

Dawson, G. D., and Scott, J. W. The recording of nerve action potentials through skin in man. *J. Neurol. Neurosurg. Psychiat.*, 1949, 12: 259–267.

de Lorenzo, A. J. Electron microscopy of the olfactory and gustatory pathways. *Ann Otol. Rhin. & Laryng.*, 1960, 69: 410–420.

―――. Studies on the ultrastructure and histophysiology of cell membranes, nerve fibers and synaptic junctions in chemoreceptors. In Y. Zotterman, ed., *Olfaction and taste.* Proceedings of the First International Symposium. New York: Macmillan, 1963. Pp. 5–18.

Dember, W. N., and Purcell, D. G. Recovery of masked visual targets by inhibition of the masking stimulus. *Science*, 1967, 157: 1335–1336.

De Reuck, A. V. S., and Knight, J., eds. *Touch, heat and pain.* Boston: Little, Brown, 1966.

De Robertis, E. Electron microscope observations on the submicroscopic organization of the retinal rods. *J. Biophys. Biochem. Cytol.*, 1956, 2: 319–330.

DeValois, R. L. Color vision mechanisms in the monkey. *J. Gen. Physiol.*, 1960, 43: Pt. 2, 115–128.

―――. Behavioral and electrophysiological studies of primate vision. In W. D. Neff, ed., *Contributions to sensory physiology.* Vol. 1. New York: Academic Press, 1965. Pp. 137–178.

DeValois, R. L.; Abramov, I.; and Jacobs, G. H. Analysis of response patterns of LGN cells. *J. Opt. Soc. Amer.*, 1966, 56: 966–977.

DeValois, R. L., and Jacobs, G. H. Primate color vision. *Science*, 1968, 162: 533–540.

DeValois, R. L.; Jacobs, G. H.; and Jones, A. E. Responses of single cells in primate red-green color vision system. *Optik*, 1963, 20: 87–98.

DeValois, R. L., and Pease, P. L. Contours and contrast: Responses of monkey lateral geniculate nucleus cells to luminance and color figures. *Science*, 1971, 171: 694–696.

DeValois, R. L.: Smith, C. J.; Kitai, S. T.; and Karoly, A. J. Response of single cells in monkey lateral geniculate nucleus to monochromatic light. *Science*, 1958, 127: 238–239.

Diamond, A. L. A theory of depression and enhancement in the brightness response. *Psych. Rev.*, 1960, 67: 168–199.

Doetsch, G. S., and Erickson, R. P. Synaptic processing of taste-quality information in the nucleus tractus solitarius of the rat. *J. Neurophysiol.*, 1970, 33: 490–507.

Doetsch, G. S.; Ganchrow, J. J.; Nelson, L. M.; and Erickson, R. P. Information processing in the taste system of the rat. In C. Pfaffmann, ed., *Olfaction and taste III.* Proceedings of the Third International Symposium. New York: Rockefeller Univ. Press, 1969. Pp. 492–511.

Døving, K. B. Experiments in olfaction. In G. E. W. Wolstenholme and J. Knight, eds., *Taste and smell in vertebrates.* London: J. & A. Churchill, 1970. Pp. 197–220.

Dowling, J. E. The site of visual adaptation. *Science,* 1967, 155: 273–279.

Dowling, J. E., and Boycott, B. B. Organization of the primate retina: Electron microscopy. *Proc. Royal Soc. Lond.,* 1966, Ser. B, 166: 80–111.

Dowling, J. E., and Werblin, F. S. Organization of retina of the mudpuppy, *Necturus maculosus.* I. Synaptic Structure. *J. Neurophysiol.,* 1969, 32: 315–354.

Dravnieks, A. Properties of receptors through molecular parameters of odorivectors. In T. Hayashi, ed., *Olfaction and taste II.* Proceedings of the Second International Symposium. Oxford: Pergamon, 1967. Pp. 89–108.

DuVerney, J. G. *Traité de l'organe de l'ouie.* Paris, 1683. Cited in E. G. Wever, *Theory of hearing.* New York: Wiley, 1949.

Dzendolet, E. A structure common to sweet-evoking compounds. *Percept. & Psychophys.,* 1968, 3: 65–68.

Easter, S. S., Jr. Excitation in the goldfish retina: Evidence for a nonlinear intensity code. *J. Physiol.,* 1968, 195: 253–271.

Eccles, J. C. *The physiology of synapses.* New York: Academic Press, 1964.

Ehrenberger, K.; Finkenzeller, P.; Keidel, W. D.; and Plattig, K. H. Electrophysiologische Korrelation der Stevensschen Potenzfunktion und objektive Schwellenmessung am Vibrationssinn des Menschen. *Pflüg. Arch. ges. Physiol.,* 1966, 290: 114–123.

Ekman, G., and Åkesson, C. Saltness, sweetness and preferences; a study of quantitative relations in individual subjects. *Scand. J. Psychol.,* 1965, 6: 241–253.

Engström, H.; Ades, H. W.; and Hawkins, J. E. Cellular pattern, nerve structures, and fluid spaces of the organ of Corti. In W. D. Neff, ed., *Contributions to sensory physiology.* New York: Academic Press, 1965. Pp. 1–38.

Erickson, R. P. Stimulus coding in topographic and nontopographic afferent modalities: On the significance of the activity of individual sensory neurons. *Psych. Rev.,* 1968, 75: 447–465.

Eriksen, C. W.; Becker, B. B.; and Hoffman, J. E. Safari to masking land: A hunt for the elusive U. *Percept. & Psychophys.,* 1970, 8: 245–250.

Eriksen, C. W., and Collins, J. F. Reinterpretation of one form of backward and forward masking in visual perception. *J. Exp. Psychol.,* 1965, 70: 343–351.

Eriksen, C. W., and Hoffman, M. Form recognition at brief durations as a function of adapting field and interval between stimulations. *J. Exp. Psychol.,* 1963, 66: 485–499.

Estes, W. K. Learning theory. *Ann. Rev. Psychol.,* 1962, 13: 107–144.

Fagot, R. F. Alternative power ions for ratio scaling. *Psychometrika,* 1966, 31: 201–214.

Farnsworth, D. Tritanomalous vision as a threshold function. *Die Farbe,* 1955, 4: 185–196.

Fechner, G. *Elements of psychophysics,* 1860. Trans. by H. E. Adler. New York: Holt, Rinehart and Winston, 1966.

Fehmi, L. G.; Adkins, J. W.; and Lindsley, D. B. Electro-physiological correlates of visual perceptual masking in monkeys. *Exp. Brain Res.,* 1969, 7: 299–316.

Feigl, H. The mental and the physical. In H. Feigl *et al.,* eds., *The Minnesota studies in the philosophy of science.* Vol. II. *Concepts, theories and the mind-body problem.* Minneapolis: University of Minnesota Press, 1958. Pp. 370–497.

Fitts, P. M.; Weinstein, M.; Rappaport, M.; Anderson, N.; and Leonard, J. A. Stimulus correlates of visual pattern recognition: A probability approach. *J. Exp. Psychol.,* 1956, 51: 1–11.

Fitzgerald, O. Discharges from sensory organs of cat's vibrissae and modification in their activity by ions. *J. Physiol.,* 1940, 98: 163–178.

Fitzgerald, R. Unpublished doctoral dissertation, University of Western Australia, Nedlands, Western Australia, 1970.

Fletcher, H. *Speech and hearing.* New York: Van Nostrand, 1929.

———. A space-time pattern theory of hearing. *J. Acoust. Soc. Amer.*, 1930, 1: 311–343.

———. Auditory patterns. *Rev. Mod. Phys.*, 1940, 12: 47–65.

Flock, Å. Sensory transduction in hair cells. In W. R. Loewenstein, ed., *Handbook of sensory physiology.* Vol. 1. New York: Springer-Verlag, 1971. Pp. 396–441.

Foster, D.; Scofield, E. H.; and Dallenbach, K. M. An olfactorium. *Amer. J. Psychol.*, 1950, 63: 431–440.

Fourier, J. B. J. Théorie du mouvement de la chauleur dans les corps solides. *Mem. Acad. Sci. Inst. Fr.*, 1824, 4 (Ser. 2): 185–525.

Fraisse, P. *The psychology of time.* New York: Harper & Row, 1963.

———. Visual perceptive simultaneity and masking of letters successively presented. *Percept. & Psychophys.*, 1966, 1: 285–287.

Frank, M., and Pfaffmann, C. Taste nerve fibers: A random distribution of sensitivities to four tastes. *Science*, 1969, 164: 1183–1185.

Frankenhaeuser, M. *Estimation of time.* Stockholm: Almquist & Hiksell, 1959.

Franzén, O., and Offenloch, K. Evoked response correlates of psychophysical magnitude estimates for tactile stimulation in man. *Exp. Brain Res.*, 1969, 8: 1–18.

Frey, M. von. Beiträge der Sinnesphysiologie der Haut (Dritte Mitteilung). Akad. Wiss. Leipzig. Math-naturw. Kl. *Berichte*, 1895, 47: 166–184.

Friedman, L., and Miller, J. G. Odor incongruity and chirality. *Science*, 1971, 172: 1044–1046.

Frommer, G. P. Gustatory afferent responses in the thalamus. In M. R. Kare and B. P. Halpern, eds., *Physiological and behavioral aspects of taste.* Chicago: Univ. of Chicago Press, 1961. Pp. 50–65.

Fuortes, M. G. F. Electric activity of cells in the eye of *Limulus. Amer. J. Ophthal.*, 1958, 46: 210–223.

Gacek, R. R., and Rasmussen, G. L. Fiber analysis of the statoacoustic nerve of guinea pig, cat, and monkey. *Anat. Record*, 1961, 139: 455–463.

Galambos, R. (with the collaboration of Davis, H.). Inhibition of activity in single auditory nerve fibers by acoustic stimulation. *J. Neurophysiol.*, 1944, 7: 287–303.

Galambos, R. Microelectrode studies on medial geniculate body of cat. III. Response to pure tones. *J. Neurophysiol.*, 1952, 15: 381–400.

Galambos, R., and Davis, H. The response of single auditory-nerve fibers to acoustic stimulation. *J. Neurophysiol.*, 1943, 6: 39–57.

Galambos, R.; Schwartzkopff, J.; and Rupert, A. Microelectrode study of superior olivary nuclei. *Amer. J. Physiol.*, 1959, 197: 527–536.

Gardner, E. P., and Spencer, W. A. Sensory funneling. I. Psychophysical observations of human subjects and responses of cutaneous mechanoreceptive afferents in the cat to patterned skin stimuli. *J. Neurophysiol.*, 1972, 35: 925–953. (a)

———. Sensory funneling. II. Cortical neuronal representation of patterned cutaneous stimuli. *J. Neurophysiol.*, 1972, 35: 954–977. (b)

Geldard, F. A. *The human senses.* New York: Wiley, 1953.

Gernandt, B., and Zotterman, Y. Intestinal pain: An electrophysical investigation on mesenteric nerves. *Acta Physiol. Scand.*, 1946, 12: 56–72.

Gesteland, R. C.; Lettvin, J. Y.; and Pitts, W. H. Chemical transmission in the nose of the frog. *J. Physiol.*, 1965, 181: 525–559.

Gibson, R. H. Electrical stimulation of pain and touch. In D. R. Kenshalo, ed., *The skin senses.* Springfield, Ill.: C. C. Thomas, 1968. Pp. 223–259.

Gilinsky, A. S., and Doherty, R. S. Interocular transfer of orientational effects. *Science*, 1969, 164: 454–455.

Gogel, W. C., and Mershon, D. H. Depth adjacency in simultaneous contrast. *Percept. & Psychophys.*, 1969, 5: 13–17.

Goldberg, J. M.; Adrian, H. O.; and Smith, F. D. Response of neurons of the superior olivary complex of the cat to acoustic stimuli of long duration. *J. Neurophysiol.*, 1964, 27: 706–749.

Goldberg, J. M., and Brown, P. B. Functional organization of the dog superior olivary complex: An anatomical and electrophysiological study. *J. Neurophysiol.*, 1968, 31: 639–656.

————. Response of binaural neurons of dog superior olivary complex to dichotic tonal stimuli: Some physiological mechanisms of sound localization. *J. Neurophysiol.*, 1969, 32: 613–636.

Goldstein, M. H., Jr.; Hall, J. L.; and Butterfield, B. L. Single-unit activity in the primary auditory cortex of unanesthetized cats. *J. Acoust. Soc. Amer.*, 1968, 43: 444–455.

Goss, C. M., ed. *Gray's anatomy of the human body*, 29th ed. Philadelphia: Lea & Febiger, 1973.

Gouras, P. Identification of cone mechanisms in monkey ganglion cells. *J. Physiol.*, 1968, 199: 533–548.

Graham, C. H., ed. *Vision and visual perception.* New York: Wiley, 1965.

Granit, R. The colour receptors of the mammalian retina. *J. Neurophysiol.*, 1945, 8: 195–210.

————. *Receptors and sensory perception.* New Haven: Yale Univ. Press, 1955.

Grassman, H. On the theory of compound colours. *Phil. Mag.*, 1854, 7: 254–264.

Gray, J. A. B., and Malcolm, J. L. Initiation of nerve impulses by mesenteric Pacinian corpuscles. *Proc. Roy. Soc. London*, 1950, Ser. B, 137: 96–114.

Gray, J. A. B., and Matthews, P. B. C. Response of Pacinian corpuscles in cat's toe. *J. Physiol.*, 1951, 113: 475–482. (a)

————. Comparison of adaptation of Pacinian corpuscles with accommodation of its own axon. *J. Physiol.*, 1951, 114: 454–464. (b)

Gray, J. A. B., and Sato, M. Properties of the receptor potential in Pacinian corpuscle. *J. Physiol.*, 1953, 122: 610–636.

Green, D. G. The contrast sensitivity of the colour mechanisms of the human eye. *J. Physiol.*, 1968, 196: 415–429.

Green, D. M., and Swets, J. A. *Signal detection theory and psychophysics.* New York: Wiley, 1966.

Greenwood, D. D. Auditory masking and the critical band. *J. Acoust. Soc. Amer.*, 1961, 33: 484–502.

Greenwood, D. D., and Maruyama, N. Excitatory and inhibitory response areas of auditory neurons in the cochlear nucleus. *J. Neurophysiol.*, 1965, 28: 863–892.

Gross, N. B. The effects of cochlear lesions on the auditory response of the guinea pig. *J. Comp. Physiol. Psychol.*, 1952, 45: 127–139.

Gross, N. B., and Thurlow, W. R. Microelectrode studies of neural auditory activity of cat. II. Medial geniculate body. *J. Neurophysiol.*, 1951, 14: 409–422.

Hagins, W. A.; Penn, R. D.; and Yoshikami, S. Dark current and photocurrent in retinal rods. *Biophys. J.*, 1970, 10: 380–410.

Hagiwara, S. On the fluctuation of the interval of the rhythmic excitation. I. The efferent impulse of the human motor unit during the voluntary contraction. *Rept. Physiograph. Sci. Inst. Tokyo Univ.*, 1949, 3: 19–24.

————. On the fluctuation of the interval of the rhythmic excitation. II. The afferent impulse from the tension receptor of the skeletal muscle. *Rept. Physiograph. Sci. Inst. Tokyo Univ.*, 1950, 4: 28–35.

Halpern, B. P. Gustatory responses in the medulla oblongata of the rat. (Doctoral dissertation, Brown University.) Ann Arbor, Mich.: University Microfilms, 1959. No. 59–4344.

Hänig, D. P. Zur Psychophysik des Geschmackssinnes. *Phil. Studien (Wundt)*, 1901, 17: 576–623.

Hardy, J. D. Method for the rapid measurement of skin temperature during exposure to intense thermal radiation. *J. Appl. Physiol.*, 1953, 5: 559–566.

Hardy, J. D.; Wolff, H. G.; and Goodell, H. *Pain sensations and reactions.* Baltimore: Williams & Wilkins, 1952.

Hartline, H. K. The response of single optic nerve fibers of the vertebrate eye to illumination of the retina. *Amer. J. Physiol.*, 1938, 121: 400–415.

Hartline, H. K., and Graham, C. H. Nerve impulses from single receptors in the eye. *J. Cell. Comp. Physiol,* 1932, 1: 277–295.

Hartline, H. K., and Ratliff, F. Inhibitory interaction of receptor units in the eye of *Limulus. J. Gen. Physiol.*, 1957, 40: 357–376.

————. Spatial summation of inhibitory influences in the eye of the *Limulus,* and the mutual interaction of receptor units. *J. Gen. Physiol.*, 1958, 41: 1049–1066.

Hartline, H.; Wagner, H.; and Ratliff, F. Inhibition in the eye of *Limulus. J. Gen. Physiol.*, 1956, 39: 651–673.

Hartridge, H. The polychromatic theory. *Documenta Ophthal.*, 1949, 3: 166–193.

Hawkins, J. E., Jr., and Stevens, S. S. The masking of pure tones and of speech by white noise. *J. Acoust. Soc. Amer.*, 1950, 22: 6–13.

Head, H. *Studies in neurology.* London: H. Frowde; Hodder & Stoughten, 1920.

Hebb, D. O. A neuropsychological theory. In S. Koch, ed., *Psychology: A study of a science.* Vol. 1. *Sensory, perceptual and physiological formulations.* New York: McGraw-Hill, 1959. Pp. 622–643.

Hecht, S. The development of Thomas Young's theory of color vision. *J. Opt. Soc. Amer.*, 1930, 20: 231–270.

————. Die physikalische Chemie und die physiologie des sehaktes. *Erg. Physiol.*, 1931, 32: 243–390.

————. Vision: II. The nature of the photoreceptor process. In C. Murchison, ed., *Handbook of general experimental psychology.* Worcester, Mass.: Clark Univ. Press, 1934. Pp. 704–828.

Hecht, S., and Shlaer, S. Intermittent stimulation by light. V. The relation between intensity and critical frequency for different parts of the spectrum. *J. Gen. Physiol.*, 1936, 19: 965–979.

Hecht, S.; Schlaer, A.; and Pirenne, M. H. Energy, quanta, and vision. *J. Gen. Physiol.*, 1942, 25: 819–840.

Heimer, L. Selective silver-impregnation of degenerating axoplasm. In W. J. H. Nauta and S. O. E. Ebbesson, eds., *Contemporaray research methods in neuroanatomy.* New York: Springer-Verlag, 1970. Pp. 106–131.

Helmholtz, H. von. *Handbuch der physiologischen Optik.* 1st ed. Hamburg and Leipzig: Voss, 1866. 3rd ed. Leipzig: Voss, 1911. English ed. J. P. C. Southall, trans., *Treatise on physiological optics.* Rochester, N.Y.: Optical Society of America, 1924–25. 3 vols.

Helmholtz, H. L. F. von. Versuch des psychophysische Gesetz auf die Farbenunterschiede trichromatischer Augen anzuwenden. *Z. Psychol. Physiol. Sinnesorg.*, 1892, 3: 1–20.

Henkin, R. I. The definition of primary and accessory areas of olfaction as the basis for a classification of decreased olfactory acuity. In T. Hayashi, ed.,

Olfaction and taste II. Proceedings of the Second International Symposium. Oxford: Pergamon, 1967. Pp. 235–252.

Henning, G. J.; Brouwer, J. N.; van der Wel, H.; and Francke, A. Miraculin, the sweetness-inducing principle from miracle fruit. In C. Pfaffmann, ed., *Olfaction and taste.* Proceedings of the Third International Symposium. New York: Rockefeller Univ. Press, 1969. Pp. 445–449.

Hensel, H. Electrophysiology of cutaneous thermoreceptors. In D. R. Kenshalo, ed., *The skin senses.* Springfield, Ill.: C. C. Thomas, 1968. Pp. 384–397.

Hensel, H., and Boman, K. K. Afferent impulses in cutaneous sensory nerves in human subjects. *J. Neurophysiol.*, 1960, 23: 564–577.

Hensel, H.; Iggo, A.; and Witt, I. Cutaneous thermoreceptors with nonmyelinated afferent fibers. *J. Physiol.*, 1960, 152: 19P. (abstract)

Hensel, H.; Ström, L.; and Zotterman, Y. Electrophysiological measurements of depth of thermoreceptors. *J. Neurophysiol.*, 1951, 14: 423–429.

Hensel, H., and Zotterman, Y. Response of mechanoreceptors to thermal stimulation. *J. Physiol.*, 1951, 115: 16–24.

Hensen, V. Zur Morphologie der Schnecke des Menschen und der Säugethiere. *Zeits. f. wiss. Zool.*, 1863, 13: 481–512. Cited in E. G. Wever, *Theory of hearing.* New York: Wiley, 1949.

Hering, E. *Zur Lehre vom Lichtsinne.* Wien: Carl Gerold's Sohn, 1878.

Hess, E. H. Attitude and pupil size. *Sci. Am.*, 1965, 212(4): 46–54.

Hill, J. W., and Carothers, W. H. Studies of polymerization and riny formation. XXI. Physical properties of macrocyclic esters and anhydrides: New types of synthetic musks. *J. Am. Chem. Soc.*, 1933, 55: 5039–5043.

Hillman, D. E., and Lewis, E. R. Morphological basis for a mechanical linkage in otolithic receptor transduction in the frog. *Science*, 1971, 174: 416–419.

Hind, J. E. (in collaboration with J. E. Rose, P. W. Davies, C. N. Woolsey, *et al.*). Unit activity in the auditory cortex. In G. L. Rasmussen and W. F. Windle, eds., *Neural mechanisms of the auditory and vestibular systems.* Springfield, Ill.: C. C. Thomas, 1960. Pp. 201–210.

Hirsh, I. J., and Sherrick, C. E. Perceived order in different sense modalities. *J. Exp. Psychol.*, 1961, 62: 423–432.

Hogg, B. M. Slow impulses from the cutaneous nerves of the frog. *J. Physiol.*, 1935, 84: 250–258.

Hubel, D. H. Tungsten microelectrode for recording from single units. *Science*, 1957, 195: 549–550.

———. Single unit activity in striate cortex of unrestrained cats. *J. Physiol.*, 1959, 147: 226–238.

Hubel, D. H., and Wiesel, T. N. Receptive fields of single neurones in the cat's striate cortex. *J. Physiol.*, 1959, 148: 574–591.

———. Receptive fields, binocular interaction and functional architecture in the cat's visual cortex. *J. Physiol.*, 1962, 160: 106–154.

———. Shape and arrangement of columns in cat's striate cortex. *J. Physiol.*, 1963, 165: 559–568.

———. Receptive fields and functional architecture in two nonstriate visual areas (18 and 19) of the cat. *J. Neurophysiol.*, 1965, 28: 229–289.

———. Receptive fields and functional architecture of monkey striate cortex. *J. Physiol.*, 1968, 195: 215–243.

Huggins, W. H., and Licklider, J. C. R. Place mechanism of auditory frequency analysis. *J. Acoust. Soc. Amer.*, 1951, 23: 290–299.

Hughes, J. R., and Hendrix, D. E. The frequency component hypothesis in relation to the coding mechanism in the olfactory bulb. In T. Hayashi, ed., *Olfaction and taste II.* Proceedings of the Second International Symposium. Oxford: Pergamon, 1967. Pp. 51–88.

Hughes, G. W., and Maffei, L. Retinal ganglion cell response to sinusoidal light stimulation. *J. Neurophysiol.*, 1966, 29: 333–352.

Hunt, C. C., and McIntyre, A. K. Properties of cutaneous touch receptors in cat. *J. Physiol.*, 1960, 153: 88–98. (a)

———. An analysis of fibre diameter and receptor characteristics of myelinated cutaneous afferent fibres in cat. *J. Physiol.*, 1960, 153: 99–112. (b)

Hurst, C. H. A new theory of hearing. *Trans. Liverpool Biol. Soc.*, 1895, 9: 321–353. (Meeting of Nov. 9, 1894.)

Hurvich, L. M., and Jameson, D. An opponent-process theory of color vision. *Psychol. Rev.*, 1957, 64: 384–404.

Iggo, A. Cutaneous mechanoreceptors with afferent C fibres. *J. Physiol.*, 1960, 152: 337–353.

———. New specific sensory structures in hairy skin. *Acta Neuroveg.*, 1963, 24: 175–180.

Iggo, A., and Muir, A. R. The structure and function of a slowly adapting touch corpuscle in hairy skin. *J. Physiol.*, 1969, 200: 763–796.

Inman, D. R., and Peruzzi, P. The effects of temperature on the responses of Pacinian corpuscles. *J. Physiol.*, 1961, 155: 280–301.

Ishiko, N., and Loewenstein, W. R. Effects of temperature on the generator and action potentials of a sense organ. *J. Gen. Physiol.*, 1961, 45: 105–124.

Iurato, S. Light microscope features. In S. Iurato, *et al.*, eds., *Submicroscopic structure of the inner ear*. Oxford: Pergamon, 1967. Pp. 18–37.

Jameson, D., and Hurvich, L. M. Some quantitative aspects of an opponent-colors theory. I. Chromatic responses and spectral saturation. *J. Opt. Soc. Amer.*, 1955, 45: 546–552.

———. Opponent-response functions related to measured cone photopigments. *J. Opt. Soc. Amer.*, 1968, 58: 429–430.

Jellinek, J. S. The effect of intermolecular forces on perceived odor. *Ann. N. Y. Acad. Sci.*, 1964, 116: 725–734.

Jenkins, W. L. Somesthesis. In S. S. Stevens, ed., *Handbook of experimental psychology*. New York: Wiley, 1951. Pp. 1172–1190.

Johnson, S. C. Hierarchical clustering schemes. *Psychometrika*, 1967, 32: 241–254.

Johnsson, L. G., and Hawkins, J. E. A direct approach to cochlear anatomy and pathology in man. *Arch. Otolaryng.*, 1967, 85: 599–613.

———. Sensory and neural degeneration with aging as seen in microdissection of the human inner ear. *Ann. Otol. Rhin. Laryng.*, 1972, 81: 179–193.

Johnstone, B. M., and Boyle, A. J. F. Basilar membrane vibration examined with the Mössbauer technique. *Science*, 1967, 158: 389–390.

Jones, R. C.; Stevens, S. S.; and Lurie, M. H. Three mechanisms of hearing by electrical stimulation. *J. Acoust. Soc. Amer.*, 1940, 12: 281–290.

Judd, D. B. Chromaticity sensibility to stimulus differences. *J. Opt. Soc. Amer.*, 1932, 22: 72–108.

———. Current views on colour blindness. *Documenta Ophthal.*, 1949, 3: 251–288.

———. Basic correlates of the visual stimulus. In S. S. Stevens, ed., *Handbook of experimental psychology*. New York: Wiley, 1951. Pp. 811–867.

Julesz, B. Binocular depth percept of computer-generated patterns. *Bell System Tech. J.*, 1960, 39: 1125–1162.

———. *Foundations of cyclopean perception*. Chicago: Univ. of Chicago Press, 1971.

Julesz, B., and Hesse, R. I. Inability to perceive the direction of rotation movement of line segments. *Nature*, 1970, 225: 243–244.

Kahneman, D. An onset-onset law for one case of apparent motion and meta-contrast. *Percept. & Psychophys.*, 1967, 2: 577–584.

――――. Method, findings, and theory in studies of visual masking. *Psychol. Bull.*, 1968, 70: 404–425.

Kahneman, D., and Beatty, J. Pupil diameter and load on memory. *Science*, 1966, 154: 1583–1585.

Kaneko, A., and Hashimoto, H. Recording site of single cone response determined by an electrode marking technique. *Vision Res.*, 1967, 7: 847–851.

Kaplan, S. The role of location processing in the perception of the environment. *Proc. Environ. Des. Res. Assoc.*, Pittsburgh, Pa., 1970.

Katsuki, Y. Neural mechanism of auditory sensation in cats. In W. A. Rosenblith, ed., *Sensory communication.* Cambridge, and New York: M.I.T. Press, Wiley, 1961. Pp. 561–584.

Katz, B. Depolarization of sensory terminals and the initiation of impulses in the muscle spindle. *J. Physiol.*, 1950, 3: 261–282.

――――. *Nerve, muscle, and synapse.* New York: McGraw-Hill, 1966.

Keidel, W. D., and Spreng, M. Neurophysiological evidence for Stevens power function in man. *J. Acoust. Soc. Amer.*, 1965, 38: 191–195.

Kenshalo, D. R. Improved method for the psychophysical study of the temperature sense. *Rev. Sci. Instr.*, 1963, 34: 883–886.

――――, ed., *The skin senses.* Springfield, Ill.: C. C. Thomas, 1968.

Kenshalo, D. R.; Duncan, D. G.; and Weymark, C. Thresholds for thermal stimulation of the inner thigh, footpad, and face of cats. *J. Comp. Physiol. Psychol.*, 1967, 63: 133–138.

Kenshalo, D. R., and Nafe, J. P. Receptive capacities of the skin. In G. R. Hawkes, ed., *Symposium on cutaneous sensitivity.* U. S. Army Medical Research Laboratory, Ft. Knox, Ky., Feb. 1960.

Kiang, N. Y.-S. *Discharge patterns of single fibers in the cat's auditory nerve.* Cambridge: M.I.T. Press, 1965.

Kibler, R. F., and Nathan, P. W. A note on warm and cold spots. *Neurol.*, 1960, 10: 874–880.

Kimura, K., and Beidler, L. M. Microelectrode study of taste receptors of rat and hamster. *J. Cell. Comp. Physiol.*, 1961, 58: 131–139.

Kinsbourne, M., and Warrington, E. The effect of an after-coming random pattern on the perception of brief visual stimuli. *Quart. J. Exp. Psychol.*, 1962, 14: 223–234. (a)

――――. Further studies on the masking of brief visual stimuli by a random pattern. *Quart. J. Exp. Psychol.*, 1962, 14: 235–245. (b)

Kistiakowsky, G. F. On the theory of odors. *Science*, 1950, 112: 154–155.

Kolers, P. A. Intensity and contour effects in visual masking. *Vision Res.*, 1962, 2: 277–294.

Kolers, P. A., and Rosner, B. S. On visual masking (metacontrast): Dichoptic observation. *Amer. J. Psychol.*, 1960, 73: 2–21.

Köllner, H. *Die Störungen des Farbensinnes.* Berlin: S. Karger, 1912.

König, A., and Dieterici, C. Die Grundempfindungen in normalen und anomalen Farben Systemen und ihre Intensitäts-Verteilung im Spectrum. *Z. Psychol. Physiol. Sinnesorg.*, 1893, 4: 241–347.

Koppitz, W. J. Mach bands and retinal interaction. Unpublished doctoral dissertation, Ohio State University, 1957.

Kozak, W.; Rodieck, R. W.; and Bishop, P. O. Responses of single units in lateral geniculate nucleus of cat to moving visual patterns. *J. Neurophysiol.*, 1965, 28: 19–47.

Krnjević, K.; Randić, M.; and Straughan, D. W. Cortical inhibition. *Nature*, 1964, 201: 1294–1296.

Kuffler, S. W. Neurons in the retina: Organization, inhibition and excitation problems. *Cold Spr. Harb. Symp. Quant. Biol.*, 1952, 17: 281–292.

——. Discharge patterns and functional organization of mammalian retina. *J. Neurophysiol.*, 1953, 16: 37–68.

Kuhn, T. S. *The structure of scientific revolutions.* 2nd ed. Chicago: Univ. of Chicago Press, 1970.

Kuile, E., ter. Die Uebertragung der Energie von der Grundmembran auf die Haarzellen. *Pflüg. Arch. ges. Physiol.*, 1900, 79: 146–157. (a)

——. Die richtige bewegungsform der membrana basilaris. *Pflüg. Arch. ges. Physiol.*, 1900, 79: 484–509. (b)

Kurihara, K.; Kurihara, Y.; and Beidler, L. M. Isolation and mechanism of taste modifiers; taste-modifying protein and gymnemic acids. In C. Pfaffmann, ed., *Olfaction and taste III.* Proceedings of the Third International Symposium. New York: Rockefeller Univ. Press, 1969. Pp. 450–469.

Lawrence, M. Dynamic range of the cochlear transducer. *Cold Spr. Harb. Symp. Quant. Biol.*, 1965, 30: 159–167.

Lee, Y. W. *Statistical theory of communication.* New York: Wiley, 1960.

Leeper, R. A study of a neglected portion of the field of learning—the development of sensory organization. *J. Genet. Psychol.*, 1935, 46: 41–75.

Legge, J. W. Mechanism of action of peripheral smell receptors. *Australian J. Sci.*, 1953, 15: 159–160.

Le Gros Clark, W. E. The laminar pattern of the lateral geniculate nucleus considered in relation to colour vision. *Documenta Ophthal.*, 1949, 3: 57–83.

Leibowitz, H.; Mote, F. A.; and Thurlow, W. R. Simultaneous contrast as a function of separation between test and inducing fields. *J. Exp. Psychol.*, 1953, 46: 453–456.

Lele, P. P., and Weddell, G. Sensory nerves of the cornea and cutaneous sensibility. *Exp. Neurol.*, 1959, 1: 334–359.

Lettvin, J. Y.; Maturana, H. R.; McCulloch, W. S.; and Pitts, W. H. What the frog's eye tells the frog's brain. *Proc. Inst. Radio Engr.*, 1959, 47: 1940–1951.

Levelt, W. J. M. Binocular brightness averaging and contour information. *Brit. J. Psychol.*, 1965, 56: 1–13.

Lichtenstein, M. Phenomenal simultaneity with irregular timing of components of the visual stimulus. *Percept. & Motor Skills*, 1961, 12: 47–66.

Lickley, J. D. *The nervous system.* New York: Longmans, 1919.

Licklider, J. C. R. A duplex theory of pitch perception. *Experientia*, 1951, 7: 128–134. (a)

——. Basic correlates of the auditory stimulus. In S. S. Stevens, ed., *Handbook of experimental psychology.* New York: Wiley, 1951. Pp. 985–1039. (b)

——. "Periodicity" pitch and "place" pitch. *J. Acoust. Soc. Amer.*, 1954, 26: 945. (abstract)

——. Three auditory theories. In S. Koch, ed., *Psychology: A study of a science.* Vol. I. *Sensory, perceptual, and physiological formulations.* New York: McGraw-Hill, 1959. Pp. 41–144.

——. Periodicity pitch and related auditory process models. *Int. Audiol.*, 1962, 1: 11–36.

Lifson, S. Potentiometric titration, association phenomena, and interaction of neighboring groups in polyelectrolytes. *J. Chem. Phys.*, 1957, 26(4): 727–734.

Lindsley, D. F.; Chow, K. L.; and Gollender, M. Dichoptic interactions of lateral geniculate neurons of cats to contralateral and ipsilateral eye stimulation. *J. Neurophysiol.*, 1967, 30: 628–644.

Linksz, A. *Essay on color vision.* New York: Grune & Stratton, 1964.

Lipetz, L. E. A mechanism of light adaptation. *Science*, 1961, 133: 639–640.

——. The relation of physiological and psychological aspects of sensory intensity. In W. R. Loewenstein, ed., *Principles of receptor physiology.* New York: Springer-Verlag, 1971. Pp. 191–225.

Bibliography

Loewenich, V., and Finkenzeller, P. Reizstärkenabhängigkeit und Stevenssche Potenzfunktion beim optisch evozierten Potential des Menschen. *Pflüg. Arch. ges. Physiol.*, 1967, 293: 256–271.

Loewenstein, W. R. Excitation and changes in adaptation by stretch of mechano-receptors. *J. Physiol.*, 1956, 133: 588–602.

———. The generation of electric activity in a nerve ending. *Ann. N.Y. Acad. Sci.*, 1959, 81: 367–387.

———. Excitation and inactivation in a receptor membrane. *Ann. N. Y. Acad. Sci.*, 1961, 94: 510–534. (a)

———. On the "specificity" of a sensory receptor. *J. Neurophysiol.*, 1961, 24: 150–157. (b)

Loewenstein, W. R., and Mendelson, M. Components of receptor adaptation in a Pacinian corpuscle. *J. Physiol.*, 1965, 177: 377–397.

Loewenstein, W. R., and Rathkamp, R. The sites for mechano-electric conversion in a Pacinian corpuscle. *J. Gen. Physiol.*, 1958, 41: 1245–1265.

Loewenstein, W. R., and Skalak, R. Mechanical transmission in a Pacinian corpuscle. An analysis and a theory. *J. Physiol.*, 1966, 182: 346–378.

Luce, R. D., and Mo, S. S. M. Magnitude estimation of heaviness by individual subjects: A test of a probabilistic response theory. *Brit. J. Math. & Stat. Psychol.*, 1965, 18 (Pt. 2): 159–174.

MacAdam, D. L. Visual sensitivities to color differences in daylight. *J. Opt. Soc. Amer.*, 1942, 32: 247–274.

Mach, E. Über die Wirkung der räumlichen vertheilung des lichtreizes auf die netzhaut. *Sitzungsber. math.-naturw. Cl. kaiserl. Akad. der Wissensch.*, 1865, Wien, 52/2: 303–322.

MacKavey, W. R.; Bartley, S. H.; and Casella, C. Disinhibition in the human visual system. *J. Opt. Soc. Amer.*, 1962, 52: 85–88.

MacKay, D. M. Interactive processes in visual perception. In W. A. Rosenblith, ed., *Sensory communication*. Cambridge, and New York: M.I.T. Press, Wiley, 1961. Pp. 339–356.

MacNichol, E. F., Jr. Visual receptors as biological transducers. In R. G. Grenell and L. J. Mullins, eds., *Molecular structure and functional activity of nerve cells*. Washington: American Institute of Biological Sciences, 1956. Pp. 34–52.

MacNichol, E. J., and Svaetichin, G. Electric responses from the isolated retinas of fishes. *Amer. J. Ophthal.*, 1958, 46(3): Pt. 2, 26–46.

Marks, W. B. Visual pigments of single goldfish cones. *J. Physiol.*, 1965, 178: 14–32.

Marks, W. B.; Dobelle, W. H.; and MacNichol, E. F. Visual pigments of single primate cones. *Science*, 1964, 143: 1181–1183.

Masterson, R. B., and Diamond, I. T. Effects of auditory cortex ablation on discrimination of small binaural time differences. *J. Neurophysiol.*, 1964, 27: 15–36.

Maturana, H. R., and Frenk, S. Directional movement and horizontal edge detectors in the pigeon retina. *Science*, 1963, 142: 977–979.

Mayzner, M. S., and Tresselt, M. E. Visual information processing with sequential inputs: A general model for sequential blanking, displacement, and overprinting phenomena. *Ann. N. Y. Acad. Sci.*, 1970, 169: 599–618.

Mayzner, M. S.; Tresselt, M. E.; and Helfer, M. S. A provisional model of visual information processing with sequential inputs. *Psychon. Monog. Suppl.*, 1967, 2(7): 91–108.

Melzack, R., and Wall, P. D. On the nature of cutaneous sensory mechanisms. *Brain*, 1962, 85: 331–352.

Mendelson, M., and Loewenstein, W. R. Mechanisms of receptor adaptation. *Science*, 1964, 144: 554–555.

Mershon, D. H., and Gogel, W. C. Effect of stereoscopic cues on perceived whiteness. *Am. J. Psychol.*, 1970, 83: 55–67.

Meyer, M. F. Über Kombinationstöne und einige hierzu in Beziehung stehende akustische Erscheinungen. *Zeits. f. Psychol.*, 1896, 11: 177–229.

Miller, G. A., and Taylor, W. G. The perception of repeated bursts of noise. *J. Acoust. Soc. Amer.*, 1948, 20: 171–182.

Miller, R. F., and Dowling, J. E. Intracellular response of the Müller (glial) cells of mudpuppy retina: Their relation to b-wave of the electroretinogram. *J. Neurophysiol.*, 1970, 33: 323–341.

Moore, G. P.; Perkel, D. H.; and Segundo, J. P. Statistical analysis and functional interpretation of neuronal spike data. *Ann. Rev. Physiol.*, 1966, 28: 493–522.

Moncrieff, R. W. What is odor? A new theory. *Essent. Oil Rev.*, 1949, 54: 453–454.

Morgan, C. T., and Stellor, E. *Physiological psychology.* 2nd ed. New York: McGraw-Hill, 1950.

Morse, R. W.; Adkins, R. H.; and Towe, A. L. Population and modality characteristics of neurons in the coronal region of somatosensory area 1 of the cat. *Exp. Neurol.*, 1965, 11: 419–440.

Moruzzi, G., and Magoun, H. W. Brain stem reticular formation and activation of the EEG. *EEG Clin. Neurophysiol.*, 1949, 1: 455–473.

Motokawa, K.; Taira, N.; and Okuda, J. Spectral responses of single units in the primate visual cortex. *Tohoku J. Exp. Med.*, 1962, 78: 320–337.

Motokawa, K.; Yamashita, E.; and Ogawa, T. Studies on receptive fields of single units with colored lights. *Tohoku J. Exp. Med.*, 1960, 71: 261–272.

Moulton, D. G. Electrical activity in the olfactory system of rabbits with indwelling electrodes. In Y. Zotterman, ed., *Olfaction and taste.* Proceedings of the First International Symposium. New York: Macmillan, 1963. Pp. 71–84.

———. Differential sensitivity to odors. *Cold Spr. Harb. Symp. Quant. Biol.*, 1965, 30: 201–206.

———. Spatio-temporal patterning of response in the olfactory system. In T. Hayashi, ed., *Olfaction and taste II.* Proceedings of the Second International Symposium. Oxford: Pergamon, 1967. Pp. 109–116.

Mountcastle, V. B. Modality and topographic properties of single neurons of cat's somatic sensory cortex. *J. Neurophysiol.*, 1957, 20: 508–534.

———. Some functional properties of the somatic afferent system. In W. A. Rosenblith, ed., *Sensory communication.* Cambridge and New York: M.I.T. Press, Wiley, 1961. Pp. 403–436.

Mountcastle, V. B.; Poggio, G. F.; and Werner, G. The relation of thalamic cell response to peripheral stimuli varied over an intensive continuum. *J. Neurophysiol.*, 1963, 26: 807–834.

Mountcastle, V. B., and Powell, P. S. Neural mechanisms subserving cutaneous sensibility, with special reference to the role of afferent inhibition in sensory perception and discrimination. *Bull. Johns Hopkins Hosp.*, 1959, 105: 201–232.

Mountcastle, V. B.; Talbot, W. H.; Darian-Smith, I.; and Kornhuber, H. H. Neural basis of the sense of flutter-vibration. *Science*, 1967, 155: 597–600.

Mountcastle, V. B.; Talbot, W. H.; Sakata, H.; and Hyvärinen, J. Cortical neuronal mechanisms in flutter-vibration studied in unanesthetized monkeys. Neuronal periodicity and frequency discrimination. *J. Neurophysiol.*, 1969, 32: 452–484.

Moushegian, G.; Rupert, A.; and Galambos, R. Microelectrode study of ventral cochlear nucleus of the cat. *J. Neurophysiol.*, 1962, 25: 515–529.

Mozell, M. M. The effect of concentration upon the spatio-temporal coding of odorants. In T. Hayashi, ed., *Olfaction and taste II.* Proceedings of the Second International Symposium. Oxford: Pergamon, 1967. Pp. 117–124.

———. Evidence for a chromatographic model of olfaction. *J. Gen. Physiol.,* 1970, 56: 46–63.

Müller, J. *Handbuch der physiologie des Menschen.* Vol. II. Coblentz: Hölscher, 1840.

Munger, B. L. Patterns of organization of peripheral sensory receptors. In W. R. Loewenstein, ed., *Principles of receptor physiology.* Vol. 1. New York: Springer-Verlag, 1971. Pp. 523–556.

Murray, R. G., and Murray, A. The anatomy and ultrastructure of taste endings. In G. E. W. Wolstenholme and J. Knight, eds., *Taste and smell in vertebrates.* London: J. & A. Churchill, 1970, pp. 3–24.

Murray, R. W. Nerve membrane properties and thermal stimulation. In A. V. S. de Reuck and J. Knight, eds., *Touch, heat and pain.* Boston: Little, Brown, 1966. Pp. 164–181.

McCullough, C. Color adaptation of edge-detectors in the human visual system. *Science,* 1965, 149: 1115–1116.

McGill, T. E. Auditory sensitivity and the magnitude of the cochlear potential. *Ann. Otol. Rhin. Laryng.,* 1959, 68: 193–207.

Nachmias, J. Effect of exposure duration on visual contrast sensitivity with square-wave gratings. *J. Opt. Soc. Amer.,* 1967, 57: 421–427.

Nafe, J. P. A quantitative theory of feeling from the psychological laboratories of Clark University. *J. Gen. Psych.,* 1929, 2: 199–210.

Naka, K. I., and Rushton, W. A. H. S-potentials from luminosity units in the retina of fish (Cyprinidae). *J. Physiol.,* 1966, 185: 587–599.

Neff, W. D. Neural mechanisms of auditory discrimination. In W. A. Rosenblith, ed., *Sensory communication.* Cambridge and New York: M.I.T. Press, Wiley, 1961.

Ness, A. R. The mechanoreceptors of the rabbit mandible incisor. *J. Physiol.,* 1954, 126: 475–493.

Norgren, R., and Leonard, C. M. Taste pathways in rat brainstem. *Science,* 1971, 173: 1136–1139.

Oakley, B., and Benjamin, R. M. Neural mechanisms of taste. *Physiol. Rev.,* 1966, 46: 199–211.

O'Connell, R. J., and Mozell, M. M. Quantitative stimulation of frog olfactory receptors. *J. Neurophysiol.,* 1969, 32: 51–63.

Ogawa, H.; Sato M.; and Yamashita, S. Multiple sensitivity of chorda tympani fibres of the rat and hamster to gustatory and thermal stimuli. *J. Physiol.,* 1968, 199: 223–240.

Ogle, K. N. *Researches in binocular vision.* Philadelphia: W. B. Saunders, 1950.

Ohm, G. S. Ueber die Definition des Tones, nebst daran Geknnüpfter Theorie der Sirene und ähnlicher tonbildener Vorrichtungen. *Ann. d. Phys.,* 1843, 59: 497–565.

Oikawa, T.; Ogawa, T.; and Motokawa, K. Origin of so-called cone action potential. *J. Neurophysiol.,* 1959, 22: 102–111.

Optical Society of America, Committee on Colorimetry. *The science of color.* Washington: Optical Society of America, 1963.

Osgood, C. E. *Method and theory in experimental psychology.* New York: Oxford Univ. Press, 1953.

Ottoson, D. Analysis of the electrical activity of the olfactory epithelium. *Acta Physiol. Scand.,* 1956, 35 (Suppl. 122): 1–83.

Ozeki, M. Hetero-electrogenesis of the gustatory cell membrane in rat. *Nature,* 1970, 228: 868–869.

Pantle, A., and Sekuler, R. Size-detecting mechanisms in human vision. *Science,* 1968, 162: 1146–1148.

Pellegrino, L. J., and Cushman, A. J. *A stereotaxic atlas of the rat brain.* New York: Appleton-Century-Crofts, 1967.

Penfield, W., and Roberts, L. *Speech and brain mechanisms.* Princeton: Princeton Univ. Press, 1959.

Perkel, D. H., and Bullock, T. H. Neural coding. *Neurosci. Res. Prog. Bull.,* 1968, 6: 221–347.

Peterson, W. W.; Birdsall, T. G.; and Fox, W. C. Theory of signal detectability. *IEEE Trans. Inf. Theory* (formerly *IRE Prof. Group on Inf. Theory*), 1954, 4: 171–212.

Pfaffmann, C. Gustatory afferent impulses. *J. Cell. Comp. Physiol.,* 1941, 17: 243–258.

———. Gustatory nerve impulses in rat, cat, and rabbit. *J. Neurophysiol.,* 1955, 18: 429–440.

———. The sense of taste. In J. Field, ed., *Handbook of physiology. Neurophysiology.* Vol. 1. Washington: American Physiological Society, 1959. Pp. 507–534.

———. Physiological and behavioral processes of the sense of taste. In G. E. W. Wolstenholme and J. Knight, eds., *Taste and smell in vertebrates.* London: J. & A. Churchill, 1970. Pp. 51–67.

Pfaffmann, C.; Fisher, G. L.; and Frank, M. K. The sensory and behavioral factors in taste preferences. In T. Hayashi, ed., *Olfaction and taste II.* Proceedings of the Second International Symposium. Oxford: Pergamon, 1967. Pp. 361–382.

Piéron, H. *The sensations.* English ed. New Haven: Yale Univ. Press, 1952.

Platt, J. R. Strong inference. *Science,* 1964, 146: 347–353.

Plattig, K. H. Über den electrischen Geschmack. *Zeitschrift für Biologie,* 1969, 116: 161–211.

Poggio, G. F., and Mountcastle, V. B. The functional properties of ventrobasal thalamic neurons studied in unanesthetized monkeys. *J. Neurophysiol.,* 1963, 26: 775–806.

Poggio, G. F., and Viernstein, L. J. Time series analysis of impulse sequences of thalamic somatic sensory neurons. *J. Neurophysiol.,* 1964, 27: 517–545.

Polyak, S. L. *The retina.* Chicago: Univ. of Chicago Press, 1941.

———. *The vertebrate visual system.* Chicago: Univ. of Chicago Press, 1957.

Pomeranz, B., and Chung, S. H. Dendritic-tree anatomy codes form-vision physiology in tadpole retina. *Science,* 1970, 170: 983–984.

Porter, K. R., and Bonneville, M. A. *Fine structure of cells and tissues.* 3rd ed. Philadelphia: Lea & Febiger, 1968.

Ranke, O. F. *Die Gleichrichter-Resonanztheorie.* München: Lehmann, 1931.

Rapoport, A. Information processing in the nervous system. *Int. Cong. Physiol. Sci., Lect. & Symp.,* 1962, 3: 16–23.

Ratliff, F. *Mach bands: Quantitative studies on neural networks in the retina.* San Francisco: Holden-Day, 1965.

Ratliff, F., and Hartline, H. K. The responses of *Limulus* optic nerve fibers to patterns of illumination on the receptor mosaic. *J. Gen. Physiol.,* 1959, 42: 1241–1255.

Ratliff, F.; Hartline, H. K.; and Miller, W. H. Spatial and temporal aspects of retinal inhibitory interaction. *J. Opt. Soc. Amer.,* 1963, 53: 110–120.

Ratliff, F., and Mueller, G. C. Synthesis of "on-off" and "off" responses in a visual-neural system. *Science,* 1957, 126: 840–841.

Reboul, J. A. *Le Phénomène de Wever et Bray.* Montpellier, 1937. Cited in E. G. Wever, *Theory of hearing.* New York: Wiley, 1949.

Rhode, W. S. Observations of the vibration of the basilar membrane in squirrel monkeys using the Mössbauer technique. *J. Acoust. Soc. Amer.*, 1971, 49: 1218–1231.

Riggs, L. A. Light as a stimulus for vision. In C. H. Graham, ed., *Vision and visual perception*. New York: Wiley, 1965. Pp. 1–38.

Riggs, L. A.; Johnson, E. P.; and Schick, A. M. L. Electrical responses of the human eye to changes in wavelength of stimulating light. *J. Opt. Soc. Amer.*, 1966, 56: 1621–1627.

Riggs, L. A.; Ratliff, F.; Cornsweet, J. C.; and Cornsweet, T. N. The disappearance of steadily fixated visual test objects. *J. Opt. Soc. Amer.*, 1953, 43: 495–501.

Ripps, H., and Weale, R. A. On seeing red. *J. Opt. Soc. Amer.*, 1964, 54: 272–273.

Rodieck, R. W.; Kiang, N. Y.-S.; and Gerstein, G. L. Some quantitative methods for the study of spontaneous activity of single neurons. *Biophys. J.*, 1962, 2: 351–368.

Rodieck, R. W., and Stone, J. Analysis of receptive fields of cat retinal ganglion cells. *J. Neurophysiol.*, 1965, 28: 833–849. (a)

———. Response of cat retinal ganglion cells to moving visual patterns. *J. Neurophysiol.*, 1965, 28: 819–832. (b)

Roeder, K. D., and Treat, A. E. The reception of bat cries by the tympanic organ of noctuid moths. In W. A. Rosenblith, ed., *Sensory communication*. Cambridge and New York: M.I.T. Press, Wiley, 1961. Pp. 545–560.

Rose, J. E.; Brugge, J. F.; Anderson, D. J.; and Hind, J. E. Phase-locked response to low-frequency tones in single auditory nerve fibers of the squirrel monkey. *J. Neurophysiol.*, 1967, 30: 769–793.

Rose, J. E.; Galambos, R.; and Hughes, J. R. Microelectrode studies of the cochlear nuclei of the cat. *Bull. Johns Hopkins Hosp.*, 1959, 104: 211–251.

Rose, J. E.; Greenwood, D. D.; Goldberg, J. M.; and Hind, J. E. Some discharge characteristics of single neurons in the inferior colliculus of the cat. I. Tonotopical organization, relation of spike-counts to tone intensity, and firing patterns of single elements. *J. Neurophysiol.*, 1963, 26: 294–320.

Rose, J. E.; Gross, N. B.; Geisler, C. D.; and Hind, J. E. Some neural mechanisms in the inferior colliculus of the cat which may be relevant to localization of a sound source. *J. Neurophysiol.*, 1966, 29: 288–314.

Rose, J. E., and Mountcastle, V. B. Touch and kinesthesis. In J. Field, ed., *Handbook of physiology. Neurophysiology*. Vol. 1. Washington: American Physiological Society, 1959. Pp. 387–429.

Rosenblith, W. A., and Vidale, E. B. A quantitative view of neuroelectric events in relation to sensory communication. In S. Koch, ed., *Psychology: A study of a science*. Vol. 4. *Biologically oriented fields: Their place in psychology and biological science*. New York: McGraw-Hill, 1962. Pp. 334–379.

Rosner, B. S. Neural factors limiting cutaneous spatio-temporal discriminations. In W. A. Rosenblith, ed., *Sensory communication*. Cambridge, and New York: M.I.T. Press, Wiley, 1961. Pp. 725–738.

Ross, J., and DiLollo, V. A consistent failure of the power law for lifted weight. *Percept. & Psychophys.*, 1970, 8: 289–290.

Rothberg, J. M. Simulation of neural nets with some applications to visual information processing. *Computers & Biomed. Res.*, 1968, 1: 435–451.

Ruch, T. C. Somatic sensation. In T. C. Ruch, H. D. Patton, I. W. Woodbury, and A. L. Lowe, eds., *Neurophysiology*. Philadelphia: Saunders, 1961. Pp. 300–322.

———. Vision. In T. C. Ruch and H. D. Patton, eds., *Physiology and biophysics*. Philadelphia: Saunders, 1965. Pp. 415–440.

Rushton, W. A. H. The difference spectrum and the photosensitivity of rhodopsin in the living human eye. *J. Physiol.*, 1956, 134: 11–29.

————. Kinetics of cone pigments measured objectively on the living human fovea. *Ann. N.Y. Acad. Sci.*, 1958, 74: 291–304.

————. Visual pigments in man. *Sci. Amer.*, 1962, 207: 120–132.

————. Interpretation of retinal densitometry. *J. Opt. Soc. Amer.*, 1964, 54: 273.

Russell, G. F., and Hills, J. I. Odor differences between enantiomeric isomers. *Science*, 1971, 172: 1043–1044.

Salzmann, M. The anatomy and physiology of the human eyeball in the normal state. Chicago: Univ. of Chicago Press, 1912.

Sato, M.; Yamashita, S.; and Ogawa, H. Afferent specificity in taste. In C. Pfaffmann, ed., *Olfaction and taste III*. Proceedings of the Third International Symposium. New York: Rockefeller Univ. Press, 1969. Pp. 470–487.

Saunders, J. C. Cochlear nucleus and auditory cortex correlates of a click stimulus-intensity discrimination in cats. *J. Comp. Physiol. Psychol.*, 1970, 72: 8–16.

Schade, O. H. Optical and photoelectric analog of the eye. *J. Opt. Soc. Amer.*, 1956, 46: 721–739.

Scharf, B. Critical bands. In J. V. Tobias, ed., *Foundations of modern auditory theory*. Vol. 1. New York: Academic Press, 1970. Pp. 157–202.

Schaumburg, H. H.; Byck, R.; Gerstl, R.; and Mashman, J. H. Monosodium L-glutamate: Its pharmacology and role in the Chinese restaurant syndrome. *Science*, 1969, 163: 826–828.

Schiller, P. H. Single unit analysis of backward visual masking and metacontrast in the cat lateral geniculate nucleus. *Vision Res.*, 1968, 8: 855–866.

Schiller, P. H. Behavioral and electrophysiological studies of visual masking. In K. N. Leibovic, ed., *Information processing in the nervous system*. New York: Springer-Verlag, 1969. Pp. 141–165.

Schiller, P., and Smith, M. A comparison of forward and backward masking. *Psychonom. Sci.*, 1965, 3: 77–78.

Schmitt, O. H., and Dubbert, D. R. Tissue stimulators utilizing radio-frequency coupling. *Rev. Sci. Instr.*, 1949, 20: 170–173.

Schneider, G. E. Two visual systems. *Science*, 1969, 163: 895–902.

Schoenberg, K. M.; Katz, M.; and Mayzner, M. S. The shape of inhibitory fields in the human visual system. *Percept. & Psychophys.*, 1970, 7: 357–359.

Schouten, J. F. The perception of subjective tones. *Proc. K. Ned. Akad. Wet.*, 1938, 41: 1086–1093.

————. The perception of pitch. *Phillips Tech. Rev.*, 1940, 5: 286–294.

Schuknecht, H. F., and Neff, W. D. Hearing losses after apical lesions in the cochlea. *Acta Oto-Laryng.*, 1952, 42: 263–274.

Schwanzara, S. A. Visual pigments of tropical freshwater fishes. *Life Sci.*, 1967, 6: 157–162.

Seebeck, A. Beobachtungen über einige Bedingungen der Entstehung von Tönen. *Ann. Phys.*, 1841, 53: Ser. 2, 417–436.

Segundo, J. P.; Moore, G. P.; Stensaas, L. J.; and Bullock, T. H. Sensitivity of neurones in *Aplysia* to temporal pattern of arriving impulses. *J. Exp. Biol.*, 1963, 40: 643–667.

Shallice, T. Temporal summation and absolute brightness thresholds. *Brit. J. Math. & Stat. Psychol.*, 1967, 20: 129–162.

Sheppard, J. J. *Human color perception. A critical study of the experimental foundation*. New York: American Elsevier, 1968.

Sherrick, C. E. Simple electromechanical vibration transducer. *Rev. Sci. Instr.*, 1965, 36: 1893–1894.

Sherrington, C. S. *Selected writings of Sir Charles Sherrington*. Ed. by D. Denny-Brown. New York: Hoeber, 1940.

Shibuya, T. Dissociation of olfactory neural response and mucosal potential. *Science*, 1964, 143: 1338–1340.

Shipley, T., and Rawlings, S. C. Sensory direction in homogenous binocular visual space. *Percept. & Psychophys.*, 1971, 9: 335–337.

Shower, E. G., and Biddulph, R. Differential pitch sensitivity of the ear. *J. Acoust. Soc. Amer.*, 1931, 3: 275–287.

Simmons, F. B. Monaural processing. In J. V. Tobias, ed., *Foundations of modern auditory theory.* Vol. 1. New York: Academic Press, 1970. Pp. 343–379.

Simmons, F. B.; Epley, J. M.; Lummis, R. C.; Guttman, N.; Frishkopf, L. S.; Harmon, L. D.; and Zwicker, E. Auditory nerve: Electrical stimulation in man. *Science,* 1965, 148: 104–106.

Sinclair, D. C. *Cutaneous sensation.* London: Oxford Univ. Press, 1967.

Sinclair, D. C., and Hinshaw, J. R. A comparison of the sensory dissociation produced by procaine and by limb compression. *Brain,* 1950, 73: 480–498.

Singer, S. J., and Nicolson, G. L. The fluid mosaic model of the structure of cell membranes. *Science,* 1972, 175: 720–731.

Singer, W., and Creutzfeldt, O. D. Reciprocal lateral inhibition of on- and off-center neurones in the lateral geniculate body of the cat. *Exp. Brain Res.,* 1970, 10: 311–330.

Skramlik, E. von. Mischungsgleichungen in Gebiete des Geschmackssinns. *Z. Sinnesphysiol.,* 1921, 53B: 36–78, 219.

Small, A. M. Periodicity pitch. In J. V. Tobias, ed., *Foundations of modern auditory theory.* Vol. 1. New York: Academic Press, 1970. Pp. 1–54.

Small, A. M., and Campbell, R. A. Masking of pulsed tones by bands of noise. *J. Acoust. Soc. Amer.,* 1961, 33: 1570–1576.

Small, A. M., and Yelen, R. D. Fatigue as an indicator of pitch channels. *J. Acoust. Soc. Amer.,* 1962, 34: 1987. (abstract)

Smith, K. R. The problem of stimulation deafness. II. Histological changes in the cochlea as a function of tonal frequency. *J. Exp. Psychol.,* 1947, 37: 304–317.

Smith, K. R., and Wever, E. G. The problem of stimulation deafness. III. The functional and histological effects of a high-frequency stimulus. *J. Exp. Psychol.,* 1949, 39: 238–241.

Sokolnikoff, I. S., and Sokolnikoff, G. S. *Higher mathematics for engineers and physicists.* New York: McGraw-Hill, 1941.

Sperling, G., and Sondhi, M. M. Model for visual luminance discrimination and flicker detection. *J. Opt. Soc. Amer.,* 1968, 58: 1133–1145.

Spinelli, D. N. Receptive field organization of ganglion cells in the cat's retina. *Exp. Neurol.,* 1967, 19: 291–315.

Spinelli, D. N., and Barrett, T. W. Visual receptive field organization of single units in the cat's visual cortex. *Exp. Neurol.,* 1969, 24: 76–98.

Stebbins, W. C., ed., *Animal psychophysics: The design and conduct of sensory experiments.* New York: Appleton-Century-Crofts, 1970.

Stebbins, W. C.; Miller, J. M.; Johnsson, L.-G.; and Hawkins, J. E. Ototoxic hearing loss and cochlear pathology in the monkey. *Ann. Otol., Rhin. & Laryng.,* 1969, 78: 1007–1026.

Stevens, C. F. *Neurophysiology: A primer.* New York: Wiley, 1966.

Stevens, S. S. The psychophysics of sensory function. In W. A. Rosenblith, ed., *Sensory communication.* Cambridge and New York: M.I.T. Press, Wiley, 1961. Pp. 1–34.

———. Neural events and the psychophysical law. *Science,* 1970, 170: 1043–1050.

———. Sensory power functions and neural events. In W. R. Loewenstein, ed., *Principles of receptor physiology.* New York: Springer-Verlag, 1971. Pp. 226–242.

Stevens, S. S., and Davis, H. *Hearing, its psychology and physiology.* New York: Wiley, 1938.

Stevens, S. S., and Newman, E. B. Localization of actual sources of sound. *Amer. J. Psychol.*, 1936, 48: 297–306.

Stigler, R. Chronophotische Studien über den Umgebungskontrast. *Pflüg. Arch. ges. Physiol.*, 1910, 134: 365–435.

Stiles, W. S. A modified Helmholtz line-element in brightness-colour space. *Proc. Phys. Soc.* (Lond.), 1946, 58: 41–65.

———. Increment thresholds and the mechanisms of human color vision. *Docum. Ophthal.*, 1949, 3: 138–163.

———. Color vision: The approach through increment-threshold sensitivity. *Proc. Nat. Acad. Sci.*, 1959, 45: 100–114.

Stretton, A. O. W., and Kravitz, E. A. Neuronal geometry: Determination with a technique of intracellular dye injection. *Science*, 1968, 162: 132–134.

Stroud, J. The fine structure of psychological time. In H. Quastler, ed., *Information theory in psychology*. Glencoe, Ill.: Free Press, 1955. Pp. 174–207.

Sumner, J. B. Problems in odor research from the viewpoint of the chemist. *Ann. N.Y. Acad. Sci.*, 1953, 58: 68–72.

Sutton, S.; Braren, M.; Zubin, J.; and John, E. R. Evoked-potential correlates of stimulus uncertainty. *Science*, 1965, 150: 1187–1188.

Svaetichin, G. Spectral responses from single cones. *Acta Physiol. Scand.*, 1956, 39 (Suppl. 134): 17–46.

Svaetichin, G., and MacNichol, E. F., Jr. Retinal mechanisms for chromatic and achromatic vision. *Ann. N.Y. Acad. Sci.*, 1958, 74: 385–404.

Sweetman, R. H., and Dallos, P. Distribution pattern of cochlear combination tones. *J. Acoust. Soc. Amer.*, 1969, 45: 58–71.

Takagi, S. F. Are OEG's generator potentials? In T. Hayashi, ed., *Olfaction and taste II*. Proceedings of the Second International Symposium. Oxford: Pergamon, 1967. Pp. 167–180.

Takagi, S. F., and Shibuya, T. "On"- and "off"-responses of the olfactory epithelium. *Nature*, 1959, 184: 60.

Takagi, S. F.; Shibuya, T.; Higashino, S.; and Arai, T. The stimulative and anaesthetic actions of ether on the olfactory epithelium of the frog and the toad. *Jap. J. Physiol.*, 1960, 10: 571–584.

Talbot, W. H.; Darian-Smith, I.; Kornhuber, H. H.; and Mountcastle, V. B. The sense of flutter-vibration: Comparison of the human capacity with response patterns of mechanoreceptive afferents from the monkey hand. *J. Neurophysiol.*, 1968, 31: 301–334.

Tanner, W. P., Jr., and Swets, J. A. A decision-making theory of visual detection. *Psychol. Rev.*, 1954, 61: 401–409.

Tasaki, I. Nerve impulses in individual auditory nerve fibers of guinea pig. *J. Neurophysiol.*, 1954, 17: 97–122.

Tasaki, I., and Davis, H. Electric responses of individual nerve elements in cochlear nucleus to sound stimulation (guinea pig). *J. Neurophysiol.*, 1955, 18: 151–158.

Tasaki, I.; Davis, H.; and Legouix, J.-P. The space-time pattern of the cochlear microphonics (guinea pig), as recorded by differential electrodes. *J. Acoust. Soc. Amer.*, 1952, 24: 502–514.

Taylor, M. M. Visual discrimination and orientation. *J. Opt. Soc. Amer.*, 1963, 53: 763–765.

Taylor, W. K. Electrical simulation of some nervous system functional activities. In C. Cherry, ed., *Information theory*. New York: Academic Press, 1956. Pp. 314–328.

Teas, D. C.; Eldredge, D. H.; and Davis, H. Cochlear responses to acoustic transients: An interpretation of whole-nerve action potentials. *J. Acoust. Soc. Amer.*, 1962, 34: 1438–1459.

Terzuolo, C. A., and Washizu, Y. Relation between stimulus strength, generator potential, and impulse frequency in stretch receptor of *Crustacea*. *J. Neurophysiol.*, 1962, 25: 56–66.

Thompson, R. F. *Foundations of physiological psychology*. New York: Harper & Row, 1967.

Thompson, R. F.; Mayers, K. S.; Robertson, R. T.; and Patterson, C. J. Number coding in association cortex of the cat. *Science*, 1970, 168: 271–273.

Thomson, L. C., and Wright, W. D. The convergence of tritanopic confusion loci derivations of the fundamental response functions. *J. Opt. Soc. Amer.*, 1953, 43: 890–894.

Thurlow, W. R., and Small, A. M. Pitch perception for certain periodic auditory stimuli. *J. Acoust. Soc. Amer.*, 1955, 27: 132–137.

Titchener, E. B. *Experimental psychology*. Vol. 1. *Qualitative experiments: Part I. Students' manual*. New York: Macmillan, 1924.

Tobias, J. V., ed. *Foundations of modern auditory theory*. Vol. 1. New York: Academic Press, 1970.

Tomita, T. Electrophysiological study of the mechanisms subserving color coding in the fish retina. *Cold Spr. Harb. Symp. Quant. Biol.*, 1965, 30: 559–566.

———. Electrical activity of vertebrate photoreceptors. *Quart. Rev. Biophys.*, 1970, 3: 179–222.

Tomita, T.; Kaneko, A.; Murakami, M.; and Pautler, E. Spectral response curves of single cones in carp. *Vision Res.*, 1967, 7: 519–531.

Tomita, T.; Murakami, M.; Hashimoto, Y.; and Sasaki, Y. Electrical activity of single neurons in the frog's retina. In R. Jung and H. Kornhuber, eds., *The visual system: Neurophysiology and psychophysics*. Berlin: Springer, 1961. Pp. 24–30.

Tonndorf, J. Time/frequency analysis along the partition of cochlear models: A modified place concept. *J. Acoust. Soc. Amer.*, 1962, 34: 1337–1350.

———. Cochlear mechanics and hydro-dynamics. In J. V. Tobias, ed., *Foundations of modern auditory theory*. Vol. 1. New York: Academic Press, 1970. Pp. 203–254.

Trevarthen, C. B. Two mechanisms of vision in primates. *Psychol. For.*, 1968, 31: 299–337.

Troland, L. T. *The principles of psycho-physiology*. New York: Van Nostrand, 1930.

Tunturi, A. R. A difference in the representation of auditory signals for the left and right ears in the iso-frequency contours of right middle ectosylvian auditory cortex of the dog. *Amer. J. Physiol.*, 1952, 168: 712–727.

Uttal, W. R. A comparison of neural and psychophysical responses in the somesthetic system. *J. Comp. Physiol. Psychol.*, 1959, 52: 485–490.

———. The three stimulus problem: A further comparison of neural and psychophysical responses in the somesthetic system. *J. Comp. Physiol. Psychol.*, 1960, 53: 42–46.

———. The effect of ischemia on the peripheral nerve action potential and its relation to somatosensory magnitude coding. *Percept. & Psychophys.*, 1967, 2: 137–140.

———. *Real time computers: Technique and applications in the psychological sciences*. New York: Harper & Row, 1968.

———. The character in the hole experiment: Interaction of forward and backward masking of alphabetic character recognition by dynamic visual noise (DVN). *Percept. & Psychophys.*, 1969, 6: 177–181. (a)

———. Emerging principles of sensory coding. *Persp. Biol. & Med.*, 1969, 12: 344–368. (b)

———. Masking of alphabetic character recognition by dynamic visual noise (DVN). *Percept. & Psychophys.*, 1969, 6: 121–127. (c)

———. On the physiological basis of masking with dotted visual noise. *Percept. & Psychophys.*, 1970, 7: 321–327.

———. The effect of interval and number on masking with dot bursts. *Percept. & Psychophys.*, 1971, 9: 469–473. (a)

———. The psychobiological silly season, or what happens when neurophysiological data become psychological theories. *J. Gen. Psychol.*, 1971, 84: 151–166. (b)

Uttal, W. R.; Bunnell, L. M.; and Corwin, S. On the detectability of straight lines in visual noise: An extension of French's paradigm into the millisecond domain. *Percept. & Psychophys.*, 1970, 8: 385–388.

Uttal, W. R., and Cook, L. Systematics of the evoked somatosensory cortical potential. *Ann. N.Y. Acad. Sci.*, 1964, 112: 60–81.

Uttal, W. R., and Hieronymus, R. Spatio-temporal effects in visual gap detection. *Percept. & Psychophys.*, 1970, 8: 321–325.

Uttal, W. R., and Kasprzak, H. The caudal photoreceptor of the crayfish: A quantitative study of responses to intensity, temporal and wavelength variables. *AFIPS Conf. Proc.*, 1962, 21: 159–169.

Uttal, W. R., and Krissoff, M. On the refractoriness of somesthetic temporal acuity. *Percept. & Psychophys.*, 1967, 2: 115–118.

———. Response of the somesthetic system to patterned trains of electrical stimuli. In D. R. Kenshalo, ed., *The skin senses*. Springfield, Ill.: C. C. Thomas, 1968. Pp. 262–303.

Uttal, W. R., and Smith, P. On the psychophysical discriminability of somatosensory nerve action potential patterns with irregular intervals. *Percept. & Psychophys.*, 1967, 2: 341–348.

———. Further studies on the psychophysics of irregular nerve action potential patterns. *Percept. & Psychophys.*, 1968, 3: 341–345.

Wagner, H. G.; MacNichol, E. F., Jr.; and Wolbarscht, M. L. The response properties of single ganglion cells in the goldfish retina. *J. Gen. Physiol.*, 1960, 43(2): Pt. 2, 45–62.

Wald, G. Vitamin A in the retina. *Nature*, 1933, 132: 316–317.

———. Human vision and the spectrum. *Science*, 1945, 101: 653–658.

———. The photoreceptor process in vision. In J. Field, ed., *Handbook of physiology. Neurophysiology*. Vol. 1. Washington: American Physiological Society, 1959. Pp. 671–692.

———. Molecular basis of visual excitation. *Science*, 1968, 162: 230–239.

———. The receptors of human color vision. *Science*, 1964, 145: 1007–1017.

———. Reflective color vision and its inheritance. *Proc. Nat. Acad. Sci.*, 1966, 55: 1347–1363.

Wall, P. D. Cord cells responding to touch, damage and temperature of skin. *J. Neurophysiol.*, 1960, 23: 197–210.

———. Two transmission systems for skin sensations. In W. A. Rosenblith, ed., *Sensory communication*. Cambridge, New York: M.I.T. Press, Wiley, 1961. Pp. 475–496.

Wall, P. D., and Cronly-Dillon, J. R. Pain, itch and vibration. *AMA Arch. Neurol.*, 1960, 2: 365–375.

Wallach, H.; Newman, E. B.; and Rosenzweig, M. R. The precedence effect in sound localization. *Amer. J. Psychol.*, 1949, 62: 315–336.

Walls, G. L. *The vertebrate eye*. Bloomfield Hills, Mich.: Cranbrook Inst. of Science, 1942.

Ward, W. D. Musical perception. In J. V. Tobias, ed., *Foundations of modern auditory theory*. Vol. 1. New York: Academic Press, 1970. Pp. 405–447.

Warren, R. M. Perceptual restoration of missing speech sounds. *Science*, 1970, 167: 392–393.

Warwick, R. Orbit, globe and its central connexions. In A. Sorsby, ed., *Modern ophthalmology* (2nd ed.). Vol. 1. *Basic aspects*. Philadelphia: Lippincott, 1972, pp. 37–170.

Weale, R. A. Photo-sensitive reactions in foveae of normal and cone-monochromatic observers. *Optica Acta*, 1959, 6: 158–174.

Weber, E. H. *De pulsa, resorptione, auditu et tactu: Annotationes anatomicae et physiologiae*, 1834. Cited in E. G. Boring, *Sensation and perception in the history of experimental psychology*. New York: Appleton-Century-Crofts, 1942. P. 513.

———. Ueber den Raumsinn und die Empfindungskreise in der Haut und im Auge. *Ber. sächs. Ges. Wiss. Leipzig, math.-phys. Cl.*, 1852, 85–164. Cited in E. G. Boring, *Sensation and perception in the history of experimental psychology*. New York: Appleton-Century-Crofts, 1942. P. 513.

Weddell, G. Somesthesis and the chemical senses. *Ann. Rev. Psychol.*, 1955, 6: 119–136.

Weddell, G., and Miller, S. Cutaneous sensibility. *Ann. Rev. Physiol.*, 1962, 24: 199–222.

Wegel, R. L., and Lane, C. E. The auditory masking of one pure tone by another and its probable relation to the dynamics of the inner ear. *Phys. Rev.*, 1924, 23: 266–285.

Weinstein, S. Intensive and extensive aspects of tactile sensitivity as a function of body part, sex, and laterality. In D. R. Kenshalo, ed., *The skin senses*. Springfield, Ill.: C. C. Thomas, 1968. Pp. 195–222.

Weintraub, D. J., and Krantz, D. H. The Poggendorf illusion: Amputations, rotations, and other perturbations. *Percept. & Psychophys*, 1971, 10: 257–264.

Weisstein, N. Backward masking and models of perceptual processing. *J. Exp. Psychol.*, 1966, 72: 232–240.

———. A Rashevsky-Landahl neural net: Stimulation of metacontrast. *Psychol. Rev.*, 1968, 75: 494–521.

———. What the frog's eye tells the human brain: Single cell analyzers in the human visual system. *Psychol. Bull.*, 1969, 72: 157–176.

———. Neural symbolic activity: A psychophysical measure. *Science*, 1970, 168: 1489–1491.

Werblin, F. S., and Dowling, J. E. Organization of the retina of the mudpuppy, *Necturus maculosus*, II. Intracellular recording. *J. Neurophysiol.*, 1969, 32: 339–355.

Werner, G., and Mountcastle, V. B. The variability of central neural activity in a sensory system, and its implications for the central reflection of sensory events. *J. Neurophysiol.*, 1963, 26: 958–977.

———. Neural activity in mechanoreceptive cutaneous afferents: Stimulus-response relations, Weber functions and information transmission. *J. Neurophysiol.*, 1965, 28: 359–397.

Wernick, J. S., and Starr, A. Binaural interaction in the superior olivary complex of the cat: An analysis of field potentials evoked by binaural-beat stimuli. *J. Neurophysiol.*, 1968, 31: 428–441.

Wersäll, J. Studies on the structure and innervation of the sensory epithelium of the cristae ampullares in the guinea pig. *Acta Oto-Laryng.*, 1956, 126: 1–85.

Wersäll, J., and Flock, Å Functional anatomy of the vestibular and lateral line organs. In W. D. Neff, ed., *Contributions to sensory physiology*. Vol. 1. New York: Academic Press, 1965. Pp. 39–62.

West, E. S., and Todd, W. R. *Textbook of biochemistry*. New York: Macmillan, 1961.

Wever, E. G. *Theory of hearing.* New York: Wiley, 1949.

Wever, E. G., and Bray, C. W. Action currents in the auditory nerve in response to acoustical stimulation. *Proc. Nat. Acad. Sci.,* 1930, 16: 344–350.

Wever, E. G.; Bray, C. W.; and Lawrence, M. The nature of cochlear activity after death. *Ann. Otol., Rhin. Laryng.,* 1941, 50: 317–329.

Wever, E. G.; Rahm, W. E.; and Strother, W. F. The lower range of the cochlear potentials. *Proc. Nat. Acad. Sci.,* 1959, 45: 1447–1449.

Whitfield, I. C., and Evans, E. F. Responses of auditory cortical neurons to stimuli of changing frequency. *J. Neurophysiol.,* 1965, 28: 655–672.

Wiener, N. *The extrapolation, interpolation, and smoothing of stationary time series with engineering applications.* New York: Wiley, 1949.

Wiesel, T. N., and Hubel, D. H. Spatial and chromatic interactions in the lateral geniculate body of the Rhesus monkey. *J. Neurophysiol.,* 1966, 29: 1115–1156.

Wilska, A. Eine Methode zur Bestimmung der Hörschwellenamplituden der Trommelfells bei verschiededen Frequenzen. *Skand. Arch. Physiol.,* 1935, 72: 161–165.

Winter, D. L. N. gracilis of cat. Functional organization and corticofugal effects. *J. Neurophysiol.,* 1965, 28: 48–70.

Witkovsky, P. The effect of chromatic adaptation on color sensitivity of the carp electroretinogram. *Vision Res.,* 1968, 8: 825–837.

———. Peripheral mechanisms of vision. *Ann. Rev. Physiol.,* 1971, 33: 257–280.

Wolbarsht, M. L. Electrical characteristics of insect mechanoreceptors. *J. Gen. Physiol.,* 1960, 44: 105–122.

Woolsey, C. N. Organization of somatic sensory and motor areas of the cerebral cortex. In H. F. Harlow and C. N. Woolsey, eds., *Biological and biochemical bases of behavior.* Madison, Wisc.: Univ. of Wisconsin Press, 1958. Pp. 63–82.

Wooten, B. R., and Wald, G. Color-vision mechanisms in the peripheral retinas of normal and dichromatic observers. *J. Gen. Physiol.,* 1973, 61: 125–145.

Wright, R. H. *The science of smell.* New York: Basic Books, 1964.

Wright, R. H., and Michels, K. M. Evaluation of far infrared relations to odor by a standards similarity method. *Ann. N.Y. Acad. Sci.,* 1964, 116: 535–551.

Wrightson, T., and Keith, A. *An enquiry into the analytical mechanism of the internal ear.* London: Macmillan, 1918.

Wyburn, G. M.; Pickford, R. W.; and Hirst, R. J. *Human senses and perception.* Toronto: Univ. of Toronto Press, 1964.

Young, R. W. The renewal of photoreceptor cell outer segments. *J. Cell Biol.,* 1967, 33: 61–72.

———. A difference between rods and cones in the renewal of outer segment protein. *Invest. Ophthalmol.,* 1969, 8: 222–231.

———. Visual cells. *Sci. Amer.,* 1970, 223(4): 80–91.

Zinnes, J. L. Scaling. *Ann. Rev. Psychol.,* 1969, 20: 447–478.

Zwicker, E. Die elementaren Grundlagen zur Bestimmung der Informationskapazität des Gehörs. *Acustica,* 1956, 6: 365–381.

INDEX OF NAMES

INDEX OF SUBJECTS